Techniques in Ophthalmic Plastic Surgery

ELSEVIER CD-ROM LICENSE AGREEMENT

Techniques in Ophthalmic Plastic Surgery

A Personal Tutorial

Jeffrey A. Nerad MD FACS

Cincinnati Eye Institute
Professor of Ophthalmology
University of Cincinnati
Cincinnati, OH
USA

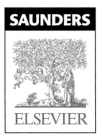

SAUNDERS

ELSEVIER

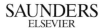

SAUNDERS an imprint of Elsevier Inc.

ISBN: 978-1-4377-0008-4

British Library Cataloguing in Publication Data
A catalogue record for this book is available from the British Library

Library of Congress Cataloging in Publication Data
A catalog record for this book is available from the Library of Congress

Notice

Medical knowledge is constantly changing. Standard safety precautions must be followed, but as new research and clinical experience broaden our knowledge, changes in treatment and drug therapy may become necessary or appropriate. Readers are advised to check the most current product information provided by the manufacturer of each drug to be administered to verify the recommended dose, the method and duration of administration, and contraindications. It is the responsibility of the practitioner, relying on experience and knowledge of the patient, to determine dosages and the best treatment for each individual patient. Neither the Publisher nor the author assume any liability for any injury and/or damage to persons or property arising from this publication.

The Publisher

ELSEVIER your source for books, journals and multimedia in the health sciences
www.elsevierhealth.com

Working together to grow libraries in developing countries
www.elsevier.com | www.bookaid.org | www.sabre.org
ELSEVIER   BOOK AID International   Sabre Foundation

Printed in China

The publisher's policy is to use paper manufactured from sustainable forests

Last digit is the print number: 9 8 7 6 5 4 3 2 1

Commissioning Editor: *Russell Gabbedy*
Development Editor: *Sharon Nash*
Project Manager: *Nayagi Athmanathan/Anne Dickie*
Design: *Stewart Larking*
Illustration Manager: *Gillian Richards*
Illustrator: *Cactus Design and Illustrations Ltd.*
Marketing Manager(s) (UK/USA): *Richard Jones/Helena Mutak*

Contents

Video Contents

Eyelid Procedures

Lacrimal Procedures

Orbital Procedures

DVD running time approximately 2 hours and 10 minutes

Preface

Thank you for your interest in *Techniques in Oculoplastic Surgery – a Personal Tutorial.*

This text is for you if you want to learn the principles and techniques of oculoplastic surgery that you can put into use in your practice every day.

This text is based on the *Requisites in Oculoplastic Surgery* textbook that I wrote in 2001. The text was written as though I was at your side there to get you through each step of the evaluation and treatment. I have followed the format here with updates and new material where appropriate. Most common disorders and procedures are included – some less common also. I suggest that you start by flipping through the chapters to get familiar with the content and layout of the text.

The book starts with an introduction to surgical technique. Being well prepared before you enter the operating room is key to your results and efficiency. Be sure to read this chapter. The second chapter is surgical anatomy. I have tried to keep the anatomy very practical and have placed clinical examples throughout. These first two chapters are important – your success as a surgeon is based on your expert technical manipulation of normal and abnormal anatomy.

The remaining chapters are topic oriented … ectropion, entropion, ptosis, and the like. All chapters begin with an outline of what is covered. A formal introduction to the chapter topic follows. A review of pertinent anatomy follows. The principles of evaluation and treatment are discussed next. Finally, surgical techniques with practical tips are outlined for you. The chapters are written in a hierarchal fashion that should make it easy for you to get the basics and then move more deeply into details on a second read. I have built in a large amount of intentional redundancy built into each chapter. Look at the summary boxes and use the checkpoints to make sure you are actually remembering what you just read. You will find over 500 diagrams and a similar number of photographs to help you understand put the principles into practice. You can check out the suggested reading list for another point of view. There are many good texts out now.

I have added a new chapter on Aesthetic Surgery. Many surgeons are including these procedures into the traditional oculoplastic practice. You will get a new appreciation of the aging process and learn the basics of skin care, resurfacing, peeling and many surgical techniques. I have included the important concepts of aesthetic forehead lifting, midface, full face and neck rhytidectomy. This is an area where an experienced mentor is helpful.

For me, learning works best in a "layered" fashion. Start with the big picture. Don't try to learn it all at once. Read and study the principles. Read again and again as many times as it might take to get the details. After you get confident in the principles and techniques, start with some easy procedures. Some of the procedures can get quite complicated. Ideally, you will have a mentor to help you put what you learn into practice. Don't forget to collaborate with colleagues outside your specialty. You will learn a good deal and make some great friendships along the way.

The techniques are described are not my own ideas, rather reflect over twenty years of practice learning from my teachers, colleagues and students. These are common approaches to the problems that you will see in your practice. The concepts and the style teaching are my own and the techniques work for me. Of course, these techniques are not the only ways to deal with a particular problem, definitely not the only way that works, but a way that does work for me. Try the techniques as written. As you get comfortable feel free to modify any part of the operation that seems to be an improvement for you.

Thanks again for reading this. If you have comments or questions, feel free to write or email me at the address below. You are on your way to a successful and rewarding surgical practice.

Jeff Nerad

Jeffrey A Nerad MD FACS
Cincinnati Eye Institute
1945 CEI Drive
Cincinnati, OH 45242
USA
Email: jnerad@cincinnatieye.com

Acknowledgements

I would like to thank the many people that helped make this book possible.

Thanks go first to my family. My parents, Frank and Blanche Nerad, made learning fun for my siblings and me. My daughters, Kristen and Elizabeth, and my wife, Jodi, offered support and encouragement throughout the whole process. Thank you very much.

My teachers, Rick Anderson, David Tse, John Wright, Richard Collins, and Dick Welham, were generous in showing me the "way" early in my career and continue to be valued friends and colleagues. Many others have taught me throughout my career. Special thanks to my colleagues, Robert Kersten, Jack Rootman, Jeff Carithers, and Keith Carter. Thanks to all the residents and fellows that have taught me so much over the last twenty plus years.

Many people helped with the production and technical aspects of the text. Thank you to my fellow, Jill Melicher, and videographer, Randy Verdick, for the work on the surgical videos. Thank you to Teresa Espy, my secretary, for managing my daily duties and correspondence. Thanks go to Susan Gilbert who made the illustrations for the original text and thanks to the art team at Elsevier for the colorizations and new illustrations. Thanks to the production team at Elsevier including Russell Gabbedy, Sharon Nash and Nayagi Athmanathan for all the direction and hard work throughout the process.

Thank you to all the readers that bought the first edition and offered suggestions and the encouragement that helped to make this book a reality. And lastly, thanks to those of you that are reading this new text. I hope that it plays some small role in your future successes.

Jeff Nerad

The Art of the Surgical Technique*

Introduction

This chapter will serve as your introduction to some theoretical and technical aspects of actually performing surgery. Successful surgery starts with planning before you enter the operating room. To be effective, you must know exactly what you are going to do and pass this information on to the operating room team. Your well-thought-out plan will inspire confidence in the operating room staff. Once in the operating room, you are the team leader. You will coordinate the setup of the operating room and necessary equipment for your procedure.

To be effective, you will need to know the tools of the trade and how to use them. We will discuss the different types of instruments and their general and special uses. We will stress some fundamental techniques, including holding and cutting the skin. We will cover the important instruments used in retraction, hemostasis, suctioning, and suturing. In the last section, we will talk about the role of the assistant, an underestimated and revealing job.

Don't labor over the details of each section in this book. Rather, read the text several times as your abilities and interest increase, each time taking in more detail.

*In recognition of Dr. Milton Edgerton's excellent text on surgical technique, a book all surgeons should read.

Preparation for the operation

Firm plan with contingencies

When you enter the operating room, you should have a firm plan in mind for the operation. In your early experience, it is worth having a set of contingency plans if things don't go as expected. As your surgical expertise increases, your need to make formal contingency plans will disappear. Early in your career, or later when you are planning a new procedure, it is worthwhile having the steps of the operation and necessary equipment written down to bring into the operating room. The nursing staff will appreciate your preparation and be confident of your abilities.

You are the team leader in the operating room. Your behavior will set the stage for how the operation goes. You set the pace and the quality of the effort. If you are operating in a new setting, be sure to introduce yourself to the nursing staff. Discuss with the operating room team your plans for surgery. Your preparation and willingness to include them in your plans will improve the overall effort and will give the team confidence in your ability to get the job done. This approach applies to every surgeon, from new residents to experienced surgeons in practice for many years.

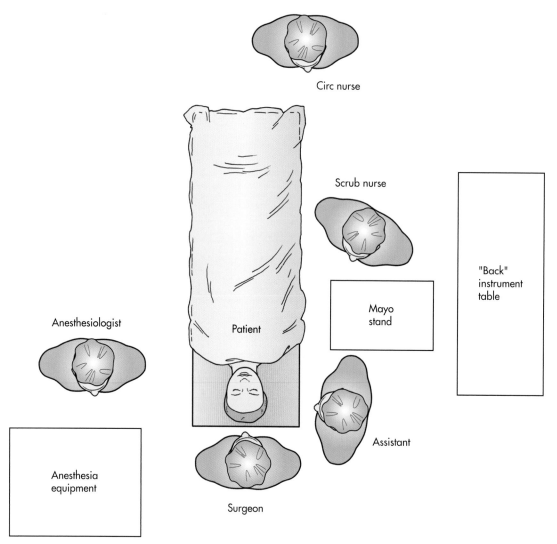

Figure 1-1 Typical operating room setup for an operation on right eye with the patient under general anesthesia.

Room setup

As part of your plan, you should know where the operating equipment will be placed. Generally, the setup is as shown in Figure 1-1. In most cases, the operated eye will be placed away from the anesthesia equipment. The surgeon will sit at the head of the bed. The assistant will sit at the side of the bed corresponding to the operated eye. For some procedures, you may find it easier to sit at the patient's side (for example, lateral tarsal strip and lateral orbitotomy). Feel free to move throughout the case and be comfortable. The nursing table will be on the same side as the assistant, but to the side of the bed.

Equipment setup

For the majority of operations that you perform, you will be in the sitting position. Adjust your chair to the appropriate height with your feet flat on the ground. If you are planning to move around the patient during the operation, as in an orbital floor exploration for a blowout fracture, you may want to stand for the operation. If so, consider step stools to make the assistant and surgeon relatively the same height.

Once you have decided whether you will be sitting or standing, you should position the operating room table. Often it is helpful to angle the head of the table away from the anesthesia equipment. Remember to consider where the operating room overhead lights are when positioning the table. Adjust the table height so that your elbows are bent slightly more than 90 degrees. Make sure that the patient's head is at the top edge of the operating table so you won't have to lean over the patient.

Do your best to position the patient for the comfort of both the patient and yourself. When operating on children, your view will improve if you place a towel roll under the patient's shoulders to hyperextend the neck, bringing the face into the same plane as the table. Older patients with neck arthritis may require a roll under the head for comfort. Markedly kyphotic patients may need a pillow under the neck and shoulders for comfort. You may have to operate standing at this patient's side with the head of the bed elevated. Do your best to maintain reasonable posture. Many older surgeons have to alter or stop their surgical practices because of the neck aches and back pains that result from years of poor body mechanics.

If you expect significant venous bleeding, as in nasal surgery, put the patient in about 10% of reverse Trendelenburg position (head up, feet down) before adjusting the table height. Once the table is at the chosen position and height, make sure that it is locked into position.

If you are using an operating microscope, this is the time to make adjustments to the scope and your chair. There are several possible positions for the operating scope base, but the most common is off the shoulder of the patient opposite to the eye you are operating on. Set the base of the scope to allow for full range of the arm. Make gross adjustments on the microscope height. Set the interpupillary distance of the microscope heads for the surgeon and the assistant. Set the focus of the microscope. If you are doing a conjunctival or canalicular procedure, set the focus of the microscope in the middle of the range. If you are doing deep orbital surgery, set the focus at the top of the travel so that you will be able to adjust the focus with the foot pedal to see deeper tissue without repositioning the operating scope as the dissection continues into the orbit. Most procedures will be performed without a wrist rest, but don't hesitate to use one if it increases your steadiness. Place any special sterile handles on the microscope before you scrub. If you plan to drape the scope, swing the microscope arm away without altering your microscope base position and have the scrub nurse drape the scope away from the operating field. Consider using sterile "baggies" over the handles rather than draping the whole scope to save time and money. Position the microscope and cautery foot pedals in the appropriate spot underneath the head of the table. If you don't do this, you will be surprised how many times you start the operation and reach for the cautery pedal, but find that it is not yet ready to use. Do all this before you leave to scrub.

Skin marking and local anesthesia

Many oculoplastic procedures require skin marking as a guide to incision placement. The majority of incisions will be *placed in natural skin creases* as in the upper lid skin crease for ptosis and blepharoplasty operations. Other skin incisions will be *placed adjacent to anatomic structures* to hide the scar. You should mark the skin before any local anesthetic is injected. Two good choices for marking eyelid skin are available: 1) gentian violet solution and 2) surgical marking pen. Gentian violet can be applied with the sharp end of a broken applicator used as a quill. With experience, you can draw a fine line that does not easily wash off with prepping, but this takes some experience to keep from making a mess. Usually, we use a thin-tipped surgical marker ("Twin-Tip" surgeon's marker, #6650-T, Hospital Marketing Services, Inc., http://www.hmsmedical.com). Be sure to degrease the skin with an alcohol wipe before marking.

You should use a local anesthetic with epinephrine for all procedures to provide some hemostasis (due to the vasoconstriction). The most common local anesthetic mixture is 2% lidocaine (Xylocaine) with 1 : 100,000 epinephrine in combination with 0.5% bupivacaine (Marcaine). Some surgeons choose to add hyaluronidase to the mix, but I have not found this necessary. For larger scalp and face procedures, you may want to consider "tumescent" anesthesia. Using this technique, a large amount of very dilute local anesthetic with epinephrine is injected into the subcutaneous tissues.

This technique firms up the tissues and makes easier to develop flaps and perform liposuction. You won't need this for periocular procedures.

Local anesthetics sting badly (if you aren't feeling sympathetic, have a colleague inject 1 cc of local anesthetic into your eyelid; you will not soon forgot how it feels). Two factors are thought to be responsible: 1) a difference in pH and 2) distention of the tissues during rapid injection. To minimize the pain, try injecting a tiny amount—about 0.1 cc—into two or three places and then massage the local anesthetic into the tissues. After a few seconds, inject more anesthetic *very slowly*. This greatly minimizes the pain. Some surgeons buffer the local anesthetic using 1 part 7.5% sodium bicarbonate in 9 parts of 2% Xylocaine with epinephrine (2 cc of bicarb in 20 cc of Xylocaine). I have not found this worth the trouble, but many swear by it. You might want to try it. If you operate with an anesthesiologist, using appropriate agents, the patient can be made totally unaware of any local injection.

Remember to inject just beneath the eyelid skin. Avoid placing the needle into the muscle to prevent a hematoma, which may make intraoperative adjustments of the eyelid difficult; this is especially true with ptosis correction. For an upper eyelid procedure, such as a blepharoplasty or ptosis repair, you should inject 1–1.5 cc of local anesthetic mix.

Topical solutions are available that provide anesthesia. You should know about these two preparations: EMLA cream and Betacaine gel. EMLA cream should be applied in a thick coating 1 hour ahead and covered with an occlusive dressing (topical lidocaine 2.5% and prilocaine 2.5%, AstraZeneca LP, http://www.astrazeneca-us.com). Betacaine gel (topical lidocaine 5%, Canderm Pharma, Inc., http://www.canderm.com) can be applied for 20–30 minutes ahead without an occlusive dressing. Both preparations provide anesthesia, but no vasoconstriction, so usually additional local injection with epinephrine is required for surgical procedures. Topical agents are also useful prior to Botox or filler injections and can be helpful in children. Overdosing with systemic reaction is unlikely, but possible. Most of the time, I do not use these preparations, but you might find them helpful in your practice.

The majority of eyelid and lacrimal operations can be easily performed under local anesthesia. If you choose to operate without the benefit of an anesthesiologist, you should consider intravenous (IV) sedation to minimize the patient's anxiety. Doses of midazolam (Versed) in 0.5–1.0 mg increments are reasonable to achieve some relaxation. I find it helpful to have a Versed drip running rather than giving intermittent doses of the medication (1–3 mg/hour). Some surgeons prefer preoperative oral sedation with 2–10 mg of oral Diazepam (Valium). Additional pain relief can be given intraoperatively using small doses of a narcotic, such as morphine (1–2 mg IV). Intravenous alfentanil (Alfenta) is useful because of its short duration, but keep in mind that this is a very potent narcotic and a highly abused drug. Avoid oversedation to the point that the patient has lost inhibitions and gets restless or is too sleepy to follow your instructions. A supportive attitude from you and the nursing staff is often as helpful, or more helpful, than intravenous sedation. I am always impressed how many postop patients comment how helpful it was to have the circulating nurse offer to hold hands during the case. The nurse can also alert you when the patient is feeling discomfort.

If your operating situation allows for the efficient use of monitored anesthesia care, your anesthesiologist can medicate your patient to the point at which there is no memory of any pain from the injection and often no memory of the entire operation. The downside of this is more staffing and increased patient cost.

Preparing and draping the patient

In most hospitals, the patient can be prepped while you scrub. This gives time for the local anesthetic to take effect. A traditional Betadine scrub applied in concentric rings away from the planned surgical excisions, repeated three times, provides adequate cleaning of the skin. A surgical stockinet can be used to keep the patient's hair out of the operating field. If the patient's hairline is particularly low or close to the operating field, tape can be used to pull the hair away from the surgical field. If the patient is awake, you will want to prep out the entire face for most procedures under local anesthesia. If the patient is asleep, prep out two eyes whenever there is a need to obtain symmetry between the two sides or if forced duction testing may be required. A good general rule is to prep out a larger area than you think you will need.

Instruments

In the next sections of the chapter, we will discuss several types of surgical instruments. These instruments include:

* Scalpel blades and other cutting tools
* Scissors
* Forceps
* Retractors
* Cautery
* Suction
* Needle holders
* Sutures

You are undoubtedly familiar with several variations of each of these instruments. I will explain the instruments that I have found most useful in my practice. You may already have your own favorite tools for specific jobs, or you may choose to use the instruments that I have suggested.

You will notice that a particular instrument is available in *different lengths and caliber*. In general, *the length of the instrument is related to the depth of the surgical incision in which the instrument will be used.* Most of the eye instruments are only 4 inches long. These instruments are not used in deep incisions and are rarely used for incisions deeper than the eyelid. Similarly delicate instruments used for neurosurgery are much longer, often measuring 12 inches. An example is the curved Yasargil scissors used in optic nerve sheath fenestration. These instruments are 9 inches long and have a finer tip than the familiar Westcott scissors that you may find for eye and cardiac surgery. Ideally, for an optic nerve procedure, we would use a 6 inch instrument, but none is currently available in this scissor type so we make do with the longer instrument. The caliber or strength of the instrument will vary, depending on what tissue is going to be manipulated or cut. We will talk more about the individual variations of each of these instrument types later in this chapter.

Cutting the skin

Hand position

Now that you are properly positioned at the head of the bed of a patient who has been prepped and draped, your next job is to make a skin incision. Remember you are positioned with your *feet flat on the ground and your elbows at your side in flexion slightly more than 90 degrees.* Hold your hands in the *functional position*, like holding a pencil with your hand in slight flexion at the wrist. This will improve your dexterity and strength.

There are three tools used for cutting the skin:

* No. 15 scalpel blade
* Colorado microdissection needle
* CO_2 laser

Most of our comments not only pertain to the traditional scalpel, but also to the cutting cautery needle and CO_2 laser. It is worth learning the traditional surgical techniques with the scalpel and scissors. As your skill increases, you will likely find that using the microdissection needle or laser shortens the operating time.

As you hold the scalpel with the *pencil grip*, you will notice that, on the scalpel handle, there is a groove or flat area where your index finger will rest. The scalpel is supported between your thumb, index finger, and middle finger (Figure 1-2).

The eyelid skin is mobile. Precision cutting requires immobilization of the skin with the help of your fingers or the assistant's fingers. Use your ring finger to rest on the patient, stabilizing the skin or guiding your hand. Learn to use the ring finger on your dominant hand and the thumb and forefinger on your nondominant hand to stabilize the skin (Figure 1-3). If the tissue is slippery, using a gauze pad for some traction will be helpful.

It is best to start the skin incision with the tip of the scalpel blade. As you move across the incision, lay the scalpel down so that you are cutting with the curved part of a no. 15 blade. As the wound edges start to separate, observe the depth of the wound. Ideally, you want to cut eyelid skin only and not extend the cut into the orbicularis. This is difficult to do, but nevertheless worthwhile. Controlling the depth

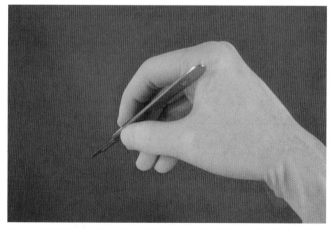

Figure 1-2 Holding the scalpel with the pencil grip. Note that the hand is in the "functional position" in slight flexion.

of any eyelid incision is critical. Remember that the eyelid is only slightly more than 1 mm thick at the skin crease, and you do not want to extend your incision into the cornea. You might find that using a corneal protector is a useful safeguard initially. With experience, you will probably find it easier not to use a corneal protector for scalpel cutting or cutting cautery incisions. Adjust the pressure to maintain the proper depth of the wound. Like driving a car, look "down the road," as you pull the scalpel across the skin. All of this is happening as you or your assistant holds steady tension on the skin. Remember, tight skin can be cut more easily and accurately than more mobile skin. Like most instruments for eye surgery, the scalpel is a "finger tool." As you bring your fingers toward your palm with the scalpel tip, you may need to reposition your hand and repeat the cutting process in lengths of the wound (Figure 1-4). As you get more experienced, you will be able to flex your fingers and move your hand at the same time.

This is a good time to remind you of your *good body position*. You should feel relaxed and at ease as you cut. Make sure your elbows remain close to your side rather than up high, which will convert the scalpel to an "arm tool" rather than a "finger tool." You will be doing many incisions in

your life, so learn to cut away from important structures such as your fingers and the eye. There are several types of scalpel blades that you should be familiar with.

Scalpel blades

- No. 11 blade: This blade has a sharp point that is good for tight angles and curves. It is not useful for longer incisions because it may cut deeper than you expect.
- No. 15 blade: This is the best all-purpose scalpel blade for eyelid and facial skin; 98% of your eyelid surgery with a scalpel will be done using a no. 15 blade.
- No. 10 blade: The no. 10 blade is shaped like a no. 15 blade except bigger. This blade is used primarily for thicker skin incisions. It is not used for periorbital incisions, but can be helpful in facial flaps.
- Beaver blades (http://www.bd.com) The #66 Beaver blade (#376600) is a special purpose right-angled blade. Its primary use is for making cuts in tight spaces. It is especially useful for nasal mucosal incisions in dacryocystorhinostomy (DCR) procedures. Angled keratomes designed for anterior segment surgery work in a similar fashion (Figure 1-5). Other useful blades are the #64 blade (#376400 rounded tip, sharp on one side), #76 blade (#376700, a mini #15 blade), both useful for delicate shaving of tissue off sclera or cornea. The needle blade #375910 is good when you need to make a microincision. Beaver handles come in a variety of lengths, the most common being 10 cm. Longer length handles (13 and 15.5 cm) are useful for deep orbitotomy or craniotomy cases.

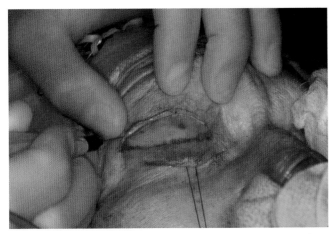

Figure 1-3 Skin stabilization. During upper eyelid blepharoplasty, the skin fold is stabilized and stretched with the surgeon's fingers while the upper eyelid is drawn downward using a lid margin traction suture. Note that a Colorado microdissection needle* is being used for the incision. With experience, the traction suture can be eliminated and the surgeon can use fingers to stretch the skin tight.

*The original micropoint electrocautery needle was called the "Colorado" needle. Other brands of true microdissection needles are now available. In this text, the terms Colorado needle and microdissection needle are considered to be the same. However, this fine tungsten microtipped needle should not be confused with the older needle point monopolar cautery tool available in many operating rooms.

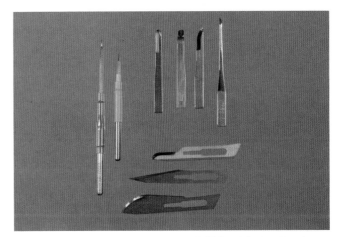

Figure 1-5 Surgical cutting instruments: Left, "Colorado" microdissection needles (blue: shorter (preferred); red: longer). Right, Beaver blades 376400, 376600, 37600, 375910. Bottom (from top), scalpel blades no. 15, no. 11, and no. 10.

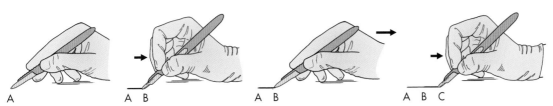

Figure 1-4 Flexion of the fingers with the scalpel blade followed by movement of the hand (adapted from Edgerton M, *The art of the surgical technique*, Baltimore, 1988, Williams & Wilkins).

Other cutting tools

Two other useful cutting tools are available for eyelid surgery: the microdissection needle and the CO_2 laser. The microdissection needle has been my choice for the majority of periocular surgical procedures in recent years. This unipolar cautery device does an excellent job of cutting and cauterizing the thin eyelid tissues. The needle is made of tungsten with an extremely fine tip. Tissue in contact with the tip is vaporized. Getting used to this instrument takes some practice. Cutting the tissue should be done with superficial light passing over the tissue in a "painting" motion with the needle slightly angled as if you are using a paint brush. If you find that carbon is building up on the tip of the instrument, you are moving too fast, you are cutting too deep, or you have the power turned up too high. The trick of using this tool is cutting only at the very tip so that there is little thermal damage to the surrounding tissues. Using a "blend" mode gives cutting and cautery. Try this for the dissection of an upper eyelid blepharoplasty skin muscle flap. Once you get used to this "bloodless" field, you will have trouble going back to scissors. You should use a smoke evacuator to eliminate the hazardous smoke produced by this tool. The patient requires grounding as with the use of other unipolar cautery equipment. The use of this unipolar cutting tool is sometimes limited to tissues anterior to the orbital septum, because the electric current is carried into the orbit and causes pain for many patients under local anesthesia. The tip works on the dry eyelid skin, but works best on tissues deep to the skin. For this reason, some surgeons prefer using a blade for the initial skin incision as the wound is sharper. I use a blade in many cosmetic cases and switch to the needle for any deeper work. You may find the Colorado needle with a foot pedal useful, but I prefer the hand switch on the cautery handle itself. Two companies make a microdissection needle (Stryker Colorado needle, Stryker Medical, http://www.stryker.com, 800 869 0770; and Tungsten microsurgical needle E1650, Valleylab, http://www.valleylab.com, 800 722 8772). The shortest length needle is the easiest to work with on periocular tissues.

The CO_2 laser is also a useful tool for cutting eyelid skin. Like the microdissection needle, tissues are vaporized with excellent cautery of capillaries and small veins. The Coherent UltraPulse 5000C CO_2 laser was introduced years ago and remains a work horse in my practice. The current model is the UltraPulse Encore made by Lumenis (Lumenis Inc., http://www.lumenis.com, 801 656 2300). These lasers remain the gold standard for laser incisional and resurfacing work. As when using a microdissection needle, large vessels are often cut with the laser rather than cauterized, so you will need a bipolar cautery tool on the operating room table as well. Both these cutting and cauterizing tools can shorten operating times considerably. If you have a CO_2 laser available, you should try this as a cutting tool. You must emphasize "pulling apart the tissues" with your forceps. There is no "touch" or "feel" involved in the cutting. It is all visual so technique is very important. Once you learn it, you will love it. Patients have less discomfort with the CO_2 laser than with the Colorado microdissection needle. Some precautions are necessary. You will need sandblasted instruments to prevent reflection of the laser energy. Metal corneal shields are a must. Surgeons and staff must wear protective goggles.

Smoke evacuation is necessary. Care with oxygen and the use of wet drapes are important to prevent fire. The majority of procedures in this text will be described with the use of the microdissection needle, but I suggest you try the laser, especially for upper blepharoplasty. The skills that you will learn using the microdissection needle and the laser are complementary; learning one will help you with the other.

Placement of skin incisions

Most skin incisions that you will make are hidden in natural creases or wrinkle lines (Figure 1-6). The *upper lid skin crease* is a natural place to make incisions in the upper lid. The upper lid skin crease will often be carried laterally into a "laugh line." If you are working away from an area where you are not familiar with the wrinkle lines, ask the patient to contract the facial muscles in that area. You will see wrinkles and folds in the skin that will show you where to place your incisions. You can anticipate these lines. Remember that the natural skin creases occur perpendicular to the direction of the muscle fibers causing this crease. Contract your frontalis muscle and you will see the furrows of the forehead perpendicular to the frontalis muscle fibers.

Other skin incisions can be camouflaged by placing them near anatomic structures such as the eyelashes or eyebrow. Adults generally have no lower lid skin crease. Skin incisions in the lower lid are usually placed *adjacent to the lower lid lashes* (subciliary incision). This incision can also be carried laterally into a "laugh line." Similarly, eyebrow incisions can be hidden by placing the incision *adjacent to the upper or lower margin of eyebrow hairs*. Incisions can be placed within the brow itself but can cause permanent visible scarring as a result of the loss of cilia roots. Other examples of camouflaging scars near facial structures include pretrichial hairline incisions, preauricular skin incisions, and incisions along the alae of the nose. Older style incisions such as the Stallard Wright lateral orbitotomy incision and the Lynch incision have been largely replaced by incisions that leave a better scar.

Anxiety and tremor

Every surgeon has a tremor to some degree or another. This tremor will be worse when you are anxious, are tired, or have drunk too much coffee. If you find that your tremor is bothersome, try to eliminate these factors. I occasionally hear of a resident who takes a beta-blocker before performing an operation. This might serve as a confidence booster, but is really not necessary once you learn to relax during surgery. A big part of being anxious when learning surgery is the feeling that you will look bad to your teacher or others observing. Consequently, you get more nervous and your tremor will increase. Don't forget, everyone in the operating room is on your side, doing everything they can to help you do your best for the patient. If you are feeling a little shaky, you might want to explain to your teacher that you are nervous. Usually, this confession will bring some deserved empathy, and your tremor will settle down a bit. Take a few deep breaths. Make sure that your chair and the table height are appropriate. Try to relax your forearms and loosen your grip on the instruments. If this does not work, consider a wrist rest. *I have yet to see a student who had a tremor that kept him or her from being a good surgeon.*

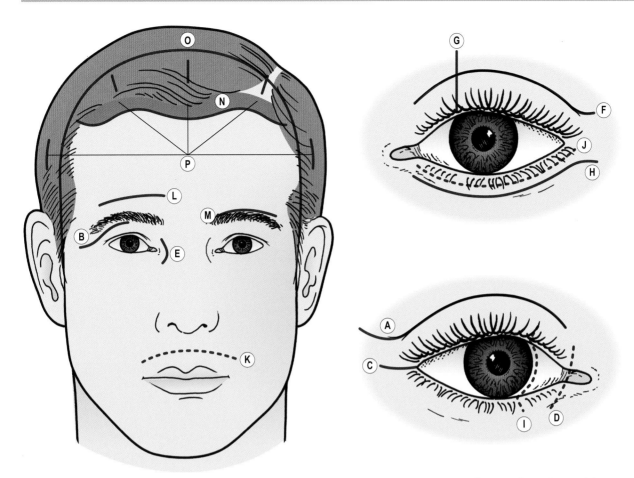

Figure 1-6 Facial incisions are typically hidden in natural skin creases or placed next to anatomic structures for camouflage. (**A**) Upper lid crease incision extended into lateral canthal laugh line for lateral orbitotomy. (**B**) Traditional Stallard Wright lateral orbitotomy incision (rarely used). (**C**) Modified Berke lateral canthotomy incision. (**D**) Transcaruncular incision. (**E**) Frontoethmoidal (Lynch) incision (rarely used). (**F**) Upper lid crease incision. (**G**) Vertical lid split incision. (**H**) Subciliary incision. (**I**) Transconjunctival incision for medial orbitotomy. (**J**) Inferior transconjunctival incision. (**K**) Gingival upper buccal incision. (**L**) Forehead furrow incision. (**M**) Suprabrow incision. (**N**) Pretrichial incision. (**O**) Transcoronal forehead incision. (**P**) Endoscopic browplasty incisions.

Checkpoint

- Remember to have a plan when you enter the operating room. Let the staff know what the plan is. Know what the room setup will be. Know the instruments. Your preparedness will inspire confidence and set the pace for the operation.
- You must have a plan for the operation and some contingencies if things don't go as planned. You would be surprised how many residents come to the operating room expecting to be "shown" what to do. As a resident, the more you know, the more you will get to do, and the faster you will learn.
- Get the patient, operating table, your stool, and your body in a comfortable position before starting. Have all the equipment prepared before you make a skin incision.
- Why should you mark the skin and inject the local anesthetic before scrubbing?

- Do you need to write down the names of special instruments, sutures, or equipment that you will be using?
- Let the operating room nurses know what you are planning, especially if you anticipate any change from the routine.
- Practice stabilizing and cutting the skin on pieces of chicken at home. It is not the perfect model, but it can be helpful. Practice everything you can at home, including cutting, suturing, and tying. Operating room time is very valuable.
- Learn to be comfortable and relaxed in the operating room. As a surgeon, it is your home and workplace for a big part of your career.

Cutting tissue with scissors

How do scissors cut?

Scissors cut by the *shearing and squeezing action* of the blades crossing so close together that tissue between the blades is separated in a controlled fashion. The majority of skin incisions, especially on thicker skin, should not be made with scissors because of this "crushing action" of the scissors blades. Some surgeons do, however, use scissors to cut the thin skin of the eyelid. Most surgeons reserve scissors for dissection of deeper tissue planes.

Types of scissors

In the Storz instrument catalog, there are 50 pages of scissors showing almost 200 types. Hopefully, after reading this section, you can make a sensible choice in selecting the right scissors for the surgical step you are doing. Scissors vary in the following characteristics:

- Length
- Caliber
- Tip sharpness
- Blade design
- Cutting motion

We will look at each of these characteristics briefly.

Length

Choose the proper length scissors for the depth of the wound that you are working in. Most of the instruments on the eye tray are 4 inches long. This size goes with the scale and depth of the usual ocular procedures. Longer instruments would be less steady and bump into the microscope. You will use many 4 inch instruments in oculoplastic surgery. Plastic surgery instruments are usually 6 inches long and fit the normal hand size better. In most cases, the longer neurosurgical instruments are not useful. For orbit surgery, on occasion, you may use a longer neurosurgical scissors for the particular tip rather than the length (Yasargil scissors).

Caliber

In general, thicker scissors blades are used for tougher tissues. This is fairly intuitive. You would not use a delicate Westcott scissors to cut through the thick dermis of the cheek. Similarly, you would not use the tough Mayo scissors to cut eyelid skin. Remember it is the blade tip size, not the length of the instrument, that you should consider for the delicacy of the tissue you want to cut. You will find that many longer delicate instruments are available.

Tip

The tip of a pair of scissors may be blunt or sharp. Blunt-tipped scissors are usually used for dissection in tissue planes. Sharp scissors are used to cut through tough tissues such as scar tissue. Face lift scissors have slightly sharpened rounded tips to facilitate flap dissection in the subcutaneous plane.

Blade design

Scissors blades are made as *straight* or *curved* (Figure 1-7). Most straight scissors are used for cutting sutures and bandages, and are sometimes called "suture scissors." It is easier to cut a straight line with straight scissors than with curved scissors. Curved scissors are useful for tissue dissections. The curved angle of the blade lifts the tissue planes apart as the tip cuts the reflected tissue, which is placed on stretch. The curve of a scissors blade is easy to palpate through tissues. You will learn to protect tissues against the convex surface of the curve. An example of this technique is separating the levator aponeurosis from the underlying Müller's muscle. As the two layers are *pulled apart*, fine tissue bands will be seen stretching between the tissue planes (learning to "pull" the layers apart is the most important surgical technical tip I can give you; more on this later). The convex surface of the scissors can slide up the fibrous bands and rest against the aponeurosis. Cutting can be performed without buttonholing the aponeurosis (Figure 1-8).

Cutting motion

Most scissors close and open with opposite hand motions. These scissors are called *iris scissors*. You can control the force when opening the blades as well as the force when closing the blades with your hands. This allows you to use the scissors tips as a dissecting tool as you spread open the tissue

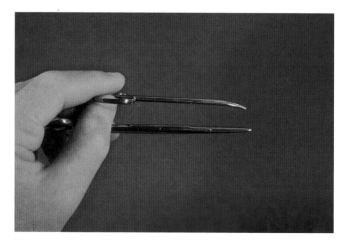

Figure 1-7 Blades of the straight Mayo scissors compared with those of the curved Stevens tenotomy scissors. Notice that the length and caliber of the scissors are also different.

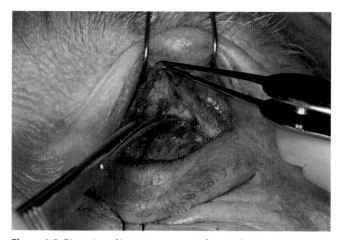

Figure 1-8 Dissection of levator aponeurosis from Müller's muscle using curved Westcott scissors. Note how "pulling" the tissues apart creates bands of tissue that are easy to see and cut. The convex side of the scissors blades should be against the tissue that is the strongest, in this case the aponeurosis (see **Figure 1-10, B**).

planes by opening the scissors. *Spring scissors* open with the recoil of a spring mechanism in the handle of the scissors. Westcott scissors are an example of this type. These scissors are generally used for fine tissues where minimal hand motion is required ("finger tools"). The spring action determines the force of the opening of the blades, making these scissors somewhat more difficult to control and less useful for dissecting tissues with the opening of the blades.

You will remember that scissors cut by a shearing action. Most iris-type scissors are designed as right-handed cutting tools. Imagine holding a pair of iris scissors in your hand. Push your thumb away from the palm and pull your fingers toward your palm. This action squeezes the blades of the scissors more tightly together, increasing the cutting power. You may recall doing this as a child playing with dull scissors. You quickly learn that squeezing the blades together increases the cutting power. This is also why left-handed children sometimes have trouble cutting with right-handed scissors. Try squeezing the blades together the next time you use a pair of scissors.

Cutting with scissors (you learned this as a child)

Spring scissors, or Westcott scissors, are held as finger tools, like a pencil. As with any scissors, you should gently squeeze the blades together in a continuous action. As the scissors cut, *watch the tissue separate. Avoid clicking or snipping the scissors closed in one quick motion* (close the scissors like you may have been taught to slowly squeeze the trigger of a gun or a camera shutter release button). Quick motions do not allow you to evaluate the depth or length of the scissors cut as you proceed. Observing how the tissues spread apart as you cut them is the very best way to stay in the correct surgical plane.

Watch less skilled surgeons or nurses cut your sutures. Often they will snip away at the suture. This type of cutting is too inaccurate for tissues.

As you proceed with cutting tissue, do not close the blades completely to the tips. You will lose your place in the wound if you close the scissors. Again, remember when you first learned to use scissors as a child. Initially, every time you cut a piece of paper, you would close the scissors blades completely. It was difficult to make a straight continuous smooth line. You had to start over each time you cut. As you learned to use the scissors better, you found that you could more effectively cut a continuous line by closing the scissors halfway to two thirds and then advancing the blades forward. This is the same technique that you should use in cutting tissue. *As the blades cut approximately halfway closed, push the blade forward in the same plane and cut again.* Don't cut with the full closure of the blade until the end of the incision.

Remember when cutting with curved scissors to position the curve of the scissors along the curve of the incision. Many of the incisions that you will be making, such as the skin crease incision, are curved.

When using an iris or ring scissors place your middle finger in one ring and your thumb in the other ring. Use this grip with the index finger providing three-point fixation of the scissors (Figure 1-9). These larger scissors are useful as a "finger and hand" tool. The same cutting motion that is described above should be used with this type of scissors. You might want to practice this technique on a piece of paper to make sure that

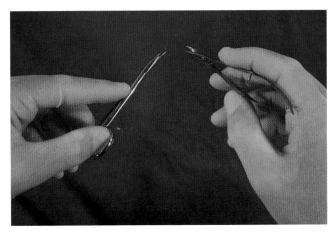

Figure 1-9 Holding scissors. *Left*, Iris or "ring" scissors (a "finger and hand tool"). *Right*, Westcott scissors, the most common spring scissors used in eyelid surgery (a finger tool).

you have the idea. Probably you may be using scissors in more than one way already. Dr. Edgerton's book nicely describes the function of scissors. Scissors can be used for cutting sutures and tissue, functioning as "shearing cutters." Scissors can be used to spread open planes as "push cutters" (Figure 1-10). Planes may be dissected using "lateral sweeps" or "pull wedges." Small vessels may be squeezed closed with the shearing action of scissors. Palpation of the curved blade of scissors can be used to help guide a deep tissue dissection.

Checkpoint

- Compare two types of scissors that you may be familiar with: straight Mayo scissors and Stevens tenotomy scissors (see Figure 1-7). Mayo scissors come in many variations, so look at the scissors pictured. This variation is almost 7 inches long and has thick straight blades with fairly pointed tips. The Stevens scissors are just over 4 inches long and have thinner curved blades with blunt tips. Which scissors would be best for cutting sutures in a deep abdominal wound? The Mayo scissors, of course. The straight, thick, pointed blades are not well suited for tissue plane dissection. The shorter, curved, blunt-tipped blades of the Stevens scissors are ideally suited for the tissue plane dissection of the relatively superficial layers of the eyelid.
- Think of which layers of the eye or eyelid Westcott scissors are suited for. Would you choose sharp or blunt Westcott scissors for a conjunctival peritomy? The soft conjunctival and episcleral tissues would tear if sharp-tipped scissors were used.
- Remind yourself how to cut tissue using a plain piece of paper. Draw a straight and a curved line. Try cutting the line in "snips." Now try cutting the line with smooth continuous strokes, not closing the blades completely. Which is easier, more accurate, and faster? Cut the straight line with a curved scissors. Cut the curved line with the curved scissors using the curve of the blades "with" the curve of the line. Now cut the curved line with the scissors blades turned "against" the curve. You should be getting the idea that learning how to use your tools correctly produces a better and faster result.

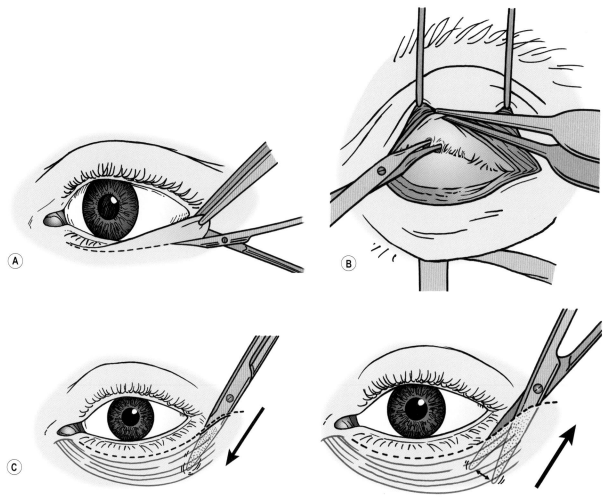

Figure 1-10 Uses of scissors. (**A**) Shearing cutters. The normal cutting action of the scissors is shown with Westcott scissors trimming redundant skin and muscle off a lower blepharoplasty flap. (**B**) Push cutters. The blades are open halfway, and the tissue is cut by pushing the scissors against the tissue. A good example is the dissecting of Müller's muscle off the levator as shown in Figure 1-8. (**C**) Lateral sweeps or pull wedges. The blades are inserted closed and opened in the wound or as they are pulled out. The action is with the outside of the scissor blade (dull side). This can be used to create a dissection plane, for example between the orbicularis muscle and the orbital septum. Scissors are typically used in this fashion to open an abscess pocket (adapted from Edgerton M, *The art of the surgical technique*, Baltimore, 1988, Williams & Wilkins).

Retraction and exposure

Fingers as retractors

One of the major differences between learning ocular surgery and oculoplastic surgery is learning how to manipulate and retract tissues. Most of the retraction done in ocular surgery is done with a lid speculum. You will learn to use a variety of tools to hold the tissues. You are already familiar with the best and most gentle retractor of all, *your fingers*. You will learn to use all the fingers on your nondominant hand to support or put the tissues on stretch. At the same time, you will be holding a cutting tool in your dominant hand with your thumb, first and second fingers while at the same time using the ring and small finger as retractors while you work (visualize holding a blade with the "pencil grip" and stretching the tissues with your other fingers—try this). A finger covered with a gauze sponge helps to stabilize slippery tissues.

Skin hooks

You may not be familiar with the use of a *skin hook*. This is one of the oldest surgical instruments and, when used correctly, one of the *most gentle retractors*. Skin hooks are available in different sizes and with varying numbers of prongs. The most useful skin hook for eyelid surgery is the *Storz double fixation hook*, a small double-pronged hook (Storz E0533) (Figure 1-11). There are also *small single-pronged hooks* that can be used for very delicate tissues (Tyrell iris hook; Storz E0548) and *rake-type skin hooks* with multiple prongs that are used for lacrimal surgery (Knapp lacrimal sac retractor; Storz E4538). A *large double-pronged skin hook*, known as the Joseph hook (Storz N4730), is useful for retraction of large tissue flaps. The Senn–Kanevel retractor (Storz N4780), or other modification of the Senn retractor, has large hooks on one end and a right-angled narrow blade retractor on the other end. This is a good all-purpose, soft tissue retractor for facial procedures. Obviously, you must be quite careful with these hooks not to pull the hook toward the eye where inadvertent puncture of the globe could occur.

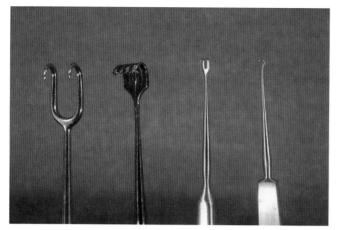

Figure 1-11 Skin hooks (left to right): large double-pronged (Joseph) skin hook, lacrimal rake, small double-pronged skin hook, small single-pronged hook (Tyrell).

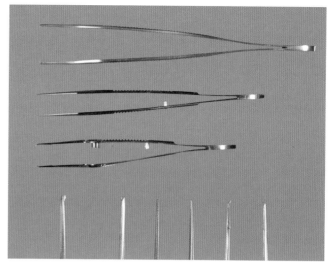

Figure 1-12 Forceps. Top: Adson forceps (large forceps with teeth, for cheek and scalp). Middle: Forceps without teeth (smooth). Bottom: Paufique forceps with teeth (the most common forceps that you will use). Forceps tips. Left: Adson forceps. Middle: smooth forceps. Right: Paufique forceps.

Forceps

The most common type of instrument to hold tissue is a forceps. All forceps work the same, using a pinching action of the fingers to grasp tissue. Forceps differ in length, caliber, and tip. Length and caliber differ for the same reasons as all instruments in general. The tips of forceps can either be *smooth* or have *teeth*.

Smooth forceps generally cause more trauma than forceps with teeth. Because there is low friction on the tip of smooth forceps, more pressure is required to hold tissue. Consequently, the tissue tends to be *crushed*. Smooth forceps (Figure 1-12) are used only on delicate tissues if concern exists over tearing the tissue with forceps with teeth. Variations of smooth forceps include diamond dusting and small serrations on the inner surface of the blades. These variations increase the friction of the forceps and reduce the pressure required to grasp the tissue.

Forceps with teeth offer a better grip with *less crushing of tissue*. You should use forceps with teeth whenever possible. Several types of forceps with teeth are available. The most common form has two teeth on one blade opposing a single tooth on the other blade. In general, forceps with multiple small teeth are more delicate than forceps with fewer and larger teeth. As you grasp the tissue with forceps you should use gentle pressure to close the tips. The teeth should not leave marks in the tissue.

As you get more facile using surgical instruments, you will use the single tooth of a toothed forceps as a skin hook to lift and sometimes unroll a skin edge. This blade is known as a *lifting jaw*. When grasping tissue, select the layer of tissue that is the least susceptible to injury. It is better to grasp the dermis or subcutaneous fat than the skin edge directly.

You will find that Paufique forceps do a great job for most periocular work. They have small teeth that grasp delicate tissues, but the blades and grip are stout enough to work with heavier tissues. You should be familiar with lighter and heavier forceps with teeth. Useful more delicate forceps include Castroviejo suturing forceps. Heavier forceps useful in the cheek, scalp, and lower face include Adson and Brown–Adson forceps (Storz N5405 and N5420).

Jeweler type forceps are the smooth pointed forceps that you are probably already using in your practice to remove delicate sutures (Storz E1947 1).

Dissection technique

Most surgery is not cutting, but separating tissue planes. This concept may be the most important in this text. The surgeon and assistant should *pull the tissues apart, as the surgeon separates the tissues with the cutting tool*. For example, to separate the orbicularis muscle from the orbital septum, the surgeon should hold the scissors in the dominant hand and grasp the muscle with forceps in the nondominant hand. The assistant should grasp the septum with another forceps. Working together, the two pairs of forceps "pull" the orbicularis muscle off the septum. You will see small fibrous bands that are easy to separate with the scissors, Colorado needle, or laser (Figure 1-13). *In a sense, your nondominant hand shows your dominant hand what to do.* You will notice that it is easy to operate with an experienced surgeon as your assistant because the layers are pulled apart for you. Use this technique whenever possible. There are a few planes that you work where this technique is not possible. For example, in the subcutaneous plane of the cheek, you will have to sharply incise the tissues. Have an experienced surgeon check your dissection technique to confirm that you are correctly *pulling the tissues apart* and *separating the planes with the cutting tool*.

Remember to avoid "snips," close the scissors slowly. Watch how the tissues open. This can be one of the most "elegant" and rewarding of surgical techniques (Box 1-1).

Retractors

There are three types of retractors:

- Self-retaining retractors
- Hand-held retractors
- Suture retractors

The *Jaffe eyelid speculum* is an excellent self-retaining retractor for eyelid surgery (Figure 1-14). This speculum was

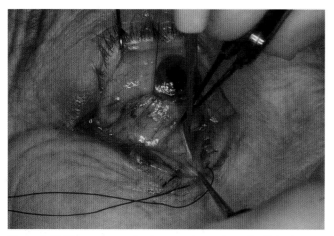

Figure 1-13 The surgeon and assistant work together to "pull" the tissues apart. Notice the bands of tissue stretched between the orbicularis muscle and the orbital septum that are easy to cut.

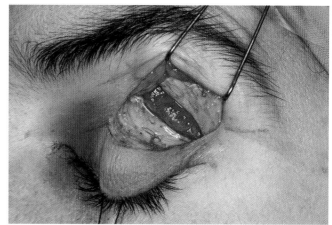

Figure 1-14 Jaffe eyelid speculum in place. The speculum can be used to open the surgical wound (as shown here for a lacrimal gland biopsy) or can be used to elevate an eyelid away from the operating site. It is a useful tool in almost every eyelid procedure.

Box 1-1

Dissection Technique That You Must Know

- Most surgery is not cutting, but separating tissue planes
- Grasp the tissue layers that you want to separate (don't hold the skin when you are separating the muscle from the septum)
- Grasp the tissues close to where you want to work on them
- Learn to "pull" the tissues apart as you cut with the scissors or Colorado needle
- Look for the fibrous bands that will show as you pull the tissues apart
- Separate the layers with controlled closure of the scissors rather than short "snips." Watch the tissues open as you close the blades

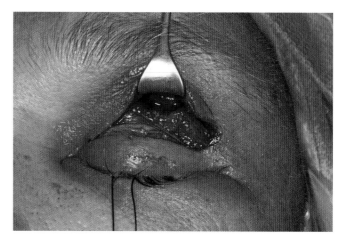

Figure 1-15 The Desmarres lid retractor is used similarly to the Jaffe lid speculum, but must be hand held. This retractor can be placed over a Jaffe lid speculum for extra retraction, a useful combination. Here, the Desmarres lid retractor is opening a skin crease incision to drain a superior orbital abscess.

originally designed for cataract surgery to retract the eyelids independently without any pressure on the globe. I use this retractor in almost every lid procedure. Self-retaining retractors are rarely used in orbital surgery because it is difficult to position the retractors adequately in the orbit. The constant pressure on the tissue with a self-retaining retractor can limit circulation to the eye. There are self-retaining retractors made for lacrimal surgery, but I have not found these instruments to be satisfactory.

Hand-held retractors are useful, but require a good assistant. The well-trained assistant will move the retractors as the surgery proceeds from area to another. When maximum retraction is not necessary, the assistant eases the pressure on the retractor to improve circulation. The most commonly used hand-held retractor for eyelid surgery is the *Desmarres lid retractor* (size 1: 13 mm; Storz E0981) (Figure 1-15). The shape of the Desmarres lid retractor is helpful to atraumatically retract tissues. Useful orbital hand-held retractors are the malleable retractors and the Sewall orbital retractors. The *flat-bladed malleable retractors* (ribbon malleable retractors, Codman, http://www.codman.com, 800 255 2500) come in different widths and can be bent to suit the particular needs of the procedure. Tapered malleable retractors are helpful in deep wounds, but require special ordering. *Sewall retractors*

are commonly used to retract orbital tissues. A disadvantage of both malleable retractors and Sewall retractors is that "towing-in" of the retractor may damage tissues, especially those deep in the orbit (experienced orbital surgeons fear the towed-in retractor as a cause of blindness more than any cutting instrument). You will find that orbital exposure is improved by lining the wound with *neurosurgical cottonoids* (similar to the lap sponges you used to pack off the bowel as a general surgery student) (Figure 1-16). The familiar *nasal speculum* is a type of hand-held retractor.

Sutures can be used as retractors. No manipulation by a surgical assistant is necessary. As many sutures as necessary can be placed to provide good tissue exposure (4-0 silk). Hand-held retractors can be placed on top of the suture retractors to give extra retraction when necessary. As with any other static or self-retaining retractor, if problems with circulation are anticipated, suture retractors should be avoided or frequently released (Figure 1-17).

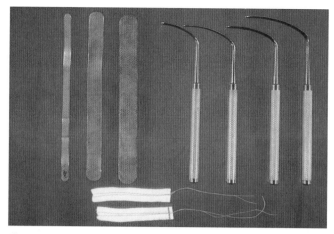

Figure 1-16 Orbital retractors (left to right): malleable retractors, Sewall retractors, and neurosurgical cottonoids (below).

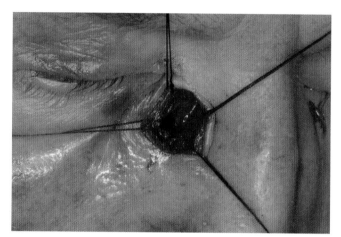

Figure 1-17 Use of 4-0 silk suture retractors for exposure of an external dacryocystorhinostomy wound.

Hemostasis

Preoperative considerations

Achieving hemostasis is another new technique to most ophthalmic surgeons. You will need to master some simple techniques for controlling bleeding if you are going to do eyelid surgery safely. Effective hemostasis technique begins with using an injection of *local anesthetic with epinephrine* (1 : 100,000) in every operation on the face. You should always inject the local anesthetic before prepping the patient and scrubbing, allowing about 10 minutes to pass to achieve maximum hemostasis.

Your time in the operating room will be shorter, and your patients will suffer less postoperative bruising if you remind them to *stop taking all anticoagulant medications* before surgery. *Warfarin* (Coumadin) should be stopped 5 days preoperatively with the consent of the patient's internist. *Aspirin-containing products* should be stopped 10–14 days before surgery. *Nonsteroidal anti-inflammatory medications* should be stopped 3–5 days before surgery. Remember that most patients do not consider aspirin and other over-the-counter medications as important when you ask what medications they are taking. You must ask specifically about these medicines. A long list of herbal remedies can affect coagulation, especially when used in combination with other anticoagulants. Among others, the 3 "G's" (garlic, ginseng, and ginkgo) should be stopped before operation. High doses of vitamin E can negatively affect coagulation as well. Under some circumstances, operating on the patient who is anticoagulated may be necessary but, to minimize the chances of hemorrhage, you should stop anticoagulants whenever possible.

Tamponade

An easy way to temporarily control bleeding is *tamponade*. Your *finger*, a gauze pad, or a Q-tip *compressing* the bleeding tissue against bone will stop most bleeding. Similarly, you can obtain hemostasis by *pinching the tissue* between your fingers or in a forceps. This is usually a temporary measure, but will minimize blood loss and facilitate your attempts to use cautery. An example of this is the bleeding that occurs after a wedge resection of the lid. The marginal artery usually bleeds. By holding the lid margin between the blades of the forceps, you can control the bleeding while you apply bipolar cautery.

If the point of bleeding cannot be identified, the wound may be *packed with a gauze sponge* to control bleeding. As the packing is removed, you may be able to isolate individual bleeding spots.

Most arteries encountered in oculoplastic surgery do not require *clamping* and *tying* to gain control of bleeding. However, placing a small hemostat on a bleeding artery may facilitate your attempts to use cautery. For larger arteries, suture ligatures or vascular clips can be used, but this is usually necessary only in large orbital procedures. You can avoid bleeding in enucleation surgery by clamping the optic nerve before cutting it. This requires some practice, but leaves a dry orbit after the removal of the eye. The stump of the optic nerve can be cauterized and the clamp removed.

Cautery

You *must* learn how to use cautery to do eyelid surgery. Three types of cautery are available:

- Heat
- Bipolar cautery
- Unipolar cautery

Battery-operated hand-held cautery units can be used for small areas of bleeding. In general, these are too inefficient for any lid surgery other than the smallest procedures, such as lid biopsies or chalazion incision and drainage. You can control the temperature of the heated wire somewhat by turning the cautery unit off and on. If you depress the finger switch on continuously while you apply cautery, the tip gets very hot and will burn through the tissue, often causing more bleeding. I also use the hot tip as a cutting and cautery tool for dissection of delicate vascular tissues as in the separation of Müller's muscle and the levator aponeurosis, which works nicely. You should remember to turn off any supplemental oxygen when using this tool. Under certain conditions, a fire can result.

Bipolar cautery

Bipolar cautery is commonly used in oculoplastic surgery. Because the current passes between the tips, there is little spreading of tissue damage. Normally, the tissue is wet enough to conduct the current between the cautery tips (this type of cautery is also referred to as a "wet field" cautery). Many surgeons accustomed to doing ocular surgery have a difficult time using bipolar cautery for eyelid surgery. The main problem is holding the cautery tips too closely together, preventing adequate amounts of tissue from being cauterized. The current has to flow through the tissue held between the cautery tips to affect coagulations. Using a bipolar cautery with a "non-stick" tip (Weck "Biceps" coagulator) works well. Like other instruments, bipolar cautery forceps are made in different lengths with different tips (the "jewelers" forceps tip is a good size for eyelid operations).

You must become adept at bipolar cautery to do eyelid surgery. Consider these three steps:

- Exposure
- Tamponade
- Cautery

Your assistant should provide exposure of the bleeding area with fingers, hand-held retractors, or forceps. If there is considerable bleeding, the assistant can provide temporary tamponade with a gauze pad while you ready a cotton-tipped applicator and the bipolar cautery tool. *Bipolar cautery technique is easiest if the surgeon, rather than the assistant, applies the tamponade* (the roles can be reversed, but the same person using the cautery tool should provide the tamponade). The surgeon places the bipolar tips in proximity to the cotton-tipped applicator. The applicator is rolled away from the bleeding site, and cautery is applied immediately. If bleeding is brisk, you may be able to provide tamponade on the tissues proximal to the bleeding site to decrease the flow of blood. If this does not work, suction can be used to provide exposure of the bleeding vessel.

Unipolar cautery

Unipolar cautery (also called monopolar cautery) can be used to provide periocular hemostasis as well. The most useful form of unipolar cautery is the microdissection or microsurgical needle discussed above. This needle provides simultaneous cutting and cautery and reduces the bleeding of soft tissues dramatically. As you may have figured out by now, this needle is often referred to as the "Colorado" needle, the proprietary name of the original product. The microdissection (or microsurgical) needle should not be confused with the cutting needle of other unipolar systems. The tungsten tip of the microdissection needle is much finer and causes less thermal damage to the surrounding tissue. Unipolar cautery with a wider flat blade is used only when all other attempts to stop bleeding fail. Remember that teamwork is necessary for efficient hemostasis techniques. A helpful assistant can make a big difference.

Bone wax

You will encounter bleeding from small perforating vessels in bone. Bipolar cautery will not stop this bleeding. Unipolar cautery can be used to provide hemostasis in bone because the current spreads directly into the bone. As a better alternative, you can use *small pieces of paraffin* or *bone wax* to plug the bleeding sites. The surrounding bone must be relatively dry to get the wax to stick.

Drugs

We have already talked about the *preoperative use of epinephrine* in the local anesthetic to decrease bleeding. You will notice the effect of the epinephrine on the surgical site by the blanching of the injected area. Similarly, injections can be used intraoperatively for additional vasoconstriction. Initially, the hydrostatic pressure effect of the injected fluid into the tissue helps control capillary bleeding as well. You can apply 0.05% oxymetazoline (Afrin) or 5% cocaine solution topically to the nasal mucosa to cause vasoconstriction. Agents such as Gelfoam, Avitene, and Surgicel can be used to promote clotting, increasing platelet activation. Thrombin (topical thrombogen) works a step later in the clotting cascade, stimulating the conversion of fibrinogen to fibrin. A small piece of Gelfoam soaked in thrombin solution as a packing material is an excellent way to stop recalcitrant bleeding from nasal mucosa (enhances platelet aggregation and fibrin formation).

If you start doing bigger flaps or reconstructive craniofacial work, you will become familiar with products that can be "lifesaving." To stop trouble bleeding or cerebrospinal fluid (CSF) leaks, FloSeal and Tisseal (http://www.baxter.com) are especially helpful. FloSeal contains bovine thrombin suspended in gelatin granules so the mechanism is similar to the Gelfoam/thrombin combination. The mix sticks to wet tissue and does not swell to the degree that Gelfoam does. Tisseal (a "fibrin glue") contain human fibrinogen, bovine thrombin, and an antifibrinolytic agent (to stabilize the clot). FloSeal tends to be more useful for cranio-orbital applications, but you should know about both. Your neurosurgical and ENT colleagues can give you tips on how to use these materials.

Occasionally, special situations occur in which hypotensive anesthesia can be used to reduce bleeding. This technique is not commonly used in the United States. In vascular tumors, preoperative intra-arterial embolization of large vessels can be used to minimize bleeding encountered during surgery.

Drains

Suction drains can be used postoperatively to increase hemostasis and decrease swelling and the risk of infection. If you are performing surgery involving large flaps, active suction devices ("grenade" type) attached to a Jackson–Pratt drain will be helpful. Some surgeons use passive drains, such as Penrose or rubber band drains, routinely for orbital surgery procedures. I rarely use these. Remember that a drain is not a substitute for intraoperative hemostasis.

Suction

Suction is a useful technique to clear unwanted blood, irrigation fluid, or other fluid from the surgical site to increase exposure of the operative wound. Three types of suction tips are used in oculoplastic surgery (Figure 1-18):

- Flexible suction catheter
- Yankauer tonsil suction tube
- Frazier and Baron suction tubes

The flexible suction catheter can be used to suction blood and irrigation fluid out of the nostril when you are perform-

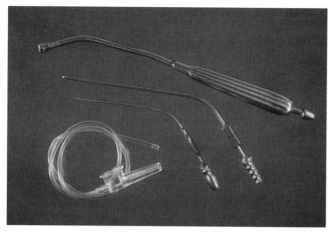

Figure 1-18 Suction types (top to bottom): Yankauer tonsil suction, Frazier suction tube, Baron suction tube, and flexible suction catheter.

ing tear duct surgery. It is also useful to pass this catheter down the nasal pharynx to remove fluid before extubation. The Yankauer tonsil suction tube is an all-purpose suction tip that is used primarily in wide surgical wounds when a large-bore general suction device is needed. The Frazier suction catheter is the most useful suction device for oculoplastic surgery. This metal angled catheter (9 French) provides directed and accurate suction to individual bleeding sites. A small version of the Frazier suction catheter is called the Baron catheter (available in 3, 5, and 7 French). Most suction catheters have a port that can be occluded to increase the suction pressure. For mild bleeding, this port does not need to be occluded. When more bleeding is present, the port may be occluded to give more suction. When dealing with tissues that are easily sucked into the catheter tip, such as orbital fat or brain, you should *suction over a gauze pad or neurosurgical cottonoid* to clear the fluid without damage to the underlying tissue.

Smaller suction tips get occluded easily and will require irrigation of the suction tube with clear fluid as necessary. You might find that clamping the suction tubing when it is not in use will make the operating room quieter.

The rigid suction tubes can also be used to provide gentle retraction of tissue. For most effective control of bleeding, the surgeon should use the suction tube and the cautery tool simultaneously, rather than the assistant and surgeon each holding one.

Suturing

Types of suture material

Suture material varies in three basic characteristics:

- Absorbable or permanent
- Monofilament or multifilament
- Natural fiber, synthetic, or metal wire

Absorbable sutures degrade naturally over time. No removal is required. Common absorbable sutures include gut (fast absorbing, plain, and chromic), Vicryl, Dexon and Monocryl and PDS (polydioxanone). These sutures vary in degradation time from 5 days to more than 30 days. Permanent sutures do not degrade in human tissue. Examples include nylon, polyester, Prolene, and stainless steel. These sutures can remain indefinitely in a deep closure, but must be removed if used on the skin.

Monofilament sutures are made of a single strand of material. *Multifilament sutures* are made of braided strands of single filaments. Monofilament sutures cause less tissue reaction and are easier to pull out than multifilament sutures. Braided sutures are easier to handle than monofilament sutures (said to have a better "*hand*"). Multifilament sutures have a higher coefficient of friction and therefore maintain tension on a wound and hold a knot better than monofilament sutures. You will find that you need to use the "3-1-1" tie with monofilament sutures, but you can usually use a "1-1-1" tie with braided sutures. Silk sutures are considered the gold standard in terms of handling and tying. Manufacturers sometimes combine characteristics to make a more versatile suture. An example of this is braided nylon sutures. These permanent sutures have little tissue reactivity and have a better hand than monofilament nylon.

Natural fibers including silk and gut are available. Chromic sutures are gut (collagen) sutures that have been treated for greater resistance to absorption. Fast absorbing gut sutures are made to be used on the skin and reabsorb in 5–7 days. *Synthetic sutures* include nylon, polyester, polypropylene (Prolene), and expanded polytetrafluoroethylene (Gore-Tex). Metal wire sutures, usually stainless steel, may be used for deep closure when a strong permanent suture is required. Wire sutures are used in some types of fracture and telecanthus repair.

You might notice that we have not mentioned glue so far. Surgical skin adhesives can be useful, but really have not "caught on" much at this point. *Dermabond* (Ethicon) is an alternative for sutures. You can use it on small lacerations in children and avoid the local anesthetic. I have used it on external DCR incisions and functional skin crease incisions with good success, and it is used in many other areas of surgery. It is helpful to put ointment on the skin around the wound where you do not want the glue to adhere. I expect we will see more use of surgical glues in the coming years. You may want to give it a try.

The choice of suture material depends largely on the surgeon's experience and individual preference. As you can see, there is no perfect suture, but rather many good materials to choose from. If you are interested in detailed closure choice, read on. If not, skip to the next section on needles.

These are the common suture choices for me. I like absorbable sutures on the eyelid skin. Patients don't like to have sutures out and it saves time postoperatively in the office. That being said, absorbable sutures tend to scar more, often untie or break, and frequently are not entirely gone at 1 week causing the patient some consternation. I no longer recommend Vicryl sutures for superficial skin closure as they take a long time to resorb and often leave tracks. For common functional surgeries, I use 5-0 fast absorbing running suture and tie with an extra throw (3-1-1-1) for the skin. I will often put an extra interrupted suture in the skin crease over a running closure. Many of my colleagues use a simple running suture with 6-0 nylon or Prolene. In cases where you are trying to get the absolute least scarring, a subcuticular Prolene removed at 5–8 days is a nice way to go (see below). For subcutaneous

closure, I use Vicryl or PDS sutures. There is a tendency for Vicryl sutures to "spit" (sterile abscesses rising to the surface as they absorb). The monofilament absorbable sutures, PDS and Monocryl, can avoid this, but require more careful knot tying as they are "more slippery." Clear sutures do not show through thin skin, but are more difficult to work with.

Types of needles

There are several types of needles available. Needles have the same parts, but vary by shape, size, and point (Figure 1-19) as follows:

- Shape
  — 3/8 circle
  — 1/2 circle
  — 1/4 circle
- Size
- Point
  — Taper
  — Cutting
  — Reverse cutting
  — Conventional cutting
  — Spatula

You will notice that the *most common shape is the 3/8 circle needle* (Figure 1-19, B). These needles are used for all general-

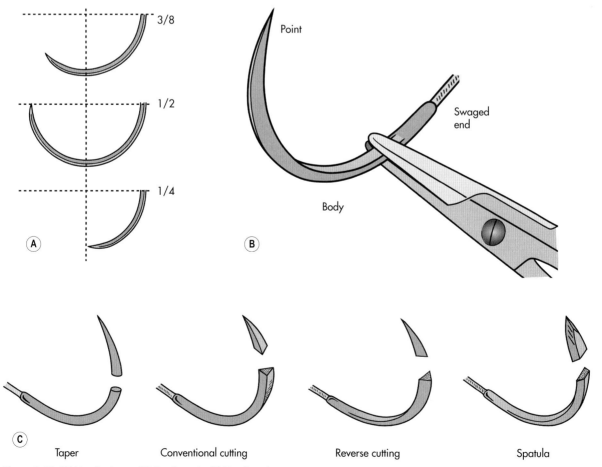

Figure 1-19 (**A**) Needle shapes. (**B**) Needle parts. (**C**) Needle points.

purpose suturing. Other shaped needles are used for special purposes.

The half-circle needle is used to suture in tight spaces. You will use these needles often. The most common use for a half-circle needle in oculoplastic surgery is to attach the lateral tarsal strip to the periosteum (4-0 Mersilene, braided polyester, Ethicon 1779G, double-armed). The sharp curve of the needle is ideal for reaching between the periosteum of the lateral orbital rim and the orbital tissues. The 4-0 Mersilene is permanent and does not cause the suture granulomas that are common with 4-0 Vicryl sutures. I use a double-armed suture that nicely "tucks in" the strip against the periosteum. The mucosal flaps of an external dacryocystorhinostomy can be closed with a half-circle needle and a chromic gut suture (Ethicon 798; 4-0 chromic gut G-2 half-circle cutting needle). The uses for this needle are similar to those for the P-2 needle. Because the mucosa heals fast and is not under tension, a chromic suture is used. In oculoplastic surgery, 5/8 inch needles are rarely used.

The *needle point* will determine how easily sutures pass through tissue. Two types of needle points are available: taper and cutting (Figure 1-19, C). *Taper point needles* come to a sharp point and *push through tissue*. There is no cutting edge of the needle. Taper needles are used in delicate tissues such as bowel. In oculoplastic surgery, taper needles are used for bridle sutures under extraocular muscles.

The majority of needles that you will use are *cutting needles*. Cutting needles have sharpened edges along the curvature of the needle. Rather than push through the tissue, these needles *cut the tissue*, facilitating penetration of the needle through the tissue. The two common types of cutting needles available are:

- Reverse cutting
- Conventional cutting

The most commonly used needle is the reverse cutting needle. This needle, when viewed on end, appears as an *up-ended triangle* (Figure 1-19, C). The sharp edges of the needle are on the *outer curvature*.

The *conventional cutting needle*, when viewed on end, is a *triangle pointed upward*. The sharp edge of the cutting needle is on the *inner curvature*. Typically, a conventional cutting needle creates a bigger hole in the tissue than a reverse cutting needle. The natural motion of passing a needle tends to pull the needle superiorly out of the wound. If the cutting blade is facing upward, the needle tends to cut superiorly as well as along the needle pass. The reverse cutting needle easily pushes through the tissue without enlarging the needle tract.

Several variations of taper needles are available. The most common variation is the *spatula needle* (Figure 1-19, C). The spatula needle is designed to pass through tissue in a lamellar fashion. The most commonly used spatula needle is used to reattach the levator aponeurosis to the tarsal plate (Ethicon 7731; 5-0 monofilament nylon S-24 spatula needle). The shape of the spatula needle facilitates a lamellar pass through the tarsus.

Many other variations of taper and cutting needle points are available. The next time you are in the operating room, ask the nursing staff to show you the suture packs. You will see a diagram of the needle shape and point on each package. You are guaranteed to be overwhelmed if you browse the Ethicon suture catalog online. You will find some good illustrations on the comparison of needle sizes and shapes that are useful when you are looking for a new suture and needle. You might find it interesting to look at some of the needle and suture brochures available from the major suture manufacturers (often they are available in the operating room). You will be impressed at the thought and the fine detail that goes into the development of these super-sharp stainless steel needles that we take for granted.

To help you appreciate the differences in needle points, compare passing a taper needle with a cutting needle of the same size and shape. Try to pass a tapered 4-0 silk suture through the lid margin as a traction suture. Repeat the same needle pass with a 4-0 silk suture on a cutting needle. You will be amazed at the difference in the way the needle is passed.

The size of the needle corresponds to the size of the suture. This choice largely depends on how much strength is required to keep the tissues sewn together. Thicker tissues under greater tension require larger sutures. Often, the choice of needles and suture size is a process of elimination. A smaller suture would break and a larger suture seems too big.

Needle holders

Two types of needle holders are used in oculoplastic surgery:

- Spring handle (Castroviejo needle holder)
- Ring handle (Webster needle holder)

The most common needle holder is the *Castroviejo needle holder*. This spring-action needle holder is excellent for the delicate work of oculoplastic surgery. The Castroviejo needle holder is held with the traditional pencil grip as this needle holder is a "finger tool" (Figure 1-20). The index finger and thumb control precise movements for delicate suturing. I prefer the locking variation of the Castroviejo needle holder. It should not be used for needles larger than 4-0, however.

The traditional plastic surgical ring handle needle holder is used for 4-0 or greater sized needles. The most commonly available ring handle needle holder is the Webster needle

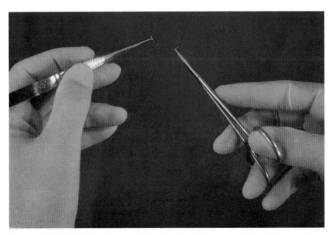

Figure 1-20 Holding the needle holder. Left, The pencil grip of the spring (Castroviejo) needle holder. This is the most common needle holder that you will use. Right, The "thumb/ring finger grip" of a ring handle (Webster) needle holder.

holder. This type of needle holder is held with the *thumb/ring finger grip*. The index finger serves to direct the tip of the needle holder. This grip allows the needle holder to be used with finger, hand, and wrist motions (Box 1-2).

The needle should be loaded on the needle holder approximately three fourths of the way back on the needle. If you look at a larger needle, you will notice that there is a flat platform that ends where the suture is swaged on to the needle (refer back to Figure 1-19, A). If you hold the needle on the round part of the needle holder, you will lose control and the needle will rotate.

Suturing technique

Passing the needle

Let's talk about the passage of a single stitch. You have selected the appropriate size, curve, and point of the needle and have positioned it properly in the needle holder. You are holding the needle holder with either the pencil grip for delicate surgery or the thumb/ring finger grip for a conventional needle holder. Now position your body comfortably facing the wound directly. If you are right-handed, it is easiest to suture from left to right so that the tail of the suture

---

Box 1-2

Sutures for Oculoplastic, Orbital, and Lacrimal Surgery

2-0 Sutures

- 2-0 Vicryl: strong stitch to use as deep anchoring sutures on cheek flaps (Ethicon J328H CT-3 taper point)
- 2-0 Vicryl: strong smaller reverse cutting needle also good for anchoring flaps (Ethicon J459H X-1 needle)
- 2-0 PDS; good anchoring suture for SMAS lift procedures, longer lasting than Vicryl (Ethicon Z317H 26 mm SH taper point, violet)

3-0 Sutures

- 3-0 Gore-Tex® CV-3: for indirect browpexy (Gore N10 PH-24 double-armed)
- 3-0 Vicryl: strong small reverse cutting needle good for anchoring flaps and deep closure in scalp and cheek (Ethicon J458H X-1 needle)
- 3-0 Vicryl: strong smaller taper needle and stitch good for anchoring sutures in tight areas for cheek or scalp flaps (Ethicon J305H RB-1 needle)
- 3-0 PDS: similar to Vicryl above, but longer lasting. Clear suture is good for anchoring facial flaps (Ethicon Z423H 19 mm FS-2 reverse cutting, clear)
- 3-0 PDS: similar to Vicryl above, but longer lasting. Violet suture is helpful in hair-bearing areas (Ethicon Z398H 19 mm FS-2 reverse cutting, violet)
- 3-0 Mayo trocar: for threading fascia during frontalis sling (Richard-Allan 216703, http://www.aspensurgical.com)

4-0 Sutures

- 4-0 chromic: long reverse cutting needle for Quickert suture and suturing oral mucosa (Ethicon 793G G-3 needle, double-armed)
- 4-0 chromic: short half-circle needle useful for suturing the flaps for external dacryocystorhinostomy (Ethicon 798G G-2 needle, double-armed)
- 4-0 Vicryl: short half-circle reverse cutting needle, useful for tight spaces that require subcutaneous closure or anchoring (cheek tissue at lateral canthus) (Ethicon J504G P-2 needle)
- 4-0 Vicryl: short reverse cutting needle for subcutaneous closure (Ethicon J464G P-3 needle)
- 4-0 Vicryl: longer reverse cutting needle for brow closure (Ethicon J682H PS-1 needle)
- 4-0 Vicryl: shorter and more sturdy than the PS-1 needle, good for tight spaces (Ethicon J496G PS-2 reverse cutting needle)
- 4-0 PDS: for subcutaneous flap suture (Ethicon Z494G 13 mm P-3 needle reverse cutting, clear)
- 4-0 PDS: anchoring suture for subcutaneous closure in hair-bearing areas (Ethicon Z513G 19 mm PS-2 needle reverse cutting 3/8 curve, violet)

- 4-0 PDS needle: anchoring suture for subcutaneous cheek or pretrichial scalp closure suture (Ethicon Z496G 19 mm PS-2 reverse cutting 3/8 curve, clear)
- 4-0 PDS P-2 needle: shorter and more sturdy than the PS-2 needle, good for tight spaces (Ethicon Z504G 8 mm P-2 needle reverse cutting, clear)
- 4-0 silk: reverse cutting needle for traction sutures (Ethicon 789G G-3 needle, single-armed)
- 4-0 silk: taper needle for bridle sutures under extraocular muscles (Ethicon K871H RB-1 needle, single-armed)
- 4-0 Mersilene S-2: short half-circle needle (S-2), braided polyester, for lateral tarsal strip operation (Ethicon 1779G, double-armed)

5-0 Sutures

- 5-0 fast absorbing gut: used as skin suture (Ethicon 1915G PC-1 needle)
- 5-0 chromic: for medial spindle operation (Ethicon 792G G-3 needle, double-armed)
- 5-0 Vicryl: for subcutaneous and orbicularis closure (Ethicon J571G S-14 needle, double-armed)
- 5-0 PDS: anchoring suture for periocular tissues. Less "spitting" than Vicryl. Clear best for nonhair-bearing tissues (Ethicon Z493G 13 mm P-3 needle reverse cutting, clear)
- 5-0 PDS: anchoring suture for periocular tissues. Less "spitting" than Vicryl. Violet best for hair-bearing tissues (Ethicon Z463G 13 mm P-3 needle reverse cutting, violet)
- 5-0 nylon: for suturing levator aponeurosis to tarsus in ptosis surgery. Periocular and brow skin closure (Ethicon 7731G S-24 spatula needle, double-armed)
- 5-0 nylon: for skin periocular and nasal skin closure (Ethicon 698G P-3 needle)
- 5-0 Prolene: periocular skin closure, blue color especially useful for repair of lacerations or incisions in hair-bearing areas. Extra knots required. Running sutures are easily removed (Ethicon 8698G P-3 needle)

6-0 Sutures

- 6-0 fast absorbing gut: for conjunctival closure or eyelid skin (Ethicon 1916G PC-1 needle)
- 6-0 Vicryl: double-armed for tarsal fracture operation and Jones' tube suture (Ethicon J-570G with S-14 needle)
- 6-0 nylon: for skin closure of eyelid and periocular skin and to tie stent used with pigtail probe for repair of canalicular lacerations (Ethicon 1698G P-3 needle)

7-0 Sutures

- 7-0 chromic gut: for conjunctival closure (Ethicon TG100-8 needle)
- 7-0 Vicryl: suture for closure of conjunctiva (Ethicon J-546 TG140-8 needle)
- 7-0 nylon: for eyelid skin closure (Ethicon 1647G P-6 needle)

is away from the site of the next needle pass. Always suture with your dominant hand. Most of the thin skin in the periocular area will require fixation with forceps to facilitate the needle pass. Efficient suturing techniques require that you "control" the tissues—get the tissues to act the way that you want them to. Grasp the tissue lightly with the tooth of the forceps very close to where you want to place the needle point. Place the point of the needle *directly adjacent* to the forceps and drive the needle through the tissue "following the curve of the needle," pushing the needle toward your chest. Take note of the depth at which the needle emerges from the wound. Grasp the near side of the wound and place the tip of the needle at the same depth. Complete the pass of the needle until the needle holder touches the skin. Regrasp *both* wound edges *directly adjacent* to the needle and begin to pull the needle out of the wound. Do not grasp the tip of the needle. Advance the needle until you can regrasp 3/4 of the way back so you can load the needle for the next suture pass (Figure 1-21).

An alternative needle passing technique is to pass the needle through the wound and then grasp the tip of the needle with the forceps and pull it out. As the needle is being pulled out, you use your needle driver to reload the needle. My preference is the former method. You might try both. The important part is not to spend a lot of time reloading the needle.

Recently, I have begun using a helpful old suturing technique. Hang a single prong Tyrell skin hook from the end of the wound. This puts the wound under some tension, stabilizes the edges for suturing, and helps with spacing. The technique works well for upper eyelid skin crease incisions.

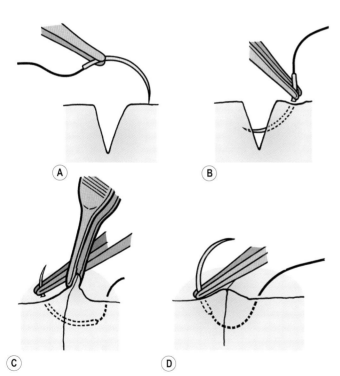

Figure 1-21 Passing the needle through the wound. (**A**) Pass the needle to enter perpendicular to the skin. (**B**) The needle should leave and enter the wound edges at the same depth. (**C**) Use the Paufique forceps to grasp both edges of the wound. Advance the needle with the needle holder, first pushing the needle, then pulling the needle out. Take care not to grasp the tip of the needle. (**D**) When the needle is advanced enough, reload it before you remove it from the tissue. You are then ready for the next needle pass.

Superficial and deep sutures

Suture placement can be considered either deep or superficial. *Deep*, or buried, sutures are used to close the subcutaneous or deeper layers of tissues. These sutures close dead space, provide wound stability, and remove tension from the final skin closure. Deep sutures are not required on the eyelid skin, but are used in the periocular area. Deep suture passes may be placed through periosteum, muscle, subcutaneous fat, or the dermis of thicker skin. Any dead space should be closed with deep sutures to prevent hematoma formation. Deep sutures may be used to anchor skin and muscle flaps and usually provide some degree of anatomic overcorrection. Long-lasting absorbable suture material (such as PDS, Vicryl, Dexon, or Monocryl) is usually used for buried sutures. My personal preference is PDS suture for most subcutaneous closure.

Superficial sutures are placed on the skin. Superficial sutures may be either *interrupted* or *running* (*continuous*). Interrupted sutures provide accurate wound alignment and appropriate eversion of the wound edges. When repairing a complex laceration, you can use interrupted sutures initially to tack together the wound in an anatomically correct alignment. When you are suturing a long wound, a good place to start is to divide the wound into halves with interrupted sutures. This prevents misalignment of the wound edges and the creation of a "dog-ear" at one end of the wound.

You can use running or continuous sutures to close incisions placed in natural skin creases or wrinkle lines as slightly more inversion of the wound may occur. Running sutures are faster to place and easier to remove than interrupted sutures. A nice healing running suture in an eyelid skin crease is a "subcuticular" suture. This suture enters the end of the wound and the trailing end is tied on itself. The needle is passed in and out of the wound edges in a plane parallel to the skin surface. The suture travels through the most superficial portion of the orbicularis muscle (there is no subcutaneous layer of the eyelid skin). At the end of the wound, the needle is brought through the skin and the suture is tied on itself. After about 1 week, the knot at one end of the wound is cut and the suture is pulled out. Prolene suture, 6-0, is ideal for this closure as it is slippery and easy to pull out. Remember that Prolene requires a 3-1-1-1 tie to ensure a secure knot.

For wounds outside of skin crease lines, it is best to use interrupted sutures to give better wound eversion, preventing a depressed scar. Two types of interrupted sutures are used to close the surgical wound:

- Simple suture
- Vertical mattress suture

Simple sutures are the most commonly used interrupted suture (Figure 1-22, A). When correctly placed, simple sutures provide good wound alignment and eversion of the wound edges. When a greater amount of wound eversion is necessary, vertical mattress sutures can be used (Figure 1-22, B). The "far–far, near–near" suture pass is especially useful to provide wound eversion of the lid margin when you are repairing a lid laceration. In skin creases, a simple running suture is used (Figure 1-22, C).

To maintain spacing of the wound closure, use the "halving" method. Successively divide the wound into halves (Figure 1-23, A). If, despite careful wound closure, redundant tissue or a "dog-ear" exists at the end of the wound,

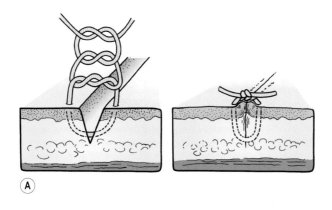

(A)

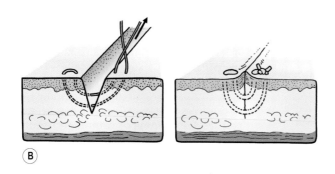

(B)

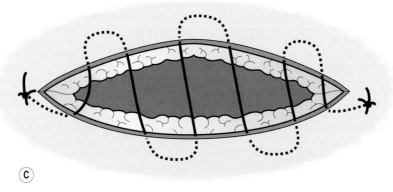

(C)

Figure 1-22 Placement of skin sutures. (**A**) Simple interrupted suture. (**B**) Vertical mattress suture used for maximum wound eversion. (**C**) Running "subcuticular" suture.

it can be excised at the expense of a slightly longer scar (Figure 1-23, B).

Tying the suture

Most sutures passed in oculoplastic surgery are tied with an *instrument tie*. There are some simple tricks that you should learn to make your knot tying secure and efficient (Figure 1-24, A). Imagine passing a suture through the wound edges. As you withdraw the needle, the two arms of the suture make a V. Place your instrument in the V and wrap the needle end of the suture around the needle holder twice (Figure 1-24, B). Grasp the end of the suture with the needle holder (grasp the suture near the end; Figure 1-24, C) and

pull your instrument toward you (Figure 1-24, D). Pull the suture down to the tissue, approximating the wound edges closed with gentle pressure. Do not apply more force than necessary to approximate the wound edges. You have created a new V in the suture arms. Repeat the wrapping of the needle holder and now reverse the pull of your hands with the needle holder being pulled away from you (Figure 1-24, E). Make sure that the knot lies down squarely on the first pass. Repeat this for a third time, completing the 2-1-1 surgeon's square knot (Figure 1-24, F).

Let's add two refining steps. When you start a tie, grasp one end of the suture with your forceps (held in your non-dominant hand) close to the end of the suture. Orient the

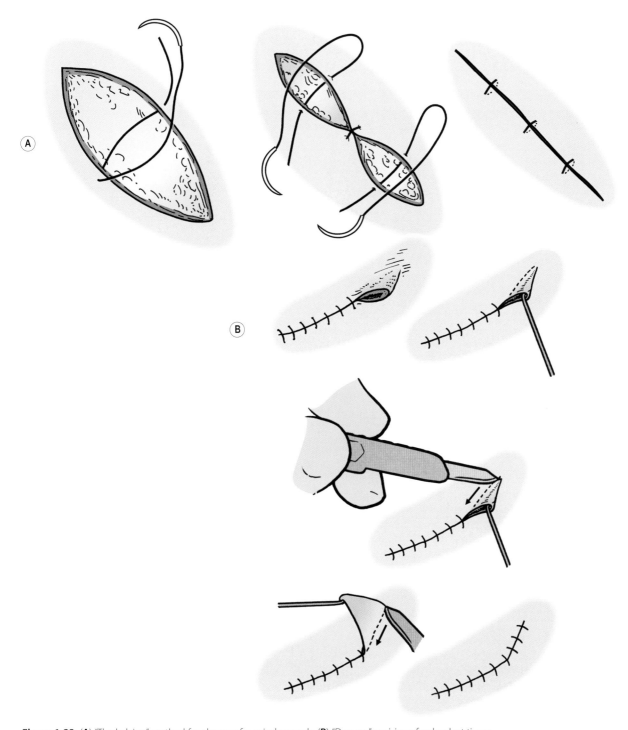

Figure 1-23 (**A**) "The halving" method for closure of surgical wounds. (**B**) "Dog-ear" excision of redundant tissue.

suture (sometimes using a gentle twist or pulling the suture) to be parallel to the needle holder. Now wind the suture around the needle holder (not the needle holder around the suture). Because the needle holder and the suture are parallel, there will be very little "spring" in the suture and little tendency for the suture to unwind from the needle holder. Be sure that you understand this. The second point to remember is that, before you wind the suture around the needle holder, place the needle holder close to the end of the suture. Avoid the tendency to bring the needle holder to the end of the free suture once the suture is wrapped around the needle holder. Practice with large sutures until you have this technique mastered. Then practice with smaller sutures. As you get better, concentrate on how to minimize your hand movements, making each tie look "easy." If you play violin or guitar, you know that minimizing your finger movements between notes is essential. *Learn to operate quickly, not by hurrying, but by moving your hands efficiently.* If each step takes twice as long as necessary, the whole operation will be twice as long as necessary.

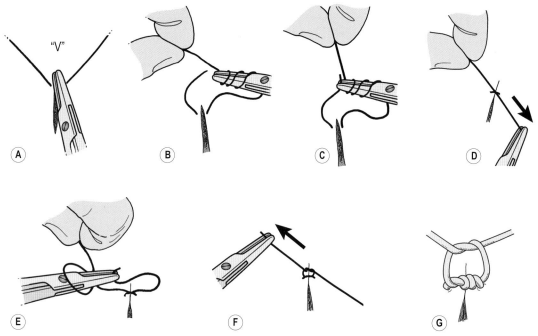

Figure 1-24 The instrument tie. (**A**) Place the needle holder in the V. (**B**) Wrap the suture around the needle holder three times. Try to make the suture and the needle holder parallel so there is not much "curl" in winding the suture. (**C**) Grasp the end of the suture (it should be near the needle holder to minimize your movements). (**D**) Pull the needle holder toward you and the suture end away from you. Notice that the knot should lie flat as you pull it down with each throw. (**E**) Put the needle holder in the V and wrap the suture around the needle holder once. Grasp the suture end and pull your hands in the opposite direction. (**F**) Repeat a third time, pulling your hands in the opposite direction again. (**G**) Each time, watch the knot tied flat.

The surgical assistant

The job of the surgical assistant is to *anticipate* and *facilitate*. It is said that good surgeons make surgery look easy, but the fact *that good assistants make surgeons look good is seldom appreciated.* If you are just learning surgery, you may not be aware of how important a good assistant is. Every day you may be operating with experienced surgeons assisting you. For you to appreciate the value of the assistant, try operating with a surgeon even less experienced than you. You will quickly realize the value of an interested and experienced assistant.

You also may not be aware of how your success as an assistant relates directly to your abilities as the primary surgeon. An experienced teacher can easily identify students with excellent surgical potential by the way they assist in surgery. Don't underestimate your value as an assistant or your ability to learn while assisting.

Checkpoint

- Do you remember the main differences between monofilament and multifilament sutures for handling and tying? Which has the better "hand?" What type of suture is the gold standard for handling?
- What are the main needle types and shapes? What is the most common needle point for sewing skin?
- Practice suturing using the "pencil grip" for the Castroviejo needle holder and the "thumb/ring finger grip" for the Webster needle holder.
- Explain the "in the V" technique for suturing to a colleague also learning to suture. Try the refinements suggested to make your ties smoother (**Box 1-3**).

Box 1-3

Instruments of Special Interest for Eyelid Operations

Retractors

- 4-0 silk traction suture (Ethicon 783 P-3 cutting needle)
- Jaffe lid retractor: recommended for all lid procedures as a self-retaining retractor (Storz E0997)
- Senn–Kanavel retractor (Storz N4780)
- Desmarres lid retractor: useful hand-held retractor for eyelids and eyelid incisions
  - Size 0: 11 mm (Storz E0980)
  - Size 1: 13 mm (Storz E0981)
  - Size 2: 15 mm (Storz E0982)
  - Size 3: 17 mm (Storz E0983)
- Skin hooks
  - Storz double fixation hook: fine double hook (Storz E0533)
  - Tyrell iris hook: fine single hook (Storz E0548)
  - Joseph double hook: larger double hook (Storz N4730)
  - Knapp lacrimal sac retractor: four-prong blunt tip (Storz E4538)

Forceps

- Paufique forceps: good all-purpose tissue forceps (Storz E1831)
- Adson forceps: cheek tissues (delicate, Storz N5405)

Box 1-3 Continued

- Brown–Adson forceps: cheek tissues (Storz N5420)
- Sanders–Castroviejo suturing forceps: delicate forceps
  - 0.12 mm teeth (Storz E1796)
  - 0.3 mm teeth (Storz E1797)
  - 0.5 mm teeth (Storz E1798)
- Bishop–Harmon straight tissue forceps: useful to thread fascia through Mayo trocar needle eye (Storz E1500)
- Lambert chalazion forceps (clamp)
  - Large, 15 mm (Storz E2632)
  - Small, 10 mm (Storz E2630)
- Halstead mosquito hemostatic forceps (Storz E3922)
- Kelly hemostatic forceps: larger than Halstead type (Storz N5511)
- Jeweler type forceps for fine suture removal (Storz E1947 1)

Needle holders

- Castroviejo needle holder: the most useful needle holder
- Straight locking, heavy, for 4-0 needles (Storz E3850)
- Straight locking, medium, for 5-0 and smaller needles (Storz E3861)
- Webster needle holder: used for 3-0 or larger needles
  - 19 mm jaw (Storz N5712)

Scissors

- Stevens tenotomy scissors
- Curved (Storz E3562)
- Straight (Storz E3560)

- Westcott tenotomy scissors: curved right, blunt tips, used for most delicate dissections (Storz E3320 R)
- Westcott stitch scissors: sharp-tipped, good for punctoplasty procedures (Storz E3321 WH)
- Mayo scissors
  - Straight (Storz N5235)
  - Curved (Storz N5236)
- Metzenbaum scissors: curved regular, useful for cheek dissections (Storz N5111)
- Facelift scissors

Elevators

- Freer septum elevator (also called a periosteal elevator)
- 4.5 mm (Storz N2348)
- 6.5 mm (Storz N2349)

Suction and hemostasis

- Frazier suction tube (9 French): general-purpose suction catheter (Storz N2421)
- Baron suction tube: small Frazier-type suction tube (Storz N0610)
- Yankauer tonsil suction tube: blunt-tipped suction catheter used for mouth and throat (Storz N7550)
- "Colorado" microdissection needle
- Bipolar cautery
- Unipolar cautery
- Disposable high-temperature cautery

Major points

- Being prepared will demonstrate your competence and instil confidence in the operating room team.
- Have the room setup in mind before you enter the operating room. Set your operating stool height first, then the operating table, and finally the microscope. Adjust the interpupillary distance on the eyepieces and set the focus of the scope. Position the necessary foot pedals before you scrub.
- Use a local anesthetic with epinephrine on all patients. Mark and inject the skin before preparing the patient.
- Learn as much as you can about the "tools of your trade":
  - Scalpel blades and other cutting instruments
  - Scissors
  - Forceps
  - Retractors
  - Cautery
  - Suction
  - Needle holders
  - Sutures
- Spread and stabilize the skin before any incision. Be aware of your body position. Always inject or cut away from the eye or your fingers. The no. 15 scalpel blade and the microdissection needle are the most useful cutting tools.
- Hide incisions in wrinkle lines or natural skin creases, when possible.

- Scissors vary in the following characteristics:
  - Length
  - Caliber
  - Tip sharpness
  - Blade design
  - Cutting motion

The scissors you will use most often are Westcott spring scissors and Stevens iris- type scissors. Use the curve of the scissors blade to your advantage. Make cutting a continuous motion. Avoid "snipping."

- Oculoplastic surgery requires skill in retracting tissues. Types of instruments use to retract tissues are the following:
  - Your fingers
  - Forceps
  - Skin hooks
  - Retractors
- Use forceps with teeth whenever possible. Learn to "pull" the tissues apart as you dissect with scissors. To separate the orbicularis muscle off the orbital septum, grasp the muscle with one forceps and the septum with another forceps (using an assistant). Gently "pull" the layers apart as you separate them with the scissors. Most surgery is not cutting, but separating tissue planes.

Major points Continued

- There are three types of retractors:
  - Self-retaining retractors
  - Hand-held retractors
  - Suture retractors
- The most useful self-retaining retractor is the Jaffe lid speculum. Hand-held retractors including the Desmarres vein retractor (for eyelids) and the Sewall and malleable ribbon retractors (for orbital retraction) are very important tools; 4-0 silk sutures are excellent suture retractors.
- Intraoperative hemostasis begins with stopping aspirin and nonsteroidal anti-inflammatory medications well in advance of surgery. Inject local anesthetic with epinephrine 10 minutes before making any incision. Learn to tamponade tissues.
- Learning effective bipolar cautery technique is a must. Consider these three steps:
  - Exposure (assistant)
  - Tamponade (surgeon)
  - Cautery (surgeon)
- The roles can be reversed.
- Three types of suction tips are used in oculoplastic surgery:
  - Flexible suction catheter
  - Yankauer tonsil suction tube
  - Frazier and Baron suction tubes
- Suture material varies in three basic characteristics:
  - Absorbable or permanent
  - Monofilament or multifilament
  - Natural fiber, synthetic, or metal wire
- Monofilament sutures are less reactive than multifilament sutures, but are more difficult to work with. Multifilament sutures hold tension and maintain a knot better than monofilament sutures.
- Needles vary by shape, size, and point. Half-circle needles are best for tight spaces (lateral canthoplasty). Reverse cutting needles are used on the skin. Spatula needles are used for most lamellar passes through tissue.
- Two types of needle holders are used in oculoplastic surgery:
  - Spring handle: Castroviejo needle holder
  - Ring handle: Webster needle holder

Use the "pencil grip" for the Castroviejo needle holder and the thumb/ring finger grip for the Webster needle holder.

- Sutures may be continuous or interrupted. Continuous sutures are used in natural skin creases or wrinkle lines (upper lid skin crease). Two types of interrupted sutures are used to close the surgical wound:
  - Simple suture
  - Vertical mattress suture
- The vertical mattress suture provides the most wound eversion.
- The job of the surgical assistant is to anticipate and facilitate. Your success as an assistant relates directly to your abilities as the primary surgeon. To be a good assistant, you need to be a part of the operation. Don't wait to be told what to do. Don't underestimate your value as an assistant or your ability to learn while assisting.
- The surgeon and the assistant work as a team. As with any team, all the players must know what the surgical plan is. As an assistant, you should be entirely familiar with the steps of the operation and any changes that the surgeon may have in mind for a particular patient. You cannot *anticipate* if you do not know the steps of the operation.
- Your job as an assistant starts with the room and equipment setup. You may be the person to administer the local anesthetic or prep and drape the patient while the surgeon scrubs. Once in the operating room, you need to *position yourself where you can see what is happening* and be a part of the operation. You would be surprised at the number of surgical students who don't do well as assistants, claiming that they can't see the operating field. If you can't see, move so you can see. If you can't get in a reasonable position to see, let the surgeon know so the situation can be changed. *To be a good assistant, you need to be a part of the operation.* Don't wait to be told what to do. If the lighting is poor, adjust the operating room lights. If there is bleeding, provide exposure and tamponade. Perhaps you can offer suction. As the dissection proceeds, move with the surgeon, constantly adjusting your retractors to provide the best exposure possible. If you cannot see the area of interest well, it is likely the surgeon cannot either. As the dissection continues, provide gentle countertraction to facilitate cutting tissue or spreading of the tissue planes. *If you don't know how to help, ask what you can do to help.*
- If you see the surgeon passing a suture, have a suture scissors ready to cut the ends of the suture. Use scissors with a straight blade and sharp tips. Hold the scissors with the tripod or thumb/ring finger grip. This allows you to stabilize the scissors with your index finger. Sometimes, it is helpful to rest the scissors on your nondominant index finger as if you were using a pool cue. The surgeon should pull the suture to the side (not straight toward you) so that you can see the full length of the suture. It is difficult to cut a suture if you are looking down the length of the suture. You may find it helpful to slide the scissors down the suture for a few inches to the knot. This gives you both visual and proprioceptive input as to where to close the scissors. Try to cut with the scissors tips to improve your accuracy. *Remember to close the scissors slowly rather than snip the suture.*
- Your efforts practicing as an assistant will help you to become a good surgeon. Take advantage of the opportunity to learn. Be interested. Ask questions. Develop a passion for the operating room. Not only will operating be how you will support your family, but it will become a part of who you are. It all starts with you as an assistant.

Suggested reading

1. Albert D, Lucarelli M, eds: Ophthalmic plastic techniques: basic considerations. In *Clinical atlas of procedures in ophthalmic surgery*, pp. 241–247, Chicago: AMA Press, 2004.

2. Christie DB, Woog JJ: Basic surgical techniques, technology, and wound repair. In Bosniak S, ed., *Principles and practice of ophthalmic plastic and reconstructive surgery*, pp. 281–293, Philadelphia: WB Saunders, 1996.

3. Edgerton MT: *The art of the surgical technique*, Balitmore: Williams and Wilkins, 1988.

4. Linberg JV, Mangano LM, Odom JV: Comparison of nonabsorbable and absorbable sutures for use in oculoplastic surgery. *Ophthal Plast Reconstr Surg* 7(1):1–7, 1991.

5. McCord C, Jr, Codner MA: Basic principles of wound closure. In McCord C, ed., *Eyelid surgery: principles and techniques*, 3rd edn, ch. 2, pp. 23–28, Philadelphia: Lippincott-Raven, 1995.

6. Nerad J: The art of the surgical technique. In *The requisites—Oculoplastic surgery*, pp. 1–24, St Louis: Mosby, 2001.

7. Sierra CA, Nesi FA, Levine MR: Basic wound repair: surgical techniques, flaps, and grafts. In Levine MR, ed., *Manual of oculoplastic surgery*, pp. 23–29, Boston: Butterworth-Heinemann, 2003.

8. Tanenbaum M: Skin and tissue techniques. In McCord CD, Tanenbaum M, Nunery WR, eds, *Oculoplastic surgery*, 3rd edn, ch. 1, pp. 1–49, New York: Raven Press, 1995.

9. Younis I, Bhutiani RP: Taking the "ouch" out—Effect of buffering commercial Xylocaine on infiltration and procedure pain—a prospective, randomized, double-blind, controlled trial. *Ann R Coll Surg Engl* 86(3):213–217, 2004.

CHAPTER 2

Clinical Anatomy

Chapter contents

Introduction

Expertise in oculoplastic and orbital surgery starts with anatomy. Learning anatomy can be very difficult. Remembering it is even harder. It's easy to get bogged down in the details without knowing why a particular anatomic feature is important in order to take care of your patients. One way to help learn anatomy is to always *understand how the anatomy makes the normal tissues function* (e.g., a certain amount of horizontal tension or "tightness" is required to hold the normal lower eyelid up against the eyeball). Then make the step to *understand how an anatomic and functional abnormality*

may be related to a clinical problem (with age, the canthal tendons lengthen, which causes the normal lower eyelid tension to be lost, allowing eversion, or ectropion, of the lower eyelid). It is not difficult to move to the final step—*understanding how to repair the anatomic abnormality and restore the function* (tightening the lower eyelid, by removing some of the redundant tendon, shortens the lax lower eyelid to correct the ectropion). These clinical anatomic correlations are not just useful teaching tools—they are the basis for most reconstructive procedures. Your real understanding of anatomy comes when you start to apply what you have read to the case that you are doing next. This is one of the thrilling parts of operating (Box 2-1).

Throughout this chapter and in the remainder of the book, we will apply the anatomy to the clinical problem and vice versa. Periocular and orbital anatomy is very complex. Understanding of anatomy comes at many levels, some of which cannot be achieved without seeing the anatomy in the "living flesh" and actually performing the surgery. In this chapter, *get the big picture. Understand the principles.* There is a tremendous amount of information in this chapter. If you are a beginner and unfamiliar with periocular anatomy and clinical oculoplastic surgery, you may be overwhelmed. If you have a working knowledge in this area, you may think this chapter is basic. In subsequent chapters, the anatomy pertinent to the clinical problem or procedure being discussed will be presented again, so don't worry about learning it all the first time through. This repetition may be unnecessary for some of you, but most of us can use it when it comes to remembering anatomy. I expect that, by the time you finish this book, this material will seem very easy to you. Remember, it is the application of the anatomy to the clinical problem that will make you a successful reconstructive surgeon. A photographic memory would be of help in learning anatomy, but that alone is not enough to get the job done for your patients.

The anatomy covered in this chapter and throughout the book is the essential material that you will need to get a good understanding of eyelid, lacrimal, and orbital surgery. Obviously, we cannot cover all of the anatomy in a text like this. I have not discussed ocular anatomy, neuroanatomy, or much anatomy related to the extraocular muscles. There are many good textbooks on periocular and orbital anatomy (see Suggested Reading at the end of this chapter). Please refer to these texts as you find necessary. Hopefully, the anatomy that is described here will be presented in a way that will be useful for you to learn the principles of oculoplastic and orbital surgery.

This chapter starts with a description of the external features of the periocular area to give a point of reference for the deeper tissues. Rather than discuss the anatomy from anterior to posterior, as is often done, we will look at the anatomy from a more functional approach. The orbital bones are covered next, as it is helpful to learn about the soft tissues relative to the bones. Most of the eyelid and orbital tissues either attach to or pass through openings in the orbital skeleton. Next, the muscles that close the eyes will be discussed, followed by a section on the muscles that open the eyes. Lastly, the nerves, vessels, and lymphatics will be covered. We will use the clinical examples as a way to learn the anatomy. In the upcoming chapters, we will spend more time on the clinical problems themselves.

Periocular anatomy

Skin creases and folds

Several lines on the skin serve to anatomically define the periocular and facial anatomy. The *upper eyelid skin crease* separates the upper eyelid skin fold from the flat pretarsal component of the upper eyelid (Figure 2-1). In your study of oculoplastic surgery, you will see that the upper eyelid crease is an anatomic landmark that is commonly referred to in oculoplastic surgery. Incisions hidden in this crease for upper eyelid ptosis repair or blepharoplasty and other procedures are among the most common incisions that you will use in oculoplastic surgery.

The *eyelid skin* above and below the crease is the thinnest in the body. The skin must be thin to allow for the spontaneous quick blinking movements of the eyelids. A *lower eyelid crease* is common in children (Figure 2-2), but is usually not visible in adults. The eyelid skin becomes thicker as you move further away from the eyelid margins toward the brow and cheek. The *nasojugal* and *malar folds* separate the thin lower eyelid skin from the thicker skin of the cheek. In younger patients, the inferior orbital rim contour is not visible or easily palpable. With age, the *malar fat pad* (sometimes called the suborbicularis oculi fat or SOOF) descends, and the rim becomes more noticeable, both visually and by palpation (compare some of your 20-year-old patients with your 50-year-old patients in this regard). The *melolabial fold* extends inferolaterally from the ala of the nose to the corner of the mouth. Subtle facial asymmetry resulting from paralysis of the facial nerve is often evident in the melolabial fold where the fold is softer or absent.

Skin creases (*rhytids* or *wrinkles*) form as a result of the movement of the underlying muscles of facial expression. The most familiar of these creases are the "crow's feet" arising at the lateral canthus caused by contraction of the orbicularis muscle. The direction of these wrinkles can be predicted by recognizing that they always form *perpendicular to the underlying muscle fibers* (Figures 2-3 and 2-16). This explains the radial orientation of the crow's feet lines to the circular orientation of the orbicularis muscle. Other prominent creases caused by underlying muscle contraction that you will see include the horizontal forehead furrows and the vertical and horizontal lines of the glabella. These lines suggest redundancy in the tissue perpendicular to the lines. That redundancy represents lax tissue that is "tightened" to reverse aging changes. The same redundancy is what you are looking for when you are trying to close a tissue defect after excision of a facial skin cancer. You will also learn to hide incisions in these creases so that the resulting scar is not easily seen.

The eyebrows

The brows, technically a part of the scalp, are divided into three anatomic parts:

- Head
- Body
- Tail

The *orientation of the brow hairs* varies in each part of the brow. The brow hairs in the head of the brow tend to be vertical. As you move toward the tail of the brow, you

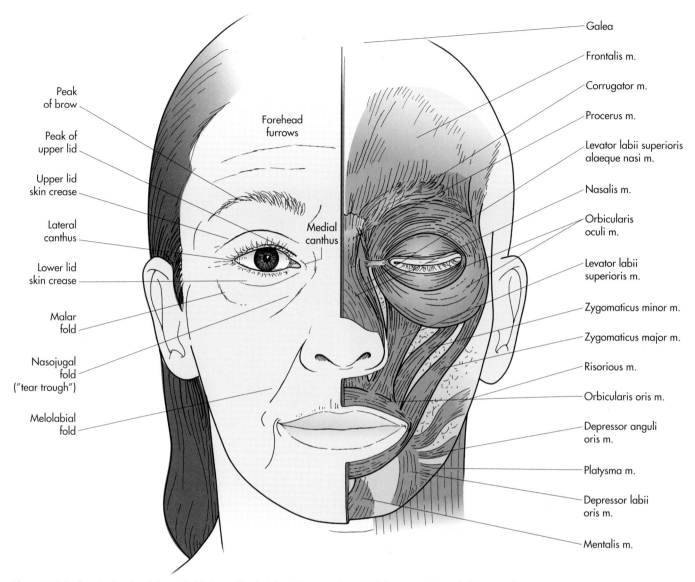

Peak of brow

Peak of upper lid

Upper lid skin crease

Lateral canthus

Lower lid skin crease

Malar fold

Nasojugal fold ("tear trough")

Melolabial fold

Forehead furrows

Medial canthus

Galea

Frontalis m.

Corrugator m.

Procerus m.

Levator labii superioris alaeque nasi m.

Nasalis m.

Orbicularis oculi m.

Levator labii superioris m.

Zygomaticus minor m.

Zygomaticus major m.

Risorious m.

Orbicularis oris m.

Depressor anguli oris m.

Platysma m.

Depressor labii oris m.

Mentalis m.

Figure 2-1 Surface landmarks of the periorbital area. The facial wrinkles are oriented 90 degrees to the underlying muscle.

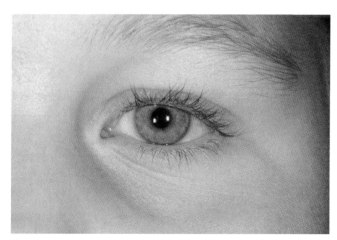

Figure 2-2 The lower eyelid crease, usually seen only in children.

will notice that the hairs tend to lie flatter or slightly downward. It has been suggested that incisions made within the brow hairs should be oriented parallel to the shafts of the hairs to minimize the number of follicles damaged. This seems reasonable, but makes closure of the wound more difficult.

The eyebrows are an important feature of an individual's facial appearance and are primary *indicators of facial expression and mood.* Look at Figure 2-3. Many texts include variations of this "happy face" eyebrow model. Look at your friends' brows carefully and you will be impressed by how the slope, shape, and position of the eyebrows give you an immediate impression of mood. You will be impressed to see that lifting a drooping tail of the brow will make a melancholic-appearing patient look happier. We will see this later in Chapter 6.

The male and female brows differ in shape and position (Figure 2-4). The normal male brow is flat and full in contrast to the thinner and more arched female brow. The supe-

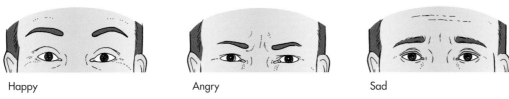

Happy   Angry   Sad

Figure 2-3 "Happy face" demonstrating how brow position reflects mood (after Ellenbogen R: Transcoronal eyebrow lift with concomitant upper blepharoplasty. *Plast Reconst Surg* 71(4):490–499, 1983).

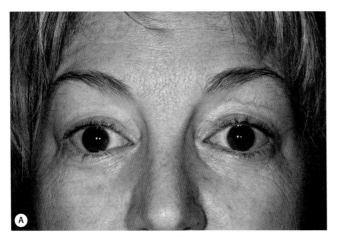

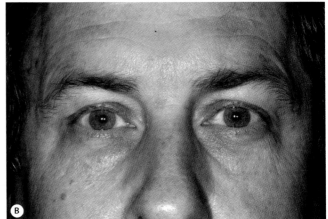

Figure 2-4 Normal eyebrow contour. (**A**) Female. (**B**) Male.

rior margin of brow hairs is "feathered" in men and smooth in women. The male brow sits squarely at the superior orbital rim. The female brow is typically arched, with the highest point being above the lateral canthus or slightly more medial. The position of the female brow is well above the rim, especially temporally, where the superior lateral part of the bony rim contour is visible and easily palpable. The male rim is generally more prominent than the female rim because of a larger frontal sinus. The male brow tends to encroach upon the otherwise hairless glabella between the brows.

The features of the brow are secondary sexual characteristics that differ in men and women. Women manicure the brows to make the female face more attractive. Epilation of the brow hairs accents differences between male and female brows in thickness, smooth margins, arched contour, and position. Although the shape and position of the brow change some with the current fashion, I suspect we all have the same image of male and female movie supermodel eyebrows. With age, the appearance of the brow changes also. The normally high arch of the young woman is lost as the brow tends to droop temporally. A ptosis of the brow accentuates the upper eyelid skin fold and fills in the deep superior sulcus of the upper eyelid seen in younger patients. Lifting a drooping eyebrow always improves the appearance of a cosmetic blepharoplasty. With a severe brow ptosis, as in facial nerve palsy, the superior visual field is obstructed. Lifting the brow will help to restore the visual field. You can see that your appreciation of the eyebrow anatomy is important for you to do cosmetic or reconstructive surgery of the face.

Checkpoint

Identify in your mind or on a patient the following features:

- Upper eyelid skin crease and skin fold
- Lower eyelid skin crease
- Thin and thick eyelid skin
- Nasojugal fold (tear trough)
- Malar fold
- Melolabial fold (also called the nasolabial fold)

Each eyebrow is divided into three parts. What are these parts? Remind yourself of the differences between male and female eyebrows.

The eyelids

The function of the eyelids is to protect the eyes and distribute the tears. It is important for you to understand the normal anatomy of the eyelids and to recognize conditions that may prevent normal function.

The lateral canthus is usually slightly higher than the medial canthus, although the slope of the eyelid fissures can vary widely among individuals (see Figure 2-1). The upper lid contour is more arched than that of the lower lid. The peak of the upper lid is just nasal to the pupil. The lowest point of the lower eyelid is below the lateral limbus. The normal contour of the eyelid must be recreated in a variety of procedures, including ptosis repair and reconstruction of the lateral canthal angle.

The horizontal length of the eyelids is 30 mm. The distance between the upper and lower eyelids, the *palpebral aperture* or *fissure*, is about 10 mm. A useful way to measure the position of the upper and lower eyelids is the *margin reflex distance*. This distance is the number of millimeters from the corneal light reflex to the lid margin. The upper lid margin reflex distance (MRD_1) usually measures 4–5 mm. That means that the upper lid margin rests slightly below the limbus. The lower lid rests at the lower limbus, making the lower lid margin reflex distance (MRD_2) 5 mm (Figure 2-5). These distances can be measured with a ruler or estimated. When you estimate the distance, keep in mind that midway between the corneal light reflex and the limbus is 2.5 mm. The eyelid aperture measurements, especially the MRD, are an essential part of the eyelid examination, one of the *eyelid vital signs*. A drooping upper eyelid is known as *ptosis* or *blepharoptosis*. An upper eyelid resting above the upper limbus or a lower eyelid resting below the lower limbus is said to have *lid retraction*. The white between the limbus and the lid is known as *scleral show*.

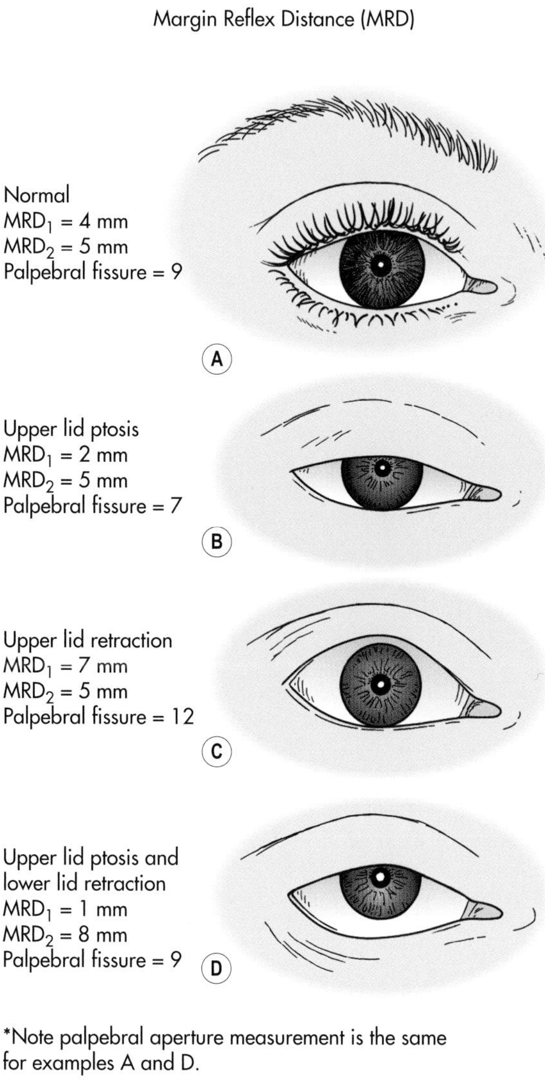

There are three or four rows of *eyelashes* along the upper lid margin and one or two rows of eyelashes along the lower lid margin. The eyelashes extend from just lateral to the puncta to the lateral canthus. Misdirection of the eyelashes against the eye, also known as *trichiasis*, causes a foreign body sensation. In some cases, trichiasis can cause severe corneal problems. Treatment is focused at redirecting or eliminating the eyelashes.

The eyelids attach to the orbital bones via the *medial* and *lateral canthal tendons*. The tendons attach to the *tarsal plates*, which are the fibrous skeleton of the eyelids. A favorite board examination question asks if the tarsal plates are made of cartilage (which they are not; they are made of fibrous tissue). The upper lid tarsal plate is about 10 mm high, corresponding with the skin crease height. The lower lid tarsal plate is about 4–6 mm high. Within the tarsal plates are the *meibomian glands*, modified sebaceous glands that secrete the majority of the oil layer of the tear film. The eyelash follicles originate on the anterior surface of the tarsal plate and exit the eyelid on the margin. The orbicularis muscle is tightly bound to the anterior surface of the tarsus.

Checkpoint

At this point, you should have a good understanding of the landmarks of the periorbital area. See if you know the answers to these questions:

- What is the definition of the margin reflex distance (MRD)?
- What are normal values for MRD_1 and MRD_2?
- Where is the peak of the upper eyelid?
- Where is the lowest point of the lower eyelid?

The orbital bones

The orbital rim

The bones of the orbital rim

Let's move from the superficial anatomy to the deep anatomy, the orbital bones. The orbit is made of a strong *bony rim* and relatively weak *orbital walls*. Several openings, *foramina*, into and out of the orbit allow the passage of the veins, arteries, and nerves that supply the orbital tissues. We will discuss the orbital rims, walls, and foramen in the paragraphs below.

The orbital rim provides protection for the eye without compromising visual field. The rim is made of thick strong bones, especially the superior and lateral rims where protection from injury is needed most. The superior orbital rim protects the eye from blows from above as well as sunlight (you will rarely see skin cancers on the upper eyelid). The lateral orbital rim curves posteriorly so that there is good peripheral vision at the sides. The inferior rim is posterior enough so that the inferior visual field is not blocked for close work and reading. The orbital rim is made of three bones, the frontal, the zygomatic, and the maxillary (Figure 2-6).

Tripod fracture

Rarely do the bones of the superior and lateral rims themselves break. More commonly, the suture lines between the bones separate. The most common facial fracture is a

Margin Reflex Distance (MRD)

Normal
MRD_1 = 4 mm
MRD_2 = 5 mm
Palpebral fissure = 9

(A)

Upper lid ptosis
MRD_1 = 2 mm
MRD_2 = 5 mm
Palpebral fissure = 7

(B)

Upper lid retraction
MRD_1 = 7 mm
MRD_2 = 5 mm
Palpebral fissure = 12

(C)

Upper lid ptosis and lower lid retraction
MRD_1 = 1 mm
MRD_2 = 8 mm
Palpebral fissure = 9 (D)

*Note palpebral aperture measurement is the same for examples A and D.

Figure 2-5 The margin reflex distance.

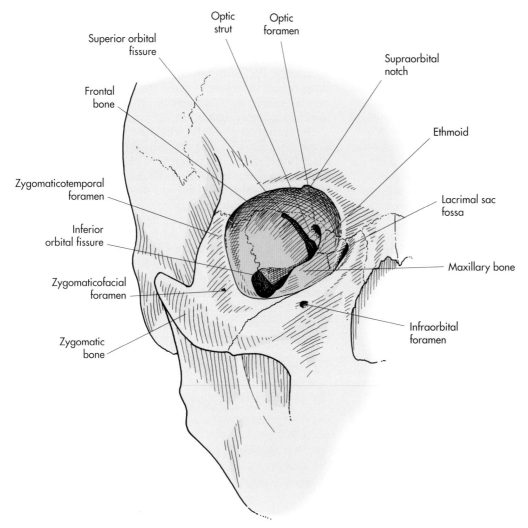

Figure 2-6 The frontal view of the orbit.

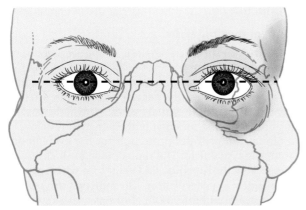

Figure 2-7 "Tripod" or zygomatic malar complex fracture (ZMC fracture). Note that the left lower lid and lateral canthus are displaced inferiorly.

zygomaticomalar complex fracture (*ZMC fracture*) (Figure 2-7). In this fracture, the zygoma is separated from the other orbital bones at the sutures connecting the zygoma to the rim. Fracture or separation occurs superiorly at the *frontozygomatic suture* and inferiorly at the *zygomaticomaxillary suture*. A fracture also occurs along the zygomatic arch posteriorly

at the suture line between the temporal bone and zygoma. Because three suture lines are fractured, this type of fracture is also known as a *tripod fracture*. The bones of the medial and inferior rims are not as strong as the superior and lateral rims. Injury to the medial and inferior rims may cause the bones to fracture in many pieces, a *comminuted fracture*.

The orbital rims provide the sites for attachment of the medial and lateral canthal tendons. Look at a skull or Figure 2-8. Follow the inferior and superior rims as they form the medial orbital rim. You will notice that the paths of the rims diverge. The superior rim moves posteriorly to form the *posterior lacrimal crest*. The inferior rim moves anteriorly to form the *anterior lacrimal crest*. The fossa between the two crests is the *lacrimal sac fossa* where the *lacrimal sac* sits. The medial canthal tendon splits into two limbs, the *anterior* and *posterior limbs*, which attach to the lacrimal crests, respectively, surrounding the lacrimal sac (Box 2-2).

The orbital walls

Boundaries of the walls

There are four orbital walls. The walls angle posteriorly to form a conical or pyramidal orbit. The orbital roof is concave in contour and forms the floor of the anterior cranial fossa.

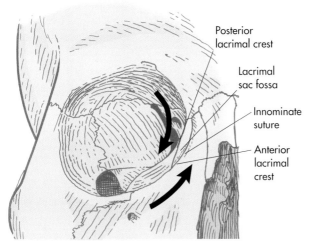

Figure 2-8 Anterior and posterior lacrimal crests diverge to form the lacrimal sac fossa.

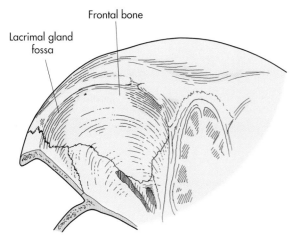

Figure 2-9 The orbital roof.

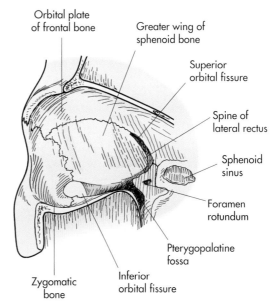

Figure 2-10 The lateral wall of the orbit.

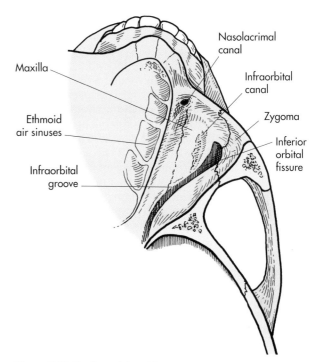

Figure 2-11 The floor of the orbit.

Box 2-2

The Orbital Rim

Superior rim
- Frontal bone

Lateral rim
- Zygomatic bone

Medial rim
- Frontal bone
- Zygomatic bone

Inferior rim
- Zygomatic bone
- Maxillary bone

The concavity of the orbital roof is particularly steep laterally and anteriorly where the lacrimal gland sits in the lacrimal gland fossa. The orbital roof is separated from the lateral orbital wall by the superior orbital fissure (Figure 2-9; see also Figure 2-7). The lateral orbital wall (Figure 2-10; see also Figure 2-6) is relatively flat on the orbital side, but curved on its exterior surface to accommodate the temporalis muscle. The inferior orbital fissure separates the lateral wall from the orbital floor (Figure 2-11). The orbital floor is the roof of the maxillary sinus. The orbital floor slopes upward posteriorly to the apex and medially toward the medial orbital wall. The medial orbital wall is the lateral wall of the ethmoid sinus. Notice that both the medial wall and the floor are normally convex. The anatomic separation of the medial wall and orbital roof is the suture line separating the ethmoid bone and the frontal bone (the frontoethmoid suture) (Figure 2-12). This suture line is easy to see because the anterior and posterior ethmoid arteries and nerves travel through the foramina in the suture line.

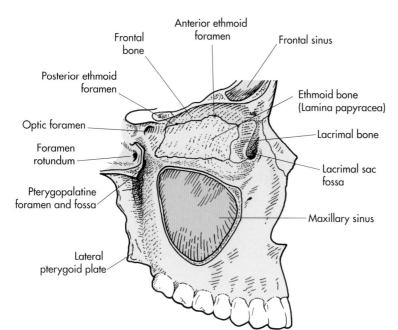

Anterior ethmoid foramen
Frontal bone
Posterior ethmoid foramen
Optic foramen
Foramen rotundum
Pterygopalatine foramen and fossa
Lateral pterygoid plate
Frontal sinus
Ethmoid bone (Lamina papyracea)
Lacrimal bone
Lacrimal sac fossa
Maxillary sinus

Figure 2-12 The medial orbital wall.

Blowout fracture

In contrast to the thick orbital rims, the orbital floor and medial wall are extremely thin. The medial wall of the orbit is made of mainly the lamina papyracea, or paper plate of the ethmoid bone, so called for the distinctively thin wall. The infraorbital nerve separates the orbital floor into a thin medial portion and a thicker lateral portion. The thin bone of the orbital floor and the medial wall is commonly fractured in trauma. The most common type of orbital fracture seen in ophthalmology is a blowout fracture. This fracture, by definition, does not involve the orbital rim. The classic blowout fracture is caused by a blow to the orbit with an object larger than the orbital diameter such as a ball or fist. The rims are not fractured, but pressure placed on the orbital contents causes the thin floor or medial wall to "blow out." Orbital tissue may become incarcerated into the fracture site, causing diplopia as a result of tethering (restriction) of the eye. Fracturing the walls into the adjacent sinus causes the size of the bony orbit to expand, which may lead to enophthalmos (remember the floor and medial wall are normally convex, bowing into the orbit). Injury to the infraorbital nerve usually accompanies a blowout fracture, causing characteristic numbness of the cheek and upper teeth. We will discuss blowout fractures in more detail in Chapter 13.

The bones of the orbital walls

Learning the bones of the orbital walls is more complicated than learning those of the orbital rims. Seven bones make up the orbit.

Roof	Frontal bone
Lateral wall	Zygoma anteriorly
	Sphenoid wing posteriorly (the greater wing)
Floor	Maxilla
Medial wall	Ethmoid bone
	Lacrimal bone (in the lacrimal fossa)
	Palatine bone (deep in the apex)

Table 2-1 Fissures, foramina, grooves, and canals

Opening	From orbit to	Contains
Superior orbital fissure	Cavernous sinus	Cranial nerves III, IV, and VI
		Superior ophthalmic vein
Inferior orbital fissure	Pterygopalatine fossa	Inferior ophthalmic vein
Foramen rotundum	Brain	Maxillary nerve (V_2)
Optic canal	Chiasm	Optic nerve (cranial nerve II)
Anterior ethmoidal foramen	Sinus mucosa	Anterior ethmoidal artery, vein, and nerve
Posterior ethmoidal foramen	Sinus mucosa	Posterior ethmoidal artery, vein, and nerve
Zygomaticotemporal foramen	Superior lateral orbital rim tissues	Nerve, artery, and vein
Zygomaticofacial foramen	Inferior lateral orbital rim tissues	Nerve, artery, and vein
Bony nasolacrimal duct	Inferior meatus of nose	Membranous nasolacrimal duct

Some important bony anatomy that we have not mentioned yet covers the orbital apex. We will discuss the apex in the next section, which deals with the openings into and out of the orbit.

Fissures, foramina, grooves, and canals

There are several openings into and out of the orbit (Table 2-1). I like to think about what these openings are for. *What spaces do the openings connect?* Once you know what spaces are connected, it's easier to remember what goes through the openings. The most obvious of these are the superior and inferior orbital fissures. These fissures form a V on the lateral side of each orbit. As we said, the superior orbital fissure separates the roof from the lateral wall, and the inferior orbital fissure separates the floor from the lateral orbital wall. See if you can visualize this (if you can't, look at Figure 2-6). Because the superior orbital fissure connects the orbit to the brain, it must carry cranial nerves to the orbit (cranial nerves III, IV, and VI). *The inferior orbital fissure connects the orbit to the infratemporal fossa and the pterygopalatine fossa* ("behind and around the maxillary sinus"—posterior and lateral to the maxillary sinus).

At the apex of the V formed by the superior and inferior orbital fissures is the *infraorbital groove* (Figure 2-11). As the groove extends anteriorly along the orbital floor, it gets a bony covering and is known as the *infraorbital canal*. The canal leaves the orbit at the *infraorbital foramen*. As you would assume, the *infraorbital nerve* travels in the infraorbital groove and through the infraorbital canal. The infraorbital nerve is the major sensory nerve of the second division of the trigeminal nerve. Go back to the apex of the V. Follow the infraorbital groove posteriorly and you will be in the *pterygopalatine fossa*. This fossa, as mentioned earlier, is the space posterior to the maxillary sinus and anterior to the skull base (the bottom of the cranial vault). The trigeminal nerve leaves the cranium through the *foramen rotundum*, entering the pterygopalatine fossa. The trigeminal nerve then crosses the fossa and enters the orbit via the posterior portion of the inferior orbital fissure, the infraorbital groove.

Let's talk about the other important opening out of the orbit into the cranium, the *optic canal*. *The optic nerve leaves the orbit via the optic canal to enter the cranial vault.* Look at Figure 2-6 or at a skull. The optic canal is the most posterior landmark in orbit. The length of the optic canal is 10 mm. Medially, the *posterior ethmoid foramen* is 4–7 mm anterior to the optic canal, an important surgical landmark when operating deeply along the posterior orbital wall (see Figure 2-12). Laterally, the optic canal is separated from the superior orbital fissure by a small piece of bone, the *optic strut*. If you follow the optic strut posteriorly and superiorly, it becomes the anterior clinoid process. Although not important for you now, if you approach the optic canal from an intracranial exposure with your neurosurgical colleagues, knowledge of this relationship may help you. (Next time you pick up a skull, look at how the optic strut extends to form the anterior clinoid process. It will help you learn some of this complicated anatomy.) When you look at a computed tomography (CT) scan, the thin piece of bone separating the optic canal from the superior orbital fissure is the optic strut. Earlier, we said that the posterior portion of the lateral orbital wall was made up of the *greater wing of the sphenoid bone* (Figure 2-13). The optic strut and the optic canal are a part of the lesser wing of the sphenoid bone. The sphenoid bone forms a large part of the skull base and posterior orbit. Its shape is complicated. For now, just remember that *the greater wing lies lateral to the superior orbital fissure and the lesser wing lies medial to the superior orbital fissure.*

Look at the CT scans shown in Figure 2-13. It is easy to recognize the superior orbital fissure because it opens into the intracranial space. Similarly, it is easy to recognize the inferior orbital fissure because it opens into the space posterior to the maxillary sinus (the pterygopalatine fossa) and

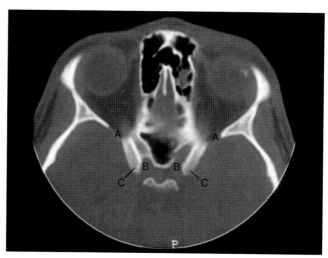

Figure 2-13 Axial CT scan of orbit. (**A**) Superior orbital fissure. (**B**) Optic canal. (**C**) Anterior clinoid process. You can see how the inferior extension of the anterior clinoid process, the optic strut, separates the optic canal from the superior orbital fissure. When you want to identify the optic canal, find the scan that shows the anterior clinoid process. Arrow points to optic canal fracture.

into the infratemporal fossa laterally. The inferior orbital fissure does not open into the brain. The optic canal is adjacent to the anterior clinoid processes (seen on the same CT cut). The optic canal also opens into the intracranial space.

There are two other sets of foramina to mention. All carry the related arteries, veins, and nerves. These foramina are:

- Anterior ethmoidal
- Posterior ethmoidal
- Zygomaticotemporal
- Zygomaticofacial

The *anterior* and *posterior ethmoidal foramina* are important surgical landmarks along the medial orbital wall. These foramina are found in the frontoethmoid suture. If you break the medial wall inferior to the suture, you will be in the ethmoid sinus. If you break the bone above the suture, you will be in the brain (causing a cerebrospinal fluid (CSF) leak). The anterior–posterior location of the foramina is a helpful indicator of how far posterior an orbital dissection along the medial wall is proceeding. The anterior ethmoidal foramen is about 24 mm posterior to the anterior lacrimal crest. The posterior ethmoidal foramen is another 10–12 mm posterior. As we already mentioned, the optic canal is 4–7 mm more posterior. A helpful way to remember is *24–12–6 mm.* During an operation, it is easy to overestimate your position on the medial orbital wall, so these numbers are surprisingly helpful as you learn orbital surgery. When you operate along the medial orbital wall, it is important to recognize the ethmoidal vessels because significant bleeding can occur if they are inadvertently torn. The ethmoidal veins are valveless and permit flow into the orbit from the ethmoid sinus. Purulent sinusitis can spread into the orbit through these vessels or directly into the orbit through the thin lamina papyracea of the medial orbital wall. We will talk more about the vessels and sensory nerves that travel in these foramina later.

The *zygomaticotemporal* and *zygomaticofacial foramina* transmit the arteries, veins, and nerves of the same name. The nerves are sensory branches of the *trigeminal nerve* (V$_2$).

The arteries are small branches that originate off the lacrimal artery (a main branch of the ophthalmic artery, which arises directly off the internal carotid artery). You will see these foramina when you lift the periorbita off the lateral wall. Cauterization is appropriate before you cut the arteries. If the artery retracts into the foramen, bleeding can be stopped by packing the foramen with a bit of bone wax. Cutting these nerves during a lateral orbitotomy results in some hypesthesia of the surrounding area that is minimal because of collateral innervation. Note that the overlap of these vessels and nerves with adjacent vessels and nerves of differing origin is typical of the collateral innervation and vascularization of the facial area. Infraorbital arterial branches (from the internal maxillary artery) medially and inferiorly overlap with the branches of the ophthalmic artery above. Anastomoses of the zygomaticotemporal nerve (from V_2) with the lacrimal nerve (from V_1) provide sensory overlap. This overlap of blood and nerve supply helps to preserve function after accidental trauma. Incisions can be made and flaps formed with relatively low risk of ischemia or sensory loss.

The periorbita

The bones of the orbit are covered with periosteum like all the other bones of body. The periosteum covering the inside of the orbit is known as the *periorbita*. The periorbita is tightly adherent to the bone at the orbital suture lines and along the orbital rims. Over the orbital walls, the periorbita is loosely adherent. You will see these differing degrees of adhesion when pus or blood accumulates under the periorbita as a result of infection or trauma. The periorbita is elevated off the orbital walls in a characteristic dome-shaped elevation ending at suture lines where the periorbita is adherent (Figure 2-14). The orbital septum is an extension of fibrous tissue continuous with the periosteum, extending from the orbital rim to lids. Where the orbital septum attaches to the rim is known as the *arcus marginalis*. Three structures meet at the arcus marginalis, the orbital septum, the periorbita, and the periosteum. We will discuss the orbital septum in more detail later.

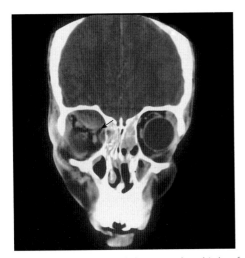

Figure 2-14 Subperiosteal abscess on the orbital roof and the medial wall of the orbit attributable to ethmoid sinus infection. Note how the abscess elevates the periorbita to form a dome. The periorbita remains fixed to the frontoethmoid suture (arrow), making two abscess spaces.

Muscles that close the eyes

The orbicularis muscle

For the eyelids to function, there must be muscles that close the eye and muscles that open the eye. The *orbicularis muscle* (Figure 2-15) is the muscle primarily responsible for closing the eyelids. The orbicularis muscle is anatomically divided into the *pretarsal* portion, the *preseptal* portion, and the *orbital* portion. The pretarsal and preseptal portions overlay the tarsus and the septum, respectively. These muscles are responsible for involuntary spontaneous blinking. The orbital portion covers the orbital rims and is responsible for forced eyelid closure. All parts of the orbicularis muscle are innervated by the facial nerve with innervation entering from the underside of the muscle like all muscles of facial expression.

The corrugator and procerus muscles

Other protractors of the eyelids (protractors being the opposite of retractors, which open the eyes) include the corrugator muscle and the procerus muscle (Figure 2-15). The corrugator muscle originates on the bone of the superonasal rim and inserts into the skin of the head of the eyebrow. Firing of the corrugator muscle pulls the heads of the eyebrows together and makes the vertical furrows of the glabella (Figure 2-16). The procerus muscle originates on the frontal bone above the glabella and inserts into the skin of the glabella. The action of these vertically oriented muscle fibers pulls the heads of the brows inferiorly and causes the horizontal furrows of the glabella.

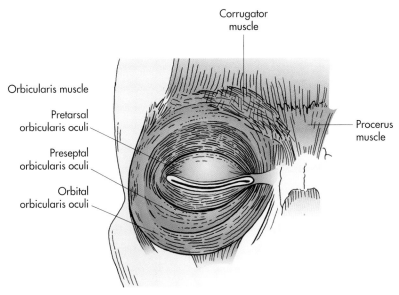

Corrugator muscle

Orbicularis muscle

Pretarsal orbicularis oculi

Preseptal orbicularis oculi

Orbital orbicularis oculi

Procerus muscle

Figure 2-15 Muscles that close the eyes.

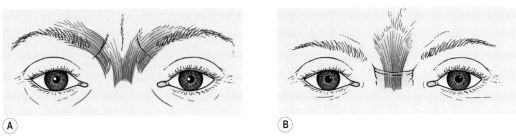

(A)

(B)

Figure 2-16 The glabellar furrows. (**A**) Corrugator muscle action causing vertical furrows in the glabella. (**B**) Procerus muscle causing horizontal furrows in the glabella.

Underactive muscles: facial nerve palsy

A number of clinical problems result from under- or overactivity of the muscles that close the eyes. Facial nerve palsy results in poor eyelid closure seen as *lagophthalmos* (the eyelids do not close with passive lid closure) or an *incomplete spontaneous blink* (quick normal blinks that do not completely cover the cornea). All the facial muscles on the affected side are also weakened, resulting in the brow ptosis, flattening of the melolabial fold, and drooping of the corner of the mouth that you have seen in patients.

Overactive muscles: orbicularis myokymia, facial tics, essential blepharospasm, and hemifacial spasm

The disorders resulting from overactivity of the orbicularis muscles are *orbicularis myokymia, facial tics, essential blepharospasm,* and *hemifacial spasm*. Probably you have suffered from orbicularis myokymia at one time or another. Hyperexcitability of the muscle, caused by stress or lack of sleep, causes a quick twitch of a few muscle fibers. Orbicularis myokymia is self-limited and usually lasts a few days or less. The other conditions involve different patterns of overactivity of the facial muscles, including the orbicularis muscle. These will be discussed in detail later in Chapter 9.

Checkpoint

The last section is straightforward. You should know:

- The muscles that close the eyes
- The muscles responsible for the horizontal and vertical glabellar furrows
- The problems associated with underactive and overactive facial muscles

You will see these conditions commonly in practice. You will learn the diagnosis and treatment of these problems in detail in Chapter 8.

The canthal tendons

The lateral canthal tendon

Before we leave the topic of the orbicularis muscle, we should discuss the canthal tendons. As we have already noted, the canthal tendons attach the eyelids to the lateral and medial orbital rims (Figure 2-17). The tendons are extensions of the orbicularis muscle that attach to the periorbita overlying the bone. The anatomy of the *lateral canthal tendon* is easy to understand (Figure 2-18, A). The pretarsal

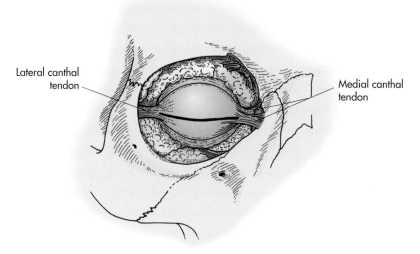

Lateral canthal
tendon

Medial canthal
tendon

Figure 2-17 The canthal tendons.

and preseptal portions of the orbicularis muscle of each eyelid taper to form the *superior* and *inferior limb of the lateral canthal tendon.* The upper and lower limbs unite to form the lateral canthal tendon, which attaches to the inner aspect of the lateral orbital rim on *Whitnall's tubercle.* Imagine the lateral canthal tendon complex as a Y lying on its side with contributions from both the upper and the lower eyelids.

The slope of the eyelid

The lateral canthal tendon is normally a few millimeters higher than the medial canthal tendon. A downward slant toward the lateral canthal tendon is known as an "anti-mongoloid slant." It is seen in a number of syndromes and is also a variation of normal. An excessive upward slant toward the lateral canthal tendon is known as a "mongoloid slant." You will want to recreate the natural slant to the eyelids when you work on the canthal tendons.

Lower eyelid laxity: the cause of ectropion

In the following chapters, you will learn that proper horizontal tension on the lower eyelid is necessary for the eyelid to maintain its position. *Laxity of the lower eyelid is the major cause of lower eyelid eversion or ectropion* (Figure 2-19). This laxity does not occur from stretching of the tarsal plate; rather, it is attributable to *lengthening of the lateral canthal tendon* with age. You may have heard of older patients stating that their eyes look smaller than they did in their youth. You have probably already noticed that, with age, the upper eyelid droops (ptosis) and the lower eyelid actually rises up a bit (stretching of the lower eyelid retractors). Less apparent, but equally common, is a horizontal narrowing of the eyelid as a result of stretching of the canthal tendons. Thus, the "small eyes" that your older patients may notice are caused by both horizontal and vertical narrowing of the palpebral fissure.

The lateral tarsal strip operation

Attributable in part to the simplicity of attachment of the lateral canthal tendon to the bone, the aim of lower eyelid

tightening operations is to shorten the lateral canthal tendon. In this procedure, known as a *lateral tarsal strip operation*, a horizontal cut is made at the lateral canthus. This incision, known as a *lateral canthotomy*, splits the Y of the lateral canthal tendon into a V. Then the lower leg of the V (the lower limb, or *crus*, of the lateral canthal tendon) is cut. This *cantholysis* releases the lower lid from the lateral orbital rim. A portion of the tendon and sometimes the tarsus itself is then shortened and resutured to the periorbita at Whitnall's tubercle. Remember that Whitnall's tubercle is on the inner aspect of the lateral rim. It is important to reattach the strip on the inside of the rim so that the lid will not pull away from the eye. Remember also to place the lateral canthal tendon slightly higher than the medial canthal tendon to recreate the normal slight upward slant to the lateral canthus.

Lateral canthal dystopia

Trauma to the orbital rims may cause displacement of the canthal tendons. The separation of the frontal and zygomatic bones seen with zygomaticomaxillary complex (tripod) fractures that we discussed above causes the lateral canthal tendon to be displaced downward.

The medial canthal tendon

The *medial canthal tendon* is much more complex than the lateral canthal tendon because of the relationship of the medial canthal tendon to the lacrimal drainage system. The pretarsal and preseptal portions of the orbicularis muscle extend medially to form the two limbs of the medial canthal tendon (Figure 2-18, B). You will recall from the discussion of the anatomy of the medial orbital rim that the anterior limb attaches to the frontal process of the maxilla along the anterior lacrimal crest. The posterior limb attaches at the posterior lacrimal crest. Remember that the two limbs of the tendon surround the lacrimal sac (Figure 2-18, C).

Medial canthal tendon laxity

Laxity of the lower eyelid is usually not caused by medial canthal tendon stretching. Occasionally, laxity of the medial

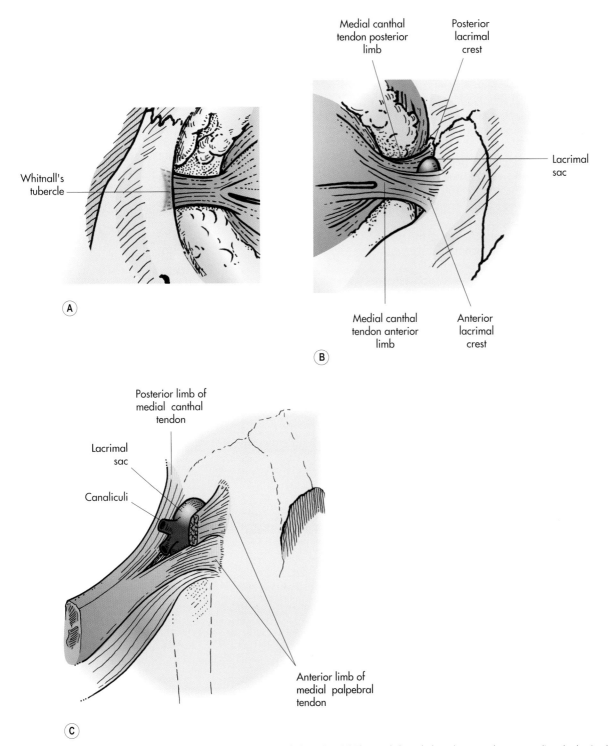

Figure 2-18 (A) The lateral canthal tendon. (B) The medial canthal tendon. (C) The medial canthal tendon complex surrounding the lacrimal sac.

canthal tendon is seen. As the lower eyelid is pulled later-ally, the lower eyelid punctum is seen to extend to or beyond the limbus. Although procedures to tighten the medial canthal tendon have been devised, they are seldom used because of the difficulty in working on the medial canthal tendon without damaging the canaliculi or the lacrimal sac.

Telecanthus

Fractures at the medial canthus generally cause the medial canthus to be displaced laterally, resulting in *telecanthus*, an increase in the distance from the canthus to the midline. The medial canthal tendon is at about the same position verti-cally as is the cribriform plate. In any operation that involves removing or repositioning bone at or superior to the medial canthal tendon, there is the risk of an inadvertent CSF leak.

You will treat many problems related to the canthal tendons. Some points to remember are:

- The lateral canthal tendon is much simpler than the medial canthal tendon. You should have an anatomic concept of what this tendon looks like to help you understand the procedures that you will be doing at the lateral canthus.
- Ectropion of the lower eyelid is one of the most common problems that you will see. Use your anatomic concept of the lateral canthal tendon to visualize canthotomy, cantholysis, and other steps in the lateral tarsal strip operation.
- Again visualize your conceptual anatomy of the medial canthal tendon surrounding the lacrimal sac. Do you remember where the anterior and posterior limbs of the medial canthal tendon insert?
- Which is more common—medial canthal tendon laxity or lateral canthal tendon laxity?
- How are lateral canthal dystopia and telecanthus similar?

Muscles that open the eyes

The levator muscle

Two muscles are responsible for opening the upper eyelids, the levator muscle and Müller's muscle. The *levator muscle* is the primary retractor of the upper eyelid. This skeletal muscle is responsible for voluntary elevation of the upper eyelid. Innervation to the levator muscle is via the superior division of the third cranial nerve (the oculomotor nerve).

One of the most common operations in oculoplastic surgery is the correction of drooping upper eyelids, so your knowledge of the anatomy and function of the levator muscle is critical to your success in oculoplastic surgery. The levator muscle originates at the orbital apex and extends forward inferior to the bone of the orbital roof (Figure 2-20). At the orbital aperture, the levator is supported by *Whitnall's*

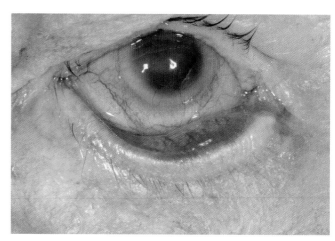

Figure 2-19 Involutional ectropion of the lower eyelid caused by horizontal lid laxity, the result of stretching of the canthal tendons.

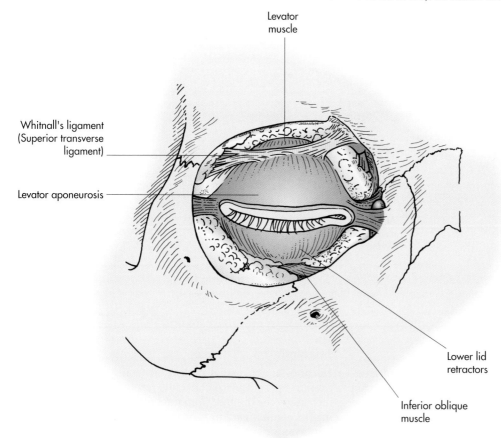

Levator muscle

Whitnall's ligament (Superior transverse ligament)

Levator aponeurosis

Lower lid retractors

Inferior oblique muscle

Figure 2-20 The levator muscle complex.

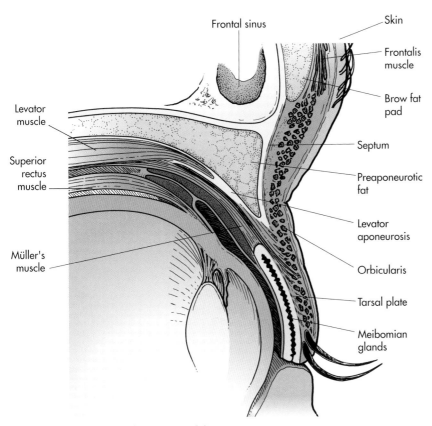

Figure 2-21 Cross-section of the upper eyelid.

Labels on figure: Frontal sinus / Skin / Frontalis muscle / Brow fat pad / Septum / Preaponeurotic fat / Levator aponeurosis / Orbicularis / Tarsal plate / Meibomian glands / Levator muscle / Superior rectus muscle / Müller's muscle

ligament. As the levator muscle travels anteriorly, it becomes a fibrous aponeurosis that extends inferiorly into the eyelid to insert on the anterior aspect of the tarsal plate. Fibrous extensions of the aponeurosis pass through the orbicularis muscle to create the *upper eyelid skin crease* (Figure 2-21).

Whitnall's ligament

Whitnall's ligament is an important anatomic landmark. The ligament extends from the fascia surrounding the lacrimal gland temporally to the trochlea medially. Whitnall's ligament is usually easy to see intraoperatively as a strong white band of fibrous tissue (Figure 2-22). Generally, the tissue superior to the ligament is muscle while the tissue inferior to the ligament is aponeurosis, although variation among individuals exists. It has been suggested that Whitnall's ligament serves as a "pulley" for the levator muscle. Although the levator muscle complex does not slide through the ligament, the concept of the ligament allowing the muscle to change direction is a helpful one.

The horns of the levator aponeurosis

As the levator aponeurosis travels from Whitnall's ligament to the tarsus, it "fans" out to form the *horns of the levator aponeurosis*. The horns are the medial and lateral flared extensions of the aponeurosis inserting into the medial and lateral canthal regions. During operations on the levator, you will see that the lateral horn of the aponeurosis is much thicker and stronger than the medial horn. This anatomic feature is said to explain the prominent *temporal flare* or retraction of the lateral third of the upper eyelid seen in Graves' disease.

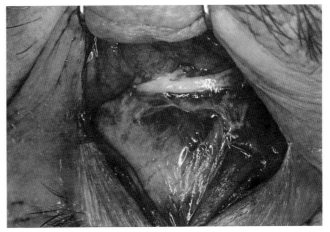

Figure 2-22 Whitnall's ligament.

Müller's muscle

Müller's muscle is responsible for the involuntary upper eyelid elevation seen in the sympathetically innervated "fight or flight" phenomenon. Müller's muscle is "sandwiched" between the conjunctiva posteriorly and the levator aponeurosis anteriorly. Müller's muscle extends from the superior margin of the upper tarsal plate to the level of Whitnall's ligament (see Figure 2-21). A prominent surgical landmark on the surface of Müller's muscle is the *peripheral arcade*, a vascular arcade extending across the muscle a few millimeters above the tarsal plate (Figure 2-23). The term *peripheral arcade* is easily confused with the *marginal arcade*, a vessel that travels on the anterior surface of the tarsus along the lid margin.

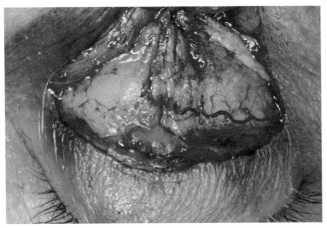

Figure 2-23 The peripheral arcade in Müller's muscle (in this case, with fatty infiltration of Müller's muscle).

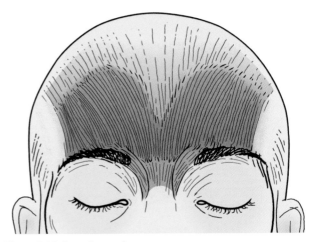

Figure 2-25 Frontalis muscle.

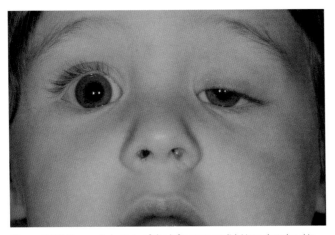

Figure 2-24 Congenital ptosis of the left upper eyelid. Note that the skin crease is absent. The eyebrows are elevated to help lift the upper eyelid above the pupil.

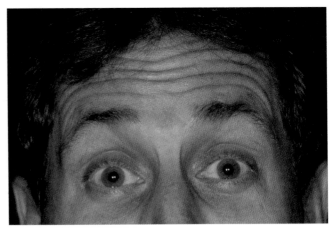

Figure 2-26 Forehead furrows form perpendicular to the direction of pull of the frontalis muscle.

Ptosis of the upper eyelid

Ptosis of the upper eyelid is one of the most commonly encountered clinical problems in oculoplastic surgery. Many causes of ptosis exist. Most cases of upper eyelid ptosis are caused by abnormalities of the levator muscle or aponeurosis. *Congenital ptosis* (Figure 2-24) results from abnormal development of the levator muscle itself. Intraoperatively, this dystrophy presents as fatty infiltration of an otherwise normal muscle. The most common type of acquired ptosis, *involutional ptosis*, is generally thought to occur as a result of stretching or thinning of the aponeurosis, rather than of the muscle itself (we will talk more about the etiology of involutional ptosis later; an entire chapter is dedicated to the evaluation and treatment of ptosis). Advancement or tightening of the aponeurosis will elevate the ptotic eyelid in most patients. Loss of sympathetic innervation to Müller's muscle will cause a mild ptosis of the upper eyelid. This problem is known as *Horner's syndrome*.

The frontalis muscle

No doubt you have already seen patients with drooping upper lids who lift their eyebrows to provide a tiny bit more upper eyelid elevation. The frontalis muscle lifts the brows and is a weak retractor of the upper eyelids. The frontalis muscle is a part of the occipitofrontalis musculofascial complex (frontalis muscle, galea aponeurotica, and occipitalis muscle) of the scalp. This broad band of tissue extends across the top of the skull from the occiput to the eyebrows (Figure 2-25). The *A* in the mnemonic for remembering the layers of the "SCALP" is this aponeurosis (*S*, scalp, *C*, subcutaneous tissue, *A*, aponeurosis, *L*, loose areolar tissue, *P*, periosteum.)

The fibrous aponeurosis becomes the frontalis muscle inferior to the hairline. Contraction of the frontalis muscle causes the *horizontal furrows in the forehead* (Figure 2-26). You may notice that the forehead furrows do not extend to the temporal hairline. The frontalis muscle thins laterally and does not extend to the tail of the brow. The lack of frontalis pull over the tail of the brow explains the temporal brow ptosis seen so commonly in older adults.

Like the other muscles of facial expression, the frontalis muscle is innervated by a branch of the facial nerve. Unlike with other branches of the facial nerve, there is no redundancy in the innervation of the frontalis muscle. A single branch, the *frontal nerve* (Figure 2-27), innervates the frontalis muscle. The path of the frontal nerve can be estimated by drawing a line from the tragus of the ear to the point 1 cm above the tail of the eyebrow. You will learn to take special care to avoid damage to the frontal nerve during any surgery near the path of the frontal branch. Damage to the nerve may leave the patient with a permanent paresis or paralysis of the frontalis muscle, resulting in a brow ptosis.

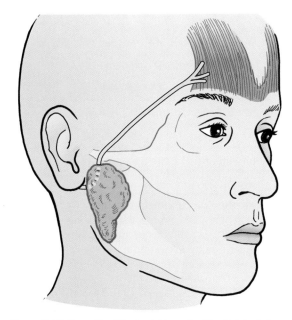

Figure 2-27 The path of the frontal branch of the facial nerve.

The lower eyelid retractors

Although we don't think about the lower eyelid moving much, there are retractors in the lower eyelid as well. The retractors of the lower eyelid are analogous to those of the upper eyelid, but are less well developed. The lower eyelid equivalent to the levator muscle is the *capsulopalpebral fascia*, which is a band of fibrous tissue that extends from the inferior rectus muscle to the inferior margin of the lower eyelid tarsus (Figure 2-28). As the capsulopalpebral fascia travels anteriorly from the inferior rectus muscle, the fascia splits to surround the inferior oblique muscle. Anterior to the inferior oblique muscle, the fascia reunites as a condensation of fibrous tissue known as *Lockwood's suspensory ligament*. This ligament is the equivalent of Whitnall's ligament in the upper eyelid.

The lower eyelid equivalent of Müller's muscle is known as the *inferior tarsal muscle*. This poorly developed smooth muscle travels from Lockwood's ligament to the inferior tarsus between the capsulopalpebral fascia and the conjunctiva. In the lower eyelid, the voluntary and autonomic portions of the retractors are not easily separated during surgery and are known collectively as the *lower eyelid retractors*.

Involutional entropion

Two clinical examples of problems with the lower eyelid retractors are worth considering. *Involutional entropion* (turning in of the lower eyelid attributable to aging) is caused by laxity of the lower eyelid retractors. The posterior and inferior pull of the normal retractors into the orbit stabilizes the inferior margin of the tarsus. In combination with other

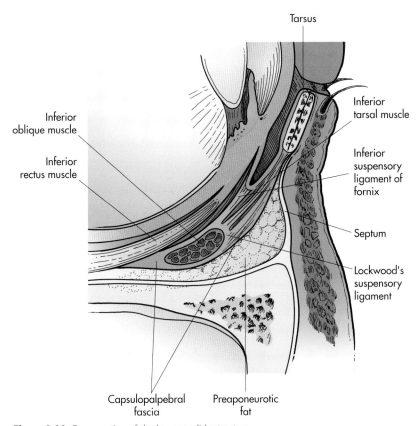

Tarsus

Inferior oblique muscle

Inferior rectus muscle

Inferior tarsal muscle

Inferior suspensory ligament of fornix

Septum

Lockwood's suspensory ligament

Capsulopalpebral fascia

Preaponeurotic fat

Figure 2-28 Cross-section of the lower eyelid retractors.

factors, loss of the tension on the tarsus as a result of stretching or "laxity" of the retractors allows the inferior margin of the retractors to rotate upward. The eyelid margin turns inward against the eyeball (Figure 2-29). An operation to tighten the lower eyelid retractors (analogous to correction of upper eyelid ptosis) corrects the entropion.

Horner's syndrome

The loss of sympathetic tone to the inferior tarsal muscle in Horner's syndrome does not result in entropion. With the loss of this tone, the lower eyelid elevates slightly, a condition described as an *upside down ptosis*. In association with the elevation of the lower eyelid are other signs of loss of sympathetic tone to the face and eye, including lack of sweating (anhidrosis) and constriction of the ipsilateral pupil (miosis).

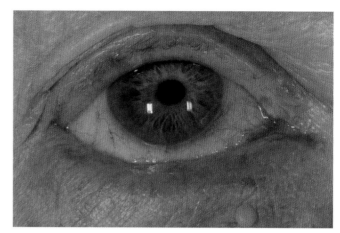

Figure 2-29 Entropion of the lower eyelid caused by laxity of the lower eyelid retractors.

Checkpoint

It is likely that you will be doing many ptosis procedures, so you will become very familiar with the anatomy of the upper lid retractors.

- What muscles are the upper lid retractors?
- Did you remember to include the frontalis? (It is not a very efficient retractor of the eyelids, however.)
- What is Whitnall's ligament? What is its purpose? How is it different from Whitnall's tubercle?
- Sketch a picture of the parts of the levator muscle (both frontal and cross-section views). Check this against the diagrams in the text.
- Now sketch the lower lid retractors. How are they different from the levator and Müller's muscles? Draw the relationship of the inferior oblique and inferior fornix ligament to the lower lid retractors.
- After you master levator advancement for repair of acquired ptosis, you can learn to recess the levator aponeurosis and extirpate Müller's muscle for the correction of upper lid retraction caused by thyroid disease (a much more difficult procedure). Similarly, you can remove the lower lid retractors to correct lower eyelid retraction.
- Remember to learn about Horner's syndrome. Keep your effort in perspective. In your office, you will see several hundred patients with routine ptosis for every one patient with Horner's syndrome. On tests, you may see more questions about Horner's syndrome than about routine ptosis. (It seems strange that we have to spend so much time preparing for the uncommon problems, rather than learning the common problems well.)

The preaponeurotic fat and the orbital septum

The preaponeurotic fat

Before we leave this topic, we should cover two other important surgical structures, the preaponeurotic fat and the orbital septum. The *preaponeurotic orbital fat* (Figure 2-30) is the surgical landmark identifying the levator aponeurosis. Every time you perform ptosis surgery from the skin approach, you will see the orbital fat. In your early experience, you will intentionally identify the fat to help you find the underlying aponeurosis. There are two fat pads that compose the upper eyelid preaponeurotic fat, the *central* and the *medial fat pads*. Later, you will learn the terms, *intraconal space* and *extraconal space*, regarding compartments in the orbit. For now, keep in mind that the preaponeurotic fat is extraconal fat, or fatty tissue lying outside the muscle cone of the orbit. The central and medial fat pads are enclosed in a thin fibrous capsule with small vessels. The medial fat pad is smaller than the central fat pad and whiter in color. No one knows why this fat is whiter. There is no lateral fat pad in the upper eyelid. The lacrimal gland is in the preaponeurotic space laterally. You will be able to differentiate the lacrimal gland from the fat because the gland is more irregular in texture and is whitish-gray in appearance rather than yellow. The fat itself is relatively avascular, whereas the lacrimal gland is well vascularized.

As in the upper eyelid, identification of the fat pads is the key to identifying the lower eyelid retractors. In the lower eyelids, there are three fat pads: the *medial, central,* and *lateral fat pads* (see Figure 2-30). As you would expect, these fat pads are found posterior to the orbital septum and anterior to the lower eyelid retractors. Prolapse, or bulging of the lower eyelid fat pads, is a common cosmetic concern. The main goal of the lower eyelid blepharoplasty operation is to eliminate this prolapse.

The orbital septum

Anterior to the preaponeurotic fat is a tough fibrous layer that extends from the orbital rims to the tarsal plates known as the *orbital septum* (Figure 2-31). The septum is the anatomic boundary between the eyelids and the orbit, lying between the orbicularis muscle and the orbital fat. Fat seen in an eyelid laceration means that the septum has been cut and that deeper tissues, including the eye or even the brain, may be injured. An intact septum means that there has been no penetration into the orbit from the anterior aspect. *Infections of the eyelid* are prevented from extending posteriorly by the orbital septum. As well as preventing infection from spreading posteriorly, the septum prevents the orbital con-

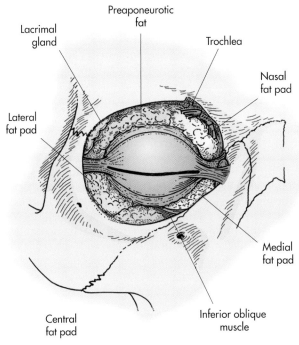

Figure 2-30 The preaponeurotic fat.

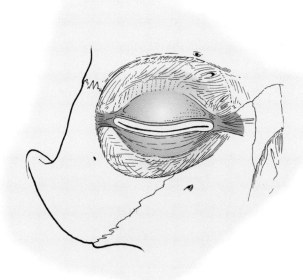

Figure 2-31 The orbital septum.

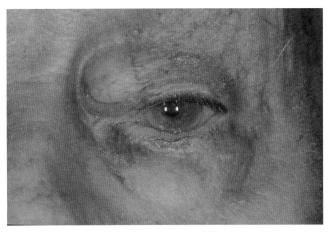

Figure 2-32 Upper eyelid fat prolapse caused by thinning of the orbital septum. Note the prominent upper eyelid nasal fat pad.

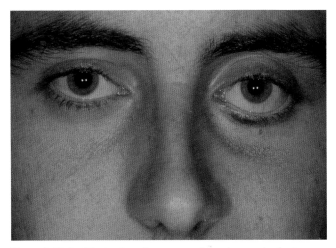

Figure 2-33 Eyelid retraction after a zygomaticomalar complex fracture.

expose the preaponeurotic fat, your landmark for the aponeurosis. The attachment of the origin of the septum along the orbital rim is called the *arcus marginalis*. A displaced orbital rim fracture may pull the eyelid out of position because of the firm attachments of the inelastic septum to the orbital rims and eyelid (Figure 2-33). You will learn to exclude the septum in closure of eyelid wounds, as the shortening of the septum can cause eyelid retraction or prevent the eyelid from closing naturally.

Checkpoint

- The orbital fat is the surgical landmark for the levator aponeurosis and the lower lid retractors, so use it during operations on these structures. Finding the fat will be especially helpful in trauma patients, where the normal anatomic structures are damaged.
- How many fat pads are there in the upper and lower eyelids?
- How does the fusion of the orbital septum to the levator aponeurosis in typical eyelids of Asians compare with that of typical eyelids of whites? Think about the presence or absence of the skin crease and the amount of fat anterior to the tarsus in each type of eyelid.

tents from bulging anteriorly. As we discussed earlier, with age, the septum thins and the orbital fat prolapses forward, accounting for some of the fullness seen in the upper and lower eyelids of adults (Figure 2-32). You will notice this difference in the thickness of the septum in pediatric and adult eyelid operations.

You will see the septum often in eyelid surgery. The eyelid incisions that you will make for ptosis correction typically start with an incision through the skin and then a cut through the orbicularis muscle to the level of the orbital septum. Once the septum is exposed, you will open the septum to

The conjunctiva

Bulbar, palpebral, and fornix conjunctiva

The conjunctiva is the mucous membrane that lines the anterior surface of the eye and posterior surface of the eyelids. The conjunctiva can be divided into *bulbar*, *palpebral*, and *fornix* locations for reference. The conjunctiva is tightly adherent to the eye at the limbus, but less adherent to the remainder of the eye. There is considerable redundancy of the conjunctiva in the fornices to allow free movement of the eye. The surface of the conjunctiva is made of non-keratinizing squamous epithelium. The main purpose of the conjunctiva is to *provide lubrication* of the eye. Goblet cells in the conjunctiva produce the mucous layer of the tear film.

Diseases of the conjunctiva

Like the skin elsewhere on the body, it is easy to take the role of the conjunctiva for granted. As you gain experience with diseases that affect the lubrication of the eye, you will develop an appreciation for the conjunctiva. You are likely to see the extremes of conjunctival disease, ranging from the patient with a mild case of dry eyes to patients with severe conjunctival problems, such as trachoma, ocular cicatricial pemphigoid, or chemical burns resulting from alkali injuries. When the ability to lubricate the eye is destroyed, you will see potentially devastating effects on the function of an otherwise healthy eye (Figure 2-34).

The anterior and posterior lamellae of the eyelid

A valuable concept is the division of the eyelid into the anterior and posterior lamellae. The *anterior lamella* of the eyelid consists of the skin and orbicularis muscle. The *posterior lamella* consists of the tarsus and conjunctiva. Physically, the anterior and posterior lamellae of the eyelid can be separated along the *gray line* of the eyelid margin (Figure 2-35). You will see many clinical examples where the concept of anterior and posterior lamellae is important. For example, the alkali burns and ocular cicatricial pemphigoid that we mentioned in the paragraph above not only destroy the

lubrication provided by the conjunctiva, but also cause scarring of the conjunctiva. This shortening of the posterior lamella causes the eyelid to turn inward, a condition known as *cicatricial entropion*. Scarring of the anterior lamella (caused by a laceration or thermal burn) causes the eyelid to turn outward, a condition known as *cicatricial ectropion*. Many other examples exist. Removal of a superficial skin cancer can leave a defect in the skin and orbicularis, the anterior lamella only. Repair will require replacing the anterior lamella with a skin graft. No repair of the posterior lamella will be required. On the other hand, a full-thickness laceration of the eyelid margin damages both the anterior and the posterior lamellae. Reconstruction requires repair of the supporting posterior lamella with deep, strong absorbable sutures, followed by suturing of the anterior lamella as well. Many of the problems that you will see in oculoplastic surgery have very mechanical origins and solutions. *The concept of anterior and posterior lamellae will help you understand the mechanical cause of and create a solution for many of the clinical problems that you will encounter.*

Checkpoint

- The next few times you examine patients look carefully at the conjunctiva. Observe what the normal bulbar, palpebral, and fornix conjunctiva look like. Compare the conjunctiva in a child with that in an older patient. Look at the difference in the thickness of the conjunctiva and the height of the tear film. When you see a patient with a known "dry eye," make the same comparisons.
- Make sure that you understand the concept of the anterior and posterior lamellae of the eyelids. You will find this very helpful for many oculoplastic surgery problems.

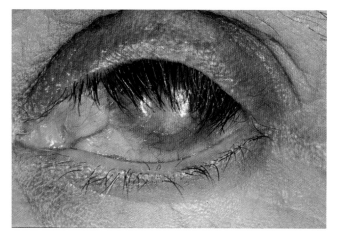

Figure 2-34 Severe dry eye from trachoma. Note the posterior lamellar shortening, which causes entropion of the upper eyelid.

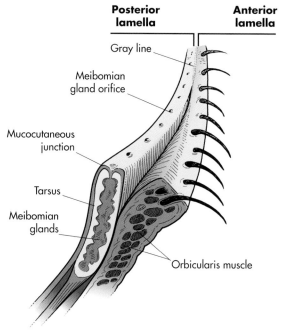

Figure 2-35 The anterior and posterior lamellae of the eyelid.

The lacrimal system

Introduction

The lacrimal system includes the lubrication of the eye and the drainage of tears. The tear film is made up of contributions from the conjunctiva, the eyelids, and the lacrimal gland. The tears are distributed across the eye by the natural spontaneous blinking of the eyelids. This blinking also functions as the "lacrimal pump," which propels tears through the lacrimal drainage system into the nose. In this section, we will discuss the anatomy, normal function, and abnormal conditions of the lacrimal system.

The tear film

The tear film is an important interface for vision as well as the health and nutrition of the cornea. Traditionally, the tear film has been considered to be composed of three layers (Figure 2-36).

- Mucous layer
- Aqueous layer
- Oil layer

More recently, it has been suggested that the mucous and aqueous layers are mixed together creating a *gel-like layer*.

There are many *mucus-producing goblet cells* throughout the conjunctiva. The mucus produced from these cells adheres to the conjunctival epithelium. The *aqueous layer is produced by the main lacrimal gland and accessory lacrimal glands* proximal to the tarsal plates (*glands of Wolfring*) and in the conjunctival fornices (*glands of Krause*) (Figure 2-37). The main *lacrimal gland* provides tears through a row of ductules that open in

the superior fornix temporally. To keep the underlying layer from evaporating, an oil layer forms the final covering. The *oil layer is provided by the sebaceous glands of the eyelids*. The most prominent sebaceous glands are the meibomian glands within the tarsal plates. In addition to the meibomian glands, oil-producing glands are found associated with the hairs in the caruncle and with the eyelashes (*glands of Zeis*). Although

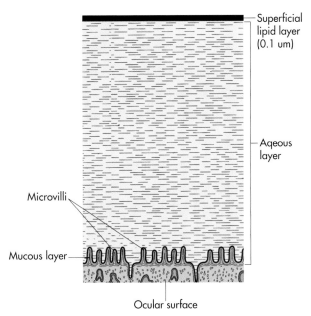

Figure 2-36 Traditional depiction of the tear film. It has been suggested that this is wrong and that the majority of the tear film thickness may exist as a mucin gel, similar to the lining of the gastrointestinal tract.

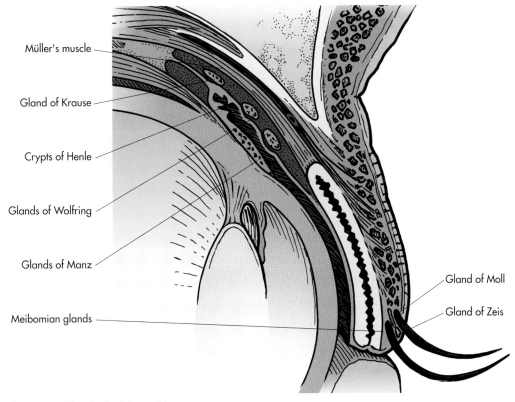

Figure 2-37 The glands of the eyelids.

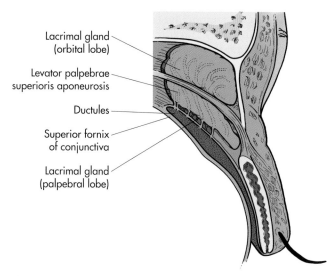

Lacrimal gland (orbital lobe)

Levator palpebrae superioris aponeurosis

Ductules

Superior fornix of conjunctiva

Lacrimal gland (palpebral lobe)

Figure 2-38 The lacrimal gland.

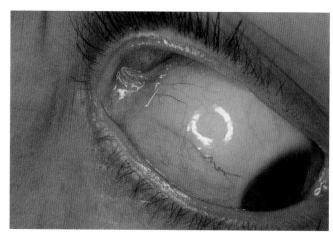

Figure 2-39 The palpebral lobe of the lacrimal gland.

the exact nature of tear film is as yet unknown, it seems reasonable to consider a role for mucous, oil- and aqueous-secreting tissues. In clinical practice, it is common to see an eye that feels "dry," but actually appears "wet"—likely due to a qualitative rather than a quantitative abnormality of the tear film. This is a concept that you will deal with many, many times in your evaluation of the treatment of the "tearing" eye. There is more on this topic in Chapter 9.

The lacrimal gland

The *lacrimal gland* sits superotemporally in the orbit in the concavity of the orbital roof known as the *lacrimal gland fossa*. The gland has two lobes, the orbital lobe and the palpebral lobe, which are divided by the lateral horn of the levator muscle (Figure 2-38). There always seems to be some confusion about the names of these lobes. The lateral horn sits at a narrowing of the gland (imagine a flattened-hourglass-shaped gland). The orbital lobe is superior to the levator and is in the orbit, actually out of the eyelid. The palpebral lobe is inferior to the levator, sitting against the superotemporal conjunctiva where the ductules of the gland enter the conjunctival cul de sac. If you evert the upper lid, you can see the palpebral lobe of the lacrimal gland in many patients (Figure 2-39). The ductules of the orbital lobe pass through the palpebral lobe to drain into the conjunctiva, so removal of the palpebral lobe blocks the drainage of the orbital lobe as well leaving a dry eye (Box 2-3).

Enlargement of the lacrimal gland is always a popular topic for test questions, so we will spend some time discussing this condition in Chapter 14. For now, remember that enlargement can be caused by cellular infiltrates (mainly lymphoid tumors) or neoplasms of the glandular tissue itself. Benign neoplasms of the gland are slow growing and cause fossa formation of the bone of the lacrimal gland fossa. Malignant neoplasms of the gland cause bone erosion. You will get a chance to learn this again later.

The lacrimal drainage system

The lacrimal drainage system consists of the *puncta, canaliculi, lacrimal sac*, and *nasolacrimal duct* (Figure 2-40). Tears

Box 2-3

The Lacrimal Gland Ductules

The exact position of the lacrimal gland ductules always seems poorly explained in most texts, but the position of these ductules, as it turns out, is quite simple to find. If you evert the upper eyelid you will see the bulge of the lacrimal gland in the temporal superior fornix in many patients. The ductules open directly from the gland into the fornix at that point (see Figure 2-38). Sometime you may find it interesting to demonstrate the flow of tears through the ductules themselves. You will need an operating microscope or a slit lamp with a cobalt blue filter in place. In a suitable patient evert the upper lid and paint the conjunctiva on the bulge of the lacrimal gland with a fluorescein strip (best to do this on a patient who has not been given preoperative medications to decrease secretions). Initially the fluorescein will not glow, but in a short time the tears flowing from the ductules will dilute the fluorescein to the point where spots of bright yellow fluorescein will be visible. After a few moments you will see a row of 10 or 12 tiny openings as the ductules appear. These openings are almost impossible to see with the microscope light alone. There may be an occasional patient for whom this location is important to know intraoperatively as incision into the conjunctiva in this area may scar the ductules.

enter the puncta and drain through the canaliculi into the lacrimal sac and down the nasolacrimal duct, which opens into the inferior meatus of the nose (under the inferior turbinate).

The puncta

The openings of the lacrimal drainage system, the *puncta*, are located on the most medial aspect of each lid margin about 5 mm from the medial canthus. Each *punctum* sits on a slight elevation of the lid margin known as the *lacrimal papilla*. You will notice that the puncta sit adjacent to the plica of the conjunctiva with the upper lid punctum slightly medial to the lower lid punctum. *The opening of the normal lower eyelid punctum sits in the tear meniscus and is not visible on slit lamp examination without slight manual eversion of the lid margin.* There are no lashes medial to the punctum.

A variety of conditions affect the punctum. The most common problem is *malposition of the punctum* caused by eyelid eversion. If the tears cannot enter the punctum, they

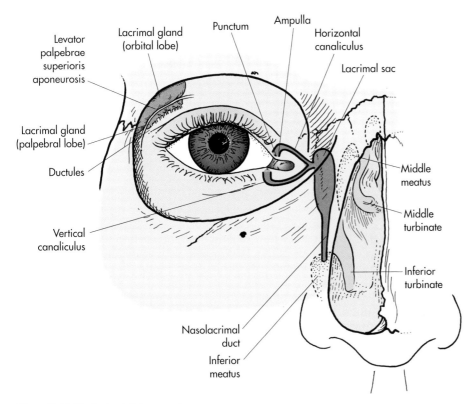

Figure 2-40 The lacrimal drainage system.

cannot drain. Other problems relate to the congenital absence of one or more puncta (*punctal atresia*) or to an acquired narrowing (*punctal stenosis*) or obstruction of the punctum.

The canaliculi

Tears enter the *canaliculus* through the punctum and travel through a short vertical portion of the canaliculus measuring 2 mm. The canaliculus turns and extends horizontally for about 8 mm. The junction of the vertical and horizontal portions is known as the *ampulla*, named after the dilated flask-like shape at this point. The horizontal portion of the canaliculus returns to the narrow diameter of 1–2 mm until it fuses with the canaliculus of the opposite lid to form the *common canaliculus*. The common canaliculus then enters the lacrimal sac through the *common internal punctum*. A minority of patients will have the upper and lower canaliculi enter the lacrimal sac independently rather than through a common canaliculus. *Obstruction of a canaliculus* may occur after infection, usually viral, or after chemotherapy. Other low-grade infections caused by anaerobic bacteria may start in the ampulla and cause a chronic discharge, *canaliculitis*. *Lacerations of the canaliculus* (Figure 2-41) are seen in association with other periocular and facial trauma. Repair of the canaliculus requires microscopic reanastomosis of the torn edges of the canaliculus over silicone stents to prevent stenosis of the repaired segment of the canaliculus. Reattachment of the anterior limb of the medial canthal tendon is often required at the same time.

The lacrimal sac

The *lacrimal sac* sits in the lacrimal sac fossa. In its resting, semi-collapsed state, the sac is only about 2 mm wide. Its length is 10–15 mm (shorter than you would think). The

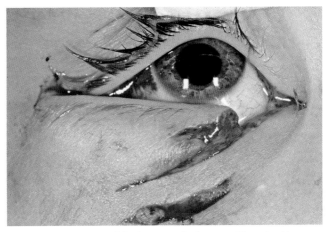

Figure 2-41 Laceration of the lower canaliculus caused by a dog bite.

inferior portion of the sac narrows to meet the *nasolacrimal duct*.

As we discussed earlier in the section on anatomy of the orbital bones, the *lacrimal sac fossa* is bounded by the anterior lacrimal crest anteriorly and the posterior lacrimal crest posteriorly. The anterior two thirds of the floor of the fossa is made up of bone from the maxilla. A suture line separates the maxillary bone contribution anteriorly from the lacrimal bone contribution. This description may seem like too much detail for such a small area of bone, but you need to become very familiar with this anatomic area before attempting surgery to correct tearing in adults. It is the easily broken, thin, lacrimal bone portion of the fossa that is initially removed when an ostium is made into the nose to redirect tear drainage.

Recall that the *anterior* and *posterior limbs of the medial canthal tendon attach to the lacrimal crests, surrounding the lacrimal sac.* The superior one third of the lacrimal sac extends above the medial canthal tendon. The canaliculi pass directly under the anterior limb of the medial canthal tendon before passing into the lacrimal sac. *Nasolacrimal duct obstruction* causes retention of fluid in the sac, sometimes creating distention of the sac. The position of the medial canthal tendon does not allow distention of the sac by fluid superior to the tendon. A *tumor within the sac*, a rare occurrence, can elevate the tendon. Any distention of the lacrimal sac superior to the medial canthal tendon should be considered to be a tumor until proven otherwise.

The nasolacrimal duct

The lacrimal sac narrows inferiorly to become the nasolacrimal duct. The membranous duct (mucosa lined) travels within the bony nasolacrimal duct into the nose. The nasolacrimal duct travels about 15 mm before it opens under the inferior turbinate into the inferior meatus of the nose (see Figures 2-40 and 2-42). It is worth remembering that the nasolacrimal duct is not long. It is easy to pass a probe too deep, beyond the valve of Hasner toward the back of the nasopharynx.

Several valves are present to prevent the retrograde flow of tears in the lacrimal drainage system. The most important valve clinically is the *valve of Hasner*, which is at the entrance of the nasolacrimal duct into the inferior meatus. *Congenital nasolacrimal duct obstruction* occurs at the valve of Hasner. This relatively common condition presents as tearing and discharge in infants. In the majority of infants, the obstruction resolves as the thin membrane causing the obstruction

ruptures spontaneously in the first year of life. Persistent obstruction of the nasolacrimal duct is treated with probing of the nasolacrimal duct using a specially designed wire probe to rupture the membrane.

Acquired nasolacrimal duct obstruction (occurring in adulthood) is caused by diffuse scarring of the membranous nasolacrimal duct, rather than obstruction at the valve of Hasner. Surgically redirecting the tears from the lacrimal sac directly into the nose, as described above, bypasses the obstruction in the duct. This procedure is called a *dacryocystorhinostomy* (abbreviated DCR, meaning "tear-sac-hole in the nose").

Other valves occur within the lacrimal drainage system. The *valve of Rosenmüller* is found at the junction of the common canaliculus into the sac. This valve will prevent retrograde flow of fluid from the sac into the eye. The effectiveness of this valve is seen with acute infection of the sac, *dacryocystitis*, which occurs as a result of obstruction of the nasolacrimal duct. Tears cannot drain into nose, nor can they drain out of the sac into the eye because the valve of Rosenmüller prevents retrograde drainage. In cases of infection, it is likely that the valve swells closed even more tightly than under normal circumstances. Recent anatomic dissections have shown that the valve of Rosenmüller is not a true valve, but an angulated entrance of the common canaliculus into the sac, functioning as a valve. Other valves are present in the nasolacrimal duct. They all have names, but are of no clinical importance. There are no valves known within the canaliculi.

The lacrimal pump

Before leaving the topic of the lacrimal system, we should discuss the *lacrimal pump* in more detail. Remember that the limbs of the medial canthal tendon surround the lacrimal sac. As the eyelids blink, the sac is compressed and expanded by the surrounding canthal limbs and fascia (the lacrimal sac fascia). This blinking action serves to fill and empty the sac in a pumping manner. The exact mechanism and specific contributions of various parts of the orbicularis muscles are debated. The concept that normal blinking is necessary for the drainage of tears is well accepted, however. Consequently, any condition that inhibits normal blinking will adversely affect tear drainage. You will see tearing in patients with *facial nerve palsy* and *scarring on the eyelids* and after *trauma or tumor reconstruction* (cases in which the normal relationship of the limbs of the medial canthal tendon to the lacrimal sac has been disrupted). You will learn to look for anatomic abnormalities that affect the *frequency* and the *quality* (completeness) of the blink, signs that *failure of the lacrimal pump* is the cause of the tearing problem.

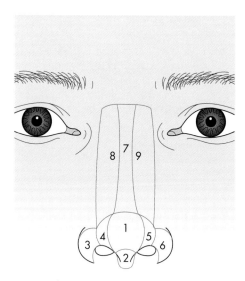

1 = Tip subunit
2 = Columellar subunit
3 = Right alar base subunit
4 = Right alar side wall subunit
5 = Right alar base subunit
6 = Left alar base subunit
7 = Dorsal subunit
8 = Right side wall subunit
9 = Left side wall subunit

Figure 2-42 The nasal subunits. The nine subunits include the dorsum, sidewalls, lobules, soft triangles, alae and the columella.

Nasal anatomy

No doubt at some time in your practice, you will put your understanding of nasal anatomy to good use. For sure, you will be inspecting the nasal anatomy and mucosa as part of your evaluation of the tearing patient. You will be reconstructing lower eyelid and midfacial defects that can extend onto the nose. You will need to know important landmarks to safely perform external and endoscopic DCR operations. You may become adept enough at endoscopic surgery to use

* What are the layers of the tear film? Where is each layer derived? Remember the traditional teaching may not be correct.
* Describe the relationship of the levator muscle to the lacrimal gland lobes. Evert an eyelid in a patient with loose upper lids to see the lacrimal gland (which lobe are you seeing?)
* Name the structures of the lacrimal drainage system. Name at least one problem associated with each structure. Can you think of the treatment for each? You may not be able to yet but, by the time you finish this text, you will.

You should have a familiarity with the concept of the "lacrimal pump." Actually understanding it will become clearer when you deal with patients that tear because they don't blink normally.

Box 2-4

The Nasal Muscles

* Elevators
  * Procerus
  * Levator labii superioris alaeque nasi
* Depressors
  * Alar nasalis
  * Depressor septi nasi
* Compressors
  * Transverse nasalis
* Dilators
  * Dilator naris anterior
  * Dilator naris posterior

---

it for orbital decompression, drainage of a subperiosteal orbital abscess, biopsy of apical orbital tumors, or transphenoidal optic canal decompression. You may not want to venture into all these areas yourself, so you should develop a good relationship with an ENT colleague who can assist you in these areas. We will discuss some of the anatomy that you should start to become familiar with. You may want to skip over the details of this and come back to it when you have a more specific need. For now, get the big picture.

The external surface of the nose is divided into subunits: the dorsum, sidewalls, tip (lobule and soft triangles), alae and the columella (See Figure 2-42). The overlying skin can be considered as vertical thirds. The skin of the upper third of the nose is thick and tapers into a thinner mid-dorsal region. The inferior third becomes thicker approaching the thickness of the upper third, mainly due to the sebaceous nature of the skin over the nasal tip. Periocular reconstructions involving the nose should be undertaken with consideration to the boundaries of the nasal subunits and associated skin thickness.

The nasal muscles are deep to the skin and comprise four principal groups: the elevators, the depressors, the compressor, and the dilators (Box 2-4). The details and names of the muscles are not so important at this point; just remember that the muscles open and close the nostrils to help with breathing. The elevators include the procerus and levator labii superioris alaeque nasi.

The depressors are made up of the alar nasalis and depressor septi nasi. The compressor of the nose is the transverse nasalis. The dilators are the dilator naris anterior and posterior. The nasal muscles are physically and functionally connected via the superficial musculoaponeurotic system (SMAS), which we will talk about later. Patients with facial palsy can suffer collapse of the nostril due to paralysis of the nasal muscles (see Figure 2-1). You may be pleasantly surprised when your facial nerve palsy patient undergoes facial sling and eyelid tightening for ectropion and tells you that his nasal breathing is improved.

The external surface of the nose is supported by underlying bone and cartilage. The nose is attached to the frontal bone at the *nasal root*. The paired nasal bones attach to the frontal bones above and extend inferiorly where the nasal cartilages form the *nasal dorsum, sidewalls,* and *tip*. The cartilaginous septum extends from the nasal bones in the midline above to the bony septum in the midline posteriorly, then down along the bony nasal floor. The *lateral nasal cartilages* support the superior portion of the lateral nasal wall. The *lateral alar cartilages* extend inferiorly to form the external nasal openings. Adjacent smaller sesamoid cartilages may be found in association the larger cartilages (see Figure 2-43).

The nasal cavity is an anatomically complex passageway that serves several functions:

* Direct airflow
* Filters, warms, and moisturizes the air
* Provides drainage for the sinuses
* Resonance of voice
* Sense of smell

The nasal aperture or *pyriform aperture* is made up of the maxillary bone on each side. The interior of the nose is divided into mirror image halves by the *nasal septum*, made of bone superiorly and cartilage inferiorly. For our purposes, the most important feature of the nasal septum to recognize is when there is significant deviation of the septum to one side that may prevent adequate visualization of the lateral walls of the nose. Turbinates or "wings" of mucosa-lined bone project from the lateral wall (Figure 2-44). There are three turbinates: the *superior, inferior,* and *middle*. The turbinates are sometimes referred to as the conchae. The space under each turbinate is know as a *meatus*, named for the turbinate above it. The shape of air passages formed by the septum and the turbinates promotes nonturbulent airflow. The large surface area of mucosa present warms and moisturizes the air. You will see that patients who have one or more turbinates removed have difficulty with nasal breathing and often develop crusting of the mucosa.

The *inferior turbinate* originates from the lateral wall of the nose and lies parallel to the floor of the nose. The bony nasolacrimal duct runs inferiorly from the lacrimal sac fossa through the lateral wall of the nose to empty in the anterior one third of the inferior meatus through the valve of Hasner. In some children, the inferior turbinate is displaced laterally, crowding the opening of the nasolacrimal duct. During a tear duct probing operation, the turbinate can be infractured, or pushed medially toward the septum, to enlarge the inferior meatus. Sometimes when you are doing a probing procedure, you may want to pass a pediatric nasal endoscope under the inferior turbinate to visualize the opening of the nasolacrimal duct. You will have to become familiar with the anatomy of the inferior turbinate and meatus in order to retrieve stents when you intubate the nasolacrimal duct in children with recurrent nasolacrimal duct obstruction.

The *middle turbinate* takes its origin superiorly from the cribriform plate. You should be careful when fracturing or removing the middle turbinate because, rarely, a CSF leak can develop. The *anterior ethmoid air* cells drain into the middle meatus. The most anterior portion of the middle meatus receives the drainage from the frontal sinus through the *nasofrontal duct*, which passes through the anterior ethmoid cells on the way to the meatus. The *frontal recess* refers to the space just inferior to the frontal sinus ostium where the nasofrontal duct forms.

The middle turbinate is an important landmark for two other anatomic structures. The attachment of the middle turbinate to the lateral wall of the nose is at the same height as the *cribriform plate*. Surgery performed to remove a portion of the middle turbinate should be done carefully to avoid a CSF leak. The anterior tip of the middle turbinate marks the *position of the lacrimal sac*. Preparation for a DCR begins with packing the tip of the middle turbinate with a topical decongestant. The opening of the lacrimal sac into the nose is made in this area. You will learn these nasal anatomic landmarks in more detail in Chapter 10.

The *middle meatus* is a complex structure that endoscopic nasal surgeons become quite familiar with. Until you start doing endoscopic DCR procedures or more complex endoscopic approaches to the orbit, you can skim over this information. On the lateral wall of the nose, just posterior to the tip of the middle turbinate, is a sickle-shaped flap of mucosa that covers the opening from the maxillary sinus, known as the *uncinate process*. A bulging anterior ethmoid air cell, known as the *ethmoid bulla*, is usually visible just posterior

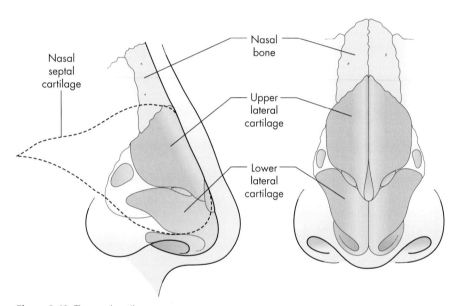

Figure 2-43 The nasal cartilages.

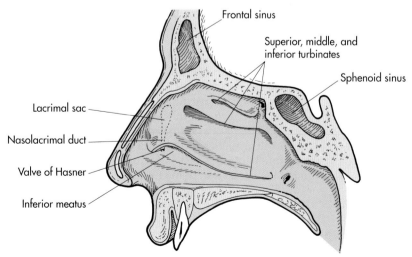

Figure 2-44 The nasal turbinates.

to the uncinate process (Figure 2-45). The initial steps of an endoscopic ethmoidectomy begin with identification and removal of the uncinate process, followed by opening the ethmoid bulla (Figure 2-46).

The *superior turbinate* is usually very small and often difficult to visualize. You won't be seeing this turbinate during lacrimal surgery unless you look for it with the endoscope. The posterior ethmoid air cells drain into the superior meatus. The sphenoid sinus is posterior to the superior turbinate. The sphenoid sinus drains into the *sphenoethmoid recess*, which is the space between the superior turbinate, the septum, and the anterior wall of the sphenoid septum. If you venture into optic canal procedures, you will have to learn this anatomy but, for now, just get the general idea. I have included some more anatomy about this in the section ahead on the sphenoid sinus (Figure 2-47).

Anatomy of the paranasal sinuses

Sinus anatomy is important to us because the majority of orbital infections and many of the tumors that invade the orbit secondarily originate in the sinus. The nose and paranasal sinuses are lined with pseudostratified ciliated columnar respiratory epithelium. The drainage of the sinus is not by gravity, but by the ciliary movement that pushes the mucous toward each sinus ostium (mucociliary clearance). If the normal drainage of the sinus is acutely blocked, sinusitis may result. If severe, the infection may spread into the orbit. If the obstruction is permanent, a mucocele can form. The mucosa of the nose and sinus may develop a number of malignancies. Because the sinuses are a "silent" area, the masses are often large before diagnosis. In many cases, these tumors will extend through the bony walls of the orbit.

The sinuses, like the nose, warm and humidify the air, lighten the weight of the skull, function as resonating chambers for the voice, and provide protection for the contents of the brain and spinal cord in cases of trauma.

The paranasal sinuses include:

- Ethmoid sinus
- Frontal sinus
- Maxillary sinus
- Sphenoid sinus

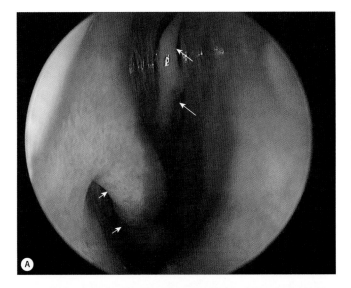

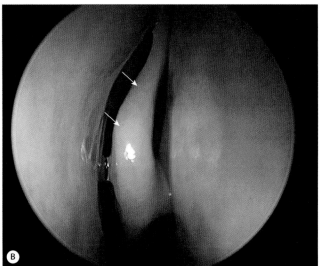

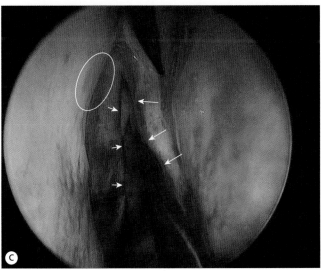

Figure 2-45 Endoscopic view of turbinates. (**A**) Endoscopic view of turbinates. Inferior turbinate (short arrows pointing to lateral side of turbinate from within the inferior meatus). Nasolacrimal duct opens in the lateral wall of the inferior meatus. Long arrows point to medial side of middle turbinate. (**B**) Endoscopic view of middle turbinate. Arrows pointing to lateral side of turbinate from within the middle meatus. (**C**) Endoscopic view of middle meatus. Long arrows point to retracted middle turbinate. Short arrows points to uncinate process. Ellipse denotes position of lacrimal sac.

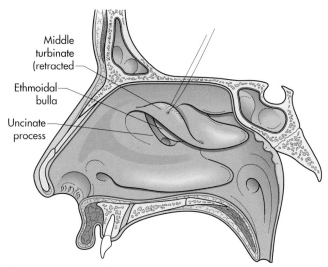

Middle
turbinate
(retracted

Ethmoidal
bulla

Uncinate
process

Figure 2-46 Lateral wall of nose from inside nose. Note retracted middle turbinate gives a view of the uncinate process.

The ethmoid sinus

The ethmoid sinus (Figure 2-48) is situated between the orbit and the nose. The ethmoid sinus is present at birth and continues to enlarge with facial development. The sinus and orbit share the thin medial orbital wall, the lamina papyracea. The ethmoid sinus is composed of many thin-walled air cells, some of which may extend anteriorly between the lacrimal sac and the nasal mucosa. You will commonly encounter a few of these cells during a DCR. As we said above, the anterior and middle air cells of the sinus drain into the middle meatus of the nose. The posterior air cells drain into the superior meatus. *Bacterial orbital cellulitis* is most commonly caused by the spread of infection in the ethmoid sinus (ethmoid sinusitis) into the orbit directly through the lamina papyracea or by traveling through the anterior and posterior ethmoid vessels.

The frontal sinus

The frontal sinus appears at the age of about 6 years and continues to enlarge until adulthood. The left and right frontal sinuses are separated by an intersinus septum. The size and shape of the frontal sinus vary greatly among individuals and, in some individuals, a frontal sinus may never form. The frontal sinus is larger in men than in women and is responsible for the prominent frontal bossing seen in many men. The drainage of the frontal sinus is through the frontonasal duct into the anterior portion of the middle meatus. The frontal sinus can be a source of orbital cellulitis, but more commonly affects the orbit with slowly progressive growth of a *frontal sinus mucocele*. Obstruction of the sinus drainage prevents drainage of sinus mucus, resulting in a sterile collection of mucus within the sinus. Frontal sinus mucoceles may get quite large, expanding the sinus cavity over a period of years. The orbital contents are displaced inferiorly and laterally (Figure 2-49). Fractures of the anterior wall of the frontal sinus are repaired when a significant deformity exists. Fractures of the posterior wall of the frontal sinus require repair to avoid meningitis.

The maxillary sinus

The *maxillary sinus* forms inferior to the orbit (Figure 2-48). The roof of the sinus forms the orbital floor, although the orbital floor extends more posteriorly than the back wall of the maxillary sinus. The maxillary sinus drains into the middle meatus with the ostium of the sinus opening into the nose on the superior aspect of the medial wall of the sinus, which may explain the high incidence of maxillary sinusitis. Because both the maxillary and the frontal sinuses drain through the anterior ethmoid air cells into the middle meatus, the health of these two sinuses is directly related to the condition of the ethmoid sinus.

The roof of the sinus contains the *infraorbital nerve*. You will commonly see fractures of the orbital floor, such as the *blowout fractures* that we discussed earlier in this chapter. These fractures can cause prolapse of orbital tissues into the sinus. Restriction of ocular movements and diplopia occur secondary to incarceration of these tissues. Hypesthesia of the cheek and upper gingiva occurs caused by contusion of the infraorbital nerve. If you suspect an orbital fracture, ask your patient to avoid nose blowing as subcutaneous emphysema may occur.

The sphenoid sinus

The *sphenoid sinus* is small at birth and continues to develop into puberty. The size of the sphenoid septum varies considerably from patient to patient. After you gain some experience in reading CT scans, note how much variability is seen from patient to patient in the size of frontal and sphenoid sinuses. The sphenoid sinus is divided by an intersinus septum as in the frontal sinus. The sphenoid sinus drains into the nose above the superior turbinate. *The lateral wall of the sphenoid sinus contains the medial wall of the optic canal and the internal carotid artery.* Because of this close anatomic relationship, *sphenoid sinusitis may cause damage to the optic nerve.* In patients with *traumatic optic neuropathy, the optic nerve can be decompressed surgically through the sphenoid sinus* by removing the bone of the medial side of the optic canal. Remember that the internal carotid artery is only a few millimeters away.

Checkpoint

You will understand the nasal and sinus anatomy when you start doing lacrimal drainage procedures, especially endoscopic surgery.

- The middle turbinate marks the approximate location of the lacrimal sac.
- The nasolacrimal duct opens into the inferior meatus. Try to see this opening (valve of Hasner) with an endoscope when the nasolacrimal duct is probed.
- The nasal subunit structure is an important consideration in periocular flaps extending onto the nose.
- Ethmoid sinusitis is the most common cause of orbital cellulitis. Look at a CT scan to locate all the sinuses. Note the variability in size and shape of the frontal and sphenoid sinuses.
- Note the relationship of the lacrimal sac to the ethmoid sinuses and the relationship of the optic canal to the sphenoid sinus.

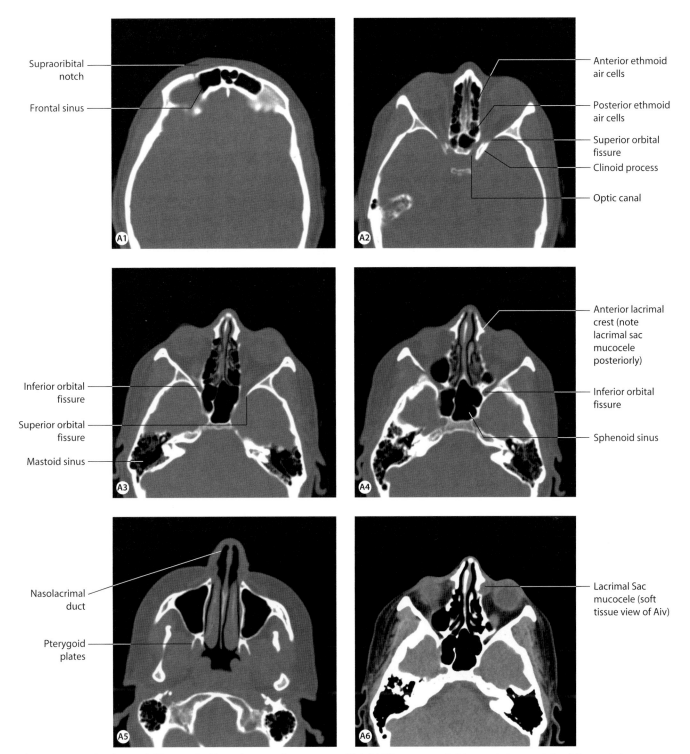

Supraoribital notch

Frontal sinus

Anterior ethmoid air cells

Posterior ethmoid air cells

Superior orbital fissure

Clinoid process

Optic canal

Inferior orbital fissure

Superior orbital fissure

Mastoid sinus

Anterior lacrimal crest (note lacrimal sac mucocele posteriorly)

Inferior orbital fissure

Sphenoid sinus

Nasolacrimal duct

Pterygoid plates

Lacrimal Sac mucocele (soft tissue view of Aiv)

Figure 2-47 Axial and coronal CT scans of orbits and surrounding structures. (**A**) Axial CT scans, parts 1–5, bone windows; part 6, soft tissue window showing better resolution of lacrimal sac mucocele. (**B**) Coronal CT scans, parts 1–6, soft tissue windows.

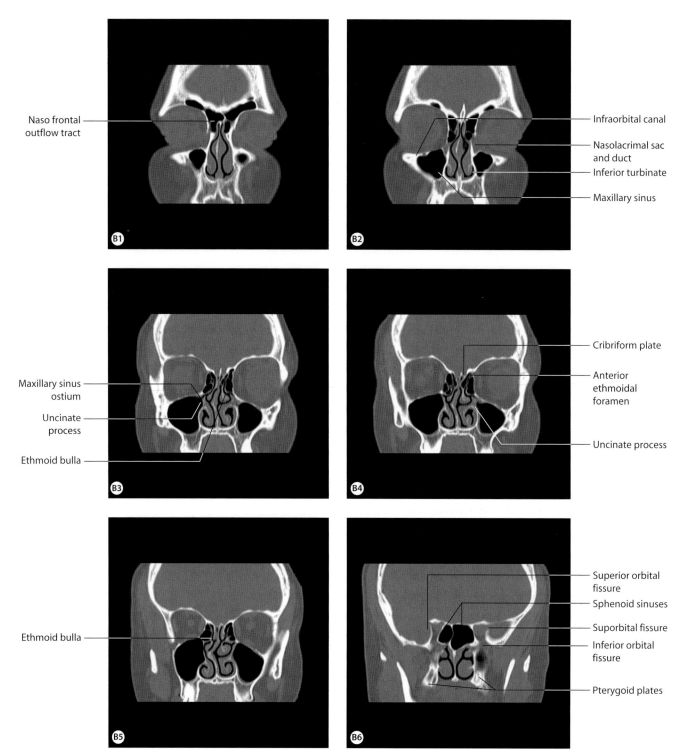

Naso frontal outflow tract

Infraorbital canal

Nasolacrimal sac and duct

Inferior turbinate

Maxillary sinus

Maxillary sinus ostium

Uncinate process

Ethmoid bulla

Cribriform plate

Anterior ethmoidal foramen

Uncinate process

Ethmoid bulla

Superior orbital fissure

Sphenoid sinuses

Suporbital fissure

Inferior orbital fissure

Pterygoid plates

Figure 2-47 Continued.

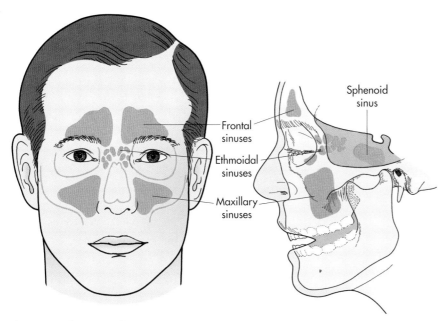

Figure 2-48 The paranasal sinuses.

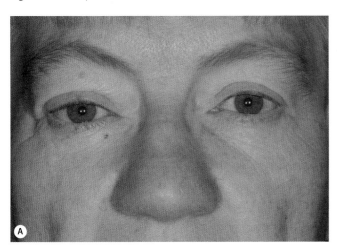
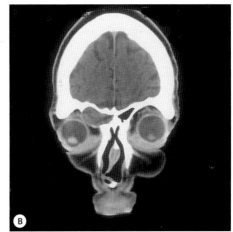

Figure 2-49 Frontal sinus mucocele. (**A**) Right globe displaced inferiorly by frontal sinus mucocele. (**B**) Coronal CT scan of frontal sinus mucocele with erosion of orbital roof.

Innervation to the periocular area

Sensory innervation

The sensory innervation to the periocular area is provided by the *ophthalmic* (V_1) and *maxillary* (V_2) *divisions of the fifth cranial nerve (the trigeminal nerve)* (Figure 2-50). Roughly speaking:

- The upper eyelid, orbit, and eye are innervated by the branches of the ophthalmic division
- The lower eyelid is innervated by the branches of the maxillary division

The *mandibular division* (V_3) of the trigeminal nerve supplies sensation to the lower part of the face. Figure 2-50 will help you understand the sensory innervation and may be all you need to concern yourself with at this point. Things get complicated quickly. If this is your first time through this chapter, you may want to skip ahead to the section "The Maxillary Division of the Trigeminal Nerve."

The ophthalmic division of the trigeminal nerve

The ophthalmic division (V_2) has three main branches:

- Frontal nerve
- Lacrimal nerve
- Nasociliary nerve

The frontal and lacrimal branches do not innervate the eyeball. The nasociliary nerve provides sensation to the eyeball (Figure 2-51).

The frontal nerve is the largest nerve of the ophthalmic division. It courses anteriorly just inferior to the orbital roof to divide into the *supraorbital nerve* (to the forehead) and the *supratrochlear nerve* (to the medial canthus). The lacrimal nerve, the smallest nerve of the ophthalmic division, has small branches that provide sensation to the skin and conjunctiva of the lateral one third of the upper lid (Figure 2-47). The lacrimal nerve also carries the postganglionic parasympathetic fibers for the reflex tearing.

The *nasociliary nerve* provides sensory innervation to the eye. Sensory branches travel alongside the short posterior

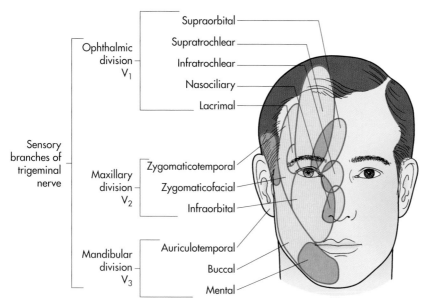

Figure 2-50 Sensory distribution of trigeminal nerve.

ciliary nerves to the back of the eye. Two long ciliary nerves branch off the nasociliary nerve to travel through the sclera to innervate the anterior portion of the eye. Other branches of the nasociliary nerve head out of the muscle cone toward the medial orbital wall as the *anterior* and *posterior ciliary nerves*, which provide sensation to the nasal and sinus mucosa. The nasociliary nerve terminates as the *infratrochlear nerve*, which emerges onto the skin inferior to the trochlea above the medial canthal tendon to provide sensory innervation to the skin of the medial canthus and lateral side of the nose, conjunctiva, and caruncle. As you know, herpes zoster infections travel along sensory nerves. Involvement of the *skin on the tip of the nose* means nasociliary nerve infection, which warns you of the possibility of infection of the eyeball as well. Severe corneal and intraocular inflammation may result in blindness if left untreated.

Because the *frontal* and *lacrimal branches do not innervate the eye*, the course of these nerves through the orbit is outside the muscle cone. These branches enter the orbit through the superior orbital fissure *outside the annulus of Zinn* because they do not have to get to the eye. The *nasociliary nerve innervates the eye*, so it enters the superior orbital fissure *inside the annulus of Zinn* with the oculomotor nerve branches (these branches will innervate the extraocular muscles on the underside of the muscle belly).

Let's go over this again: the branches of the ophthalmic division of the trigeminal nerve are the *frontal* (supraorbital and supratrochlear nerves), *lacrimal*, and *nasociliary* (ciliary, ethmoidal, and infratrochlear nerves). These nerves provide sensory innervation to:

- *Medial canthus* via the *supratrochlear nerve* (superior portion of the medial canthus) and the *infratrochlear nerve* (inferior portion of the medial canthus)
- *Upper lid* via the *supratrochlear nerve* (*medial lid*) and *lacrimal nerve* (*lateral lid*)
- *Forehead* and *scalp* via the *supraorbital nerve*
- *Eyeball* via the *ciliary nerves*

- *Nasal* and *sinus mucosa* via the anterior and posterior ethmoidal nerves

The maxillary division of the trigeminal nerve

The *maxillary division of the trigeminal nerve* (V_2) has one main branch, the infraorbital nerve (see Figures 2-50 and 2-51), which innervates the lower eyelid. We discussed the path of the infraorbital nerve earlier in the section on the bony anatomy of the orbit. In review, the infraorbital nerve leaves the skull base through the foramen rotundum, travels along the floor of the orbit in the *infraorbital groove*, then enters the infraorbital canal and, finally, emerges out of the *infraorbital foramen* 1 cm below the infraorbital rim (refer back to Figures 2-6 and 2-11).

The infraorbital nerve supplies sensation to the lower eyelid, the cheek, and the upper gingiva and teeth. The infraorbital nerve lies outside the periorbita and so provides no innervation of the orbital tissues proper. As we discussed earlier in the section on the anatomy of the maxillary sinus, an important clinical sign of an orbital floor fracture is hypesthesia of the lower lid, cheek, and teeth secondary to contusion of the infraorbital nerve. You will see this clinical sign commonly in trauma patients.

Two other small cutaneous nerve branches arise from the maxillary V_2 division of the trigeminal nerve, the *zygomaticotemporal* and *zygomaticofacial nerves* (see Figure 2-51). These nerves supply sensation to the skin over the malar region and the lateral orbital rim. We discussed the foramina with the same names on the lateral orbital wall. These nerves communicate with the small branches of the lacrimal nerve superiorly to complete the innervation to the lateral portion of the upper eyelid.

The lower face is innervated by branches of the mandibular V_3 nerve. The nerve leaves the skull through the foramen ovale. Major branches include the *lingual nerve*, the *inferior alveolar nerve*, and *auriculotemporal* nerve. The terminal branch of the lingual nerve, the *mental nerve*, exits the mandible through the mental foramen, which is found in a line inferior to the infraorbital and supraorbital nerves. Motor

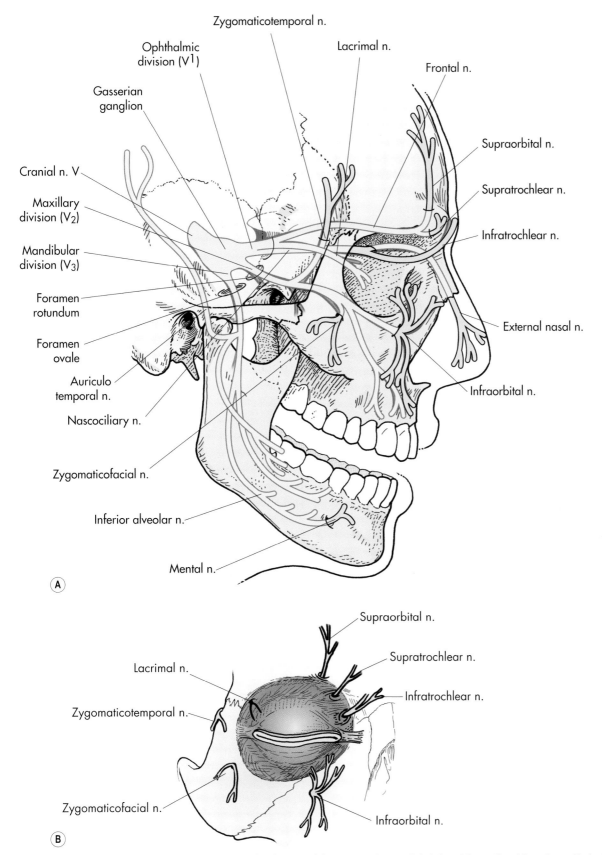

Zygomaticotemporal n.

Ophthalmic division (V¹)

Lacrimal n.

Frontal n.

Gasserian ganglion

Supraorbital n.

Cranial n. V

Supratrochlear n.

Maxillary division (V₂)

Infratrochlear n.

Mandibular division (V₃)

Foramen rotundum

Foramen ovale

External nasal n.

Auriculo temporal n.

Infraorbital n.

Nascociliary n.

Zygomaticofacial n.

Inferior alveolar n.

Mental n.

(A)

Supraorbital n.

Supratrochlear n.

Lacrimal n.

Infratrochlear n.

Zygomaticotemporal n.

Zygomaticofacial n.

Infraorbital n.

(B)

Figure 2-51 The branches of the trigeminal nerve. (**A**) The divisions of the trigeminal nerve: Ophthalmic (V₁), maxillary (V₂), and mandibular (V₃). (**B**) The terminal branches of the ophthalmic (V₁) and maxillary (V₂) divisions of the trigeminal nerve.

branches to muscles of mastication are associated with the sensory branches of V₃.

As you can see there is tremendous overlap of the sensory nerves. The redundancy of innervation makes permanent loss of sensation after accidental or surgical trauma uncommon. The overlapping innervation makes the use of regional nerve blocks less effective for eyelid surgery. You may find that supraorbital, infraorbital, and mental nerve blocks can be a useful addition to a generalized local infiltration for effective facial anesthesia.

Innervation to the muscles of facial expression

The facial nerve

Innervation to the orbicularis muscle and the other muscles of facial expression is supplied by the *facial nerve*, cranial nerve VII. The facial nerve exits the skull at the *stylomastoid foramen* deep to the tragus of the ear. The nerve enters the parotid gland where it divides into five peripheral branches, each headed for a different area of the face (Figures 2-52 and 2-53). From superior to inferior, the branches of the facial nerve are:

- Temporal branch
- Zygomatic branch
- Buccal branch
- Mandibular branch
- Cervical branch

The *temporal branch* supplies the orbicularis, procerus, corrugator, and frontalis muscles. The *zygomatic branch* innervates the orbicularis of the lower lid. The lower branches innervate the remaining facial muscles, including the platysma of the neck. All the facial muscles are innervated from the posterior aspect of the muscle, so dissection anterior to the muscle will not cause motor nerve damage. With the exception of the temporal branch, there is significant arborization of the named branches of the facial nerve. Trauma to the smaller peripheral branches is compensated for by adjacent intact nerve fibers. Remember that the closer to the nerve trunk an injury occurs, as is the case with a laceration, the more widespread the paralysis will be.

The *temporal branch*, in contrast to the other branches, supplies innervation to the forehead via a *single nerve branch. Loss of the temporal branch of the facial nerve results in total paralysis of the brow, creating a brow ptosis. The path of the temporal branch can be approximated by drawing a line from the tragus to a point 1 cm above the tail of the brow* (see Figure 2-52). You should draw this line when doing any dissections in this area. You must also *consider the depth of the nerve* in the area where you are working. Immediately anterior to the tragus, the facial nerve trunk is deep within the parotid gland. It is difficult to damage the nerve in this area when you are creating any facial flaps or harvesting preauricular skin. *The nerve becomes most superficial as it crosses the zygomatic arch, so be careful in this area.* In the temple, the frontal branch of the facial nerve lies deeper in the loose areolar

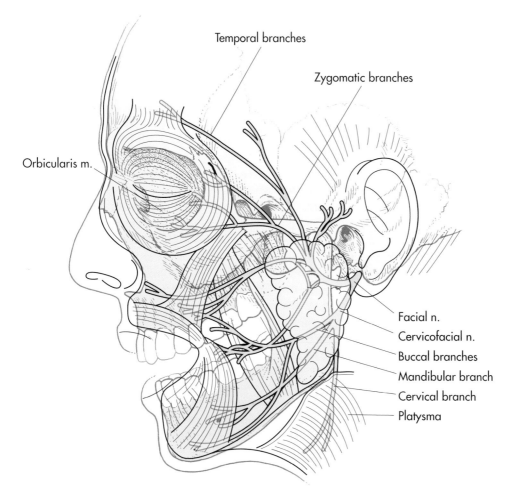

Figure 2-52 The branches of the facial nerve.

Temporal branches

Zygomatic branches

Orbicularis m.

Facial n.

Cervicofacial n.

Buccal branches

Mandibular branch

Cervical branch

Platysma

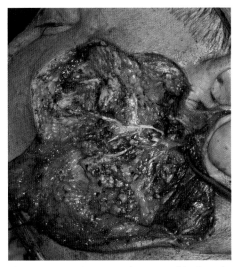

Figure 2-53 Intraoperative dissection of the branches of the facial nerve during parotidectomy. In this case, the facial nerve has been preserved and the surrounding parotid gland has been removed (courtesy of Henry Hoffman, MD).

tissue anterior the temporalis muscle. If you are dissecting in this area, you must be superficial to the nerve (in the fat of the subcutaneous layer) or deep to the nerve (directly on or under the deep fascia of the temporalis muscle). The nomenclature of the fascial planes over the temporalis muscle are somewhat complicated, so for now just remember that this is a danger zone. Later in this chapter, you will learn the difference between what is called the deep temporalis fascia and the temporoparietal fascia. This is important clinical anatomy that you should learn if you are planning to perform coronal flaps or other reconstructive procedures outside the lateral canthus.

In the neck, the cervical branch of the facial nerve gives rise to a branch called the *ramus mandibularis*. This terminal branch has a variable course along the ramus of the mandible and can be damaged during mobilization of the platysma muscle during neck lift or liposuction procedures. Damage to this nerve can cause drooling and an asymmetric smile.

Innervation to the extraocular muscles

Innervation to the extraocular muscles including the levator muscle is by the *third, fourth,* and *sixth cranial nerves.* The third nerve, the *oculomotor nerve,* has two divisions. The *upper division* innervates the levator muscle and the superior and medial rectus muscles. The *lower division* innervates the inferior rectus and the inferior oblique muscles. The sixth cranial nerve, the *abducens nerve,* innervates the lateral rectus. The fourth cranial nerve, the *trochlear nerve,* innervates the inferior oblique muscle.

No doubt at some time you will be faced with learning the complicated arrangement of nerves within the superior orbital fissure. This is a good time to look at this arrangement because the nerves to all the extraocular muscles enter the orbit through the superior fissure.

Imagine the bony orbit as a funnel. As you look into the funnel toward its neck, you will see the optic canal and the V shape of the superior and inferior orbital fissures just temporal to the canal. A ring of connective tissue, known as

the *annulus of Zinn,* surrounds the optic canal and a portion of the superior fissure (Figure 2-54). The rectus muscles originate from the annulus and extend anteriorly. Because the rectus muscles are innervated on the "inner" side of the muscle belly, all the nerves to the rectus muscles must enter the orbit through the annulus of Zinn. These nerves include both divisions of the oculomotor nerve and the abducens nerve. *The trochlear nerve enters the orbit through the superior orbital fissure like the other cranial nerves to the extraocular muscles, but it does not go through the annulus because the superior oblique muscle lies outside the muscle cone defined by the rectus muscles.*

Look at the sensory nerves in Figure 2-51 and remind yourself of their paths in the orbit. The *frontal* and *lacrimal sensory nerves* (V_1) do not pass through the annulus because they travel outside the muscle cone adjacent to the orbital roof. The branches of the nasociliary nerve provide the sensory innervation to the eye, so it does enter the muscle cone through the annulus. The *optic nerve* enters through the optic canal directly into the annulus and extends anteriorly to the eye. You should note not only that the optic nerve enters through the annulus, but also that the dura of the optic canal is fused with the annulus on all sides except laterally. *The lateral rectus origin forms the lateral part of the annulus.* The superior oblique and the levator muscles originate superior to the annulus. The remaining extraocular muscle, the inferior oblique, originates anteriorly adjacent to the lacrimal sac.

When the apical optic nerve is approached surgically after removal of the orbital roof through a craniotomy (known as a *transcranial orbitotomy*), these structures can be visualized (see Figure 2-54). Once the periorbita is opened, the frontal nerve is easily seen because of its large size and extraconal position. The trochlear nerve is small, but it can usually be seen in the apex as it crosses from its lateral entrance into the orbit (superior orbital fissure) to its medial point of innervation in the superior oblique muscle. The apical optic nerve can be visualized only when the levator muscle origin is cut and reflected laterally. The annulus should then be opened on the superior *medial* aspect to avoid damage to the nerves and vessels entering laterally through the superior orbital fissure. All this may be a bit advanced for now. It becomes important if you are doing complicated orbital apex surgery.

Anterior orbital surgical approaches rarely damage the innervation to the rectus muscles because the motor nerves enter the muscle in the posterior one third of the muscle belly. Likewise, *surgical approaches outside the muscle cone rarely damage innervation* because the extraocular muscles are innervated from within the muscle cone.

Autonomic innervation

The exact route of the autonomic nerves within the orbit is complex and not clinically important, so aim to get the overall picture. It is easy to get confused here. A helpful point is to remember that the parasympathetic innervation is via the short posterior ciliary nerves. Sensory and sympathetic nerves travel through the ciliary ganglion and alongside the short posterior ciliary nerves, but do not synapse in the ciliary ganglion.

The *sympathetic innervation* to the eye originates in the *hypothalamus* with the first synapse occurring in the spinal cord. These nerve fibers leave the spinal cord to synapse in

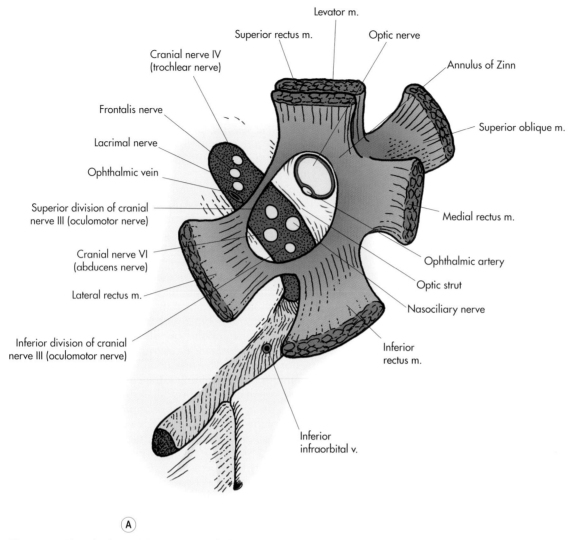

Levator m.

Superior rectus m.

Optic nerve

Cranial nerve IV
(trochlear nerve)

Annulus of Zinn

Frontalis nerve

Superior oblique m.

Lacrimal nerve

Ophthalmic vein

Superior division of cranial
nerve III (oculomotor nerve)

Medial rectus m.

Cranial nerve VI
(abducens nerve)

Ophthalmic artery

Optic strut

Lateral rectus m.

Nasociliary nerve

Inferior division of cranial
nerve III (oculomotor nerve)

Inferior
rectus m.

Inferior
infraorbital v.

(A)

Figure 2-54 The orbital apex. (**A**) Anterior view of orbital apex showing the distribution of nerves as they enter through the superior orbital fissure and optic canal. (**B**) Superior view of the orbital apex.

the *superior cervical ganglion*. Fibers then travel with branches of the external carotid artery to the face and with branches of the internal carotid artery (carotid plexus) to the orbit and eye. The path of the nerves entering and traveling in the orbit is not well understood. Once in the orbit, some of the sympathetic fibers pass through the *ciliary ganglion*, which is lateral to the optic nerve in the orbital apex (remember that the ciliary ganglion has synapses only for parasympathetic nerves). The sympathetic nerves travel to the back of the eye together with the short *posterior ciliary nerves* (to innervate the uveal blood vessels). Other sympathetic nerves bypass the ganglion, enter the eye near the optic nerve, and travel with the long posterior ciliary nerves (remember these are the sensory nerves to the eye) within the sclera to the front of the eye to provide innervation to the dilator of the iris. The path of the sympathetic nerves to Müller's muscle is variable.

Earlier in this chapter, we talked about the loss of sympathetic tone to the face, causing *Horner's syndrome* (*upper lid ptosis, lower lid elevation, miosis, and anhidrosis of the ipsilateral side of the face*). Horner's syndrome is rare, but presents an interesting clinicoanatomic correlation that every resident needs to know. Understanding the sympathetic pathway and

simple testing with eye drops (discussed in Chapter 8) will help to determine if a patient with Horner's syndrome has a life-threatening problem or just an annoying asymmetry.

Interruption of sympathetic innervation may occur within the central nervous system (first-order neurons), between the spinal cord and superior cervical ganglion (second-order neurons), or between the superior cervical ganglion and the orbit (third-order neurons). A central nervous system cause of Horner's syndrome is accompanied by other signs of disease in the brainstem or spinal cord. Second-order neuron damage (so-called *preganglionic Horner's syndrome* because the interruption is before the superior cervical ganglion) may be caused by apical lung cancer, mediastinal lymphoma, other tumors, cervical trauma, or congenital abnormalities ("cervical rib"). Third-order neuron damage (so-called *postganglionic Horner's syndrome* because the interruption is after the superior cervical ganglion) is usually not attributable to malignancy.

Less is known about the *parasympathetic innervation* of the eye and orbit. Parasympathetic innervation of the eye and orbit originate at the Edinger–Westphal nucleus (within the oculomotor nucleus). These fibers follow the third nerve to

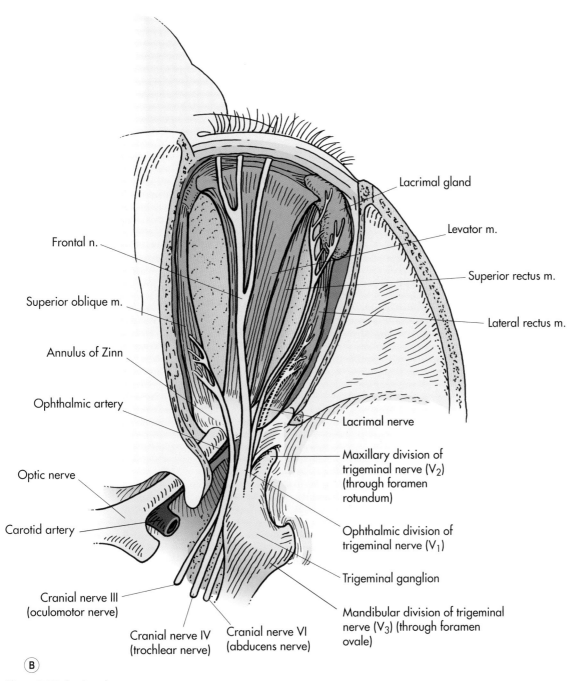

Frontal n.

Superior oblique m.

Annulus of Zinn

Ophthalmic artery

Optic nerve

Carotid artery

Cranial nerve III
(oculomotor nerve)

Cranial nerve IV
(trochlear nerve)

Cranial nerve VI
(abducens nerve)

Lacrimal gland

Levator m.

Superior rectus m.

Lateral rectus m.

Lacrimal nerve

Maxillary division of
trigeminal nerve (V$_2$)
(through foramen
rotundum)

Ophthalmic division of
trigeminal nerve (V$_1$)

Trigeminal ganglion

Mandibular division of trigeminal
nerve (V$_3$) (through foramen
ovale)

(B)

Figure 2-54 Continued.

enter the muscle cone where they synapse in the *ciliary ganglion* lateral to the optic nerve near the orbital apex (you may recall that the first parasympathetic synapse is always outside the central nervous system in a distant ganglion). Postganglionic fibers head to the back of the eye and penetrate the sclera as four to six *short posterior ciliary nerves,* most of which travel anteriorly to the ciliary body. The remaining fibers travel to innervate the sphincter of the iris. Damage to these nerves causes a *tonic pupil,* also called *Adie's pupil,* which shows no immediate constriction to bright light. Other parasympathetic pathways exist, of which the most important provides innervation to the lacrimal gland.

Checkpoint

- What is the innervation of the eye?
- Short posterior ciliary nerves
- Parasympathetic tone to the ciliary body and sphincter of iris
- Long ciliary nerves
- Sensation to the eye

The arterial supply to the orbit and periocular tissues

The basics

Let's start with some basics. *The carotid artery is the main source of the blood supply to all the structures of the head. The internal carotid artery supplies the brain, eye, and orbit. The external carotid artery supplies the remainder of the head including the face, scalp, and parts of the neck.* There are rich anastomoses between the branches derived from the branches of the internal and external carotid arteries. In the periocular area, these areas of anastomosis and overlap occur mainly in the lids and anterior orbit. Remembering these few facts forms a basis for understanding the rest of the blood supply to the orbit and eye.

The external carotid artery

With that background, let's get more specific. In the neck, the common carotid artery divides into the internal and external carotid arteries. The internal carotid artery has no branches in the neck. The external carotid has many named branches arising in the neck (eight branches). The three branches important for our purposes are:

- Facial artery
- Internal maxillary artery
- Superficial temporal artery

Before the discussion gets too complicated, remember that the external carotid supplies the tissues of the face, scalp, and neck, but not the eye or orbit:

- The tissues anterior to the orbit are supplied by the facial artery
- The tissues inferior to the orbit are supplied by the internal maxillary artery
- The tissues superior and temporal to the orbit are supplied by the superficial temporal artery

This is a good place to stop unless you want more detail (Figure 2-55), which is provided in the following paragraphs.

The *facial artery* passes between the submandibular gland and the mandible and heads for the melolabial fold (you should be able to feel the pulse of the facial artery on the inferior edge of your own mandible slightly more than half of the way back to the angle of the mandible). The artery follows the side of the nose toward the medial canthus, where the facial artery terminal branch, the *angular artery*, is found. You will occasionally encounter brisk bleeding from

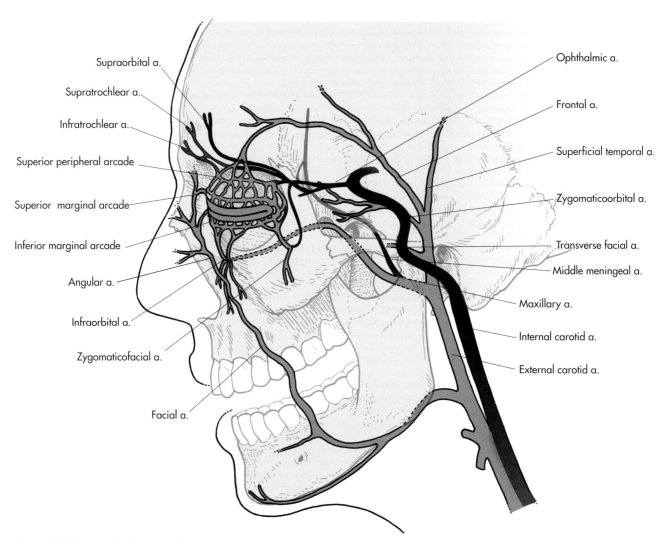

Figure 2-55 The superficial arteries of the face.

the angular artery during an *external DCR operation* as you dissect through the orbicularis on your way to the anterior lacrimal crest. The angular artery perforates the orbital septum to anastomose with branches of the internal carotid artery in the superomedial orbit. Some texts refer to the facial artery as the external maxillary artery.

The *internal maxillary artery (IMA)* arises from the external carotid artery near the upper part of the jaw and runs forward. Its branches supply the jaws, the palate, and the interior of the nose. You might remember from medical school the IMA ligation for severe nosebleeds that could not otherwise be controlled. In the pterygopalatine fossa, the IMA sends a branch anteriorly, the *infraorbital artery*. You are already familiar with this path as the artery follows the infraorbital nerve into the orbit through the inferior orbital fissure, groove, and canal to emerge onto the cheek through the infraorbital foramen. You will see branches of this artery during dissections of the orbital floor or the cheek. The infraorbital artery supplies the cheek, lower eyelid, and conjunctiva.

The *superficial temporal artery* is the terminal branch of the external carotid artery. The artery is first seen on the face anterior to the ear (feel your own superficial temporal artery pulse). The superficial temporal artery travels superiorly into the scalp where it lies in the same plane as the temporal branch of the facial nerve. The superficial temporal artery branches supply the temple and surrounding areas. From superior to inferior, the branches of the superficial temporal artery are (Table 2-2):

- Frontal artery
- Zygomatic artery
- Transverse facial artery

The names of these branches are less important than the concept of their distribution to the temple and lateral orbit. We will discuss the anastomoses with the internal carotid branches in the next section.

The internal carotid artery

The ophthalmic artery

Let's start with the *basics*. The blood supply to the eye and orbit is from the internal carotid artery. For practical purposes, this entire blood supply to the eye is provided by the first named branch of the internal carotid artery, the *ophthalmic artery*. You need to learn about this important artery. On the way to the orbit, the internal carotid artery ascends the neck, enters the skull, traverses the cavernous sinus, and then

pierces the dura adjacent to the intracranial opening of the optic canal. *At that point, the ophthalmic artery branches off the internal carotid artery and travels in the optic canal to enter the orbit.* Once in the orbit, the branching gets complicated. An easy way to look at the branches of the ophthalmic artery is to think about what structures are being supplied. All structures within the orbit and eye will receive blood from a branch of the ophthalmic artery. In his excellent anatomy text, Jon Dutton divides the branches into three groups:

- Branches to the eye
- Branches to the nonocular orbital tissues
- Branches to the periocular tissues

Although we are still at a fairly basic level, we have covered a lot of information. Let's review the arterial supply that we have covered thus far.

Make sure that you know these points:

- The external and internal carotid arteries supply the head.
- The external carotid artery has many branches in the neck, which supply the neck, face, sinuses, and scalp.
- The internal carotid artery supplies the eye, orbit, and brain.
- The only branch of the internal carotid artery that goes to the eye and orbit is the ophthalmic artery. All structures in the eye or orbit will be supplied by branches of the ophthalmic artery.
- The terminal branches of the ophthalmic artery (you can learn these later) will anastomose with terminal branches of the external carotid artery to form a rich arterial network of collateral circulation in the periocular area.

There are exceptions to these generalizations in individual patients, but this information will be what you need to know for most patients. *Don't spend a lot of time learning the branches of the ophthalmic artery, but make sure you understand and can repeat to yourself the above concepts. This is a good place to stop unless you want the details.*

The ophthalmic artery branches to the eye

Here are the *details*. The branches of the ophthalmic artery that supply the contents of the eye and the optic nerve are the central retinal artery and the ciliary arteries. The *central retinal artery* branches off the ophthalmic artery and travels anteriorly where it enters the optic nerve, eventually branching into the arterioles of the retina that you examine regularly with indirect ophthalmoscopy. Posterior ciliary arteries branch off the ophthalmic artery in two forms. Two *long posterior ciliary arteries* travel within the sclera to supply the ciliary muscle and iris. As many as 20 small *short posterior ciliary arteries* supply the optic nerve head and choroid. *Anterior ciliary arteries* arise from the branches of the ophthalmic artery that supply the rectus muscles. The anterior ciliary arteries leave the muscle near its insertion to enter the sclera, anastomosing with the posterior ciliary circulation. Other small branches of the ophthalmic artery penetrate the dura directly to supply the optic nerve.

The branches of the ophthalmic artery to the nonocular orbit

The *branches of the ophthalmic artery* that supply the structures in the orbit other than the eye and optic nerve are the muscular branches, the lacrimal artery, and the supraorbital

Table 2-2 Branches of superficial temporal artery

Branch	Tissue supplied	Internal carotid artery anastomoses
Frontal artery	Frontalis, orbicularis muscles	Supraorbital and lacrimal arteries
Zygomaticofacial	Lateral portion of lids	Lacrimal, zygomaticofacial and zygomaticotemporal arteries
Transverse facial artery	Lateral portion of lower lids and cheek	Infraorbital and lacrimal arteries

artery. The *muscular branches* enter the extraocular muscles posteriorly and travel within the muscle itself. As we said above, the anterior extensions of the muscular branches are the anterior ciliary arteries to the anterior segment. Each rectus muscle has two anterior ciliary arteries with the exception of the lateral rectus, which has only one artery. The lacrimal gland is supplied by the *lacrimal artery*. Upon leaving the lacrimal gland, the lacrimal artery gives rise to the *zygomaticofacial* and *zygomaticotemporal arteries*, which exit the orbit via foramina of the same names in the lateral orbital wall. The lacrimal artery also divides to form the *lateral palpebral arteries*, which leave the orbit to supply the lids. The *supraorbital artery* travels anteriorly in the orbit to supply parts of the levator, superior oblique, and superior rectus muscles on its way out of the orbit.

The branches of the ophthalmic artery to the periocular tissues

The branches of the ophthalmic artery that supply tissues outside the orbit include the ethmoid arteries and the nasofrontal artery. The *posterior ethmoid artery* is found deep in the orbital apex headed for the mucosa of the posterior ethmoid air cells. You will find the posterior ethmoid foramen in the frontoethmoid suture line 4–7 mm anterior to the optic canal. As is the case for many of the extraorbital branches of the ophthalmic artery, the posterior ethmoid artery provides some arterial blood to deep orbital structures via accessory muscular branches. The *anterior ethmoid artery* supplies the mucosa of the anterior ethmoid air cells, the frontal sinus, and the lateral wall of the nose and nasal septum. The ante-

rior ethmoid artery exits the orbit through the anterior ethmoid foramen. Both the anterior and the posterior ethmoid arteries are important surgical landmarks.

Although somewhat variable among individuals, the identification of these arteries is a good indicator of your position in the orbit along the medial orbital wall. We have already discussed that the rule of thumb for these landmarks is the *"24–12–6 mm"* rule. The anterior ethmoid artery is 24 mm from the anterior orbital rim; the posterior ethmoid artery is 12 mm more posterior and 6 mm from the optic canal. These vessels are also accurate indicators of the position of the cribriform plate, so care should be taken to avoid damage to the bone superior to the frontoethmoid suture to avoid a *CSF leak*. Inadvertent tearing of these anterior or posterior arteries during orbitotomy causes brisk bleeding and may lead to an orbital hematoma.

Other branches originate from the ophthalmic artery within the orbit and penetrate the orbital septum anteriorly to supply the periocular tissues. The names of these arteries are not as important as the idea that the arteries arise posteriorly and eventually emerge anteriorly (Figure 2-56). The *nasofrontal artery* is the main extension of the ophthalmic artery branching anteriorly to form the supratrochlear and dorsal nasal arteries. The *supratrochlear artery* supplies the medial forehead and eyebrow. The *dorsal nasal artery* supplies the nasal bridge, forehead, and scalp. Some important arteries that you will likely encounter during lid surgery arise from the dorsal nasal artery are the *medial palpebral arteries* (we will discuss these below). The last of the branches of the

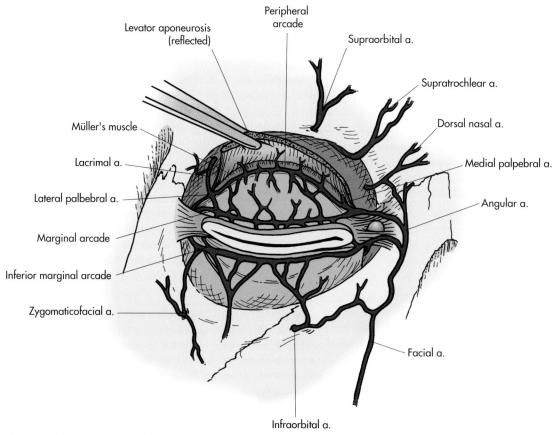

Figure 2-56 The anastomoses of the anterior orbital and facial arteries.

ophthalmic artery that emerge from the orbit anteriorly is the *supraorbital artery*. On the way out of the orbit, the artery supplements the blood supply to the levator, superior rectus, and superior oblique muscles. The supraorbital artery leaves the orbit through the supraorbital notch or foramen as the main blood supply of the scalp and forehead. The predictable vascular pattern and long straight orientation of this artery and the supratrochlear artery *allow flaps of the forehead to be rotated into medial canthal defects after skin cancer removal* (we will talk about the difference between "random" flaps and these "axial" flaps below).

The rich anastomoses of the internal and external carotid arteries

We talked about the extensive anastomoses of internal and external carotid arteries in the periocular region. Let's look at the lids themselves. Each eyelid has a *marginal arcade*, which is found on the surface of the tarsus along the eyelid margin. The upper eyelid has an additional arterial supply known as the *peripheral arcade*, which lies between the levator aponeurosis and Müller's muscle (Figure 2-56). You will see these arcades during lid surgery. The peripheral arcade is always seen during eyelid ptosis repair. Each arcade is formed from medial and lateral branches known as the *medial* and *lateral palpebral arteries*. The medial palpebral artery is a branch of the dorsal nasal artery (see paragraph above). The lateral palpebral artery is a branch of the lacrimal artery. Remember, it is not so important to memorize all these branches, but rather to understand the extensive anastomoses that are present. If the lid margin is cut, the marginal arcade is interrupted, but blood will still flow to the tissues from both medial and lateral palpebral arteries.

Other collateral vessels form between branches of the internal carotid as well as anastomoses between branches of the internal and external carotid arteries (Figure 2-56). I will abbreviate the origin of each branch to jog your memory: OA is ophthalmic artery, ECA is external carotid artery, and ICA is internal carotid artery. Laterally, the zygomaticofacial and zygomaticotemporal branches (OA) meet the frontal and zygomatic arteries of the superficial temporal artery (ECA). Medially, the dorsal nasal artery (OA) shares collateral circulation with the angular branch of the facial artery (ECA) and the infraorbital artery (ECA). Inferiorly, branches of the infraorbital artery meet branches off the inferior arcade (OA), the angular artery (ECA), and the transverse facial artery (ECA). Superiorly, overlap between branches of the supraorbital artery (OA), the supratrochlear artery (OA), and the lacrimal artery (OA) occurs.

Reconstructive flaps in the periocular area are "forgiving," rarely failing because of ischemia. The vascular supply to flaps can be described as either *axial* or *random*. Axial flaps are designed based on a specific single arterial supply. An example of this is the *median or paramedian forehead flap* for medial canthal reconstruction, in which the supraorbital and/or supratrochlear artery provides the main blood supply (Figure 2-57). Random flaps are not based on a specific artery. The *glabellar flap* is an example of a random flap that is also used for medial canthal reconstruction. The extensive blood supply of the periocular tissues allows incision and mobilization of the tissues of the glabellar flap without a specific arterial supply.

These extensive anastomoses provide a rich blood supply to the tissues of the periocular area, which prevents infection and promotes healing after trauma. Some evening when you are on call, you will see a serious lid laceration where a large area of tissue, perhaps almost an entire eyelid, will be nearly torn free. You should attempt to sew the tissue back into place. In many cases, this tissue will survive without signs of infection. You will be surprised how resistant the periocular tissues are to ischemia (Box 2-5).

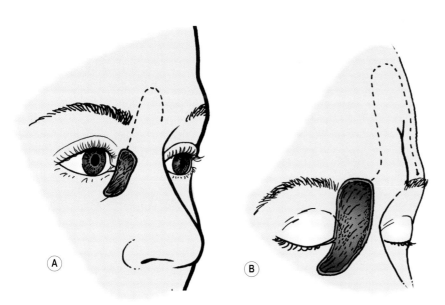

Figure 2-57 Axial and random flaps. (**A**) Glabellar flap with random vascular blood supply from surrounding tissues. (**B**) Median or paramedian forehead flap based on the supratrochlear and/or supratrochlear artery (axial flap).

This is a complicated section. Don't try to get all the details the first time through. Important points to remember are:

- The external and internal carotid arteries supply the head.
- The external carotid artery has many branches in the neck, which supply the neck, face, sinuses, and scalp.
- The internal carotid artery supplies the eye, orbit, and brain.
- The only branch of the internal carotid artery to the eye and orbit is the ophthalmic artery. All structures in the eye or orbit will be supplied by branches of the ophthalmic artery.
- The terminal branches of the ophthalmic artery (you can learn these later) will anastomose with terminal branches of the external carotid artery to form a rich arterial network of collateral circulation in the periocular area.

If you have all that, try to name the terminal branches of the ophthalmic artery. (Remember, "to the eye," "to the nonocular orbit," and "to the periorbital tissues".)

The venous drainage of the orbit and periocular tissues

Unlike elsewhere in the body, the veins of the periocular region do not closely follow the arterial supply. There is a high degree of variability among individuals. We won't spend much time on this topic. You should know that the drainage of the orbit is primarily by the *superior ophthalmic vein* out of the superior orbital fissure into the *cavernous sinus*. Many other paths of venous drainage occur. The *inferior ophthalmic vein* exits the orbit through the inferior orbital fissure into the pterygopalatine plexus of veins behind the maxillary sinus (Figure 2-58). Anteriorly, the veins drain into the *veins of the face* and eventually into the external jugular vein. The veins in the orbit have no valves, a fact thought to be responsible, in part, for the spread of bacterial infection from the ethmoid sinus into the orbit.

The superior ophthalmic vein courses in the superior orbit from the anterior medial corner to the posterior lateral wall to enter the superior orbital fissure where the vein drains into the cavernous sinus (Figure 2-59). You can almost always see a normal superior ophthalmic vein on an axial CT scan series. In the section above, we didn't mention that there are small branches of the internal carotid artery coursing through the venous lakes of the cavernous sinus, the dura, and surrounding structures. As a consequence of trauma or atherosclerosis, one of these small arterial branches of the intracavernous internal carotid artery may connect directly to a venous space in the cavernous sinus. This *arteriovenous shunt* is known a *carotid cavernous fistula* (CCF). Arterial blood will flow into the veins, reversing the flow of the venous blood back into the orbit. Clinically, the fistula is recognized as dilated conjunctival vessels, chemosis, slight proptosis, and increased

---

Box 2-5

Branches of the Ophthalmic Artery

To eye and optic nerve

- Central retinal artery
- Posterior ciliary arteries
  - Two long posterior ciliary arteries to the ciliary muscle and iris
  - Many short posterior ciliary arteries to the optic nerve head and choroid
  - Anterior ciliary branches arising from the muscular branches to the anterior segment with the posterior ciliary circulation
  - Small branches to the dura of the nerve

To orbital tissues

- Muscular arteries to supply the extraocular muscles
  - Anterior extensions as the anterior ciliary muscles
  - Two anterior ciliary arteries for each rectus muscle except the lateral rectus, which has only one
- Lacrimal artery to the lacrimal gland
  - Zygomaticofacial and zygomaticotemporal branches leaving the orbit in foramina of the same name
  - Inferior and superior lateral palpebral arteries
  - Supraorbital artery travels anteriorly in the orbit to supply parts of the levator, superior oblique, and superior rectus muscles; main blood supply to the forehead and eyebrows

To tissues outside the orbit

- Posterior ethmoid artery to the mucosa of the posterior ethmoid air cells with smaller accessory branches to the muscles in the apex
- Anterior ethmoid artery to the mucosa of the anterior ethmoid air cells, frontal sinus, lateral wall, and septum of the nose
- Nasofrontal artery main extension anteriorly
  - Supratrochlear artery to medial forehead and eyebrows
  - Dorsal nasal artery to nasal bridge, forehead, and scalp
  - Inferior and superior medial palpebral arteries to form arcades in the lids anastomosing with the lateral palpebral contributions
- Supraorbital artery supplying the forehead through the supraorbital notch or foramen

---

intraocular pressure (caused by venous engorgement preventing the aqueous fluid from draining properly into the veins). The dilated superior ophthalmic vein can be seen on a CT scan (Figure 2-60). If the flow is high (usually only seen after trauma), venous congestion will be severe and can result in serious damage to he eye.

- What vessel carries the main venous drainage out of the orbit? Where does this vessel drain? Visualize its path on a CT scan.
- What does a CCF do to the drainage of the orbit? Clinically, what do you see?

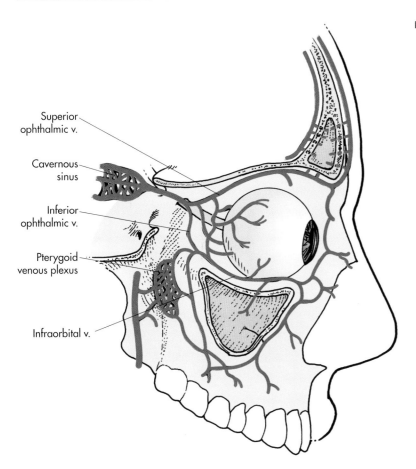

Figure 2-58 The venous drainage of the orbit.

Superior ophthalmic v.

Cavernous sinus

Inferior ophthalmic v.

Pterygoid venous plexus

Infraorbital v.

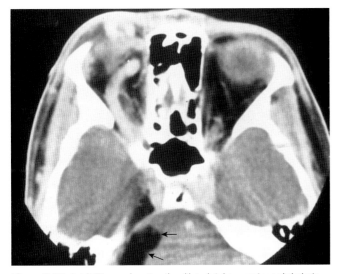

Figure 2-59 Axial CT scan showing the dilated right superior ophthalmic vein, a result of venous obstruction caused by compression of the cavernous sinus by a lipoma of the skull base (arrows point to the radiolucent mass). This is a rare cause of enlargement of the superior ophthalmic vein, but a good illustration of orbital venous drainage into the cavernous sinus (from Howard G, Nerad J, Carter K: Superior ophthalmic vein enlargement and proptosis due to middle cranial fossa lipoma. *Am J Ophthalmol* 110(6): 705–706, 1990).

Lymphatic drainage

The drainage of the extracellular fluid from the eyelids is into the preauricular or submandibular nodes (Figure 2-61). The lateral two thirds of the upper eyelid, the lateral one third of the lower eyelid, and the lateral half of the conjunctiva drain into the *preauricular nodes*. The remaining tissues drain deeply into the *submandibular nodes*. Lymph drainage from these two regions continues into the anterior and deep cervical nodes. Regional metastases of eyelid tumors are rare for basal cell and squamous cell carcinoma, but may occur more commonly with sebaceous cell carcinoma (Figure 2-62).

The path of drainage of lymphatic fluid in the orbit remains a mystery. No lymphatic channels or lymph nodes have been discovered. Presumably, the posterior fluid drains toward the cavernous sinus and the anterior fluid drains into the lymphatic system of conjunctiva and eyelids. Despite the absence of true lymphatic channels in the orbit, tumors of lymphatic tissue (lymphangiomas) are seen in the orbit. These benign tumors are congenital lesions, probably choristomas (normal tissue in an abnormal place). A reversible change in proptosis occurs during upper respiratory infections. Hemorrhage of vessels in the thin-walled lymph spaces may cause sudden proptosis. Because of their infiltrative nature, lymphangiomas are not amenable to complete surgical excision.

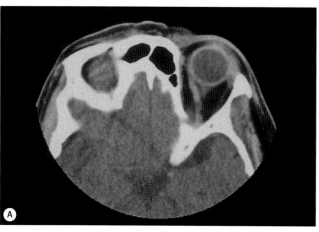

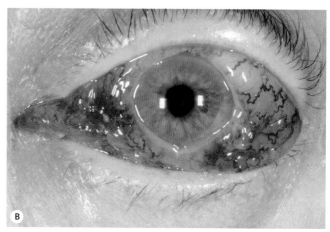

Figure 2-60 Carotid cavernous fistula. (**A**) Dilated left superior ophthalmic vein caused by a carotid cavernous fistula. (**B**) Chemosis and injected conjunctiva are seen as a result of venous congestion from arterial flow into the venous system.

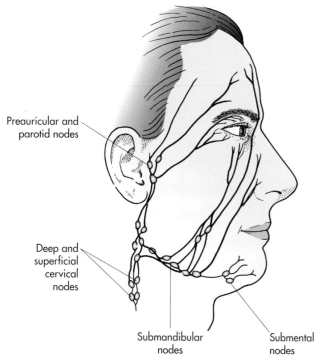

Figure 2-61 The lymphatic drainage of the eyelids.

Preauricular and parotid nodes

Deep and superficial cervical nodes

Submandibular nodes

Submental nodes

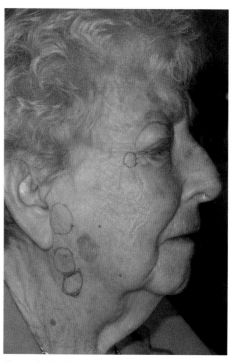

Figure 2-62 Sebaceous cell carcinoma of the eyelid with "in transit" (skin lymphatic veins at lateral canthus) and regional metastases to preauricular and cervical lymph nodes.

Checkpoint

- What parts of the eyelid drain into the preauricular nodes?
- What parts of the eyelid drain into the submandibular nodes?
- Remember to check these lymph nodes for patients with melanoma, sebaceous cell carcinoma, and squamous cell carcinoma of the eyelids and face.

Facial anatomy

Introduction to facial anatomy

So far, we have spent a great deal of time discussing mainly periorbital anatomy. Now, we'll move lower in the face to discuss the anatomy of the middle and lower face, as well as the superficial layers of the neck. I have chosen to look at these layers from the perspective of function to prepare you to do rejuvenation procedures of the aging face. You should get an idea of the *descent and deflation* process of the face that is responsible for the *sags, bags and wrinkles* that occur with aging.

This is very complicated anatomy and, when looked at in detail, takes years to learn well. As always, the *big picture* is important so, rather than focus on the detail, I will try to leave a general impression of the structure and function of each layer. We will talk about the layers from the superficial layers inward toward the bones. The next step is for you to pick up a few clinically important anatomic details that you need to know as the basis of effective and safe facial surgery. Later, in Chapters 6, *Involutional Changes of the Periocular Region*, and 7, *Aesthetic Surgery of the Face*, we will discuss some of the current treatments for aging in more detail. There are many good texts and articles, some of which are listed in the suggested readings that you may want to refer to as you get beyond the big picture.

Layers of the face

The face has both functional and expressive roles. Seeing, smelling, breathing, and chewing are some of these basic functions. The muscles of the face and the supporting tissues blink the eyes, open and close the nostrils, and help us to manage the food in our mouth. But for now let's look at the expressive role of the face. As we saw how simple changes of the eyebrow position change the "happy face" to the "sad face," the other facial muscles are indicators of mood and feeling as well. All of this seems pretty obvious, but will help you to understand how the layers are arranged and work. An oversimplified anatomic scheme of the layers of the face is:

* Skin
* Muscles of facial expression
* Bone

Now make a big smile. As you smile, you feel your lips elevate, your nostrils open and, if you pay attention, you can feel or imagine that your ears perk up and your neck and forehead may even tense a bit. Your facial muscles act simultaneously with a controlled co-innervation of the facial nerve branches. Beyond that, the muscles work together because they are physically connected with a broad connective tissue layer. In the face, this is known as the superficial musculoaponeurotic system (SMAS). There is a continuation of this layer across the whole face and skull. All these muscles are physically interconnected. This is an extremely important concept because the correction of the "sags and bags" of aging has to do with tightening this layer of tissue extending across the face, skull, and neck. The principle is simple, but the names get complicated. Although the layer is continuous (the major concept we are trying to get across), the name is different depending where you are talking about on the head. You already know most of the names of the layers. In the:

* Face — SMAS
* Forehead — Galea
* Temple — Temporoparietal fascia
* Neck — Platysma

As far as correcting the "sags and bags" of aging, you tighten:

* SMAS and platysma for a face and neck lift
* Galea and temporoparietal fascia for a brow lift

Obviously, there is more to it than this, but it is a good start to get you interested in understanding the anatomy. Let's look at the action of the muscles of facial expression some more. The facial muscles originate on the underlying bone and insert into the skin. That is how the skin moves. There are "ligaments" that extend through the SMAS (and its equivalent layer) from the bone to the skin. These ligaments, known as *retaining ligaments*, serve as support for the facial soft tissues and link one layer to another. You will see that the position of the ligaments has a lot to do with the characteristic sags that develop when a loose area of tissue hangs over a more tightly bound tissue (for example the jowls and melolabial fold).

The strongest of the retaining ligaments are at the zygoma (zygomatic, orbitomalar and mandibular retaining ligaments) and along the mandible. To help understand this supporting system, think of an analogy in the eyelid—levator palpebrae superiorus system. This thin levator muscle is not so dissimilar in shape to each facial muscle and has many anatomic similarities to the system of support and action of the muscles of facial expression. A thin band of levator muscle originates at the orbital apex and travels forward where it spreads into a broad band, also an aponeurosis. The levator muscle is supported superiorly at the bony rim by Whitnall's ligament (with attachments at the trochlea and lacrimal gland). The levator aponeurosis is also tightly bound to the bone through the attachments of the "horns" at the medial and lateral canthi. When the eye moves, the levator moves in a coordinated fashion due to the simultaneous innervation of the superior rectus and physical connection provided by the fascial connections between the two muscles. The levator aponeurosis terminates with its fibers attaching into the skin forming the skin crease. You can see the similarities of the levator system to the muscles of facial expression. The levator muscle is supported via several attachments to the skeleton and adjacent muscles. Movements are coordinated by co-contraction and physical connections. The actions are spread to the overlying skin. The same principle applies to the facial muscles and the SMAS.

As the SMAS is so important in understanding facial anatomy, we started there, albeit is an oversimplification. Aside from the SMAS, there are fascial planes that allow tissues to slide over one another, important nerves and vessels (that often travel in the fascial planes), deeper muscles (mainly for mastication), all covered with fat pads softening the facial contours. Now let's go back to the layer approach starting superficially. We will consider the following layers:

* Skin
* Subcutaneous fat
* Muscles of facial expression
* SMAS and related layers
* Retaining ligaments
* Deeper muscles and fat pads

Once you have a feel for these layers, it is worth following the course of the facial nerve and describing important "safe and danger zones" for dissection.

The skin

The skin has two layers, the epidermis and dermis. The *epidermis* turns over rapidly, within 2 weeks, providing a new protective layer against the environment. There are four layers of the epithelium: the basal, spinous, granular, and cornified layers. Cells at the junction of the epidermis and dermis (basal layer) mature and move toward the skin surface, eventually losing their nuclei and producing keratin. Remember that the two most common skin cancers, basal cell and squamous cell carcinoma, arise from the epidermis.

The *dermis* lies beneath the epidermis. The dermis is a connective tissue layer that contains the adnexae—the hair follicles, oil, and sweat glands. Blood vessels, lymphatics, and nerves travel within the dermis. There are two layers of the dermis: the more superficial papillary and the deeper reticular dermis. These layers become important in understanding the repair of wrinkles.

The dermis is made up of largely *collagen*, predominantly type I. Mixed in with the collagen are *elastin fibers* and a cellular component. A *"ground substance,"* a watery matrix largely containing plasma proteins and mucopolysaccharides, fills in the spaces between the fibers of the dermis. *Hyaluronic acid* is the major component of the embryonic ground substance. The skin acts as a viscoelastic tissue. When healthy, it is relatively noncompressible (viscous) and, when stretched, it returns to its normal length (elastic). It is the ground substance (mainly water) that is responsible for the plumpness (viscosity) of the skin and the collagen and elastin that are responsible for the elasticity. The dermis also contains nerves, vessels, and the ocular adnexae—the eccrine and apocrine sweat glands and the pilosebaceous apparatus. Healthy adnexal tissues are important as new epithelial cells arise from these glandular tissues. You may already know prior to any facial resurfacing procedure that your patient must stop acne treatment with Accutane (isotretinoin) for at least 6 months prior to treatment. Accutane works to decrease the size and productivity of the sebaceous glands and can drastically affect the production of a new skin surface.

The *ultraviolet (UV) damage* we see as part of aging affects both the plumpness and the elasticity of the skin. Loss of collagen results in thinning of the dermis and some of the "deflation" changes that we see in the face. Fat injection or other "volumizing" filler agents, most commonly containing hyaluronic acid, act to plump up the thinning dermis. Loss of the elastin fibers results in less skin elasticity and more wrinkling.

Laser resurfacing and chemical peeling remove the epithelium and cause injury to the dermis. The healing process induces a "remodeling" of the dermis with increased fibroblasts and new elastin fibers. As the epidermis heals, the melanocytes (found in the basal layer) do not return in the same density and you will see a lighter skin. The result is a smoother, tighter skin with fewer dyschromias. In general, the deeper the injury, the more profound and long-lasting the result will be. Injury to the papillary dermis improves superficial and mild wrinkling. Deeper wrinkles require treatment beyond the papillary dermis into the reticular dermis. After some experience, you can get comfortable with how much treatment is required for a desired improvement. Deeper treatment gives a more pronounced effect, but at the same time you must realize that deeper treatment means longer healing and more risk of complication.

The role of botulinum toxin for reducing wrinkles is well known. Just to remind you, Botox is used to decrease the muscle contraction that is causing the overlying wrinkles (so-called *dynamic wrinkles*). Wrinkles at rest (*static wrinkles*) result from changes in the dermis.

Subcutaneous fat

Except in the eyelid, there is a plane of subcutaneous fat beneath the skin. The fat layer is thickest in the cheeks and temples. The subcutaneous fat is septate due to ingrowth of fibrous tissue from the dermis, creating a dense adhesion that requires sharp dissection. You will be safe creating wide dissections in the subcutaneous plane because of a well-formed "subdermal" vascular plexus. This broad blood supply is the basis for the large "random" reconstructive flaps that you will use after removal of extensive skin cancer resection.

You need to know about two other pockets, or planes, of fat in the midface—the malar fat pad and the suborbicularis oculi fat pads (the SOOF and ROOF). These pads are not part of the subcutaneous fat plane and are discussed in the next section.

Muscles of facial expression—and function

Let's think about the muscles of facial expression in terms of function rather than expression. We have already discussed the functioning of muscles of the upper third of the face—the eyelid opening and closing muscles. The "opening muscles" of the eyes are the levator, Müller's, and the frontalis muscles. The closing muscles are the orbicularis oculi and, to a lesser degree, the eyebrow depressors, the corrugator and procerus muscles. We are familiar with the periocular consequences of facial nerve palsy—lagophthalmos and brow ptosis. We will take a similar functional approach to other facial muscles. I suggest that you don't memorize all these muscles, but gain an understanding of the muscle groups. A couple of comments that will help you:

- Although the muscles are named individually, they work as group facilitated by the investing layer of SMAS.
- Most have a related muscle that does the opposite function. Get an overview from Figure 2-1.
- All the muscles of facial expression are innervated by branches of the facial nerve.
- All the muscles are innervated from the posterior surface
  — Important for safe dissection
  — Exceptions are the buccinator, mentalis, and levator anguli oris
- The zygomaticus muscle will be an important landmark for you as you learn facelift procedures that mobilize and tighten the SMAS.

There is a group of muscles that help with *nasal breathing*. Opening of the nostrils is caused by the nasalis dilator, the levator superioris alae nasi, and the depressor septi muscles. Closing the nostrils is caused by the nasalis compressor. Facial nerve palsy allows nasal alar collapse on inspiration. For the patient with facial palsy, this can be a problem. Aside from improvement in facial symmetric after a static facial sling is an improvement in nasal breathing (what the over-the-counter nasal strips claim to do).

Looking at Figure 2-1, you can imagine which muscles work on your lips. Again, at this point, there is no need to memorize these muscles, just get the idea of the orientation and function of the muscle groups. The muscles that move the lip are:

- Elevators
  - Risorius
  - Zygomaticus major and minor
  - Levator anguli oris
  - Levator labii superioris
- Depressors
  - Depressor anguli oris
  - Depressor labii inferioris
  - Mentalis
  - Platysmus
- Closing
  - Orbicularis oris

Because of its variable course along the inferior border of the mandible, the marginal branch of the mandibular portion of the facial nerve can be damaged with mobilization of the platysma. Damage to this nerve results in loss of lip depressor function and creates an asymmetric smile. You may be wondering what the major functional role of the platysmus muscle is. This muscle does contribute to lip depression. Its primary role seems to be related to that seen in other animal species, for example horses flicking flies off the neck.

The superficial musculoaponeurotic system (SMAS)

Hopefully by now, you have an overall idea of what the SMAS is and how it works. We'll discuss some of its related anatomic counterparts (temporoparietal fascia, galea, and platysma), the associated fat pads (SOOF and ROOF), and some clinical points of interest. In the next section, we will discuss how the SMAS anchors to the facial skeleton and how laxity of the facial tissues typically appears related to these attachments.

Inferiorly, the SMAS is continuous with the *platysma muscle* as the muscle crosses over the mandible. The platysma consists of two flat muscles that join centrally in the neck in an inverted V pattern (Figure 2-63). A layer of fat is present anterior and posterior to the platysma (you will see an analogy with the fat pads anterior and posterior to the orbicularis—SOOF and ROOF). Laxity of the central platysma causes the familiar *vertical banding* in the neck. Commonly, a separation of the platysma in the midline causes the posterior fat pad to prolapse forward. The laxity and fat herniation cause a blunting of the *cervicomental angle* and the familiar *turkey gobble*. You will see later that tightening of the platysma (remember, the equivalent of tightening the SMAS in the midface), repair of any central dehiscence, and liposuction, primarily of the posterior fat pad, can greatly sharpen the angle. You may be surprised to learn that, after a "facelift," it is the improvement in the neck that patients often appreciate most.

The platysma extends inferiorly overlying the clavicles and onto the chest. Posteriorly, the platysma crosses over the posterior margin of the sternocleidomastoid muscle. Here, at Erb's point, the *greater auricular nerve* emerges and runs superiorly to give sensory innervation to the ear. This nerve is the most commonly injured nerve in the facelift procedure so you must be careful working in this area.

The galea and temporoparietal fascia

Just as an SMAS-like layer extends inferiorly into the neck, there are analogous structures extending superiorly and laterally. Superiorly, the SMAS invests the orbicularis and frontalis muscle to become continuous with the *galea*. The galea extends superiorly across the skull to fuse with the occipitalis muscle. Laterally, the galea is continuous with the *temporoparietal fascia*, which is in turn continuous with the SMAS into the face (Figure 2-64).

By now, you should be getting the idea that there is this extensive plane of tissue investing the facial muscles from the clavicles all the way across the top of the head. As you can see from the description above, the temporal extension of the SMAS plane is known as the temporoparietal fascia (TPF). Unlike elsewhere, this SMAS-equivalent layer does

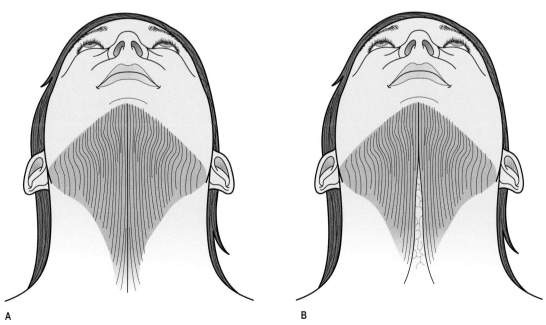

A   B

Figure 2-63 The platysma muscle. The bellies of the platysma form an inverted V in the superficial plane of the neck. Loss of the normal central decussation of the muscle fibers contributes to the vertical bands that occur in the neck due to aging.

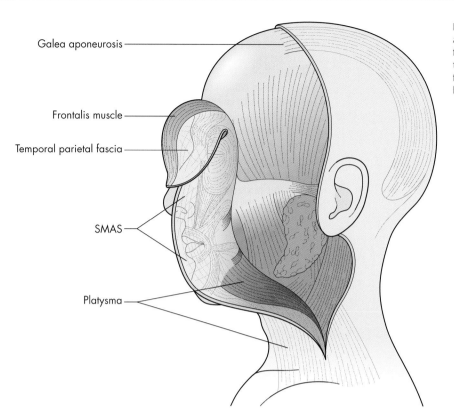

Figure 2-64 The SMAS and the analogous anatomic layers—a fibromuscular layer covers the face and skull. The SMAS (face) is continuous with the platysma in the neck, the temporoparietal fascia in the temple, and the galea forehead and head.

Galea aponeurosis

Frontalis muscle

Temporal parietal fascia

SMAS

Platysma

not contain any facial muscles. The TPF *overlies* the temporalis muscle (which is not a muscle of facial expression, rather a muscle of mastication), but *does not invest* the temporalis muscle. The *frontal branch* of the facial nerve lies within the TPS so this anatomy is important for safe browplasty procedures. *Unless you are ready to focus on brow lifting, skip the anatomic details of the temple for now and just remember the concept of the SMAS and its counterparts, the platysma, the galea, and the TPF, extending across the face and skull.* The concept of a strong continuous layer of facial tissue that can be tightened to lift the sags and bags of aging is essential for modern rejuvenation surgery.

The temporoparietal fascia and the galea

Again, you may want to skip this part, unless you are ready to do some of the more complex brow elevation operations. If this is new material to you, it will take several readings to really understand this.

The anatomy of the temporal region is easiest to understand if you start deeply with the temporalis muscle (Figure 2-65). Most surgeons new to temporal anatomy get bogged down with the confusing nomenclature of the temporal fascial layers. Like the masseter muscle, the temporalis muscle pulls the mandible closed. Also like the masseter muscle, there is a layer of tough fascia covering the muscle itself. The fascia on the external surface of the temporalis muscle is called the *deep temporalis fascia*. A thin layer of fat separates this fascia from the overlying *temporoparietal fascia*. Easy so far (deep temporalis fascia over chewing muscles, TPF more related to the mimetic muscles), but here is where things get confusing. As the temporalis muscle extends inferiorly toward the zygomatic arch, its fascia (the *deep temporalis fascia*) splits into two layers called the *superficial and deep layers of the **deep** temporalis fascia* (don't get hung up on

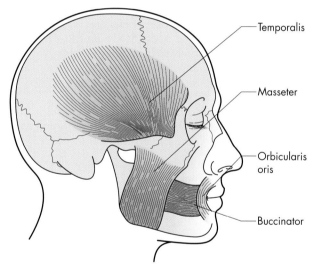

Temporalis

Masseter

Orbicularis oris

Buccinator

Figure 2-65 Deep muscles of the face.

the names at this point). Between these two layers of fascia is a pocket of fat called the *temporal fat pad*. Aside from trying to sort out the confusion of these named layers, the main reason to know about this split in the fascia and its attachments on each side of the arch is for easy access to repair of a depressed zygomatic arch fracture. You can slip an elevator under the deep layer of the temporalis fascia over the muscle and slide the elevator inferiorly to the arch and elevate a depressed zygomatic arch fracture. You are in a safe plane because you are in the temporal fat pad superior to the arch and *deep to the frontal branch* of the facial nerve.

Remember that the frontal branch of the facial nerve is most superficial over the zygomatic arch just deep to the SMAS over the arch. If you operate in the area of the arch, you must be careful in this "danger" area and stay either deep to the nerve as described above or superficial to the nerve in the subcutaneous fat plane (see checkpoint below).

Clinically, these are important surgical planes. As you learn to operate at any location in the face, temple, or neck, you should always know where the branches of the facial nerve are relative to your position. *In the lower two thirds of the face, your dissection plane will usually be anterior to the facial nerve branches. In the forehead and temple, you will usually be deep to the facial nerve branches.*

Let's talk about the transition point from the galea over the forehead to the TPF in the temple. Imagine a coronal incision from ear to ear through skin, subcutaneous fat, and the galea. In the center of the incision, you are in a plane of loose areolar tissue (allows the galea to move), and you can easily elevate the scalp off the bone (the "scalping plane"). The facial nerve branches are superficial to you, the periosteum is posterior. As you sweep inferiorly and laterally toward the temple, you will run into a point where you cannot easily lift the scalp off the bone. This is the anterior edge of attachment of the temporalis muscle to the skull (*the temporal line*). Now imagine the same wound, but starting your dissection laterally. You are over the temporalis muscle. As you cut though the layers, you will come upon a white fascial layer. To be sure that you are at the deep temporal fascia, cut through this layer and you will see the underlying temporalis muscle. If you stay on top of this fascia, you can easily create a plane. Where is the SMAS equivalent, the TPF? It is directly superficial in the scalp flap. As you move centrally, you will encounter the temporal line again—the line of fusion of all the layers we have been discussing. The fusion of the deep temporal fascia, the TPF, and the galea with the periosteum here is called the *conjoined tendon*. When you cut the conjoined tendon, you free the galea and TPF from the bone and create one continuous plane (SMAS equivalent). The release of this tendon all the way inferiorly to the lateral canthus allows you to freely lift the eyebrows (forehead lift). Later, in Chapter 6, you will learn how to cut the conjoined tendon using an endoscope though a scalp incision or directly from below through an upper eyelid skin crease incision (The endoscopic lifts that you will learn are performed in the subperiosteal plane. The relationship at the conjoined tendon remains the same.)

One more detail, as you elevate the TPF off the deep temporal fascia, the frontal branch of the facial nerve is in the tissue superficial to your dissection plane, so don't pull really hard with any retractor. As you dissect inferiorly in this plane toward the arch, the thin layer of fat just deep to the TPF that we mentioned earlier is a warning that you are near the frontal branch of the facial nerve. You might see a larger vein nearby called the *sentinel vein*. Sounds complex now, but like most anatomy, when you get some experience, it is easy to appreciate and remember. This is a good dissection to do in the anatomy lab.

The SMAS and associated fat pads

We have devoted a lot of attention to the concept of the SMAS and the related structures of the galea, TPF, and platysma. Now we'll go into a bit more detail on the SMAS itself. Remember that the SMAS is a fibromuscular layer that invests the muscles of facial expression. It is a true anatomic structure, but not as distinct as other planes that you may

- What are the structures analogous to the SMAS in the forehead, temple, and neck?
- Follow the path of the frontal branch of the facial nerve from the tragus to the lateral aspect of the eyebrow. What is the depth:
  — At the tragus—deep to the parotid fascia
  — Over the arch—superficial to the bone
  — Over the temporalis muscle
  — 1 cm superior to the brow—deep to the frontalis muscle
- What are the safe planes of dissection:
  — At the tragus—anterior to the parotid gland (nerve is deep)
  — At the arch—in the subcutaneous fat layer (nerve is deep)
  — 1 cm superior to the arch—in the subcutaneous layer (nerve is deep) or deep to the superficial layer of the deep temporal fascia (nerve is superficial)
  — Over the temporalis muscle—directly superficial to the deep temporal fascia (nerve is superficial in TPF)
  — Over the frontalis muscle—in the subcutaneous fat layer (nerve is deep) or deep to the galea (nerve is superficial)

be more familiar with. In some patients, it is more distinct than others. The thickness of the SMAS varies with regard to the location in the face. The SMAS is well formed over the parotid gland and fuses with the parotid fascia. As you move toward the melolabial fold, the SMAS becomes thinner. (As a reminder, the melolabial fold is also known as the nasolabial fold. Many facial anatomists prefer the term melolabial fold because the term more accurately describes involution facial anatomy (melo = cheek, labial = lip). The fold forms as lax, redundant cheek tissue falls over the more rigidly fixed lip tissue. Consequently, we will use the term melolabial fold throughout the text.) In the perioral area, the SMAS is very thin. The melolabial fold forms where condensations of the fascia overlying the masseter extend through the SMAS attaching to the skin. Inferiorly, the SMAS is continuous with the platysma muscle as it crosses the mandible.

Pads of fat exist anterior and posterior to the SMAS overlying the zygoma. The *malar fat pad* is a collection of fat on and within the anterior surface of the SMAS over the malar eminence. A full normally positioned malar fat pad contributes to the high full cheek in children and young adults.

A deeper plane of fat exists behind the orbicularis muscle overlying the inferior rim (*suborbicularis oculi fat pad*—SOOF) and extending superiorly over the lateral rim to overlie the superior orbital rim (*retroorbicularis fat pad*—ROOF) (Figure 2-66). The fullness of the lateral portion of the superior orbital rim seen in youth is due to the ROOF.

The malar fat pad, the ROOF, and SOOF allow the SMAS to move freely while maintaining an attachment with the underlying bone. For this reason, I consider them to be a part of the SMAS. Lifting of the forehead by tightening the galea repositions the ROOF. Lifting the midface (cheek) by tightening the SMAS has a similar action elevating the SOOF and malar fat pads. Both procedures are part of rejuvenation surgery.

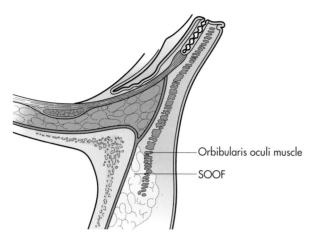

Figure 2-66 The SOOF, ROOF, and malar fat pads. The SMAS and its analogous anatomic layers are surrounded by layers of fatty tissue that allow the SMAS to move.

The retaining ligaments

There are areas where the SMAS is particularly well attached to the underlying and overlying tissues. These "anchor" points tend to stay fixed with aging. Over time, neighboring less well-anchored tissues tend to sag over these fixed points creating the characteristic facial folds of aging. In the midface, the SMAS is tightly attached to the parotid gland, along the inferior and lateral orbital rim and near the frontozygomatic (FZ) suture. These regions of attachment are referred as retaining ligaments, somewhat of a misnomer as they do not connect bone to bone. Rather, osseocutaneous ligaments attach the SMAS and skin to the underlying bone. At the melolabial fold, the ligaments extend from the fascia overlying the masseter muscle to the skin.

- Midface
  — Orbitomalar osseocutaneous ligaments
  — Orbital ligaments near FZ suture suspending the eyebrow
  — Zygomatic osseocutaneous ligaments (Figure 2-67, McGregor's patch) at the junction of zygoma and arch
- Lower face
  — Buccomaxillary ligament
  — Mandibular ligaments

In the forehead, galea laxity allows the ROOF and the eyebrow to droop over the superior orbital rim creating the typical temporal brow droop. In the lateral midface, the malar and the suborbicularis fat pads descend in a characteristic manner creating the *malar triangle* laterally (Figure 2-68). Medially, the cheek drops, the inferior orbital rim loses its soft tissue padding, and the characteristic deepening of the nasojugal fold occurs (so-called "tear trough" deformity). As the cheek tissues descend inferiorly and medially, the melolabial fold deepens. As the orbital septum thins, fat prolapses forward. With this characteristic midfacial aging, the youthful cherubic single soft curve of the cheek falls and forms the "double convexity" (Figure 2-69) of the eyelid cheek profile.

In the lower face, the descending cheek hangs over the retaining ligaments along the mandible forming *jowls*. From the corner of the mouth moving inferiorly, redundant tissues droop over the more tightly attached tissue at the chin forming *marionette lines* (Box 2-6).

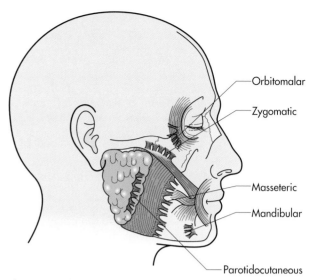

Figure 2-67 The osseocutaneous retaining ligaments. In the midface: orbitomalar osseocutaneous, the orbital ligaments (near the frontozygomatic suture suspending the eyebrow), and the zygomatic osseocutaneous ligaments ("McGregor's patch" at the junction of zygoma and arch). In the lower face: the buccomaxillary ligament and mandibular ligaments.

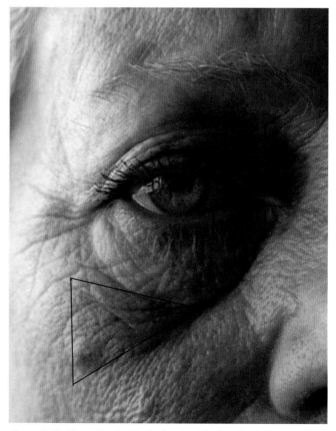

Figure 2-68 The malar triangle. As the cheek "deflates" a characteristic "malar triangle" forms. This change occurs when cheek tissues overhang the underlying anchoring orbito-malar osseocutaneous ligaments located at the inferior margin of the triangle.

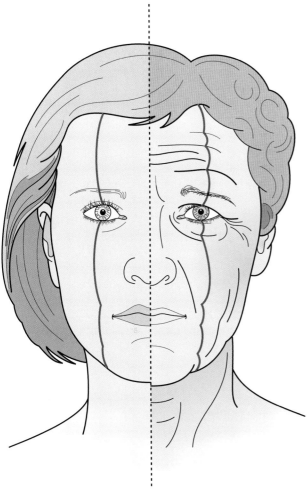

Figure 2-69 The "double convexity" of the lower eyelid. As the cheek descends and the eyelid fat prolapses forward, the normal smooth contour of the lower eyelid is lost and the "double convexity" forms. Note the other associated convexity changes in the lower face.

Box 2-6

SMAS—Clinicopathologic Correlations

A fibromuscular layer containing the mimetic muscles of the face continuous with the:

- Temporoparietal fascia superolaterally
- Frontalis muscle and galea superiorly
- Platysma inferiorly
  Strong over parotid, thin over zygoma and perioral area.

Anchor points

- Midface anchor points
  - Orbitomalar
  - Orbital
  - Zygomatic (McGregor's patch)
- Lower face anchor points
  - Buccomaxillary
  - Mandibular

Aging changes

- Midface
  - Malar mound
  - Double convexity
  - Melolabial fold
- Lower face
  - Jowling
  - Marionette lines

Attachments to the skin, underlying bone, and surrounding tissues

- Skin—at the nasolabial fold and oromandibular fold
  - Leading to deepening of melolabial fold and marionette lines
- Bone
  - Zygomatic retaining ligament
  - Orbitomalar retaining ligament
  - Orbital retaining ligament
  - Mandibular retaining ligament

Checkpoint

- Refresh in your mind the positions of the SOOF, ROOF, and malar fat pads.
- The SMAS and the temporoparietal fascia are analogous anatomic structures. How do they differ with regard to mimetic muscles?

- Describe the physical basis of the double convexity of the eyelid cheek profile. Think of this as the "textbook" example of facial descent and deflation.
- What is the anatomic name for the "tear trough"?
- Recall another name for the melolabial fold.

Major points

There is a great deal of information in this chapter. Don't try to learn it all at once. You will forget what you learned at the beginning of the chapter by the time you get to the end. This is a good chapter to reread after you have read a chapter on a particular clinical problem.

Learn the anatomic principles. Use the clinical examples to help remember the anatomy.

Important surface landmarks include:

- The upper eyelid skin crease (and the lower crease in children)
- The upper eyelid skin fold

- Nasojugal and malar folds (and malar fat pad)
- Melolabial fold
- The eyebrow (head, body, and tail)
- The slope of the eyelid
- Margin reflex distance (MRD_1 and MRD_2)

The orbital rim is made of three bones, the frontal, zygomatic, and maxillary bones. A ZMC fracture breaks the rims at the suture lines. The nasolacrimal sac is formed as the medial rim moves posteriorly and the inferior rim moves anteriorly.

Major points Continued

In contrast to the orbital rims, the medial orbital wall and the orbital floor are thin. A blowout fracture of the medial wall or floor does not break the rims. Diplopia and enophthalmos are common findings.

The openings of the orbit include:

- Superior and inferior orbital fissures
- Infraorbital groove, canal, and foramen
- Optic canal
- Anterior and posterior ethmoidal foramina
- Zygomaticofacial and zygomaticotemporal foramina

You should know what anatomic spaces these "openings" connect and what structures pass through them.

The periorbita is the periosteum lining the orbit. The line of fusion of the periorbita to the periosteum is called the arcus marginalis.

The orbicularis is the main muscle responsible for eyelid closure. The procerus and corrugator muscles are lesser protractors (responsible for the horizontal and vertical furrows of the glabella, respectively). All are innervated by branches of the facial nerve.

The medial and lateral canthal tendons attach the tarsal plates to the periorbita of the orbital rims. The lateral canthal tendon attaches to Whitnall's ligament. Laxity of the lateral canthal tendon is the major cause of lower eyelid ectropion. The medial canthal tendon has anterior and posterior limbs that surround the lacrimal sac. Blinking of the eyelids contributes to the "lacrimal pumping" of the tears out of the eye.

The retractors of the upper eyelid include:

- The levator muscle complex
- Müller's muscle
- The frontalis muscle

The levator muscle is the major retractor of the upper eyelid. It is innervated by cranial nerve III. The parts of the levator include the muscle belly, the fibrous aponeurosis, the horns of the aponeurosis, and Whitnall's ligament.

Müller's muscle is innervated by the sympathetic nervous system and is responsible for 1–2 mm of upper eyelid elevation. Loss of sympathetic tone to the face results in a mild ptosis of the upper lid, a part of Horner's syndrome.

The frontalis muscle raises the eyebrows, elevating the eyelids a small amount. The frontalis muscle is innervated by cranial nerve VII. The horizontal furrows of the brow are created by the frontalis muscle action.

The lower eyelid retractors are less well developed than the levator, but also consist of voluntary and involuntary components. Laxity of the lower lid retractors is the main etiologic factor in lower lid involutional entropion.

The orbital septum is a fibrous layer of tissue that separates the eyelid from the orbit. The orbital septum attaches to the periosteum at the arcus marginalis along the orbital rims.

Posterior to the septum is the preaponeurotic fat. The upper lid contains two fat pads (central and medial). The lower lid contains three fat pads (medial, central, and lateral).

The fat pads are the surgical landmark for the aponeurosis and lower lid retractors.

Lamellae of the eyelid

- The anterior lamella of the eyelid consists of the skin and orbicularis muscle.
- The posterior lamella of the eyelid consists of the tarsus and conjunctiva.
- The concepts of the anterior and posterior lamellae of the eyelids are important for understanding cicatricial diseases of the eyelids.
  - Cicatricial changes in the posterior lamella cause entropion.
  - Cicatricial changes in the anterior lamella cause ectropion.

These principles are also useful in lid reconstruction.

The lacrimal gland has two lobes, the orbital and palpebral lobes. The aqueous layer of the tear film flows into the superior conjunctival cul de sac through the lacrimal ductules.

The lacrimal drainage system consists of:

- The puncta
- The canaliculi
- The lacrimal sac
- The nasolacrimal duct

Obstruction can occur at any point, resulting in tearing. Pertinent nasal anatomy includes:

- The turbinates (superior, middle, and inferior)
- The middle turbinate is the landmark for the cribriform plate and the lacrimal sac
- The uncinate process, seen in the middle meatus, is the landmark for the maxillary ostium
- The space under each turbinate (meatus)
- The nasolacrimal duct opens in the inferior meatus

Understanding the anatomy of the nose and paranasal sinuses is important in treating lacrimal and orbital disease. The sinuses include:

- Ethmoid sinus
- Frontal sinus
- Maxillary sinus
- Sphenoid sinus

Sensory innervation to the periocular region is from:

- The upper eyelid, orbit, and eye are innervated by the branches of the ophthalmic division (V_1).
- The lower eyelid is innervated by the branches of the maxillary division (V_2).

Motor innervation to the muscles of facial expression is from the facial nerve (VII). From superior to inferior, the branches of the facial nerve are:

- Temporal branch
- Zygomatic branch

Major points Continued

- Buccal branch
- Mandibular branch
- Cervical branch

Innervation to the extraocular muscles including the levator muscle is by the oculomotor (III), trochlear (IV), and abducens (VI) cranial nerves.

The arterial supply to the eye, orbit, and periocular regions is complex. Learn these basic principles:

- The external and internal carotid arteries supply the head.
- The external carotid artery has many branches in the neck, which supply the neck, face, sinuses, and scalp.
- The internal carotid artery supplies the eye, orbit, and brain.
- The only branch of the internal carotid to the eye and orbit is the ophthalmic artery. All structures in the eye and orbit will be supplied by branches of the ophthalmic artery.
- The terminal branches of the ophthalmic artery (you can learn these later) will anastomose with terminal branches of the external carotid artery to form a rich arterial network of collateral circulation in the periocular area.

The venous drainage of the orbit is through:

- The superior orbital fissure to the cavernous sinus
- The inferior orbital fissure to the pterygopalatine plexus
  The lymphatic drainage of the eyelids is summarized as:
- The lateral two thirds of the upper eyelid, one third of the lower eyelid, and half of the conjunctiva drain into the preauricular nodes.
- The remaining tissues drain deeply into the submandibular nodes. Lymphoid tissue exists in the lacrimal gland and the conjunctiva, common sites of orbital lymphoma.

UV changes result in loss of the viscoelastic properties of the skin—the plumpness (ground substance and collagen) and elasticity (elastin fibers) of youthful skin.

Fat pads are found posterior to the orbicularis muscle known as the SOOF and ROOF (sub- and retroorbicularis fat pads). The malar fat pad is found superficial to the orbicularis at the zygoma. Equivalent fat pads are found surrounding the other facial muscles.

The "double convexity" of the eyelid cheek profile occurs as the cheek descends and the eyelid fat prolapses forward. The eyelid becomes "longer" and loses its single curve.

The SMAS (superficial musculoaponeurotic system) is a layer of tissue that invests the muscles of facial expression physically responsible for the coordinated movements we see. Equivalent structures exist across the face and skull and are continuous with the SMAS. The structures analogous to the superficial musculoaponeurotic system are:

- Temporoparietal fascia in the temple
- Galea over the skull
- Platysma in the neck

The retaining ligaments extend from the facial bones to the skin. These anchor the soft tissues to the facial skeleton. The typical facial "sags" of facial aging are the looser tissues hanging over tissues held in place by the retaining ligaments—jowls, melolabial fold.

The melolabial fold is a more appropriate name than the nasolabial fold as it more accurately describes the lax cheek (melo) tissues drooping over the more adherent lip (labial) tissues.

Follow the path of the frontal branch of the facial nerve from the tragus to the lateral aspect of the eyebrow. What is the depth?

- At the tragus—deep to the parotid fascia
- Over the arch—superficial to the bone
- Over the temporalis muscle
- 1 cm superior to the brow—deep to the frontalis muscle

As you learn to operate at any location in the face, temple, or neck, you should always know where the branches of the facial nerve are relative to your position. In the lower two thirds of the face, your dissection plane will usually be anterior to the facial nerve branches. In the forehead and temple, you will usually be deep to the facial nerve branches.

The temporal line is the anterior edge of attachment of the temporalis muscle to the skull. The deep temporal fascia, the temporoparietal fascia (TPF), and the galea fuse with the periosteum here—the conjoined tendon.

Unless you are ready to focus on brow lifting, skip the anatomic details of the temple for now and just remember the concept of the SMAS and its counterparts, the platysma, the galea, and the TPF, extending across the face and skull.

Suggested reading

1. Aiache AE, Ramirez OH: The suborbicularis oculi fat pads: an anatomic and clinical study. *Plast Reconstr Surg* 95:37–42, 1995.

2. Albert D, Lucarelli M, eds: Anatomy of the eyelids, lacrimal system and orbit. In *Clinical atlas of procedures in ophthalmic surgery*, pp. 230–241, Chicago: AMA Press, 2004.

3. American Academy of Ophthalmology: *Basic and clinical science course: orbit, eyelids and lacrimal system*, sect. 7, pp. 7–21, 135–145, 253–257, San Francisco: The American Academy of Ophthalmology, 2006/2007.

4. Anderson RL, Beard C: The levator aponeurosis. *Arch Ophthalmol* 95:1437–1441, 1977.

5. Bergen MP, Los JA: The vascular system in the orbit: special relationships. *Orbit* 2:33, 1983.

6. Bergin DJ: Anatomy of the eyelids, lacrimal system and orbit. In McCord CD, Tanenbaum M, Nunery WR, eds, *Oculoplastic surgery*, 3rd edn, ch. 2, pp. 51–83, New York: Raven Press, 1995.

7. Blaylock WK, Moore CA, Linberg JV: Anterior ethmoid anatomy facilitates dacryocystorhinostomy. *Arch Ophthalmol* 108(12):1774–1777, 1990.

8. Bron AJ: Lacrimal streams: the demonstration of human lacrimal fluid secretion and the lacrimal ductules. *Br J Ophthalmol* 70:241–245, 1986.

9. Burget GC, Menick FJ: The subunit principle in nasal reconstruction. *Plast Reconstr Surg* 76(2): 239–247, 1985.

10. Chen WPD, Khan JA: Eyelid anatomy. In Chen WPD, Khan JA, McCord CD, eds. *The color atlas of cosmetic oculofacial surgery*, pp. 5–18, Philadelphia: Butterworth and Heinemann, 2004.

11. Doxanas MT, Anderson RL: *Clinical orbital anatomy.* Baltimore: Williams & Wilkins, 1984.

12. Dutton JJ: Clinical anatomy of the eyelids. In Yanoff M, Duker J, eds. *Ophthalmology*, pp. 637–640, Mosby, 2004.

13. Dutton JJ: *Atlas of clinical and surgical orbital anatomy*, Philadelphia: WB Saunders, 1994.

14. Dutton JJ: Clinical anatomy of the orbit. In Yanoff M, Duker J, eds. *Ophthalmology*, pp. 641–648, Mosby, 2004.

15. Gioia VM, Linberg JV, McCormick SA: The anatomy of the lateral canthal tendon. *Arch Ophthalmol* 105(4):529–532, 1987.

16. Hawes MJ, Dortzbach RK: The microscopic anatomy of the lower eyelid retractors. *Arch Ophthalmol* 100:1313–1318, 1982.

17. Honrado CP, Bradley DT, Larrabee WF: Facial embryology and anatomy. In Azizzadeh B, Murphy MR, Johnson CM, eds. *Master techniques in facial rejuvenation*, pp. 17–32, Philadelphia: Elsevier, 2007.

18. Housepian EM: Microsurgical anatomy of the orbital apex and principles of transcranial orbital exploration. *Clin Neurosurg* 25:556–573, 1978.

19. Johnson CM, Alsarraf R: Surgical anatomy of the aging face. In *The aging face, a systematic approach*, pp. 27–36, Saunders Elsevier, 2002.

20. Jordan DR, Anderson RL: The facial nerve in eyelid surgery. *Arch Ophthalmol* 107:1114–1115, 1989.

21. Kikkawa DO, Lemke BN: Orbital anatomy and embryology. In Bosniak S et al, eds. *Principles and practice of ophthalmic plastic and reconstructive surgery*, vol. 2, ch. 80, pp. 837–852, Philadelphia: WB Saunders, 1996.

22. Knize DM, ed: *The forehead and temporal fossa: anatomy and technique.* Philadelphia: Williams & Wilkins, 2001.

23. Koornneef L: Orbital septa: anatomy and functions. *Ophthalmology* 86:876–880, 1979.

24. Lemke BN, Lucarelli MJ, Rose JG Jr.: Cosmetic facial anatomy. In *Gladstone and Nesi's oculoplastic surgery atlas.* New York: Springer, 2005.

25. Lemke BN, Stasior OG: The anatomy of eyebrow ptosis. *Arch Ophthalmol* 100:981–986, 1982.

26. Lucarelli MJ, Khwarg S: The anatomy of midfacial ptosis. In Lemke BN, Kozel JS, Dortzbach RK, eds. *Ophthalmic plastic and reconstructive surgery* 16, 2000.

27. Lyon DB, Lemke BN, Wallow IH, Dortzbach RK: Sympathetic nerve anatomy in the cavernous sinus and retrobulbar orbit of the cynomolgus monkey. *Ophthal Plast Reconstr Surg* 8:1–12, 1992.

28. McGetrick JJ, Wilson DG, Dortzbach RK et al: A search for lymphatic drainage of the monkey orbit. *Arch Ophthalmol* 107:255–260, 1990.

29. Meyer DR, Linberg JV, Wobig JL, McCormick SA: Anatomy of the orbital septum and associated eyelid connective tissues. Implications for ptosis surgery. *Ophthal Plast Reconstr Surg* 7(2):104–113, 1991.

30. Moss CJ, Mendelson BC, Taylor GI: Surgical anatomy of the ligamentous attachments in the temple and periorbital regions. *Plast Reconstr Surg* 105:1475–1490, 2000.

31. Mendelson BC, Muzaffer AR, Adams WP: Surgical anatomy of the midcheek and malar mounds. *Plast Reconstr Surg* 110:885–986, 2002.

32. Nerad J: Clinical anatomy. In: *The requisites—Oculoplastic surgery*, pp. 25–70. St Louis: Mosby, 2001.

33. Nowinski TS: Anatomy and physiology of lacrimal system. In Bosniak S et al, eds. *Principles and practice of ophthalmic plastic and reconstructive surgery*, vol. 2, ch. 73, pp. 731–747, Philadelphia: WB Saunders, 1996.

34. Rootman J, Stewart B, Goldberg RA, eds: Orbital anatomy. In *Orbital surgery, a conceptual approach*, ch. 7, pp. 79–146, Philadelphia, Lippincott-Raven, 1995.

35. Rootman J, Stewart B, Nugent R, Robertson W: Anatomy of the orbit. In Rootman J, ed. *Diseases of the orbit*, pp. 1–48, Philadelphia: JB Lippincott, 1988.

36. Sherman DD, Gonnering RS, et al: Identification of orbital lymphatics: enzyme histochemical light microscopic and electron microscopic studies. *Ophthal Plast Reconstr Surg* 9:153–169, 1993.

37. Shovlin JP, Lemke BN: Clinical eyelid anatomy. In Bosniak S et al, eds. *Principles and practice of ophthalmic plastic and reconstructive surgery*, vol. 2, ch. 26, pp. 261–280, Philadelphia, WB Saunders, 1996.

38. Tolhurst DE, Carstens MH et al: The surgical anatomy of the scalp. *Plast Reconstr Surg* 87:603–612, 1991 [Discussion, pp. 613–614].

39. Tucker NA, Tucker SM, Linberg JV: The anatomy of the common canaliculus. *Arch Ophthalmol* 114(10):1231–1234, 1996.

40. Tucker SM, Linberg JV: Vascular anatomy of the eyelids. *Ophthalmology* 101(6):1118–1121, 1994.

41. Wobig JL, Dailey RA, eds: *Oculofacial Plastic surgery: face, lacrimal system, and orbit*, pp. 3–29, 129–137 and 192–212. New York: Thieme, 2004.

42. Wulc AE, Dryden RM et al: Where is the gray line? *Arch Ophthalmol* 105:1092–1098, 1987.

43. Zide BM, Jelks GW: *Surgical anatomy of the orbit.* New York: Raven Press, 1985.

44. Zide BM, Jelks GW: *Surgical anatomy around the orbit: the system of zones.* Philadelphia: Williams & Wilkins, 2006.

Diagnosis and Treatment of Ectropion

Introduction

Ectropion of the eyelid occurs *when the lid margin everts* or turns away from the eyeball. Lower lid ectropion is a common problem. Patients may complain of *irritation* or *mattering, erythema of the lid margin*, or *tearing*. Three types of lower lid ectropion occur:

- Cicatricial
- Paralytic
- Involutional

Cicatricial ectropion is caused by shortening of the anterior lamella as a result of either trauma or cicatricial skin disease. *Involutional ectropion* is caused by horizontal laxity of the eyelid. *Paralytic ectropion* is caused by loss of orbicularis muscle support of the lower eyelid. Associated lower facial paralysis and brow ptosis usually accompany paralytic ectropion. The type and cause of the ectropion are usually obvious from the history and the examination.

After the etiology of the ectropion is identified, a treatment plan can be made. The *lateral tarsal strip operation* is used to correct horizontal lid laxity. The lower eyelid is shortened at the lateral canthus. The lateral tarsal strip operation is the procedure of choice for repairing involutional eyelid ectropion. Paralytic ectropion is usually treated with a lateral tarsal strip procedure also. You will find that the lateral tarsal strip procedure is probably the most useful operation to learn in all of oculoplastic surgery. Paralytic ectropion is somewhat more complicated to treat than involutional ectropion because corneal exposure and brow ptosis may also require treatment.

Cicatricial ectropion is treated by lengthening the shortened anterior lamella with a *full-thickness graft*. Frequently, a lateral tarsal strip operation will be used in conjunction with a full-thickness skin graft to treat any associated lid laxity.

Cicatricial ectropion of the upper eyelid may also occur. There is no upper eyelid equivalent for paralytic or involutional ectropion.

Congenital ectropion or eversion of the upper or lower eyelid can occur, but is extremely rare. Some texts include a mechanical form of ectropion. This is said to occur when a large tumor occurs on the eyelid, pulling the eyelid off the eye. I consider this to be more of a tumor problem than a lid malposition and so have not included discussion of a mechanical ectropion in this chapter. An unusual, but not extremely uncommon, form of upper eyelid eversion occurs during sleep. This is known as *floppy eyelid syndrome*. Irritation and mattering occur. Floppy eyelid syndrome will be discussed later under "Physical Examination."

Ectropion is common and easy to diagnose. The mechanisms are understandable, and the cause is recognizable during the history and physical examination. Appropriate treatment can be chosen based on the type of ectropion identified. Surgical correction is successful in most cases.

Anatomic considerations

Normal eyelid anatomy

The normal lower lid rests at the limbus (Figure 3-1; also see Figure 2-1). There is normally no sclera visible between the lower lid margin and the limbus. The lower eyelid apposes the eye for the entire length of the eyelid. There should be no separation of the posterior lid margin from the eye. The lateral canthus is slightly higher than the medial canthus. The lower lid punctum sits in the tear lake at the conjunctival plica. The next time you look at a patient with the slit lamp, notice that the normally positioned punctum is not visible at the slit lamp without using your finger to slightly evert the punctum. Normal tear drainage will not occur if the punctum

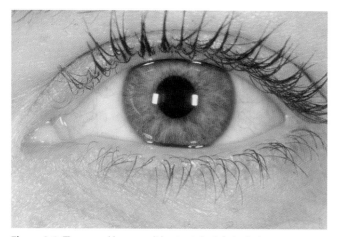

Figure 3-1 The normal lower eyelid rests at the inferior limbus.

is vertical or upright. The normal tear lake should be approximately 1 mm high. You will see examples of excessive and inadequate tear lakes.

Abnormal eyelid anatomy

Horizontal eyelid laxity

The tarsal plates are attached to the bony orbital rims by the lateral and medial canthal tendons. Lengthening of the tendons occurs with age. This increase in the horizontal length of the eyelid is responsible for the *eyelid laxity* that causes involutional ectropion. The tarsal plates do not lengthen with time. The insertion of the lateral canthal tendon is on the inner aspect of the lateral orbital rim at Whitnall's tubercle. This slightly elevated area of the lateral orbital rim is approximately 10 mm inferior to the frontozygomatic suture. Remember when you reattach the lateral canthal tendon using the lateral tarsal strip procedure to place the tendon on the inner aspect of the rim to prevent lid distraction from the globe.

Midfacial hypoplasia

The bony architecture of the inferior orbital rim provides support for the lower eyelid. Individual and racial variations occur. Patients with higher cheekbones or prominent malar bones tend to have less ectropion. Asian patients tend to have a flat face with more prominent malar bones. Black patients tend to have less prominent malar bones. The bony architecture of white patients is intermediate. Patients with the so-called *hypoplastic midface* or *maxilla* have an inferior orbital rim that is somewhat posterior in relationship to the eyeball (Figure 3-2). These patients tend to have less support for the lower lid and may have lower lid retraction or ectropion. Another term for the hypoplastic maxilla is "*hemiproptosis*." I like this term because it emphasizes the fact that the inferior half of the eye is more anterior than the orbital rim. Tightening of the lower lid in a patient with hemiproptosis may cause the eyelid to slide under the eye, so be careful in tightening any lower eyelid in a patient with hemiproptosis. The relationship of the maxilla to the inferior rim should be considered in patients undergoing lower eyelid blepharoplasty in order to avoid the common complication of eyelid retraction or "rounding" of the lower eyelid. You will see later that the term "hemiproptosis" is also referred to as a

"negative vector" eyelid, especially in the context of lower eyelid cosmetic surgery.

Anterior lamellar shortening

The skin, orbicularis muscle, and orbital septum are normally flexible enough that spontaneous movement of the eyelids can occur. You are already familiar with the terms anterior lamella (skin and muscle) and posterior lamella (tarsus and conjunctiva). *Scarring of the anterior lamella* can cause a cicatricial ectropion (Figure 3-3). Lengthening of the shortened lamella by adding a *full-thickness skin graft is the treatment for cicatricial ectropion*. As you know, scarring of the posterior lamella also causes a cicatricial entropion.

Middle lamella

Recently, the term *middle lamella* has been used to describe the tissues between the anterior and posterior lamellae of the eyelid inferior to the tarsal plate. These tissues include the orbital septum, the preaponeurotic fat, and the lower lid retractors. Scarring of the middle lamella may tether the eyelid, which causes cicatricial ectropion, lid retraction, or even cicatricial entropion, depending on how the scar tissue forms. This middle lamella scarring occurs most commonly after eyelid trauma or surgery.

Paralysis of the orbicularis muscle

The resting tone of the orbicularis muscle supports the tarsal plate and canthal tendons, helping to support the lower eyelid in the normal position. *In patients with paralytic ectropion, the resting tone of the orbicularis muscle is reduced or absent* (Figure 3-4). Ectropion occurs primarily in older patients who have an underlying element of lid laxity. In younger patients with facial nerve palsy, ectropion generally does not occur because there is no underlying lid laxity.

Normal lid position and function are necessary for tear drainage. Any type of ectropion may cause tearing as a result of reflex tearing, punctal eversion, or loss of the lacrimal pump. Interestingly, many older patients with ectropion do not complain of tearing. This is probably because tear production decreases with age.

Checkpoint

At this point you should:
- Know the types of ectropion
- State the anatomic cause for each type of ectropion
- Explain the term *hemiproptosis*
- Understand why younger patients with facial nerve palsy may not have ectropion
- Understand the reasons for tearing resulting from ectropion

History

Symptoms

The history in ectropion is straightforward. You will want to understand what bothers the patient about the ectropion. Patients with ectropion usually complain of *irritation, redness,*

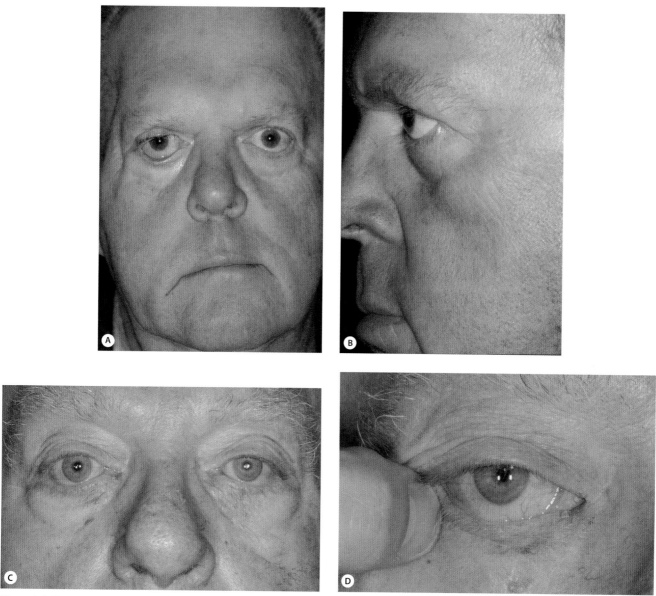

Figure 3-2 "Hemiproptosis" or hypoplastic midface associated with lid retraction. Facial nerve paralysis after parotidectomy. (**A**) Note lower eyelid retraction on both sides and ectropion of right lower eyelid. (**B**) Inferior orbital rim is posterior to the front of the globe which complicates ectropion repair. (**C**) Note lower lid retraction in a second patient with hemiproptosis. (**D**) Simulated horizontal tightening of the lower eyelid increases the retraction.

or *tearing*. As the lower eyelid everts, the normally moist conjunctival tissues become exposed to air and dry out. The conjunctiva becomes erythematous and may cause a slight discharge. The irritation is usually mild, and some patients may choose to ignore recommended treatment for the ectropion. This is in contrast to entropion in which the irritation is more severe, and patients seldom refuse treatment. For some patients, the main complaint about the ectropion is the erythematous appearance of the lid margin. Tearing may accompany the ectropion. The cause of tearing may be punctal malposition or inadequate lacrimal pump function. Tearing is more severe in young patients than in older patients. A young patient with mild punctal eversion may complain of severe tearing, whereas an older patient with complete ectropion may have no complaints of epiphora. If tearing is present, you need to pay particular attention to the position of the punctum when you are correcting the eyelid position.

Etiologic factors

Look for causes of anterior lamellar shortening

A history of *trauma* or *cicatricial skin disease* may explain why a patient has *cicatricial ectropion*. Previous excision of *skin cancer* or repair of a laceration in the periocular area may cause anterior lamellar shortening. The most common cause of anterior lamellar shortening is *actinic damage* in fair-skinned whites. Rarely, a patient may have a cicatricial skin disease such as ichthyosis that may cause the eyelid skin to shorten.

Is there any history of facial nerve paralysis?

Even a patient who has no obvious facial asymmetry may recollect a "resolved" *Bell's palsy*. This mild orbicularis weakness may combine with horizontal laxity to cause *paralytic ectropion*.

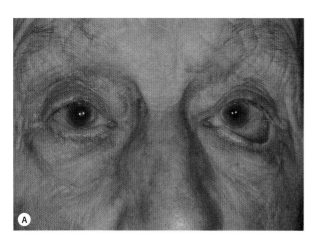
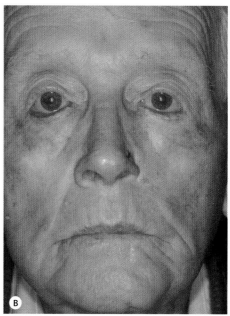

Figure 3-3 Cicatricial ectropion caused by anterior lamellar shortening. (**A**) Trauma to the skin over the zygoma, resulting in a scar that pulls the eyelid down. (**B**) Chronic sun-damaged skin causing a generalized tightness of the facial skin. In both cases, surgical correction requires lengthening of the anterior lamella, usually with a full-thickness skin graft and lower eyelid tightening.

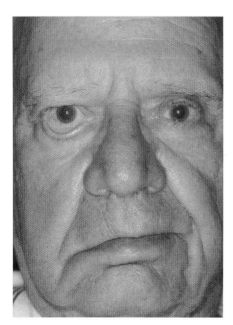

Figure 3-4 Paralytic ectropion caused by right facial nerve palsy. Note the flattened nasolabial fold and brow ptosis accompanying the ectropion.

Physical examination

Location and severity

The purpose of the physical examination is to identify the presence, location, and severity of the ectropion, as well as the underlying etiology. Any eversion of the lid margin off the eyeball is considered ectropion. The lid distraction may be mild and relatively asymptomatic. Only the punctum may be everted, with tearing as the complaint rather than ectropion. The ectropion may be lateral or medial or involve the entire lower eyelid. The ectropion may be severe with the entire lid everted to the degree that the eyelid is turned inside out. This condition is known as *tarsal ectropion*.

Etiology

Are cicatricial changes present?

The etiology of the ectropion is usually apparent. The first question to ask is *Is the ectropion cicatricial? Is there scar tissue pulling the eyelid away from the eyeball?* Look for any specific scarring of the periocular area that would indicate previous accidental or surgical trauma. Look to see if the patient has tight skin on the whole face. Some patients, despite their age, may have tight skin with very few wrinkles. These patients may have generalized skin shrinkage as a cause of the cicatricial ectropion. Cicatricial ectropion is less common than involutional ectropion (see Figure 3-3).

Is there facial asymmetry?

If there are no cicatricial changes, ask the question, *Is there evidence of facial asymmetry suggesting paralytic ectropion?* Patients with facial nerve palsy have associated flattening of the nasolabial fold and coexisting brow ptosis. Patients with paralytic ectropion have significant laxity of the involved lower eyelid. Be sure to check for evidence of corneal exposure that would require additional medical or surgical treatment aside from repair of the paralytic ectropion (Figure 3-4). The additional procedures used in the management of facial nerve palsy will be covered in Chapter 9.

Horizontal eyelid laxity

If the ectropion is not cicatricial and not paralytic, it must be involutional. Involutional ectropion occurs in older patients with eyelid laxity (Figure 3-5). The eyelid laxity can be demonstrated by the *eyelid distraction test* and the *eyelid snap test*.

The eyelid distraction test

The eyelid distraction test is performed by manually pulling the eyelid away from the eyeball. The lower lid should not move more than 6 mm off the eyeball (Figure 3-6).

The eyelid snap test

The eyelid snap test is performed by pulling the lower eyelid inferiorly toward the inferior orbital rim. An eyelid without lower eyelid laxity will spring back into position without a blink. The lax lower eyelid will remain away from the eye for a period of time. The amount of laxity can be grossly quantified by asking the patient to blink and counting the number of blinks required to return the lid to normal position. I note in the chart something like, "eyelid returns with two blinks." You will find the eyelid distraction and eyelid snap tests very helpful (Figure 3-7). The amount of laxity is directly related to the treatment—shortening the eyelid with

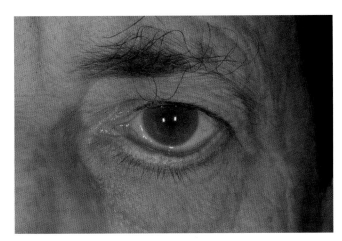

Figure 3-5 Involutional ectropion resulting from horizontal lower eyelid laxity.

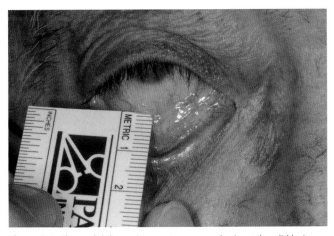

Figure 3-6 The eyelid distraction test to measure horizontal eyelid laxity. The eyelid should not pull away from the globe more than 6 mm.

a lateral tarsal strip operation. Remember that involutional ectropion is one of the most common oculoplastic conditions you will see.

Considerations for treatment

The aim of the last portion of the physical examination is to determine what treatment will be required to repair the ectropion. In patients with cicatricial ectropion, the position and severity of the scarring should be estimated. The location and size of the full-thickness skin graft required to lengthen the anterior lamellar shortage can be estimated. In general, the horizontal length of the graft should extend slightly beyond the areas of involved scarring. You should also estimate if lid laxity is present. In most cases, an eyelid tightening procedure (almost always a lateral tarsal strip procedure) is used in conjunction with a full-thickness skin graft.

In patients with involutional ectropion, the effect of lower eyelid tightening can be estimated at the slit lamp. Using your index finger, pull the eyelid laterally and watch how the eyelid margin fits against the eyeball. In many cases, tightening the eyelid at the lateral canthus will return the punctum to the normal position. If the punctum remains everted, additional treatment of the punctal eversion should be considered in conjunction with the lateral tarsal strip operation. The most useful operation to correct punctal eversion is the *medial spindle operation*.

Rarely with involutional ectropion, the punctum will be everted in the absence of lower eyelid laxity. In these patients, the medial spindle operation alone may be sufficient.

Many texts suggest evaluating the eyelid for the presence of medial canthal tendon laxity. If lateral traction of the lower eyelid displaces the punctum to or beyond the limbus, medial canthal tendon laxity exists. Several procedures have been devised to tighten or plicate the medial canthal tendon. All are complicated by the presence of the lower canaliculus. None of these procedures works consistently well for me. Horizontal lower eyelid tightening with the standard lateral tarsal strip procedure is effective in most of these patients.

In patients with paralytic ectropion, the effect of lower lid tightening can also be estimated during the slit lamp examination. Often the lateral tarsal strip procedure alone will reposition the lower lid nicely. For paralytic ectropion, other factors should be considered as discussed above. Lubricating drops and ointment may be needed to correct corneal exposure. Additional procedures to improve blinking or protect the cornea may be necessary. Consideration should be given to elevating the ptotic eyebrow.

Floppy eyelid syndrome

This is a good place to talk about the *floppy eyelid syndrome*. Patients with this syndrome complain of unilateral or bilateral irritation and ocular injection. On examination, a papillary conjunctivitis present. No obvious upper or lower eyelid ectropion is present. The main diagnostic finding is an enormous amount of upper eyelid laxity, so much so that the eyelid can be folded on itself and easily turned inside out (Figure 3-8). The cause of the irritation seems to be nocturnal eversion of the extremely lax upper eyelid rubbing on the pillow. Even more interesting is the fact that the majority of these patients are obese men with obstructive sleep apnea caused by similarly lax tissue in the upper airway. If the sleep

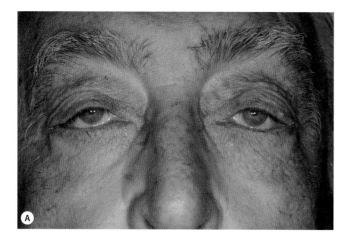

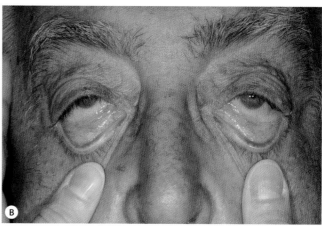

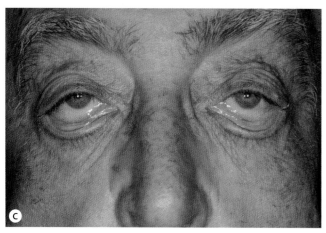

Figure 3-7 The eyelid snap test to measure horizontal lower eyelid laxity. (**A**) The eyelid at rest. (**B**) The lower eyelids manually retracted. (**C**) The normal eyelid should return to normal position in one blink. In this case, the eyelids do not return to normal with several blinks.

apnea has already been recognized, the patient is usually wearing a continuous positive airway pressure (CPAP) mask at night or has had a uveopalatoplasty to tighten the airway. If the patient does not have a diagnosis of sleep apnea, ask about snoring, sleepless nights, and daytime fatigue. If any of these symptoms are present, refer the patient to a sleep specialist, and you may save the patient from some serious cardiopulmonary consequences. The treatment for floppy eyelid syndrome is horizontal lid tightening of the upper eyelid (usually a pentagonal wedge resection).

Checkpoint

At this point you should:
- Know the questions to ask yourself during the physical examination to determine the type of ectropion
- Understand and be able to perform
  - The eyelid snap test
  - The eyelid distraction test
  - Describe the floppy eyelid syndrome

Treatment of ectropion

Treatment of lower eyelid involutional ectropion

As we said, the *most common type* of ectropion is involutional ectropion. Correction of the lower eyelid laxity using the

lower lid-tightening procedure, the lateral tarsal strip operation, will correct the ectropion. *The lateral tarsal strip operation is one of the most useful operations you will encounter in oculoplastic surgery. Make sure that you learn how to do this operation.*

The lateral tarsal strip operation

The lateral tarsal strip operation involves shortening the lower lid at the lateral canthus. The lower lid is released from the lateral orbital rim. A tab, or strip, of lower lid tarsus is fashioned and denuded of conjunctival epithelium and skin. The strip is shortened to provide appropriate tension. The strip is then reattached to the inner aspect of the orbital rim. Many patients benefit from 1–2 weeks of ointment lubrication before correction of the ectropion if there is conjunctival thickening. The lubrication eliminates some of the roughness of the conjunctival mucosa that will be against the eye again.

To complete a lateral tarsal strip procedure, you will:
- Perform a lateral canthotomy
- Perform a cantholysis
- Form the strip
- Shorten the strip
- Reattach the strip
- Trim redundant anterior lamella
- Close the canthotomy

The steps of the tarsal strip procedure are:

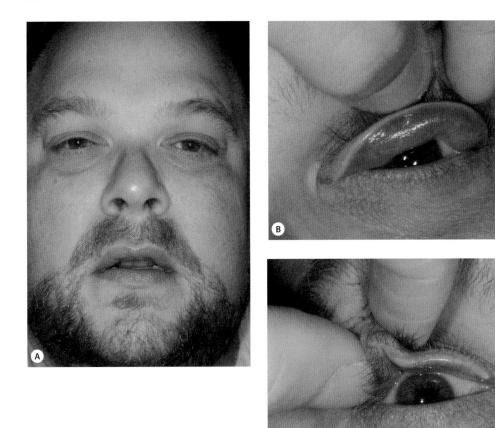

Figure 3-8 Floppy eyelid syndrome. (**A**) Overweight man complaining of eye irritation. (**B**) Note how easily you can pull the lax upper eyelid away from globe. The conjunctiva is erythematous. (**C**) The redundant upper eyelid can be easily folded on itself.

1. Prepare the patient
   A. Instill topical anesthetic drops.
   B. Inject a *local anesthesic* with epinephrine into
      (1) The lateral canthal skin.
      (2) On the inner aspect of the orbital rim against the bone.
      (3) The lateral third of the lower lid skin and conjunctiva (Figure 3-9, A).
2. Perform a lateral canthotomy
   A. Perform a *lateral canthotomy* using the Colorado microdissection needle or Westcott scissors. In most cases, I use the needle for this portion.
   B. Cautery may be necessary to stop the small amount of bleeding if you use scissors.
   C. Take a few extra seconds to dissect through the orbicularis overlying the lateral orbital rim to actually visualize the periosteum. This will make reattachment of the strip much easier. Do not cut the periosteum off the bone (Figure 3-9, B).
3. Perform a cantholysis
   A. Cut the lower limb of the lateral canthal tendon off the inferior orbital rim. This maneuver is known as a *cantholysis*.
   B. Pull the lateral aspect of the lid margin laterally and toward the ceiling of the operating room. You will notice that the eyelid does not pull away much from

the rim. Using Westcott scissors or the needle, identify the fibrous tissues holding the eyelid on the rim. A *strumming action* across the tissue will help you to find the taut tissues to be cut.
   C. As you cut these tissues, *the lid should release from the rim.* Although we say we are cutting the lower limb of the lateral canthal tendon, we are also cutting some of the septum and the lower eyelid retractors that attach to the tendon at the lateral canthus.
   D. Make your goal to complete the cantholysis in one or two cuts. Some bleeding usually occurs with each cut (Figure 3-9, C and D). For the first several procedures, you will want to use the Westcott scissors for this. After you get the strumming idea, you may want to do the canthotomy and cantholysis with the microdissection needle. Strumming is a little more difficult.
4. Form the strip
   A. Split the anterior and posterior lamellae.
      (1) Form a tarsal strip by splitting the anterior lamellae off the posterior lamellae for approximately 5 mm (you will learn to estimate the appropriate amount) (Figure 3-9, E).
      (2) Slide a Westcott scissors between the tarsal plate and the orbicularis muscle. Skin, muscle, and lashes are freed from the tarsus.

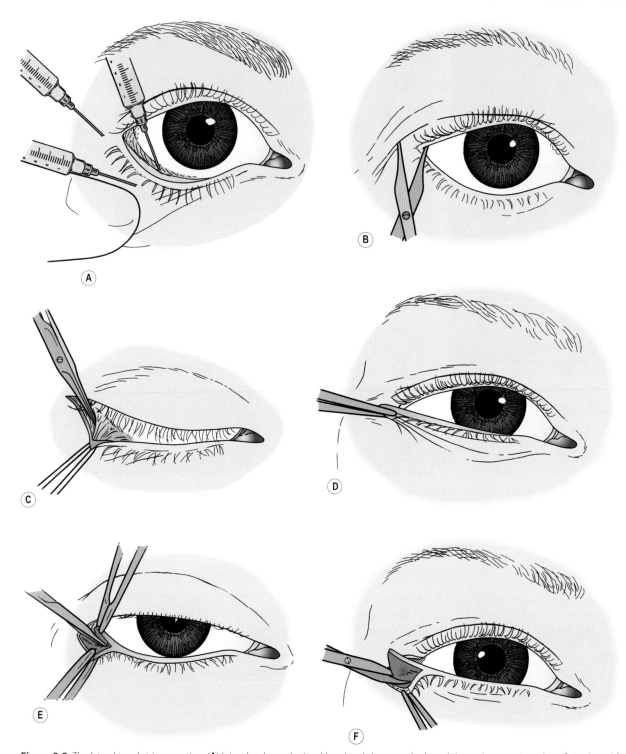

Figure 3-9 The lateral tarsal strip operation. (**A**) Inject local anesthetic with epinephrine over the lateral rim periosteum, into the inferior lateral fornix, and into the lateral lower lid skin. (**B**) Make a small lateral canthotomy, but deep enough to extend to the rim. (**C**) Strum the tissues and perform a lateral cantholysis, freeing the eyelid from the attachments to the rim. (**D**) The eyelid should release laterally. (**E**) Form the strip: split the anterior and posterior lamellae. (**F**) Form the strip: separate the inferior margin of the tarsus from the conjunctiva and lower lid retractors. (**G**) Form the strip: remove the conjunctival epithelium from the posterior tarsus and the margin of the lid. (**H**) Estimate the amount of eyelid to be shortened and trim the excess off the strip. (**I**) Reattach the strip to the inner aspect of the periosteum using a 4-0 Vicryl suture on a P-2 needle. (**J**) Note that the strip is on the inner aspect of the rim. (**K**) Excise the lashes and redundant anterior lamella. (**L**) Close the canthotomy with two or three absorbable sutures.

(3) Make sure that the plane of the scissors blades is *parallel to the plane of the tarsus.*

B. Cut along the inferior margin of the tarsus.

   (1) *Cauterize* along the inferior margin of the tarsus.

   (2) Then *cut* where you have just cauterized, freeing the tarsus from the conjunctiva and retractors.

Additional cautery is often necessary at this point (**Figure 3-9, F**).

C. Remove the skin and conjunctiva from the strip.

   (1) *Denude the conjunctival epithelium* off the posterior surface of the tarsal plate using a no. 15 blade.

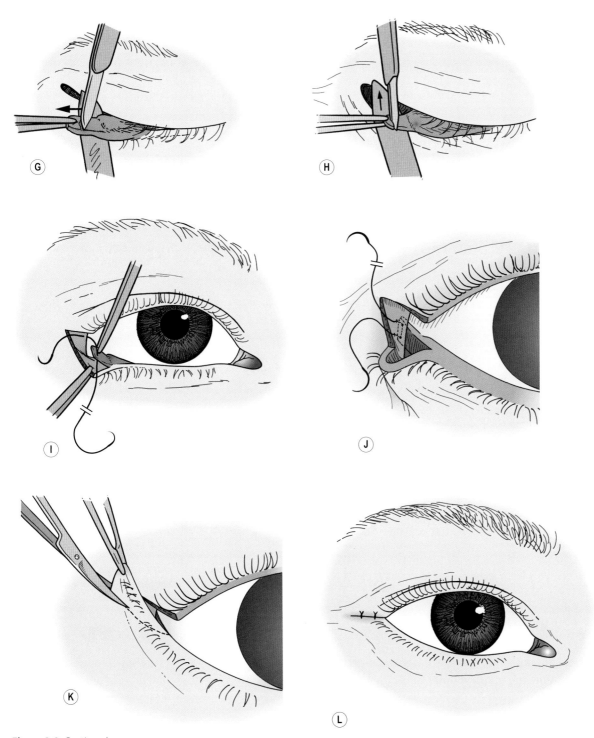

Figure 3-9 Continued.

(2) *Cut the skin off the lid margin* using Westcott scissors.

(3) The strip is now complete (Figure 3-9, G).

5. Shorten the strip
   A. Pull the tarsal strip to the periosteum and estimate the *amount of tarsus to be shortened.* This amount should be *conservative.* In some cases, no removal is necessary (Figure 3-9, H).

6. Reattach the strip
   A. Reattach the strip to the inner aspect of the lateral orbital rim with a double-armed 4-0 Mersilene suture on a P-2 half-circle needle. Use moderate tightness and slight superior placement of the lateral canthal tendon. Remember the precaution about the patient with hemiproptosis, in whom lid tightening can exacerbate lid retraction.

(1) This particular step is difficult for surgeons learning the lateral tarsal strip operation. It is made much easier by cleaning the soft tissues off the periosteum well during the canthotomy as explained above.

(2) Remember: do not clean the periosteum off the bone. If you do, there will be no way to suture the tarsal strip to the bone.

(3) Pass the double-armed 4-0 Mersilene suture (Ethicon 1779G), entering from the anterior surface at the upper third of the strip. Next pass the same needle from the posterior surface of the strip, at the inferior third of the strip. Use the same needle to pass the inferior bite of the periosteum.

(4) *Load the needle as far back as possible* while staying on the flat part of the needle. *Back the needle into the wound*, keeping the needle tip pointed toward the ceiling. It will help to push any orbital fat away from the rim. *Rotate the needle through the periosteum.* Do not move your hand up toward the ceiling, just rotate. Do not try to push the needle into the bone.

    a) If you have trouble passing the suture, make sure that you are seeing the periosteum well. If necessary, clean the periosteum again by scraping the rim with a Freer elevator.

    b) Sometimes it can be helpful to have an assistant use Tyrell skin hooks to pull the wound open.

    c) A Freer elevator can be used to retract the orbital tissues away from the rim.

    d) This step takes practice, but after several tries with an emphasis on the technique of rotating the suture, it will be easy and you won't need any help with retraction.

(5) Have a Paufique forceps handy to grasp the needle and rotate it out of the wound. Use moderate tightness and slight superior placement of the lateral canthal tendon.

(6) The appropriate point to reattach the strip is immediately inferior to the intact superior crus of the lateral canthal tendon. You will find that this recreates the slope of the eyelid naturally.

(7) Repeat the suture pass with the superior arm of the suture. Pull both arms out of the wound and watch the strip insert itself on the inner aspect of the rim (Figure 3-9, I).

B. Once you have placed the sutures, they can be *temporarily tied and the tension of the eyelid can be checked.* When you pull the lower lid off the eye, there should be minimal movement of the eyelid. This is a good time to remind you not to overtighten the eyelid in a patient with hemiproptosis.

C. *Be conservative.* If the eyelid is too lax, a little more tarsus can be trimmed and the sutures can be repassed.

D. Once the tension is correct, tie the sutures (Figure 3-9, J).

7. Trim redundant anterior lamella

A. *Trim redundant anterior lamella* including eyelashes. I try to excise enough anterior lamellar tissue so that lashes do not extend into the lateral canthus (Figure 3-9, K).

8. Close the canthotomy

A. If you have separated the anterior lamella from the tarsus more medially than necessary, use a single suture to reattach the separated anterior lamella to the tarsal plate. If you estimate the amount of lamellar split correctly, this step is not necessary.

B. The usual skin closure is with interrupted 5-0 fast absorbing sutures. Use a minimal number of sutures. Usually two interrupted sutures are passed in the skin beyond the lateral canthus to close the canthotomy.

    (1) Do not pull the upper lid down (creating "hooding") by putting too many sutures in the canthotomy closure.

    (2) The canthotomy will almost close itself with the natural blinking so don't be concerned if the wound gapes a bit (Figure 3-9, L). Some surgeons add an extra intermarginal suture through the meibomian glands of the upper and lower eyelid margin at the most lateral extent of the wound. This helps to "tuck" in the relatively longer upper eyelid.

C. At the conclusion of the lateral tarsal strip operation, the lower lid should be drawn up tightly with the lateral canthal height overcorrected.

9. Provide instructions for postoperative care

A. Postoperative care after the lateral tarsal strip procedure is routine—topical antibiotic ointment, no patch. Ice for 48 hours then warm, wet compresses for a few days as needed.

Discontinue use of the antibiotic ointment after 1 week. If you have corrected a severe ectropion, you will notice that the lower eyelashes will remain pointed upward for a few weeks postoperatively but will eventually return to a normal position. In the past, we used two single armed 4-0 Vicryl sutures at the lateral orbital rim. This occasionally caused a sterile suture granuloma which required debridement. The permanent suture avoids this problem. The double-armed suture positions the lid against the eye better than the single-armed technique (Box 3-1).

Review the steps of the lateral tarsal strip operation and commit them to memory. You will use them over and over again.

The pentagonal wedge resection

An alternative but less appropriate way to tighten a lower lid to correct ectropion is the traditional *wedge resection* of the lid margin. A pentagonal wedge of eyelid is excised, usually at the junction of the lateral one third and medial two thirds of the eyelid. *There are several advantages of the lateral tarsal strip operation over the pentagonal wedge resection of the eyelid in patients with involutional ectropion.* Remember that the pathologic problem is at the lateral canthal tendon. In an older patient, the lateral canthus is often blunted or rounded as a result of stretching of the lateral canthal tendon. Performing a lateral tarsal strip operation recreates the lateral canthus and pulls the lid laterally into the natural position. This lengthens the palpebral aperture. The tarsal strip sharpens the lateral canthal angle. The pentagonal wedge resection does the opposite. It shortens the palpebral aperture and blunts the lateral canthal angle more. The pentagonal wedge resection requires precise alignment and reconstruction of the lid margin. The lateral tarsal strip operation requires no lid margin sutures and is somewhat simpler.

Box 3-1

The Lateral Tarsal Strip Operation

Prepare the patient

- Use local anesthesia

Perform a lateral canthotomy

- Clean the soft tissue off the periosteum

Perform a lateral cantholysis

- Strum and cut the lower crus
- The lid should "release" from the rim

Form the strip

- Split the anterior and posterior lamellae
- Cut along the inferior margin of the tarsus
- Remove the skin and conjunctiva from the strip

Shorten the strip

- Be conservative

Reattach the strip

- Use a double-armed 4-0 Mersilene suture on a P-2 needle
- Remember to "back" the needle into the wound and rotate through the periorbita into position

Trim redundant anterior lamella

Close the canthotomy

- Consider reattaching the anterior lamella to the tarsus
- Use a minimal closure to prevent "hooding" of the upper lid (5-0 fast absorbing gut)

The pentagonal wedge resection of the upper eyelid is *the treatment for floppy eyelid syndrome*. Protecting the eye with a fox shield at night for a few weeks is a good test to see if lid tightening will improve the irritation. If use of the shield is successful, some patients may choose to continue with its use. Most patients proceed with upper eyelid resection. A generous amount of the upper lid is removed at the junction of the lateral one third and medial two thirds of the upper eyelid. The exact amount varies from patient to patient, but 10 mm or more is a good place to start. Remember, the lengthened lower eyelid in involutional ectropion is caused by tendon laxity, making the lateral tarsal strip operation an appropriate technique to shorten the eyelid. In floppy eyelid syndrome, the tarsal plate is lengthened. Consequently, a pentagonal wedge resection of the tarsus and lid margin is appropriate. Usually only upper eyelid shortening is necessary. The pentagonal wedge resection technique is described in Chapter 13 (see Figure 13-8).

The medial spindle operation

If you have determined preoperatively that a lateral tarsal strip operation alone will not reposition the punctum perfectly into the tear lake, perform the *medial spindle operation* before starting the lateral tarsal strip procedure. The medial spindle operation involves excision of a diamond of conjunctiva inferior to the lower punctum and closure with a suture, causing mechanical inversion of the punctum.

The medial spindle operation includes:

- Excision of a diamond of conjunctiva inferior to the lower punctum
- Closure of the conjunctiva to provide inversion of the punctum

The steps of the medial spindle operation are:

1. Prepare the patient
   A. Instill topical anesthetic drops.
   B. Inject local anesthetic into the inferior fornix of the medial conjunctiva.
   C. Inject local anesthetic under the skin at the orbital rim inferior to the punctum.
2. Excise a diamond of conjunctiva inferior to the lower punctum
   A. Place a no. 1 Bowman probe into the canaliculus and evert the lid margin.
      (1) Excise a "diamond" *of conjunctiva* (and theoretically lower eyelid retractors) inferior to the punctum and the tarsal plate (3–4 mm by 3–4 mm).
      (2) The diamond-shaped excision can be made by grasping the conjunctiva with a Paufique forceps and using Westcott scissors to excise a V of conjunctiva inferiorly. A similar V of conjunctiva is cut superiorly so the two incisions form a diamond (Figure 3-10, A). The excision of conjunctiva will be closed vertically, shortening the posterior lamella and turning the punctum inward.
      (3) Take care not to cut the vertical portion of the canaliculus when performing the excision.
3. Close the conjunctiva to provide inversion of the punctum
   A. Use a double-armed *5-0 chromic suture* (Ethicon 792 G-3 needle double-armed) to close the diamond, incorporating a pass through the lower lid retractors in the center of the diamond excision. (You will not always be able to recognize retractors.)
   B. Next, pass the two arms of the suture backhanded through the apex of the diamond adjacent to the punctum. This part of the operation theoretically advances the lower lid retractors to the top of the diamond.
   C. The remainder of the closure involves collapsing the diamond and passing the sutures out through the eyelid. Pass each suture arm through the inferior apex of the diamond and continue the full-thickness pass through the lid, exiting at the junction of the eyelid and cheek skin. The suture pass can be visualized as a *spiral* if viewed laterally (Figure 3-10, B). The conjunctival suture passes close to the posterior lamella, resulting in posterior lamellar shortening. The full-thickness pass of the suture through the eyelid, emerging inferiorly, causes a mechanical inversion of the punctum. A significant mechanical inversion of the punctum will occur when the sutures are pulled tightly on the skin side of the eyelid.
4. Do a lateral tarsal strip operation (usually)
   A. Cut the needles of the spindle suture off and clamp the suture ends out of the way. If a lateral tarsal strip operation is also being done (as is usually the case), it should be performed at this point.
   B. The medial spindle suture should be tied after the strip is sewn into position (Figure 3-10, C). The amount of inversion can be titrated by tying the

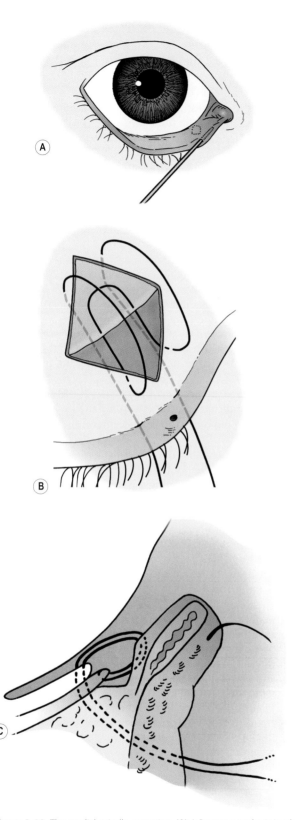

Figure 3-10 The medial spindle operation. (**A**) A Bowman probe is in place. Excise a diamond of conjunctiva and lower lid retractors. (**B**) The spiral suture. Pass sutures through the retractors, through the superior edge of the diamond, through the inferior edge of the diamond, and finally full thickness through the eyelid. Use a double-armed 5-0 chromic suture. (**C**) Tie the sutures to provide a slight inversion of the punctum (lateral view).

suture with more or less tension. At the conclusion of the medial spindle procedure, a *slight overcorrection (inversion) is desired.*

5. Provide postoperative care
   A. No special care is required after the medial spindle operation.
   B. The chromic suture will fall out on its own in approximately 7 days.
   C. The overcorrection will reduce spontaneously, leaving the punctum in its normal position. Overcorrection is rare, but undercorrection can occur, leaving the punctum vertical. If the patient is asymptomatic, no reoperation is required.

Remember that the medial spindle operation must be performed before the eyelid is tightened with a lateral tarsal strip operation. Once the lateral tarsal strip sutures are tied, the medial eyelid cannot be everted to perform the medial spindle operation (Box 3-2).

Treatment of paralytic lower eyelid ectropion

The treatment of paralytic ectropion is essentially the same as that for involutional ectropion. In paralytic ectropion, more tightening is usually necessary. The medial spindle operation is often used as well. An additional anchoring suture can be used to lift the cheek laterally. Read Chapter 9 before you perform a lateral tarsal strip operation on a patient with a paralytic ectropion because alternative or additional procedures may be required.

Treatment of cicatricial ectropion

Full-thickness skin grafting

Cicatricial ectropion is caused by a shortage of the anterior lamella. Lengthening of the anterior lamella, usually with a full-thickness skin graft, returns the scarred lid to normal position (Figure 3-11). Frequently, a lateral tarsal strip operation is used in conjunction with a full-thickness skin graft. The procedure begins with cutting the scar tissue in the anterior lamella to allow the posterior lamella of the eyelid to return to its normal position. The lateral tarsal strip operation is performed next. Lastly, a full-thickness skin graft is harvested and sewn into the defect created by cutting the scar

---

Box 3-2

The Medial Spindle Operation

Prepare the patient

- Instill a topical anesthetic
- Inject local anesthetic into the conjunctiva and skin on the medial one third of the lid

Excise a diamond of conjunctiva

- Evert the lid margin with a Bowman probe
- Excise a diamond of conjunctiva and lower lid retractors

Close the diamond

- Pass double-armed 5-0 chromic suture through the lower lid retractors, then apex near the punctum, then the apex inferiorly, and out full thickness through the lid

Do a lateral tarsal strip operation for most patients

- Tie the sutures to invert the punctum slightly

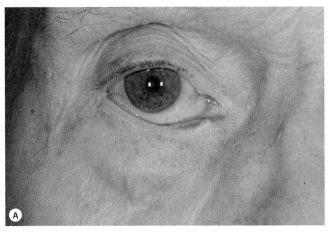
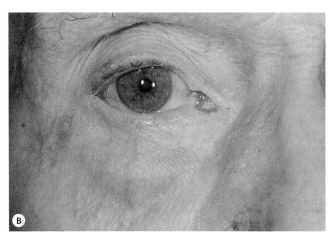

Figure 3-11 Repair of cicatricial ectropion using a full-thickness skin graft. (**A**) The punctum and medial lid are pulled away from the eye. (**B**) A full-thickness skin graft, harvested from the preauricular area, has been used to restore the length of the anterior lamella. Note the excellent tissue match and normal position of the punctum. No lower eyelid tightening was performed in this case since ectropion was medial and no laxity was present.

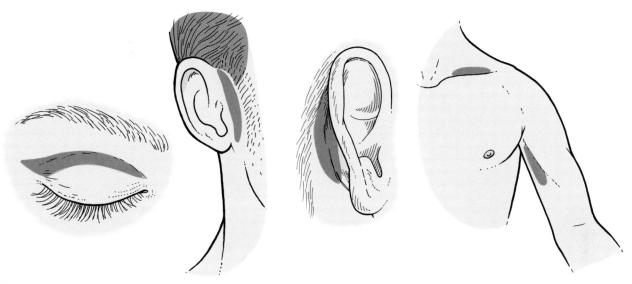

Figure 3-12 Donor sites for full-thickness skin grafting. In order of preference: upper eyelid, preauricular, retroauricular, supraclavicular, and upper arm.

tissue. Similar principles apply to the treatment of cicatricial ectropion of the upper eyelid.

Several *donor sites for full-thickness skin grafts* are available. Remember, full-thickness skin harvesting means that you will take all the layers of the skin from the donor site down to the subcutaneous fat. The donor site will require closure, and any hair will be transferred with the graft.

The eyelid skin is the thinnest skin in the body so only other eyelid skin is an exact match. Always consider using *redundant upper eyelid* skin as a donor. Sometimes you can use extra tissue from both upper eyelids to get enough skin. The most practical choice is the *preauricular skin*. You might be surprised at the amount of skin available there. In the average man, you can harvest a piece of skin 15 mm by 40 mm between the sideburn whiskers and the tragus, often just the right amount and shape for repair of lower eyelid cicatricial ectropion. The *retroauricular area* is the next best site. The skin is thin and is a good color match. You can harvest a wider piece of skin, but working behind the ear is difficult, and patients are bothered by the sutures postoperatively. Other sites include the supraclavicular area, inner

upper arm, inguinal area, or the inframammary fold. These sites do not provide a good match and are used only if no better choice is available (Figure 3-12).

Harvesting a split-thickness skin graft leaves some of the dermis so that the donor site heals spontaneously, and no hair is transferred. Larger areas of split-thickness skin can be harvested because no closure is required. The color match is poor, and shrinkage is high, making split-thickness grafting a poor choice for most repairs of cicatricial ectropion.

Full-thickness skin grafting for cicatricial ectropion requires that you:

- Mark the skin for incision
- Release the cicatricial forces
- Harvest the full-thickness skin graft
- Suture the full-thickness skin graft in place

The steps of full-thickness skin grafting for cicatricial ectropion are:

1. Mark the skin for incision
    A. Instill topical anesthetic drops.

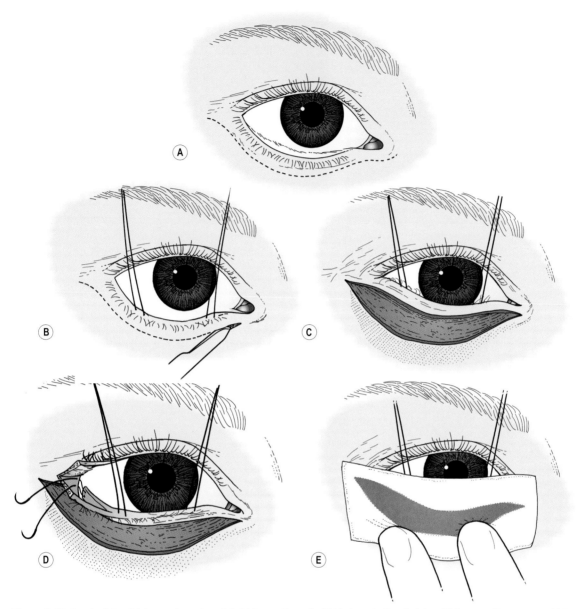

Figure 3-13 Repair of cicatricial ectropion using a full-thickness skin graft. (**A**) Mark a subciliary incision. (**B**) Pass two Frost sutures. Make a subciliary incision with a no. 15 blade or Colorado needle. Release the scar tissue to allow the lid to return to the normal position. (**C, D**) Tighten the lower lid using a lateral tarsal strip type of procedure. (**E**) Make a template by pressing a piece of Gelfoam against the wound. (**F, G**) Harvest a full-thickness skin graft from the preauricular or retroauricular area and sew the graft in place. (**H**) Tie a bolster in place to immobilize the graft. Place a tight eye patch over the eye for 1 week.

B. Identify the cicatricial bands to be cut.
   (1) For diffuse cicatricial skin changes, mark a *subciliary incision* that extends approximately 5 mm horizontally beyond the canthi (or any involved cicatricial change) (Figure 3-13, A).
   (2) If a localized area of scar tissue exists, mark a skin incision to release this scar tissue (don't forget to extend beyond the scar tissue).
C. Inject local anesthetic with epinephrine into the area of the planned incision.
D. The patient is prepped and draped while you scrub.
2. Release the cicatricial forces
  A. Place two 4-0 silk sutures in the lid margin and clamp them to the drape to stabilize the lid in a superior direction.

B. *Make a subciliary incision* with a no. 15 blade (Figure 3-13, B and C).
   (1) You will notice that the skin edges separate as the incision is made.
C. *Use a blade or the Westcott scissors to continue sharp dissection of the scar tissue* until the eyelid margin easily returns to its normal position apposing the globe. Usually you will cut skin, muscle, and scar tissue. You will know when you are finished because the plane of dissection will start to go deep to the skin and muscle without any further release of the eyelid.
D. Next perform a *lateral tarsal strip procedure*.
   (1) This will help to prevent the lid from developing ectropion again as the skin graft shrinks with healing.

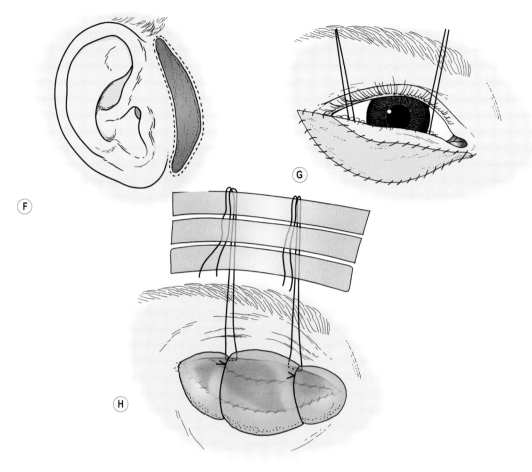

Figure 3-13 Continued.

(2) Remember to reattach the strip to the lateral orbital rim slightly high to overcorrect the height at the lateral canthus (Figure 3-13, D).

3. Harvest the full-thickness skin graft
   A. Draw a *template* indicating the size of the defect to be repaired.
      (1) The template can be made by tracing the area onto a piece of the clear plastic surgical drape.
      (2) A clever alternative method is to use a piece of Gelfoam pressed into the surgical defect. Blood in the defect stains the Gelfoam in the precise size and shape of the defect.
   B. The template is then cut, and its outline is transferred onto the skin of the preauricular area or other donor site. The *graft should be slightly oversized.* By tracing the proposed graft size on the outside of the template, some oversizing is accomplished (Figure 3-13, E).

4. Harvest the full-thickness skin graft
   A. Use *a no. 15 blade to cut full thickness through the skin* along the mark of the template.
   B. Use a *Westcott scissors to separate the subcutaneous fat from the dermis* of the skin. Try to leave as little "yellow" on the dermis as possible.
   C. *Close the donor bed* using subcutaneous interrupted 4-0 Vicryl or PDS sutures. Generally, little or no undermining is required.
   D. Close the skin with a running 5-0 Prolene suture.

5. Suture the graft into place
   A. Before transferring the graft, remove any remaining fat from the posterior surface of the graft. In most cases, you will want the thinnest graft possible.
   B. Suture the skin graft into position using an absorbable skin suture, usually 5-0 fast absorbing gut (Figure 3-13, F and G).
   C. Place topical antibiotic ointment over the graft.
   D. No pie-crusting is necessary.
   E. Tape the two 4-0 silk lid margin sutures to the forehead to place the graft on stretch.
   F. Use four 4-0 silk sutures at the perimeter of the graft to tie a bolster into position over the graft. Tape a patch over the eye. For effective healing, the graft must not move (Figure 3-13, H).

No postoperative oral antibiotics are prescribed. The patch and bolster are removed after 1 week. Postoperatively, the graft often looks dark, and the lower lid position appears overcorrected. With time, the normal color of the full-thickness skin graft returns and the lid assumes a normal position.

Start massage of the lid after 2 weeks to help prevent shrinkage of the graft. Full-thickness grafts in the periocular area rarely fail. Color and texture are usually good after healing over 3–4 months. Over a period of many years, repeat grafting may be required if the cicatricial process continues.

Checkpoint

At this point you should:

- Memorize the steps of the lateral tarsal strip and medial spindle
- Understand the treatment of paralytic ectropion and cicatricial ectropion
- Know the donor sites for full-thickness skin grafting of the eyelid
- Be able to compare full-thickness grafting to split-thickness skin grafting
- Know the advantages of a lateral tarsal strip procedure over a pentagonal wedge resection for most types of ectropion (Box 3-3)

Box 3-3

Full-Thickness Skin Grafting for Cicatricial Ectropion

Identify the cicatricial forces

- Mark a subciliary incision
- Use topical and local anesthetics

Release the cicatricial forces

- Use 4-0 silk to stabilize the lid margin
- Make a subciliary incision to release scarring
- Continue sharp dissection until the posterior lamella returns to normal position
- Consider horizontal eyelid tightening with a lateral tarsal strip procedure

Harvest the full-thickness skin graft

- Draw a template outlining the size and shape of the graft
- Transfer the template to the donor site
- Harvest and thin the graft
- Cauterize and close the donor site

Suture the graft into position

- Use absorbable skin sutures
- Use 4-0 silk sutures to tie a bolster in place
- Tape a patch over the eye

Major points

Ectropion of the eyelid is said to occur when the eyelid margin is everted off the eyeball.

Three types of ectropion occur:

- Involutional
- Cicatricial
- Paralytic

Involutional ectropion is the most commonly seen form of ectropion. Lower lid laxity is the cause of the involutional ectropion. Lower lid laxity often accompanies cicatricial and paralytic ectropion as well.

Cicatricial ectropion is caused by shortening of the anterior lamella.

Paralytic ectropion is caused by a loss of orbicularis muscle tone associated with facial nerve paralysis.

The history and physical examination will determine the etiology and best treatment of the ectropion.

Involutional ectropion is treated with lower lid tightening using the lateral tarsal strip operation.

- The lateral tarsal strip operation is the most useful operation that you can learn in oculoplastic surgery

- The medial spindle operation is a helpful adjunct to the lateral tarsal strip operation for correcting punctal eversion

Cicatricial ectropion is treated with full-thickness skin grafting, often in conjunction with the lateral tarsal strip procedure.

Paralytic ectropion is treated with a lateral tarsal strip operation.

- Other considerations, including treatment of corneal exposure and brow ptosis, are necessary in the treatment of facial nerve palsy

The eversion of the upper eyelid that occurs in floppy eyelid syndrome is caused by extreme upper eyelid laxity.

- Patients are usually obese men
- Obstructive sleep apnea is associated with this syndrome
- Treatment is a generous pentagonal wedge resection of the lateral upper eyelid

Suggested reading

1. American Academy of Ophthalmology: *Basic and clinical science course: orbit, eyelids, and lacrimal system*, sect. 7, pp. 195–201, San Francisco: The American Academy of Ophthalmology, 2006/2007.

2. Albert DM, Lucarelli MJ: Ectropion. In *Clinical atlas of procedures in ophthalmic surgery*, pp. 251–256, Chicago: AMA Press, 2004.

3. Anderson RL, Gordy DD: The tarsal strip procedure. *Arch Ophthalmol* 97:2192–2196, 1979.

4. Culbertson WW, Ostler HB: The floppy eyelid syndrome. *Am J Ophthalmol* 92(4):568–575, 1981.

5. Dutton JJ: Ectropion. In *Atlas of ophthalmic surgery*, vol. 2, pp. 94–113, St Louis: Mosby Year Book, Inc., 1992.

6. Dutton JJ: Surgical management of floppy eyelid syndrome. *Am J Ophthalmol* 99(5):557–560, 1985.

7. Hawes MJ: Cicatricial ectropion. In Levine MR, ed. *Manual of oculoplastic surgery*, 3rd edn, pp. 173–179, Boston: Butterworth-Heinemann, 2003.

8. Jordan DR, Anderson RL: The lateral tarsal strip revisited: the enhanced tarsal strip. *Arch Ophthalmol* 107:604–606, 1989.

9. McNab AA: The eye and sleep. *Clin Exp Ophthalmol* 33(2):117–125, 2005.

10. Nerad J: Diagnosis and treatment of ectropion. In *The requisites—Oculoplastic surgery*, pp. 71–88. St Louis: Mosby, 2001.

11. Nerad JA: Eyelid causes of tearing. In Bosniak S, ed. *Principles and practice of ophthalmic plastic and reconstructive surgery*, vol. 2, Philadelphia: WB Saunders, 1996.

12. Nerad JA: Eyelid malpositions. In Linberg JV, ed. *Contemporary issues in ophthalmology: lacrimal surgery*, ch. 4, pp. 62-89, New York: Churchill Livingstone, 1988.

13. Nerad JA, Carter KD, Alford MA: Ectropion. In *Rapid diagnosis in ophthalmology—oculoplastic and reconstructive surgery*, pp. 80–91, Philadelphia: Mosby Elsevier, 2008.

14. Nowinski TS, Anderson RL: The medial spindle procedure for involutional medial ectropion. *Arch Ophthalmol* 103(11):1750–1753, 1985.

15. Penne, Robert B: Ectropion. In *Color atlas & synopsis of clinical ophthalmology: oculoplastics*, pp. 62–69, New York: McGraw-Hill, 2003.

16. Robinson FO, Collin JRO: Ectropion. In Yanoff M, Duker J, eds. *Ophthalmology*, pp. 676–683, Mosby, 2004.

17. Schlotzer-Schrehardt U, Stojkovic M, Hofmann-Rummelt C et al: The pathogenesis of floppy eyelid syndrome: involvement of matrix metalloproteinases in elastic fiber degradation. *Ophthalmology* 112(4):694–704, 2005.

18. Swartz NG, Murphy M, Cohen MS: Lower eyelid retraction and cicatricial ectropion. In Bosniak S, ed. *Principles and practice of ophthalmic plastic and reconstructive surgery*, vol. 1, ch. 40, pp. 438–451, Philadelphia: WB Saunders, 1996.

19. Tse DT: Involutional ectropion repair. In Levine MR, ed. *Manual of oculoplastic surgery*, 3rd edn, pp. 163–172, Boston: Butterworth-Heinemann, 2003.

20. Wesley RE: Ectropion repair. In McCord CD, Tanenbaum M, Nunery WR, eds. *Oculoplastic surgery*, 3rd edn, ch. 9, pp. 249–261, New York: Raven Press, 1995.

21. Goldberg et al: Ectropion repair. In Wobig JL, Dailey RA, eds. *Oculofacial plastic surgery: face, lacrimal system, and orbit*, pp. 97–102, New York: Thieme, 2004.

22. Woog JJ: Obstructive sleep apnea and the floppy eyelid syndrome. *Am J Ophthalmol* 110(3):314–316, 1990.

The Diagnosis and Treatment of Entropion

Introduction

Entropion of the eyelid occurs when the *lid margin inverts* or turns against the eyeball. The keratinized skin of the eyelid margin and eyelashes rub against the cornea and conjunctiva, causing irritation. Unlike with ectropion, the irritation is troublesome enough so that most patients seek medical treatment early. Entropion is common, but less common than ectropion of the lids.

There are four types of entropion (Box 4-1). A congenital form of entropion exists, but it is so rare that it is hardly worth mentioning.

We will discuss the *anatomy* of the lower eyelid as it relates to the causes of entropion in some detail. The two most important causes of involutional entropion are *horizontal lid laxity* and *disinsertion* or *laxity of the lower eyelid retractors*. As discussed in Chapter 3, any horizontal laxity of the eyelid contributes to instability. Without the normal tension of the lower eyelid retractors pulling the lower edge of the tarsus inferiorly and posteriorly, the eyelid may invert. The concepts of *anterior* and *posterior lamellar shortening* are also important in the discussion of entropion. Scarring of the posterior lamella, conjunctiva, and tarsus causes a cicatricial entropion.

The *history and physical examination* will show the etiology of entropion to be either lax tissues (seen with involutional and spastic entropion types) or shortening of the posterior lamellar tissues (seen with cicatricial and marginal entropion types). Lower eyelid entropion is most commonly involutional. The symptoms of irritation are *intermittent*, and you will see lower eyelid horizontal laxity. Upper eyelid entropion is always cicatricial and is a source of *constant* irritation. When you evert the lid, you will see cicatricial changes. Cicatricial forms of lower lid entropion do occur, so it is important to look for scarring of the posterior lamella

in the lower lid also. Spastic entropion occurs when the eye is irritated and inflamed. Marginal entropion is often perceived by the patient as an eyelash problem.

Involutional entropion is the most common type of entropion seen in the United States so you should be familiar with its management. The aim of surgical treatment is to restore the normal tension of the lower lid retractors and to correct any coexisting horizontal lid laxity. We will discuss the *retractor reinsertion operation* and the *lateral tarsal strip operation* to correct involutional entropion. Learn these operations well.

Cicatricial entropion is less common than involutional entropion. Trachoma is the "textbook" cause of posterior lamellar scarring that leads to cicatricial entropion. Trachoma is rarely seen in the United States. The typical patient with cicatricial entropion has severe conjunctival scarring with the eyelid margin inverted, causing skin and lashes to rub against the eye. In reality, the patient with the most commonly seen type of cicatricial entropion has a mild form, called *marginal entropion*. The eyelid margin is turned in slightly, bringing the lashes against the eye. We will spend a considerable amount of time covering marginal entropion in Chapter 5. The aim of treatment of all forms of cicatricial entropion is to restore the normal length of the posterior lamella using either incisions alone or incisions with grafts. The *tarsal fracture operation* is a great procedure to add to your list of competencies for repair of marginal entropion or mild degrees of cicatricial entropion of the lower eyelid. We will also talk about an upper eyelid everting incisional procedure called the terminal tarsal rotation operation. When the entropion is too severe for incisional lengthening, *mucous membrane grafts* are necessary. You should learn to recognize patients with severe entropion who will need the more advanced operations involving grafting. It is not likely that you will do many of these grafts.

Spastic entropion is an unusual form of eyelid entropion. You will occasionally see this form of entropion occurring with squeezing of the lids in association with ocular pain or inflammation, often after eye surgery. Frequently, the entropion resolves as the postoperative discomfort disappears. If corneal irritation is severe, treatment with *Quickert sutures* will return the lid to its normal position. Although you won't see many patients with spastic entropion, Quickert sutures are easy to learn and are an easy solution for spastic entropion.

Anatomic considerations

The normal eyelid margin

Understanding exactly how the eyelid sits against the eyeball is important for understanding cicatricial entropion. We take the eyelid margin for granted, but there is a very specific relationship between the mucosal tissues on the back of the lid and the keratinized skin on the lid margin. The next time you are performing a slit lamp examination, start to become familiar with this eyelid margin anatomy. The normal eyelid margin is flat, ending at right angles anteriorly and posteriorly to form a long thin rectangle of tissue (Figure 4-1). The most posterior aspect of the normal lid margin is the *mucocutaneous junction*. It is at this point that the mucosa of the palpebral conjunctiva stops and the keratinized skin of the eyelid margin begins. Look at several normal patients to see this junction. The next time you see a patient with cicatricial entropion, you may be able to appreciate the fact that the

mucocutaneous junction moves forward as the eyelid margin inverts (Box 4-2).

Just anterior to the mucocutaneous junction are the *meibomian gland orifices* extending out from the tarsal plate. Evert the eyelid during the slit lamp examination, and you will see the faint vertical lines of the meibomian glands visible in the tarsal plate. Anterior to the meibomian gland orifices is the *gray line*. Initially, this line was thought to result from the fusion of the anterior and posterior lamella. In reality, the gray line is a specialized muscle of the pretarsal orbicularis, known as the muscle of Riolan. The gray line is still used as a landmark to surgically separate the anterior and posterior lamella of the eyelid in some procedures. You will recall that posterior to the gray line is the posterior lamella (the tarsus and the conjunctiva). Anterior to the gray line is the anterior lamella (the skin and muscle). The *eyelashes* arise anterior to the gray line, usually in one or two irregular rows in the lower lid and three or four irregular rows in the upper lid. The eyelash follicles originate on the surface of the tarsal plate. Learn these subtle anatomic features of the eyelid. They are especially important when you are evaluating patients with mild cicatricial entropion or trichiasis. We will emphasize the changes that occur in the lid margin later in this chapter and more completely in Chapter 5.

The stable lower eyelid

Let's go over the anatomic factors that are important for understanding and treating entropion. Remind yourself of the layers of the eyelid inferior to the tarsal plate (see Figure 2-28). Starting at a point below the tarsus from anterior to posterior, the layers of the eyelid are:

- Skin
- Orbicularis muscle
- Septum
- Preaponeurotic fat (the landmark for the lower lid retractors)
- Retractors
- Conjunctiva

The lid margin remains normally apposed to the eye during eye movements through a combination of forces holding the lid in position. Watch the lid during the slit lamp examination as the eye moves up and down. You will see that the pretarsal eyelid and the eyelid margin move as a unit. *Remember that the pretarsal orbicularis is firmly adherent to the anterior surface of the tarsus, creating a block of tissue. The lid margin does not change its position relative to the eyeball.*

Several factors contribute to the stability of the lid. *In general, a tight lower eyelid, without horizontal lid laxity, is a stable lid. Laxity predisposes the lower lid to either ectropion or entropion, as we have seen in Chapter 3.* Think about what the lower eyelid retractors do. As the eye looks down, the

---

Box 4-1

Types of Entropion
- Involutional
- Spastic
- Cicatricial
- Marginal

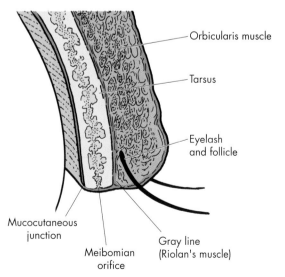

Mucocutaneous junction

Meibomian orifice

Gray line (Riolan's muscle)

Eyelash and follicle

Tarsus

Orbicularis muscle

Figure 4-1 Normal eyelid margin architecture. Note the position of the gray line, the meibomian glands, and the mucocutaneous junction.

Box 4-2

Eyelid Margin Architecture
- Mucocutaneous junction
- Meibomian gland orifices
- Gray line
- Eyelashes

---

lower lid retractors pull the lower eyelid downward. If the retractors did not work in synchrony with the eyeball, the eyelid would block the pupil in downgaze. This synchronous movement results from the connection of the capsulopalpebral fascia portion of the lower eyelid retractors with the inferior rectus muscle.

The lower eyelid retractors also help to keep the eyelid margin in normal position. The retractors pull the lower margin of the tarsus inferiorly and posteriorly, in the direction of the pull of the inferior rectus muscle. This keeps the lower edge of the tarsal plate "tucked in" against the eye with the eyelid margin in the normal position. *Normal tension on the lower eyelid retractors is essential for maintaining a stable eyelid and preventing entropion* (Box 4-3).

In the normal eyelid, the anterior and posterior lamella both have enough redundancy and flexibility so that normal movement does not alter the position of the lid margin. There is no "pull" or cicatricial force turning the eyelid inward or outward.

Involutional entropion

Involutional entropion occurs only in the lower lid. Three anatomic factors play a role in involutional entropion:

- Laxity of lower eyelid retractors
- Horizontal lid eyelid laxity
- Overriding preseptal orbicularis muscle

Laxity of the lower lid retractors is the primary cause of involutional entropion (Figure 4-2). Lower lid horizontal laxity is usually present, making the lid unstable. *Laxity of the lower lid retractors* allows the inferior edge of the tarsus to rotate away from the eye. This allows the lid margin to invert (Figure 4-3). In many cases, the preseptal orbicularis muscle actually seems to "push" the lower eyelid margin inward. Variations of Figure 4-2 are shown in all texts discussing entropion. Make sure that you understand this figure.

For many years, enophthalmos was considered to be an etiologic factor in involutional entropion. Recently, this has been disproved. The presence of enophthalmos has been shown to be no different in age-matched patients with or without entropion.

As an aside, many older patients have the appearance of small eyes. This is caused by a narrowing of the eyelid aperture both vertically and horizontally. As the retractors relax with age, the position of the lower eyelid elevates a bit. This "upside-down ptosis" of the lower eyelid is common in elderly patients with entropion. The upper eyelid becomes

somewhat ptotic. The horizontal length of the palpebral aperture decreases and the canthi become rounded as the canthal tendons lengthen; this condition is known as *phimosis* of the aperture. Look for this in your elderly patients. It is an apparent, but unappreciated, feature of aging. When you lift the upper eyelids and recreate the sharp lateral canthal angle with a lid-tightening procedure, you will notice that the patient's eyes (and face) look younger.

Spastic entropion

Spastic entropion occurs when the eyelids are held in a closed or "guarded" position. The sustained "squinting" of the lower lid is the initiating force for the entropion. The

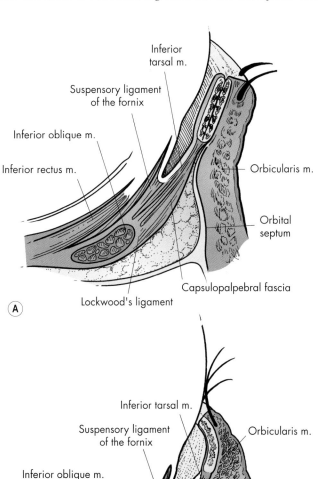

Figure 4-2 (**A**) Normal lower eyelid anatomy. The retractors pull the lower margin of the tarsus inferiorly and posteriorly, stabilizing the eyelid. (**B**) Involutional entropion: laxity of the lower lid retractors is the primary cause of involutional entropion.

most common situation for this reflex blepharospasm is after surgery, usually an anterior segment trauma repair or an extensive posterior segment procedure. The spasm or squeezing of the lid seems to push the lid margin against the eye. This condition most often occurs in patients who have predisposing factors to involutional entropion, such as horizontal laxity and lax lower lid retractors. The retractors cannot hold the lid in normal position against the forceful "overriding orbicularis" pushing the lid margin inward.

Cicatricial entropion

Cicatricial entropion is caused by shortening of the posterior lamella, which pulls the eyelid margin inward (Figure 4-4). Cicatricial entropion is common throughout the world, especially where trachoma is endemic. Cicatricial entropion is less common than involutional entropion, but it is still seen in the United States. Any problem that causes scarring of the conjunctiva may cause a cicatricial entropion (Box 4-4). Common causes include:

- Ocular cicatricial pemphigoid (OCP)
- Alkali burns
- Surgical or accidental trauma
- Recurrent chalazia or blepharitis
- Stevens–Johnson syndrome
- Trachoma

In most patients with cicatricial entropion, the conjunctival scarring is easy to see and the etiology is usually obvious (Figure 4-5). As I said earlier, all instances of upper lid entropion are cicatricial. There is no upper lid involutional entropion.

Marginal entropion

Patients with cicatricial entropion have eyelashes against the eye. The problem is classified as entropion, not trichiasis,

---

Box 4-4

Anatomic Factors Contributing to Involutional Entropion
- Laxity of lower lid retractors
- Horizontal lid laxity
- Overriding preseptal orbicularis muscle

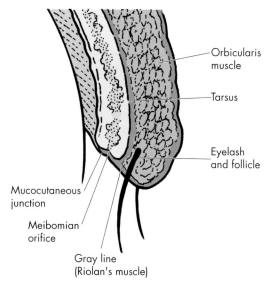

Orbicularis muscle

Tarsus

Eyelash and follicle

Mucocutaneous junction

Meibomian orifice

Gray line (Riolan's muscle)

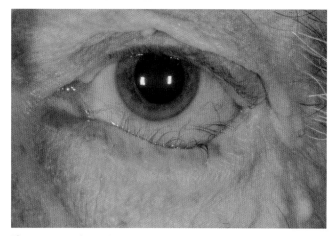

Figure 4-3 Involutional entropion. Lax lower eyelid retractors allow the lid margin to turn inward.

Figure 4-4 Cicatricial entropion. Note that the posterior lamellar shortening pulls the eyelid inward.

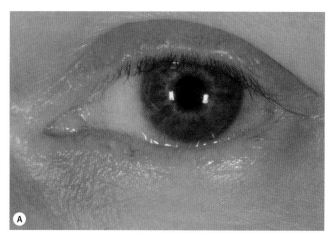

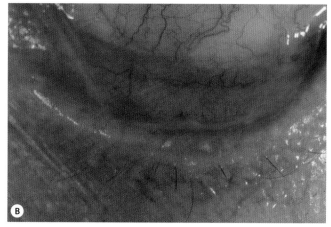

Figure 4-5 Mild cicatricial entropion caused by the Stevens–Johnson syndrome. (**A**) Note subtle inversion of eyelid margin. (**B**) Mild conjunctival scarring and shortening of the fornix are present. The scarring pulls the lid margin inward, causing the cicatricial entropion.

because the eyelid margin is obviously inverted. Most patients diagnosed with "trichiasis" have a subtle form of cicatricial entropion known as *marginal entropion*. Slit lamp examination of these patients shows that the lid margin is no longer a flat platform with well-defined right-angled anterior and posterior edges. The posterior angle of the lid margin has a *slightly rolled* appearance with the mucocutaneous junction being more anterior than normal. There may be subtle scarring or inflammation of the posterior surface of the conjunctiva and tarsus. This subtle shortening brings the eyelashes against the cornea. The diagnosis and management of marginal entropion will be discussed in the next chapter. This is an important concept, so don't ignore it.

Checkpoint

At this point you should:
· Understand the definition of entropion
· Be able to recognize entropion in a patient
· Know the normal anatomic appearance of the eyelid margin as seen with the slit lamp. This will be very important in understanding trichiasis
· Know the anatomic factors responsible for a stable eyelid
· Understand the anatomic factors responsible for
  — Involutional entropion
  — Cicatricial entropion

History

Patients with entropion complain of eye irritation. You may be able to identify the type of entropion based on the features of the irritation. *Intermittent symptoms suggest an involutional cause.* The patient often recognizes that the eyelid is inverting and causing the symptoms. The patient may have discovered that manual eversion of the eyelid temporarily improves the irritation. Occasionally, a patient will come to the office with tape on the cheek to prevent the involutional entropion. *Constant symptoms of irritation suggest a cicatricial cause.* Manual repositioning of the lid does not offer any relief because the lid immediately returns to its inverted position on release. The patient with cicatricial entropion may identify a specific onset of the entropion after an injury or infection.

Physical examination

Etiology of the entropion

Is the entropion cicatricial?

The goal of the eyelid examination in the patient with entropion is to determine the type of entropion and the most appropriate treatment. First, look to see if the lid margin is in the normal position. If the eyelid margin is inverted, the patient has entropion. Now ask yourself a few questions to determine the etiology of the entropion. Ask *Is the entropion cicatricial?* With your finger, return the inverted lid to its normal position. Is there resistance to placing the lid in the

normal position? See if it springs back to the inverted position when you release it. If cicatricial changes are present, it will not be easy to return the lid to its normal position. After you release the lid, it will return to the inverted position. Reposition the lid and observe the eyelid margin during the slit lamp examination to see where scar tissue might be causing the lid to pull inward. Evaluate the conjunctiva and tarsal plate for signs of shrinkage or scarring. You will usually be able to see some obvious conjunctival scarring that is the cause of the entropion (Figure 4-6).

If not cicatricial, the entropion must be involutional

With involutional entropion, you can return the lid to the normal position with your finger and it will remain there for a blink or two. If the entropion does not recur with a few blinks, ask the patient to squeeze the lids closed for a moment and the entropion will often return. If the history suggests episodic inversion of the eyelid, but none is present at the time of the examination, ask the patient to squeeze the lids tightly. Frequently the entropion will appear. Watch the patient blink normally. In some patients, you will notice the preseptal orbicularis muscle roll upward, starting to push the lid margin inward (the so-called "overriding preseptal orbicularis"). In some cases, it seems that laying the examination chair downward helps to elicit the entropion with forced eyelid closure.

There is no clinically reliable diagnostic sign that shows that the lower lid retractors are lax. Some texts describe a white line of retractors that is visible through the palpebral conjunctiva, signifying a "disinsertion" of the retractors. I have never been convinced that this sign is present. Often the lower eyelid rides above the lower limbus, suggesting some laxity of the lower eyelid retractors.

Planning the treatment of entropion

Involutional entropion: is there associated lower lid laxity?

The typical patient with lower lid involutional entropion is elderly and will have horizontal lower eyelid laxity associated. Once you have established that the entropion is

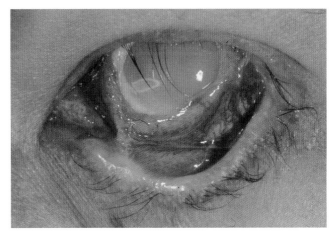

Figure 4-6 Cicatricial entropion. Note conjunctival scarring, caused by a chemical burn in this patient, causing the entropion. Note upper eyelashes turned against the cornea. The lower eyelid is being manually everted to demonstrate inferior fornix scarring.

involutional, check for horizontal lid laxity using the *eyelid distraction and eyelid snap tests* (explained in Chapter 3). Although the mainstay of surgical correction of lower lid involutional entropion is to tighten the lower lid retractors, any horizontal lid laxity should be corrected as well.

Cicatricial entropion: characterize the scar tissue

If the entropion is cicatricial, the scarring is usually obvious. The goal of the repair of cicatricial entropion is to restore the posterior lamella to its normal length. Think about how this might be done as you are assessing the scar tissue. Is the scarring localized or widespread? Is the contracture minimal or extensive? *The easiest way to evaluate the degree of scarring is to identify the position of the meibomian gland orifices.* Start evaluating the position of the meibomian glands in the least inverted part of the lid and follow them to the most inverted part. With severe cicatricial entropion, you will see the meibomian glands opening on the posterior surface of the tarsus (Figure 4-7). *With subtle cicatricial entropion, visualization of the line of meibomian gland orifices and the relationship to the mucocutaneous junction is especially important.* You will often see that the mucocutaneous junction is near, or sometimes anterior, to the meibomian glands.

The diagnosis of entropion is usually straightforward. Identifying the cause becomes easy with experience. Once you have identified the type of entropion, selection of the appropriate treatment follows (Box 4-5).

Treatment of entropion

Treatment of involutional entropion

As discussed above, involutional entropion is associated with:

- Horizontal lower lid laxity
- Laxity of lower lid retractors
- Overriding preseptal orbicularis

The ideal operation to repair involutional entropion should correct as many of these etiologic factors as possible.

The *retractor reinsertion operation is the procedure of choice for correction of lower lid involutional entropion.* Tightening of the lower lid retractors pulls the inferior edge of the tarsus

inferiorly, providing a powerful eversion of the lid margin. The retractor reinsertion operation is so powerful that overcorrection of the entropion is possible when lid laxity is present. Overcorrection can actually cause the lid to be everted postoperatively (Figure 4-8). Performing a lateral tarsal strip operation in addition to the retractor reinsertion procedure adds stability to the eyelid and prevents an overcorrection. I use the lateral tarsal strip procedure for nearly all patients with lower lid involutional entropion. The preseptal orbicularis muscle is prevented from "overriding" superiorly on the tarsus by the subciliary incision scar. Enophthalmos is no longer considered an etiologic factor so we don't need to worry about that.

The retractor reinsertion operation

The goal of the retractor reinsertion operation is to correct the laxity of the lower lid retractors. During this procedure, the retractors are identified and advanced onto the

---

Box 4-5

Entropion Evaluation: Ask Yourself These Questions

Is the entropion cicatricial?

- Reposition the eyelid
- Is eversion difficult?
- Does the lid return to the inverted position immediately?

If yes, it is probably cicatricial

- Look for scarring of posterior lamella
- Determine the location and the severity of the scarring
- Will a graft be necessary or is a tarsal fracture operation enough?

If not cicatricial, then it must be involutional

- Reposition the eyelid
- Does the eyelid easily evert with your finger?
- Does the eyelid remain in position?
- Does forceful lid closure cause the entropion to return?
- If yes, the entropion is involutional

Is there lid laxity present?

- Do eyelid distraction and eyelid snap tests
- Plan retractor reinsertion, usually with a lateral tarsal strip operation

---

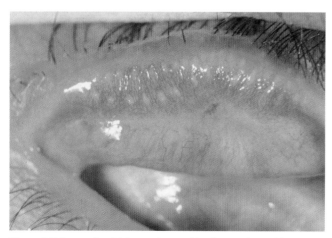

Figure 4-7 Severe cicatricial entropion resulting from trachoma. Note meibomian glands opening as slits on the back of the tarsus.

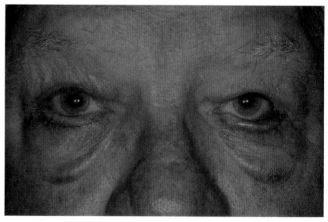

Figure 4-8 Postoperative ectropion after retractor reinsertion. Note that a lateral tarsal strip was done on the right side, but not on the left side.

lower lid tarsus. This provides a greater inferior and posterior pull on the inferior edge of the tarsal plate and an eversion of the lid margin.

The lower lid anatomy is similar to the upper lid anatomy. Let's preview the steps of the retractor reinsertion operation. The lower lid retractors are approached through a lower lid subciliary incision. *The landmark for the lower lid retractors is the preaponeurotic fat.* The fat is dissected off the anterior surface of the retractors. The posterior surface of the retractors is dissected free from the underlying conjunctiva. The retractors are pulled superiorly and sutured to the inferior tarsal margin. A slight eversion of the lid margin is recommended. This slight intraoperative overcorrection usually resolves postoperatively. *Using a lateral tarsal strip operation in combination with the retractor reinsertion operation eliminates overcorrection from a practical point of view.*

To perform a retractor reinsertion operation, you will:

- Make a subciliary incision
- Identify the lower lid retractors
- Dissect the retractors off the conjunctiva
- Advance the lower lid retractors onto the tarsus
- Add a lateral tarsal strip operation if necessary
- Close the skin

The steps of the retractor reinsertion operation are:

1. Prep the patient
   A. Instill topical anesthetic.
   B. Mark for the subciliary incision.
   C. Inject local anesthetic containing epinephrine into the lower lid fornix and anteriorly under the skin (Figure 4-9, A).
2. Make a subciliary incision
   A. Stabilize the lower lid with a 4-0 silk traction suture (Ethicon no. 783 P-3 cutting needle) and clamp to the drape. As you get more experience, you will find the traction suture not necessary for many procedures but, for the retractor reinsertion, I use it routinely.
   B. Cut along the mark with a no. 15 blade or Colorado microdissection needle through the skin (Figure 4-9, B).
   C. Use a Colorado microdissection needle (or Westcott scissors) to cut the orbicularis muscle. Usually the subciliary incision is superior to the inferior edge of the tarsus.
   D. After cutting into the pretarsal orbicularis muscle stay anterior to the septum, if possible, and dissect inferiorly toward the inferior orbital rim (Figure 4-9, C).
3. Identify the lower lid retractors
   A. Remember that the preaponeurotic fat is the landmark for the lower lid retractors. Open the orbital septum to find the preaponeurotic fat. In many older patients, the fat will be retracted and difficult to see. Frequently the white layer of the retractors will be visible before the fat is seen. If you are not sure that these are the retractors, have the patient look way up and way down to see if the retractors move. Don't expect the lower lid retractors to move as much as the levator aponeurosis in the upper lid (Figure 4-10, A).

4. Dissect the retractors off the conjunctiva
   A. After you have identified the retractors, use Westcott scissors to free the fat from the anterior surface of the retractors (Figure 4-9, D).
   B. Next free up the posterior aspect of the retractors from the underlying conjunctiva (Figure 4-9, E).
   C. Start a few millimeters below the inferior edge of the tarsus. Cutting through the retractors causes some bleeding. Dissect a plane between the conjunctiva and the retractors. It is helpful to inject some local posteriorly to "hydro dissect" the conjunctiva off the lower eyelid retractors.
      (1) It is not possible or necessary to separate the retractors into the voluntary and involuntary parts. The full thickness of the retractors should be advanced as a whole.
      (2) If you buttonhole the conjunctiva, it is not a problem.
   D. Free up 5–10 mm of the retractors (Figure 4-10, A).
   E. Note that most patients do not have a disinsertion of the retractors. You have to create an edge of retractors to reattach onto the tarsus.
5. Advance the lower lid retractors onto the tarsus
   A. Reattach the edge of the retractors to the inferior margin of the tarsus using three interrupted 5-0 Vicryl sutures on a spatula needle (Ethicon J571 5-0 Vicryl S-14 needle) (Figures 4-9, F, and 4-10, B).
   B. Release the traction suture and you will immediately notice that the lid margin is turned outward slightly. If the retractors do not seem tight enough, advance them a bit more. It is ideal to have a small amount of overcorrection (Figure 4-9, G).
   C. If you are not going to add a lateral tarsal strip operation (LTS) to the procedure, be careful not to overcorrect much.
6. LTS is usually necessary
   A. If there is associated lower lid laxity, this is the time to do the LTS procedure. The LTS procedure is performed in the same way as in any ectropion repair. When the lid is tightened appropriately, you will see the lid well apposed to the globe.
7. Close the skin
   A. Close the subciliary skin incision with a running 5-0 fast-absorbing gut suture (Figure 4-9, H).
   B. During the skin closure, combine the canthotomy with the subciliary incision closure, reforming the lateral canthal angle.
8. Provide postoperative care. Instil topical antibiotic ointment.

The retractor reinsertion operation is a very powerful procedure. Recurrence of entropion is rare, because the procedure addresses all the factors contributing to entropion. Adding the lateral tarsal strip procedure corrects the etiologic factor of lid laxity and prevents overcorrection (Box 4-6).

Treatment of spastic entropion

Quickert sutures

Spastic entropion occurs when the lids are held in a guarded position (protective blepharospasm) in response to eye pain

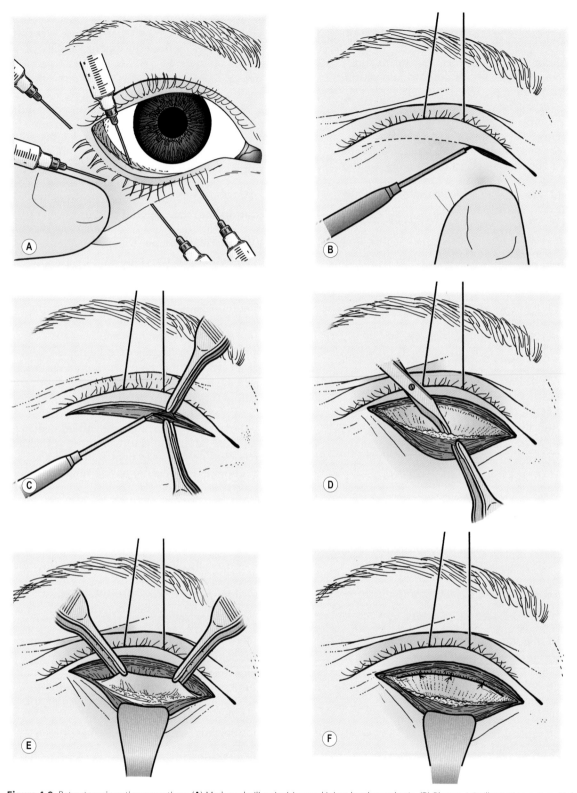

Figure 4-9 Retractor reinsertion operations. (**A**) Mark a subciliary incision and inject local anesthetic. (**B**) Place a 4-0 silk traction suture. Make a skin incision with Colorado needle or no. 15 blade. (**C**) Dissect a skin muscle flap inferiorly. (**D**) Open the orbital septum to find the preaponeurotic fat. Use the Westcott scissors to dissect the fat off the anterior surface of the lower lid retractors. (**E**) Dissect the lower lid retractors off the conjunctiva. (**F**) Advance the lower eyelid retractors onto the tarsus. (**G**) Lateral view of the lower lid retractors reattached. (**H**) Close the skin with absorbable sutures. Note that a LTS procedure has been performed.

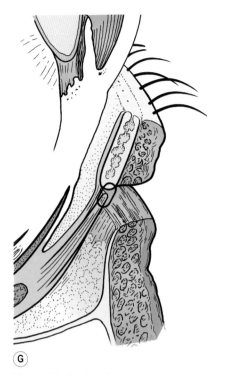

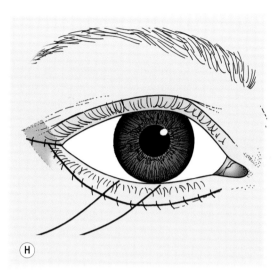

Figure 4-9 Continued.

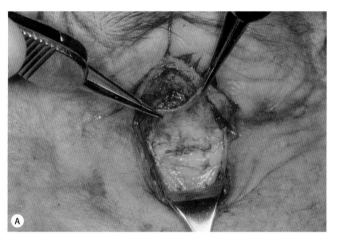

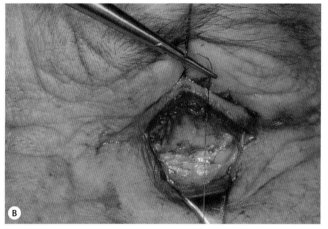

Figure 4-10 Retractor reinsertion operation. (**A**) 5–10 mm of lower lid retractors have been freed up from the underlying conjunctiva. Note the preaponeurotic fat anterior to the lower lid retractors. (**B**) The retractors have been advanced onto the tarsus.

Box 4-6

The Retractor Reinsertion Operation
- Instill local anesthetic with epinephrine
- Use 4-0 silk traction suture to stabilize the lower lid margin
- Make a subciliary incision
- Identify the retractors
- Dissect the preaponeurotic fat off the retractors
- Dissect the retractors off the conjunctiva
- Advance the retractors onto the tarsus using 5-0 Vicryl sutures (Ethicon J571 5-0 Vicryl S-14 needle)
- Consider adding the lateral tarsal strip operation to stabilize the lid
- Close the skin

---

or inflammation. The constant spasm of the lids causes an entropion. The exact mechanical factors are poorly understood, but are probably the same as those causing involutional entropion. If the cause of the underlying spasm can be eliminated, the spastic entropion will resolve. If it is not possible to eliminate the irritation, a cycle of spasm, irritation, and more spasm follows. A quick solution to spastic entropion is the use of *Quickert sutures*.

Quickert sutures are used to mechanically tighten the lower lid retractors without any skin incision. After administration of local anesthetic, double-armed sutures are passed full thickness through the lid, entering the conjunctiva posteriorly low in the fornix and exiting on the anterior surface of the lid just inferior to the lashes. Medial, central, and lateral double-armed sutures are placed. The sutures are tied to give a slight overcorrection. The sutures are not removed, but left to dissolve over 7–10 days. In theory, the sutures plicate the retractors, making them stronger. The scar tissue that forms as the suture dissolves holds the retractors in position. A scar forms where the sutures leave the skin, creating a barrier to the overriding preseptal orbicularis.

The steps of the Quickert suture procedure are:

1. Instill local anesthesia
   A. Instill topical anesthetic, inject local anesthetic with epinephrine in the conjunctival fornix and the skin.
2. Pass double-armed sutures from the fornix through the lid to emerge under the lashes
   A. Load a double-armed 4-0 chromic (Ethicon 793, G-3 needle) suture back-handed.
   B. Pass each arm of the suture through the lid from deep in the conjunctival fornix, passing anteriorly and superiorly to emerge from the skin just inferior to the eyelashes (Figure 4-11, A). Repeat, placing medial, central, and lateral sutures in position (Figure 4-11, B).
3. Tie the sutures
   A. Tie the sutures on the skin, creating a slight eversion of the eyelid margin. Remember that you will not be correcting any horizontal lid laxity if it is present, so be conservative with the overcorrection (Box 4-7).

A few surgeons use Quickert sutures as a primary method of repair for all instances of involutional entropion. In many patients, this technique will provide a long-term cure for the entropion. However, any lower lid laxity is not addressed, and the advancement of the retractors is not as secure. In theory, recurrence is more likely to occur. The main indication for Quickert sutures is spastic entropion, in which the irritation is likely to resolve, or the rare situation for which a retractor reinsertion operation is not practical in debilitated patients. For those patients, Quickert sutures can be performed at the bedside or in the examination chair.

Treatment of cicatricial entropion

Cicatricial entropion is treated by lengthening of the posterior lamella. If the posterior lamellar shortening is mild, as with marginal entropion of the lower eyelid, the *tarsal fracture operation* (also called a *tarsotomy*) is used. This procedure can also be used for mild cases of contracture in the upper eyelid; however, your patient will need to wear a soft contact lens for a few weeks after surgery to avoid the irritation of the cut tarsus. For upper eyelid cases where the contracture is worse, but not severe, a similar lengthening procedure, known as the *terminal tarsal rotation operation*, is used. If the cicatricial changes are severe, lysis of the scar tissue and lengthening of the posterior lamella are necessary using *mucous membrane grafts*.

You will find the tarsal fracture operation to be very successful for patients with mild lower lid cicatricial changes. The more advanced procedures have variable results and secondary procedures are often required.

Mild cicatricial entropion of the lower eyelid: the tarsal fracture operation

The tarsal fracture operation lengthens and reorients the scarred posterior lamella by a small amount. A horizontal

---

Box 4-7

Quickert Sutures Operation

- Instill topical and local anesthetic
- Load a double-armed 4-0 chromic suture (Ethicon no. 793, G-3 needle) back-handed
- Pass the arms of the suture through the lid from deep in the conjunctival fornix, passing anteriorly and superiorly to emerge from the skin just below the eyelashes
- Repeat so that there are medial, central, and lateral sutures in position
- Tie the sutures so that there is a slight overcorrection

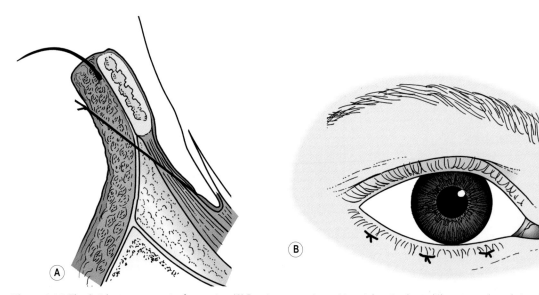

Figure 4-11 The Quickert suture repair of entropion. (**A**) Everting sutures in position, tightening lower lid retractors, lateral view. (**B**) Everting sutures in position, front view.

incision across the lower tarsus is made. The lid is then "fractured" or bent out. The surgical wound spreads apart. The wound is stabilized in an open position with double-armed 6-0 Vicryl sutures (Figure 4-12). Keep in mind that this procedure is only good for mild cicatricial entropion because the posterior lamella is lengthened only minimally. The tarsal fracture operation is most often used in the lower eyelid. If you have a patient with mild entropion of the upper eyelid, the tarsal fracture operation can be used, but you must be careful to place the conjunctival pass of the

suture in the fracture wound to avoid sutures rubbing against the cornea (a bandage soft contact lens is appropriate). The tarsal fracture operation will be discussed in more detail in Chapter 5.

Mild to moderate cicatricial entropion of the upper eyelid: the terminal tarsal rotation operation

The terminal tarsal rotation operation is similar to the tarsal fracture procedure. Both operations lengthen the posterior

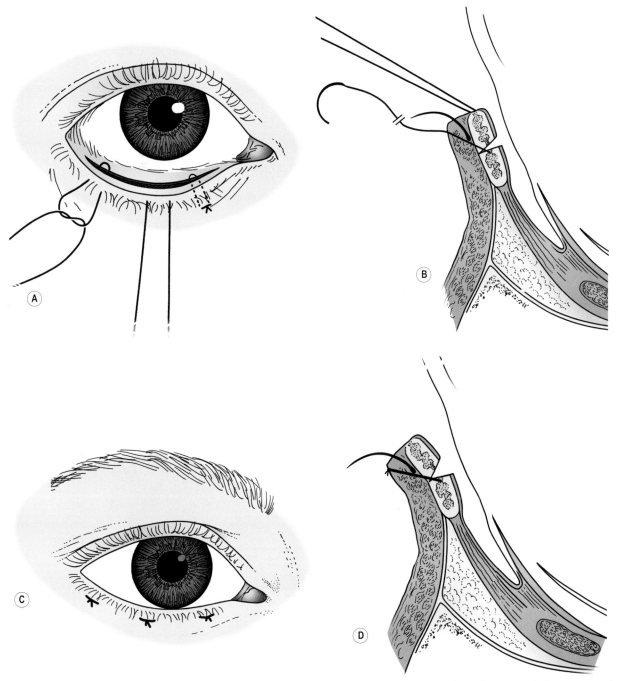

Figure 4-12 Tarsal fracture operation. (**A**) Pass a traction suture. Evert the eyelid. Make a horizontal incision full thickness through the posterior surface of the tarsus. The Colorado needle is useful for minimizing bleeding. (**B**) Pass double-armed 6-0 Vicryl sutures below the inferior margin of the tarsus to emerge immediately inferior to the eyelashes, lateral view. (**C**) Pass and tie three or four double-armed sutures. (**D**) Leave the lid margin in a slightly everted position, lateral view.

lamella and reorient the lid margin by incision and suturing rather than grafting. The terminal tarsal rotation operation gives a greater degree of rotation than the tarsal fracture operation. For mild cases of either upper or lower lid entropion, I use the tarsal fracture operation.

The terminal tarsal operation starts with a horizontal incision across the upper tarsus as in the tarsal fracture operation. The posterior lamella of the distal lid (basically the lid margin) is dissected away from the orbicularis and rotated 180 degrees. The margin is sutured into position (Figure 4-13). The terminal tarsal operation requires more dissection and creates more eversion of the lid margin. The sutures are not on the conjunctival side of the eyelid, so there is little worry about corneal irritation even in the upper eyelid. The terminal tarsal rotation procedure is more powerful than the tarsal fracture procedure, but is more difficult to perform and has more variable results. The operated eyelid margin can be irregular so I use this procedure sparingly.

Moderate or severe cicatricial entropion: mucous membrane grafting

Moderate or severe shortening of the posterior lamella cannot be repaired with excision of the scar tissue alone. Mucous membrane grafts must be placed to prevent the scarring of the posterior lamella from returning. Correction of the entropion starts with lysis of the scarred conjunctiva so that the lid margin can return to its normal position. After the scar has been released, mucous membrane is sewn over the defect (Figures 4-14 and 4-15).

Mucous membrane can be harvested from the side of the mouth, from the buccal mucosa, or from the labial mucosa of the lower lip. Buccal mucosa wounds can be closed primarily, whereas labial mucosal donor sites must granulate in.

Anterior lamellar eyelash excision can be used in patients with moderate degrees of cicatricial entropion of the upper eyelid if a somewhat ptotic eyelid exists. This procedure is easier to do and heals more comfortably than the tarsal fracture type procedure. The patient has to agree to lose all the eyelashes completely, however. Under local anesthesia, you can split the eyelid at the gray line and excise the inferior 2–3 mm of anterior lamella containing the eyelash follicles. Suture the remaining anterior lamellar edge to the tarsus with vertical mattress sutures in a recessed position. In some cases, the eyelid skin will eventually be pulled inward and a further operation may be necessary.

More advanced forms of cicatricial entropion are difficult to treat. Reoperations are often required. Despite repositioning of the lid margin and eyelashes, many patients will still complain of eye irritation because of the poor lubrication associated with loss of healthy conjunctiva or scarring of the lacrimal ductules. Do not be overly optimistic and promise complete anatomic and functional rehabilitation to patients with moderate or severe cicatricial entropion.

Checkpoint

You should be able to:

- Describe the typical presentation of
  - A patient with involutional entropion
  - A patient with cicatricial entropion
- How do the history and physical examination for cicatricial entropion differ from those for involutional entropion?
  - Remember the questions to ask yourself in the physical examination (can the lid be everted easily? etc.)
- State by memory the steps of the retractor reinsertion operation
- State by memory the steps of the Quickert suture procedure
- Understand the principles of repair of cicatricial entropion and when a graft might be needed

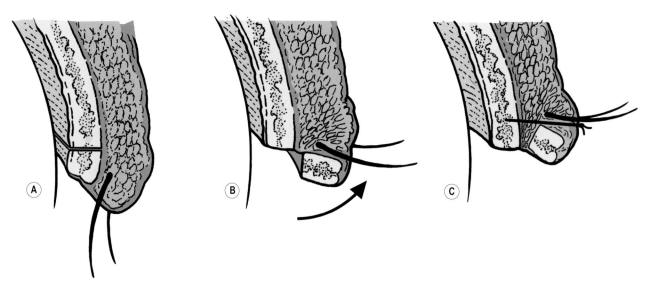

Figure 4-13 The terminal tarsal rotation operation for moderate cicatricial entropion. (**A**) Make a full-thickness horizontal incision across the shortened tarsus. (**B**) Rotate the lid margin 180 degrees. (**C**) Hold it in place with mattress sutures.

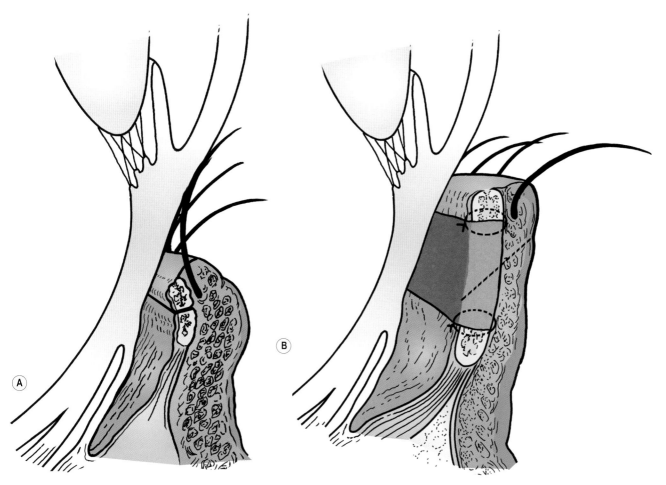

Figure 4-14 Mucous membrane grafting to lengthen the posterior lamella in cicatricial entropion (see **Figure 4-15**). (**A**) Cut the scar tissue using a horizontal incision through the posterior surface of the tarsus to return the eyelid margin to normal position. This will create a posterior lamellar defect. (**B**) Repair the posterior lamellar defect using a mucous membrane graft to prevent contracture.

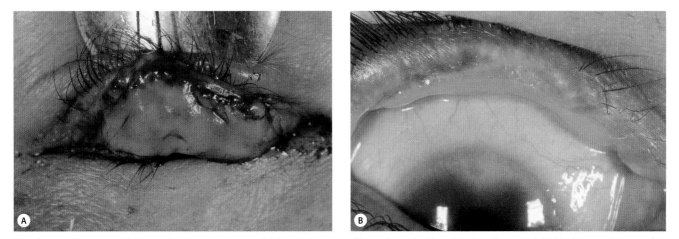

Figure 4-15 Mucous membrane graft to repair severe cicatricial entropion, caused by trachoma in this patient (see **Figure 4-7**). (**A**) Mucous membrane graft sewn in position, lengthening the posterior lamella. (**B**) Following healing, the eyelid margin is no longer inverted. A thin line of the graft is visible.

Major points

Entropion of the eyelid occurs when the lid margin inverts or turns against the eyeball. There are four main types of entropion:

- Involutional
- Spastic
- Cicatricial
- Marginal

Factors contributing to lower lid involutional entropion include:

- Laxity of lower lid retractors
- Horizontal lid laxity
- Overriding preseptal orbicularis muscle

Shortening of the posterior lamella causes cicatricial entropion.

Identification of the cause of the entropion is the key to defining treatment.

Treatment of lower lid involutional entropion is:

- The retractor reinsertion operation
- Usually with a lateral tarsal strip operation

Treatment of mild cicatricial entropion uses incisions with sutures to stabilize the lid while healing occurs, restoring the length of the posterior lamella:

- For mild lower lid entropion—the tarsal fracture operation
- For mild upper lid entropion—the terminal tarsal rotation operation (some surgeons prefer the tarsal fracture procedure; if you use this, be sure to bury the sutures to protect the cornea. A bandage contact lens may be required for a few weeks)

For mild to moderate upper eyelid entropion, excision of the anterior lamella containing the eyelash follicles is an alternative to rotation procedures. This procedure shortens the anterior lamella to match the posterior lamella length and removes all eyelashes.

Treatment of moderate or severe cicatricial entropion requires lysis of the scar tissue and mucous membrane grafts to lengthen the posterior lamella.

Suggested reading

1. American Academy of Ophthalmology: *Basic and clinical science course: orbit, eyelids, and lacrimal system*, sect. 7, pp. 201–205, San Francisco: The American Academy of Ophthalmology, 2006/2007.

2. Albert DM, Lucarelli MJ: Entropion. In *Clinical atlas of procedures in ophthalmic surgery*, pp. 257–260, Chicago: AMA Press, 2004.

3. Anderson RL, Gordy DD: The tarsal strip procedure. *Arch Ophthalmol* 97:2192–2196, 1979.

4. Barber K, Dabbs T: Morphologic observations on patients with presumed trichiasis. *Br J Ophthalmol* 72:17–22, 1988.

5. Collin JR, Rathbun JE: Involutional entropion: a review with evaluation of a procedure. *Arch Ophthalmol* 96(6):1058–1064, 1978.

6. Dutton JJ: Entropion. In *Atlas of ophthalmic surgery*, vol. 2, pp. 114–143, St Louis: Mosby Year Book, 1992.

7. Jones LT, Reeh MJ, Wobig JL: Senile entropion: a new concept for correction. *Am J Ophthalmol* 74(2):327–329, 1972.

8. Katowitz JA, Heher KL, Hollsten DA: Involutional entropion. In Levine MR, ed., *Manual of oculoplastic surgery*, 3rd edn, pp. 137–144, Boston: Butterworth-Heinemann, 2003.

9. Kersten RC, Kleiner FP, Kulwin DR: Tarsotomy for the treatment of cicatricial entropion with trichiasis. *Arch Ophthalmol* 110:714, 1992.

10. Martin RT, Nunery WR, Tanenbaum M: Entropion, trichiasis, and distichiasis. In McCord CD, Tanenbaum M, Nunery WR, eds, *Oculoplastic surgery*, 3rd edn, ch. 8, pp. 221–248, New York: Raven Press, 1995.

11. Nerad J: The diagnosis and treatment of entropion. In *The requisites—Oculoplastic surgery*, pp. 89–103, St Louis: Mosby, 2001.

12. Nerad JA: Eyelid causes of tearing. In Bosniak S, ed., *Principles and practice of ophthalmic plastic and reconstructive surgery*, vol. 2, Philadelphia: WB Saunders, 1996.

13. Nerad JA: Eyelid malpositions. In Linberg JV, ed., *Contemporary issues in ophthalmology: lacrimal surgery*, ch. 4, pp. 62–89, New York: Churchill Livingstone, 1988.

14. Nerad JA, Carter KD, Alford MA: Entropion. In *Rapid diagnosis in ophthalmology—oculoplastic and reconstructive surgery*, pp. 92–95, Philadelphia: Mosby Elsevier, 2008.

15. Penne RB: Entropion. In *Color atlas & synopsis of clinical ophthalmology: oculoplastics*, pp. 56–61, New York: McGraw-Hill, 2003.

16. Wesley RE: Cicatricial entropion. In Levine MR, ed., *Manual of oculoplastic surgery*, 3rd edn, pp. 145–150, Boston: Butterworth-Heinemann, 2003.

17. Goldberg et al, Entropion repair. In Wobig JL, Dailey RA, eds, *Oculofacial plastic surgery: face, lacrimal system, and orbit*, pp. 91–97, New York: Thieme, 2004.

CHAPTER 5

The Diagnosis and Management of Misdirected Eyelashes

Introduction

Trichiasis is said to exist when the eyelashes are misdirected against the eye. You will see trichiasis often in your practice. Patients complain of a foreign body sensation. Discharge or conjunctival injection is rarely present. Let's preview what we will be discussing in this chapter.

The most common cause of trichiasis is a form of mild cicatricial entropion known as *marginal entropion*. Subtle cicatricial changes of the posterior lamella pull the eyelid margin inward, misdirecting the eyelashes. The concept that most instances of misdirected lashes result from mild posterior lamellar shortening is relatively new.

Accidental trauma may tear the lid margin. Frequently the lacerations are not sharp, and the tissue is swollen at the time of repair. Poor healing or inadequate alignment may cause misdirection of the eyelashes. *Surgical trauma*, such as a wedge resection, also leads to misdirected lashes if the lid margin alignment is not exact.

Two congenital conditions cause the eyelashes to rub against the eye:

- Epiblepharon
- Distichiasis

Epiblepharon is an unusual condition in which an extra roll of eyelid skin pushes the eyelashes against the cornea. Epiblepharon is most commonly seen in Asian children. *Distichiasis* is a rare congenital condition in which an extra row of eyelashes arises from the meibomian gland orifices. Although both these conditions are unusual, they are worth knowing about.

An understanding of the *anatomy of the lid margin* is necessary to identify the specific cause of the trichiasis. We have discussed this in Chapter 4 and will review it again in this chapter. The *history* and *physical examination* will identify the exact cause of the misdirected lashes and point to the appropriate treatment. Marginal entropion of the lower eyelid is usually treated with an incisional lengthening of the posterior lamella. The *tarsal fracture operation* works well for redirecting the lower eyelashes. Individual or small numbers of misdirected lashes may be ablated using *cryotherapy, electrolysis,* or *laser epilation.* Larger segments of misdirected lashes may be excised using the *pentagonal wedge resection* followed by meticulous lid margin repair. The misdirected lashes of epiblepharon are reoriented by removing an ellipse of skin and muscle under the eyelashes. The extra row of eyelashes seen in distichiasis is removed by a lid-splitting operation with cryotherapy for the abnormal lashes (Box 5-1).

The understanding of trichiasis has come a long way in the last 15 years. There has been a *major shift away from destructive procedures,* such as cryotherapy, *toward reconstructive procedures that reorient the lashes* or at least provide a continuous row of lashes on a newly reconstructed lid margin. The concepts in this chapter will help you treat many patients. With the exception of the operations for epiblepharon and distichiasis, all the procedures discussed are useful on a routine basis.

Anatomic considerations

The normal eyelid margin

In Chapter 4, we introduced the anatomy of the lid margin. You will need to learn this anatomy well and pay close attention to anatomic details when evaluating a patient with misdirected lashes. We will review the normal lid margin architecture before further discussion of trichiasis.

The lid margin is a thin, flat platform ending at right angles anteriorly and posteriorly (Figure 5-1). The most posterior aspect of the normal lid margin is covered with conjunctiva. Anterior to this is the *mucocutaneous junction*. It is at this point that the mucosa of the palpebral conjunctiva stops and the keratinized skin of the eyelid margin begins. In Chapter 4, I suggested that you look at several normal patients to see this junction. If you are not certain what this junction looks like, review it again when you examine one of your normal patients. It is important to be able to see these landmarks.

Just anterior to the mucocutaneous junction are the *meibomian gland orifices* extending out from the tarsal plate. Anterior to the meibomian gland orifices is the *gray line*. Anterior to the gray line is the anterior lamella, which includes the skin and muscle. The *eyelashes* arise anterior to the gray line, usually in one or two irregular rows in the lower lid and three or four irregular rows in the upper lid. Learn these anatomic landmarks during a slit lamp examination.

The anatomic abnormalities causing misdirected eyelashes

The causes of trichiasis are easy to understand on an anatomic basis:

- *Marginal entropion*: Posterior lamellar shortening pulls the eyelashes posteriorly toward the eye (Figure 5-2)
- *Traumatic misdirection of eyelashes*: The position of eyelash follicles or surrounding tissues is physically altered, which causes the eyelashes to grow in an irregular manner, pointing in different directions and sometimes toward the eye (Figure 5-3)

Box 5-1

Causes of Misdirected Eyelashes

- Marginal entropion
- Trauma
- Epiblepharon
- Distichiasis

- *Epiblepharon*: A roll of extra skin pushes the normal eyelashes against the eye (Figure 5-4)
- *Distichiasis*: An incomplete row of eyelashes arises abnormally from the meibomian glands (Figure 5-5)

Many older textbooks define "trichiasis" as a condition in which the eyelashes are misdirected, and *the lid margin is in normal position*. This definition stressed that the condition was an eyelash problem, not an abnormality of the eyelid. Eyelid malpositions such as involutional entropion and cicatricial entropion were not (and generally still are not) considered to be causes of trichiasis because the lid margin was obviously inverted (Figure 5-6). Now that we have a greater appreciation of the lid margin architecture, we realize that *many (probably most) cases of trichiasis are actually the result of subtle inversion of the lid margin, marginal entropion*. The definition of trichiasis is not as important as understanding the mechanics of the misdirected lashes. As you have seen, epiblepharon and distichiasis are usually included in the discussion of trichiasis because the lid margin is in a normal position. In this book, the terms "misdirected eyelashes" and "trichiasis" are used interchangeably.

Checkpoint

- Review the anatomic landmarks of the eyelid margin. What are the four causes of misdirected eyelashes (Boxes 5-1 and 5-2)?
- You should understand the mechanics of each cause. Describe the changes in the anatomic landmarks of the lid margin for each cause.
- Remember that the most common cause of trichiasis is marginal entropion.

History

Most adults with misdirected lashes complain of foreign body sensation. Often they epilate the lashes themselves to eliminate the symptoms. Usually patients cannot remember

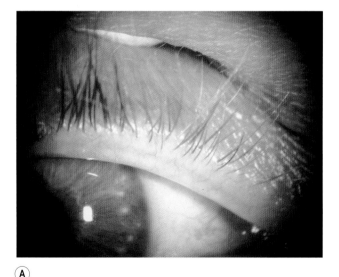

(A)

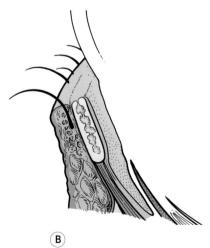

(B)

Figure 5-1 Normal eyelid margin. The lid margin is a flat platform with a sharp right-angled posterior edge. Normal landmarks (from posterior to anterior) are: mucocutaneous junction, meibomian gland orifices, gray line, and eyelashes.

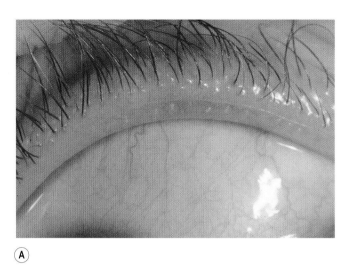
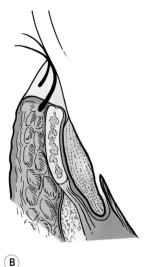

(A)

(B)

Figure 5-2 Marginal entropion. Mild posterior lamellar shortening causes rounding of lid margin and anterior migration of mucocutaneous junction.

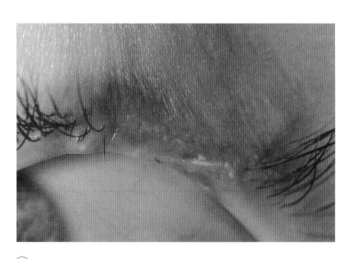
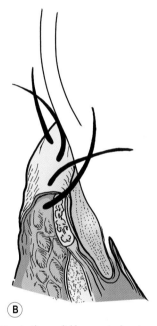

(A)

(B)

Figure 5-3 Traumatic misdirection of the eyelashes (aberrant eyelashes). A laceration to the eyelid has created an irregular eyelid margin with eyelash loss. The soft tissue scarring causes a random orientation of the eyelashes.

Box 5-2

Causes of Misdirected Lashes

- Marginal entropion: Posterior lamellar shortening pulls the eyelashes posteriorly toward the eye
- Traumatic misdirection of eyelashes: The position of eyelash follicles or surrounding tissues is physically altered, causing the eyelashes to grow in an irregular manner pointing in different directions, sometimes toward the eye
- Epiblepharon: A roll of extra skin pushes the normal eyelashes against the eye
- Distichiasis: An incomplete row of eyelashes arises abnormally from the meibomian glands

---

when the symptoms started or what caused the problem. Some patients will tell you that the problem started after trauma, an infection, or an operation.

With epiblepharon and distichiasis, the age of presentation varies, but is often not until age 4 or 5. Children may complain of irritation. More commonly, children rub the eye or have associated tearing and mild discharge. Photophobia suggests significant corneal irritation. I use the presence of symptoms of photophobia as a strong indication for treatment.

Physical examination

The physical examination will tell you the cause and extent of the trichiasis. Given this information, you will be able to plan a treatment. Usually the diagnosis will be clear but, if

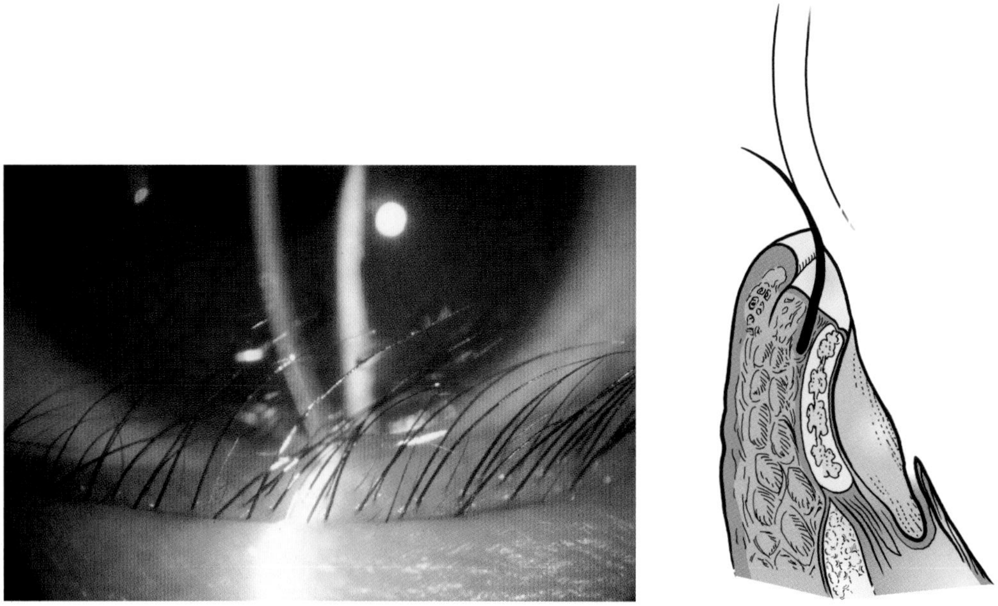

A B

Figure 5-4 Epiblepharon. A redundant roll of skin pushes the eyelashes upward against the cornea in a parallel orientation.

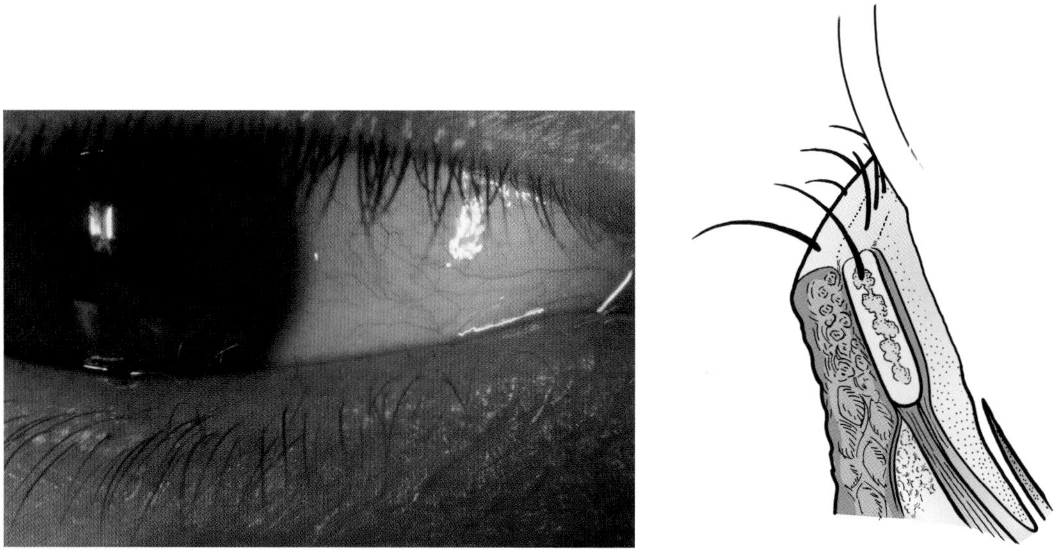

A B

Figure 5-5 Distichiasis. An incomplete row of eyelashes arises from the meibomian gland orifices.

the patient has recently had the lashes epilated, the cause or extent of the trichiasis may not be clear. Ask the patient to return in about 2 weeks for a repeat examination. In the interim, the patient should not have any epilation. As the lashes grow back, they may be extremely irritating because they are short and stiff so ask your patients to use lubricating ointment if necessary. You will be able to determine the problem when you can see the abnormal lashes.

Marginal entropion

I have told you that the most common cause of trichiasis is *marginal entropion*. Usually you will see several lashes or a whole area of lashes pointed against the cornea. Although the lashes are misdirected, they maintain their parallel orientation to one another. Probably there will be corneal staining consistent with the lash position. Rarely will you see ulceration. *The subtle inversion of the lid margin will go unnoticed without a careful examination of the lid margin anatomy.* Start your examination on the most normal part of the lid margin and identify the normal landmarks. As you move toward the areas of trichiasis, you will see that the *posterior lid margin loses its square edge and becomes rounded* (Figure 5-7, A and B). The rounding indicates that the lid margin is being pulled posteriorly. Go back to the normal part of the eyelid margin and look at the mucocutaneous junction. Follow this junction toward the involved lashes, noting the position of the junction related to the

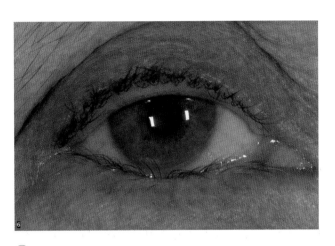

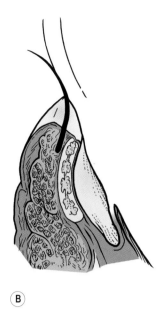

(A)   (B)

Figure 5-6 Involutional entropion for comparison. The lid margin is turned inward, indicating entropion rather than trichiasis. Laxity of the lower eyelid retractors, horizontal eyelid laxity, and an overriding preseptal orbicularis muscle are etiologic factors.

eyelashes. You will see that the mucocutaneous junction has migrated anteriorly and is at or beyond the meibomian gland orifices. *Anterior migration of the mucocutaneous junction indicates the diagnosis of marginal entropion* (Figure 5-7, B–D). As the lid margin moves into the tear lake, the normal relationship of the mucocutaneous junction to the meibomian glands changes. The conjunctiva migrates onto the wet part of the lid margin covered with tears. It may take some practice to see the mucocutaneous junction (use the position of the meibomian glands to help you if the mucocutaneous junction is normal). If you are having trouble with this concept, look at some more normal patients during a slit lamp examination.

Next look at the conjunctiva of the tarsal plate to see if there is any abnormality that would explain why the lid is being tugged inward. In most patients with marginal entropion, there is no obvious abnormality. Some inflammation consistent with blepharitis or meibomianitis may be present. Occasionally, you will see scar tissue where a chalazion has been excised. You may see some obvious scar tissue without an identifiable cause. Note the length of the involved lid margin so that you can plan the extent of the treatment that will be required.

Traumatic misdirection of the eyelashes

If the lash problem occurs after trauma, you will usually see an area of misdirected lashes associated with scarring of the lid margin. In these patients, the lashes are erratically positioned, pointing in different directions. In trauma patients, the misdirected lashes lose their parallel orientation to one another, a diagnostic feature differing from marginal entropion. Often there will be lashes arising anteriorly from the skin away from the margin. Sometimes areas of lashes will be missing (see Figure 5-3). During a slit lamp examination, you can imagine that the individual eyelash follicles have become disoriented, repositioned, or damaged as a result of the trauma. The irregular misdirection of these lashes appears different than that associated with marginal entropion in

which the involved lashes are all misdirected in a similar manner, more or less parallel to one another (see Figure 5-3, A and B). The number of lashes and the length of the margin involved dictate the treatment. If the lid margin is discontinuous, surgical excision of the abnormal lashes and lid margin may improve the appearance and the trichiasis.

Epiblepharon

Epiblepharon is a relatively rare condition in which the eyelashes are pushed against the cornea by a roll of skin arising from the eyelid. The roll of skin is easy to see from the lateral view (Figure 5-8; see also Figure 5-4). Epiblepharon most commonly involves the lower eyelid of Asian children. Often half or more of the eyelid is involved. You may be surprised to see the number of lashes in contact with the eye. Sometimes 20 or more lashes will be seen brushing across the cornea. Signs of corneal exposure are usually present but are less severe than you would predict by the number of lashes on the cornea. It has been said that children often outgrow this condition as adult facial features develop, but I don't know if this is true. The treatment is an elliptical excision of the redundant skin and muscle.

Distichiasis

Distichiasis is a rare condition in which an extra row of lashes arises from the meibomian gland orifices (see Figure 5-5). When you first hear this word, you may think that it is "dys-trichiasis." But don't be confused. The word, distichiasis, is derived from the Greek words, *di* and *stichos*, meaning "two rows." As you probably recall, the meibomian glands are specialized sebaceous glands. Throughout the body, the sebaceous glands are associated with hair follicles: the pilosebaceous apparatus. Presumably, in distichiasis, the meibomian glands have dedifferentiated, or retained, the associated hair. Often you will see only a few lashes arising from the posterior lamella. In almost all patients, the row of lashes is incomplete. If the patient is symptomatic (photophobia is a

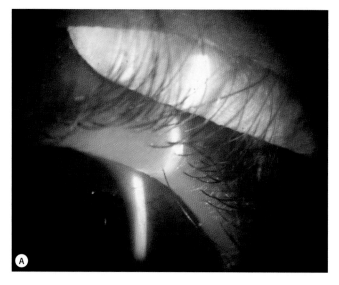

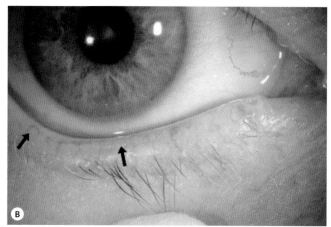

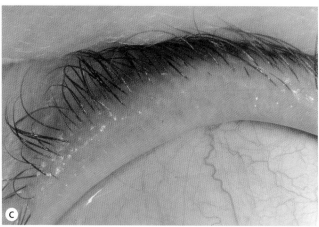

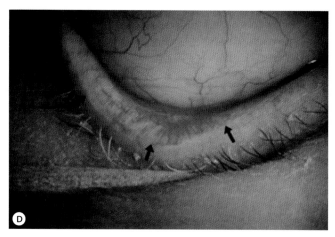

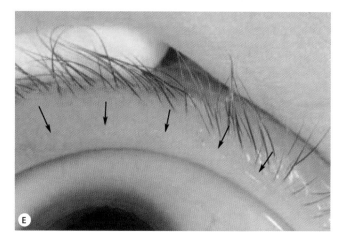

Figure 5-7 Marginal entropion. (**A**) Note the rounded lid margin with lashes pulled posteriorly. (**B**) Note rolled lower eyelid margin. Anterior migration of mucocutaneous junction noted by arrows. (**C**) Anterior migration of the mucocutaneous junction with meibomian glands opening as slits on the posterior aspect of the lid margin. (**D**) Everted lower eyelid margin. Follow mucocutaneous junction move anteriorly toward lash roots. Meibomian glands are dilated suggesting blepharitis as a cause of the marginal entropion. (**E**) To identify anterior migration of the mucocutaneous junction, follow the normal mucocutaneous junction (thin arrow) as it moves anteriorly in the area of rounded lid margin (thick arrows).

good clue) and corneal exposure is present, treatment is recommended.

Treatment of trichiasis

Goals of treatment

The indications for treatment of any misdirected lash depend on the patients' symptoms and the degree of corneal expo-

sure present. You will choose the appropriate treatment based upon the cause of the misdirected lashes and the number of lashes involved. *Epilation of lashes* is a temporizing measure. In almost all patients, the lashes will grow back within a month. Often, as the lashes grow back, the irritation will be more severe when they are short and stiff. If you remove the lashes in anticipation of a more permanent procedure, try to perform it within 3 weeks.

In adults, the trichiasis will be caused by either marginal entropion or trauma. Some patients have no history of

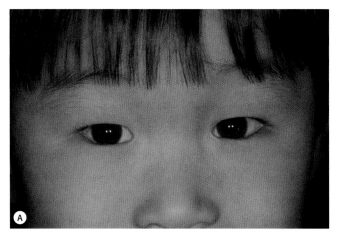
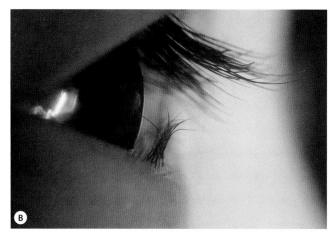

Figure 5-8 Epiblepharon. (**A**) Front view. Note the redundant fold of lid skin. (**B**) Lateral view. The lashes are "pushed" against the cornea.

trauma or physical findings consistent with marginal entropion. These are unusual patients. Regardless, the principles of treatment discussed in this section can be applied to all patients even if the diagnosis does not fit neatly into one category.

The treatment of misdirected lashes has moved away from destructive procedures, such as cryotherapy, to more reconstructive procedures, which redirect or remove the abnormal lashes, while at the same time preserve the normal lid margin and lashes. The *goals* of the treatment of misdirected lashes are to:

- Reposition the misdirected lashes, if possible
- Eliminate those lashes that cannot be repositioned
- Create a continuous row of lashes on the lid margin
- Reconstruct the lid margin if irregularities exist

The misdirected lashes seen in marginal entropion can be repositioned with the tarsal fracture operation.

Treatment of marginal entropion of the lower eyelid: the tarsal fracture operation

The tarsal fracture operation returns the lid to a more normal position. Its use has dramatically changed my approach to the treatment of trichiasis and has almost eliminated cryotherapy from my practice. This operation has not found its way into the hands of most ophthalmologists. *You should learn the tarsal fracture operation.* A horizontal incision is made across the posterior surface of the tarsus. This incision allows the lid to "bend" or "fracture" anteriorly. Sutures are placed through the eyelid to hold the eyelid margin in an everted position.

The tarsal fracture operation includes:

- Stabilizing the lid
- Making a horizontal tarsal incision
- Passing double-armed 6-0 Vicryl sutures
- Tying the sutures to evert the margin

The steps of the tarsal fracture operation are:

1. Prep the patient
   A. Instill topical anesthetic.
   B. Inject local anesthetic with epinephrine under the skin and conjunctiva of the eyelid.

2. Stabilize the lower eyelid
   A. Pass a 4-0 silk suture through the lid margin.
   B. Evert the lid over a Jaeger lid speculum ("shoehorn").

3. Make a horizontal tarsal incision
   A. Use a no. 15 blade to make a full-thickness horizontal incision *through the tarsus* 2–3 mm laterally beyond the area of entropion (Figure 5-9, A). A Colorado needle works nicely for this.
   B. Try to avoid cutting the marginal artery by making the incision at least halfway down on the tarsal plate.
   C. Bleeding usually occurs if you are using a scalpel blade, so have a cautery device ready.

4. Pass double-armed 6-0 Vicryl sutures
   A. Pass double-armed 6-0 Vicryl sutures full thickness through the lid (Ethicon J-570 with S-14 needle). Start with a "back-handed" pass entering the inferior edge of the wound and exiting just under the lashes anteriorly (Figure 5-9, B).
   B. Pass as many pairs of double-armed sutures as required to evert the length of the lid margin involved. Usually the majority of the tarsus is incised and three pairs of sutures are used (Figure 5-9, C).

5. Tie the sutures to evert the margin
   A. *Tie the sutures* as you pass them or wait until all are passed.
   B. *Aim for a slight overcorrection.* Recognize that some inversion will occur with healing (Figure 5-9, D).

6. Provide postoperative care
   A. Apply topical antibiotic ointment.
   B. You do not need to remove the sutures. They will absorb over 6 weeks, allowing the eyelid to heal in normal position.

You will find the tarsal fracture operation to be an effective technique for repositioning the lashes. The procedure is quick to perform and easy to learn (Figure 5-10).

The tarsal fracture operation can be used for the upper eyelid. The suture must be buried in the tarsal incision (you may need a bandage lens). The *terminal tarsal rotation operation,* as described in Chapter 4 (see Figure 4-13, A–C), can be

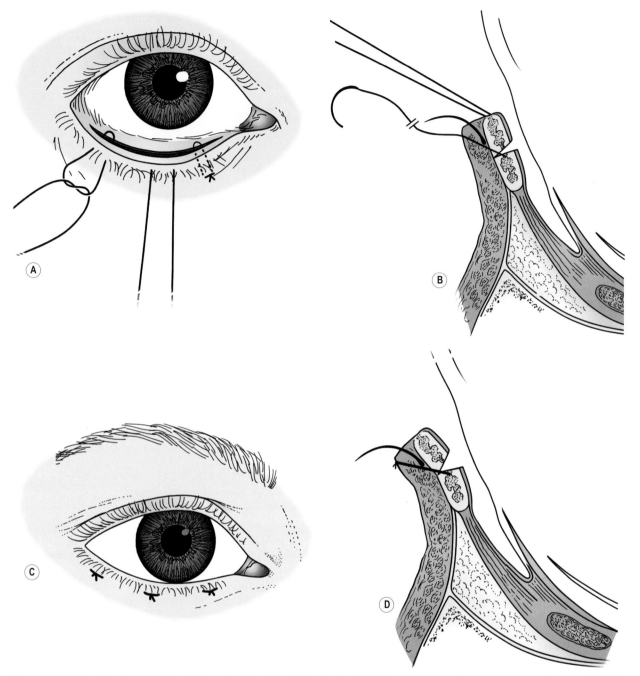

Figure 5-9 The tarsal fracture operation. (**A**) Pass a traction suture. Make a horizontal incision full thickness through the tarsus using a no. 15 blade or Colorado needle. (**B**) Pass double-armed 6-0 Vicryl sutures below the inferior margin of the tarsus to emerge immediately inferior to the eyelashes (lateral view). Tie the suture. (**C**) Repeat, using three double-armed sutures. (**D**) Leave the lid margin in a slightly everted position (lateral view).

used to evert the upper eyelid margin for more severe entropion. In this procedure, a horizontal incision across the posterior aspect of the tarsal plate is made. Further dissection is performed to totally evert the lid margin (180 degrees). Sutures are placed to hold the lid margin in an everted position. The terminal tarsal rotation operation is effective in most patients, but the procedure is more difficult than the tarsal fracture procedure, and healing is much slower with lid margin abnormalities sometimes resulting. Master the tarsal fracture procedure before taking on the terminal tarsal rotation operation (Box 5-3).

Treatment of traumatic causes of eyelash misdirection

Misdirected lashes may occur after accidental trauma or after surgical resection of a portion of the eyelid. In most patients, the misdirected lashes cannot be repositioned. Elimination of the abnormal lashes is required. Frequently, areas of lashes are missing. In some patients, the lid margin may be irregular.

Elimination of abnormal lashes can be accomplished in several ways:

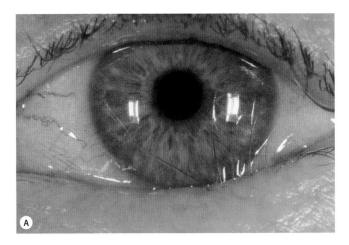

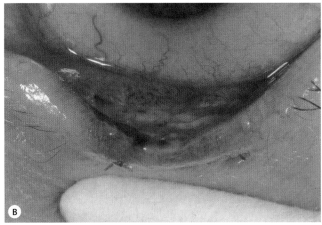

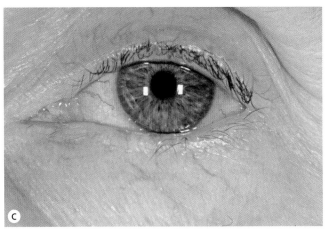

Figure 5-10 The tarsal fracture operation. (**A**) Preoperative marginal entropion. (**B**) Intraoperative view showing the horizontal incision through the tarsus. (**C**) Postoperative result.

Box 5-3

The Tarsal Fracture Operation

- Topical anesthetic is instilled. Local anesthetic with epinephrine is injected under the skin and conjunctiva
- Prep and drape the patient
- Stabilize the lower lid margin
- Pass a 4-0 silk suture through the lid margin
- Evert the lid over a Jaeger lid speculum ("shoehorn")
- Use a no. 15 blade or Colorado microdissection needle to make a full-thickness horizontal incision through the posterior surface of the tarsus
- Pass three double-armed 6-0 Vicryl sutures full thickness through the lid starting below the tarsal cut posteriorly emerging just inferior to the lashes anteriorly (Ethicon J-570 with S-14 needle)
- Tie the sutures on the skin. Aim for a slight overcorrection

---

- Manual epilation
- Hyfrecation
- Electrolysis
- Laser epilation
- Pentagonal wedge resection
- Cryotherapy

Manual epilation is a *short-term solution*. The lashes grow back in almost all situations (about 4 weeks). Epilation can give patients some relief while they wait for a more definitive procedure, but be sure to carefully note the exact position

of the abnormal lashes if you are planning surgery before the lashes grow back. Epilation can also be a useful way to see if permanent removal of the lashes will eliminate the patient's symptoms if the benefit of surgery is questionable (try to epilate before using any topical anesthetic). Often when the short stubby eyelashes grow in, they cause more irritation than the longer softer eyelashes did prior to epilation.

For a fairly effective treatment of a few eyelashes, I prefer *hyfrecation* over electrolysis or laser epilation. After injecting local anesthetic, a thin hyfrecator wire is slid into the eyelash follicle. Start at low settings and increase the power until the lash appears to coagulate, then remove the eyelash. A battery-operated *electrolysis unit* can be used in a similar way. A thin wire is used to send a unipolar current down the shaft of the hair follicle. The heat generated kills the follicle. Hyfrecation seems to have a higher success rate than electrolysis.

Laser epilation has also been used when a small number of lashes are to be removed. This procedure, like electrolysis, has a low success rate, so it has largely been abandoned. I have not used it for several years. If you choose to try it for a few lashes, aim the beam of the argon laser parallel to the hair shaft by everting the lid margin. Start with 300 mW for 0.5 second with a 50 µ spot size. Increase the power as necessary. Burn a hole 1–2 mm deep with the goal of destroying the follicle without damaging the surrounding lid margin. Although this technique still has advocates, the hyfrecator seems to do a better job.

If more than three or four lashes are present in a localized area, cryotherapy or pentagonal wedge resection can be used. Cryotherapy is a quick easy treatment, but destroys healthy eyelid tissue, so I reserve it for broad areas of treatment. Local wedge resection is covered after cryotherapy.

Cryotherapy using a liquid nitrogen probe will permanently destroy the lash follicles. Its main indication is for *broad areas of misdirected lashes* where individual lash destruction is not a practical solution. In most patients, the diagnosis is actually marginal entropion, and you should consider the tarsal fracture procedure as a better alternative. However, some patients may prefer a "freezing" operation over a "cutting" operation. The main advantage of cryotherapy is its ability to destroy large numbers of lashes quickly. The procedure is easy to learn and quick to perform. A *double freeze–thaw* application of cryotherapy shows the highest success rate.

Cryotherapy includes:

- Local anesthetic with epinephrine to promote freezing
- Fast freeze followed by slow thaw
- Repeat fast freeze followed by slow thaw, using a slight overlap of the freeze spots
- Epilation

The steps of cryotherapy are:

1. Prep the patient
   A. Instill topical anesthesic.
   B. Inject *local anesthetic with epinephrine under the skin and conjunctiva and wait 10 minutes.* The vasoconstriction decreases the blood flow promoting a *fast freeze and slow thaw*, which gives the best result.
   C. Prep the patient, usually with no drape.
2. Apply the cryoprobe
   A. Protect the eye with a *plastic* lid plate (it must be plastic to insulate the eyeball from the cold).
   B. Place the cryoprobe onto the skin inferior to the misdirected lashes.
   C. Leave the probe in position for *30 seconds on the upper lid or 25 seconds on the lower lid to give an ice ball that surrounds the probe for 2–3 mm* (Figure 5-11).
   D. Let the probe *warm slowly* until it releases from the tissue.

E. Avoid the temptation to irrigate for faster warming.
F. Move to the adjacent tissue and repeat the application as needed along the lid. I use a *slight overlap of the ice ball edges.*

3. Let the tissues thaw slowly
4. After the tissue is thawed, repeat the freeze
   A. You will notice that the tissue freezes much more quickly, and a slightly shorter freezing time is required to get the same sized ice ball to form. This is not a precise procedure. It will take a few times to get the feel of how much overlap to apply and how long to leave the probe in place for each patient.
5. Epilate the misdirected lashes
   A. You will notice that the lashes "slide" out rather than "pop" out, suggesting that you have damaged the lash root.
6. Provide postoperative care
   A. Apply an antibiotic ointment.
   B. *Warn the patient* that there will be significant swelling. The freezing creates a mild frostbite with some associated burning pain. Postoperative narcotic treatment is appropriate for most patients.

Cryotherapy is easy to administer and destroys about 75% of the lashes treated. Some reoperations will be necessary. Most patients are surprised by the postoperative pain and swelling. You should warn them about this.

Although the freezing damages the lashes more than the surrounding soft tissue, cryotherapy can also damage the lid margin, leaving a *thinned lid margin.* Overaggressive freezing can kill the soft tissue, creating *lid notching* or another deformity. *Depigmentation* of the skin occurs and is noticeable in patients who are not white. Recurrence of the misdirected lashes after cryotherapy is low, but repeat freezing is sometimes required.

There is a theoretic possibility of *reactivation of ocular cicatricial pemphigoid* when cryotherapy is used. My personal feeling is that this is not true. Rather, these patients have a disease that is progressing rapidly, causing problems that require treatment. Nevertheless, I have any patient with active ocular cicatricial pemphigoid take 60 mg of prednisone a few days before and after the cryotherapy.

The most common use of cryotherapy in the past was for patients with many misdirected lashes. We now recognize that most of these patients have marginal entropion. With the use of the tarsal fracture procedure and other operations to redirect or excise lashes, the use of cryotherapy has decreased markedly (Box 5-4).

Pentagonal wedge resection for a segment of eyelash misdirection

Pentagonal wedge resection is a useful solution for removing a *localized segment of lashes.* This situation usually occurs after trauma. In many patients, a coexisting lid deformity, such as an eyelid margin notch, can be repaired.

The abnormal lashes are excised with a full-thickness pentagonal wedge resection of the eyelid. In most patients, you will remove less than one quarter of the eyelid. The reconstruction of the lid margin follows the same principles outlined in Chapter 13. Repair begins with *identifying the appropriate anatomic landmarks* of the eyelid, especially the

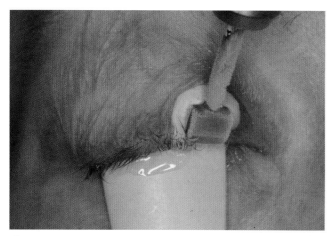

Figure 5-11 Cryotherapy. Form an ice ball 2–3 mm beyond the cryoprobe (usually 25–30 seconds). Use a double freeze–thaw cycle.

Box 5-4

Cryotherapy

- Inject local anesthetic with epinephrine; wait 10 minutes. You want a fast freeze and slow thaw
- Prep the patient, usually with no drape
- Protect the eye with a *plastic* shoehorn
- Apply the cryoprobe to the skin just inferior to the misdirected lashes:
  - 30 seconds on the upper lid or
  - 25 seconds on the lower lid
  - Allow an ice ball that surrounds the probe for 2–3 mm to form
- Move to the adjacent tissue and repeat the application
- Let the tissues thaw slowly. Repeat the freeze with slight overlap
- Epilate the misdirected lashes. Note that the lashes "slide" out
- Apply an antibiotic ointment
- Warn the patient of pain and swelling
- Prescribe a narcotic

landmarks of the lid margin. The *strength of the closure is in the sutures placed in the tarsal plate. Eyelid margin eversion* is necessary to prevent lid notching.

Pentagonal wedge resection and repair include:

- Excising the abnormal segment of lashes
- Aligning the lid margin
- Suturing the tarsal plate
- Suturing the lid margin
- Closing the skin

The steps of the pentagonal wedge resection and eyelid margin repair are:

1. Excise the abnormal segment of lashes
   A. Repair can be done with local anesthesia, unless excessive scarring exists.
   B. Mark a pentagonal wedge excision on the eyelid to include the abnormal lashes and 2–3 mm of normal margin on each side (Figure 5-12, A).
      (1) Extend the vertical marking to the superior edge of the tarsus.
      (2) Angle the markings to meet at the apex of the pentagon.
   C. Instill topical anesthetic drops and inject local anesthetic with epinephrine into the wound.
   D. Use a no. 15 scalpel blade to make the initial lid margin cut so that the wound edges will be sharp and close easily.
   E. Use scissors, preferably with straight blades, to excise the pentagonal wedge (Figure 5-12, B).
2. Align the lid margin
   A. Use a 7-0 Vicryl suture passed through the meibomian gland orifices to align the lid margin (Figure 5-12, C). Evert the wound edges slightly, using a vertical mattress suture pass. Keep this suture long.
3. Suture the tarsal plate
   A. Use two or three interrupted 5-0 Vicryl sutures passed in a lamellar fashion to align the tarsal plate

(Figure 5-12, D). The initial lid margin suture will help with the positioning of your tarsal sutures.
   B. If the wound is under considerable tension, you may want to place one or two 5-0 Vicryl sutures in the tarsal plate before passing the eyelid margin sutures. This can be a little more difficult as you will have to estimate the suture placement that properly aligns the eyelid margin.
4. Suture the lid margin
   A. Go back to the lid margin and place a 7-0 Vicryl suture in a *vertical mattress* fashion at the base of the eyelashes (Figure 5-12, E). This suture should provide *eversion* of the lid margin.
   B. If you are unhappy with the alignment of the lid margin, replace the margin sutures.
   C. An additional suture may be used to help align the eyelid margin.
   D. I prefer to use *7-0 Vicryl sutures for the eyelid margin.* Traditional teaching suggests the use of 6-0 or 8-0 silk sutures, which are left long and require removal later. The 7-0 Vicryl sutures can be cut on the knot and allowed to absorb.
   E. Don't tie the margin sutures very tightly because the tissue may die, resulting in a lid margin notch.
5. Close the skin
   A. The skin can be closed with an interrupted simple or vertical mattress suture using permanent or absorbable sutures (usually 5-0 fast absorbing gut) (Figure 5-12, G).
   B. If the wound seems to be under tension, you may want to place 5-0 Vicryl sutures through the orbicularis muscle before closing the skin (Figure 5-12, F).
6. Provide postoperative care
   A. Postoperative care is routine. Occasionally the sutures will rub against the cornea and require removal.

Careful realignment of the wound corrects the eyelash misdirection and creates a continuous row of lashes. Although a somewhat unusual situation, when you see a localized segment of misdirected lashes, consider this technique. It works very well (Box 5-5, Figure 5-13).

Treatment of epiblepharon

Children with epiblepharon are usually too young to complain about the lashes. More commonly, the children rub their eyes or have mild mattering. If the symptoms are mild and the cornea has little or no staining, I will treat with lubricating ointment and follow the child. If the child has photophobia or significant corneal staining, I recommend surgical excision of the redundant skin fold. In most cases, the lower lid is involved.

With the child under general anesthesia, the redundant lower lid skin is outlined with a marker. This is the most important part of the operation—too little excision means recurrence of the problem; too much excision means ectropion. The superior incision line is placed close to the eyelashes. The lower incision line should be positioned so that most of the fold is included within the marks (Figure 5-14). Moving the lid inferiorly and superiorly will help to identify

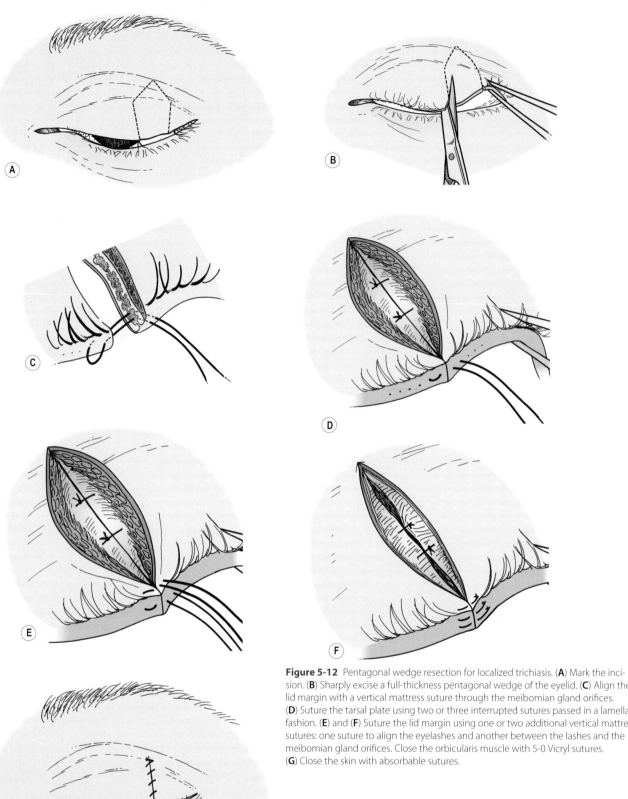

Figure 5-12 Pentagonal wedge resection for localized trichiasis. (**A**) Mark the incision. (**B**) Sharply excise a full-thickness pentagonal wedge of the eyelid. (**C**) Align the lid margin with a vertical mattress suture through the meibomian gland orifices. (**D**) Suture the tarsal plate using two or three interrupted sutures passed in a lamellar fashion. (**E**) and (**F**) Suture the lid margin using one or two additional vertical mattress sutures: one suture to align the eyelashes and another between the lashes and the meibomian gland orifices. Close the orbicularis muscle with 5-0 Vicryl sutures. (**G**) Close the skin with absorbable sutures.

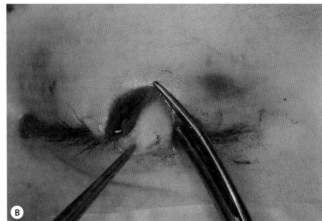

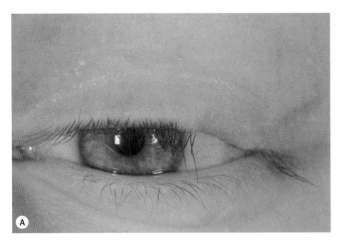

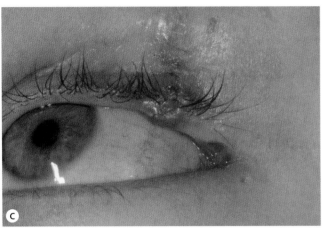

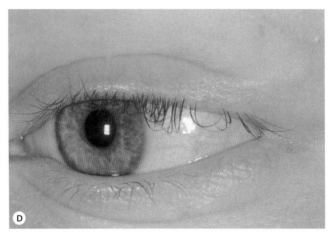

Figure 5-13 Pentagonal wedge resection of localized trichiasis. (**A**) Note the irregular lid margin and misdirected eyelashes. (**B**) Pentagonal wedge excision of the lid margin. (**C**) View of the lid margin 1 week postoperatively. Note elevation of the lid margin. (**D**) View of the lid margin 4 months postoperatively. Note the smooth lid margin and improvement of misdirected eyelashes.

Box 5-5

Pentagonal Wedge Resection

Excise the eyelid margin containing the abnormal lashes

- Mark a pentagon 2–3 mm beyond the abnormal lashes
- Use a no. 15 blade to excise the lid margin
- Use straight scissors to excise the pentagon wedge

Align the lid margin

- Use a vertical mattress 7-0 Vicryl suture through the meibomian gland orifices to align the lid margin

Suture the tarsal plate

- Use 5-0 Vicryl sutures to suture the lid margin
- Make lamellar passes

Suture the lid margin

- Use a 7-0 Vicryl suture at the base of the eyelashes
- Use a vertical mattress pass
- In some patients, an additional margin suture may be required
- Create slight eversion of the wound edges

Close the skin

- Pass absorbable skin sutures
- Consider 5-0 Vicryl sutures in the orbicularis muscle if the closure is under tension

---

the redundant tissue. "Pinching" the excess tissue with smooth forceps will help you to identify the amount of skin and muscle that can be safely excised. Be sure to extend the marking medially and laterally to include the full width of the excess fold. Inject local anesthetic with epinephrine and prep and drape the patient. Use a 4-0 silk suture as a traction suture in the lid margin. Incise the skin with a no. 15 blade. Use Westcott scissors to excise the skin and muscle (the Colorado needle works well also). Try not to cut the marginal arcade, which will be close to the superior incision. Close the skin edges with an absorbable suture such as 7-0 Vicryl or 5-0 fast absorbing gut. Some surgeons use a closure that incorporates the deeper tissues (tarsus or retractors) into the wound. I have found this to be unnecessary. The excision of the redundant skin fold is successful in most cases. Reoperations are infrequent but, as always when undertaking a new procedure, be conservative when you perform your first few operations.

Repair of upper lid epiblepharon is more difficult. Excision of the skin and muscle is difficult to do without forming an upper eyelid crease, which will change the appearance of the eyelid. This should be discussed with the patient preoperatively. The line of excision must blend into any medial epicanthal fold that is present.

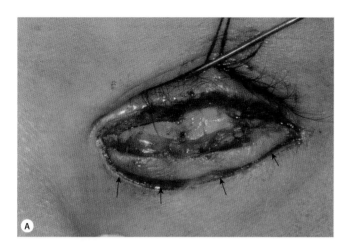

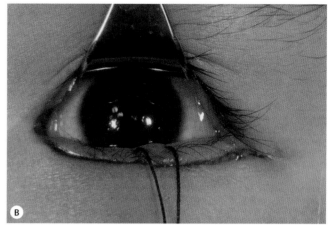

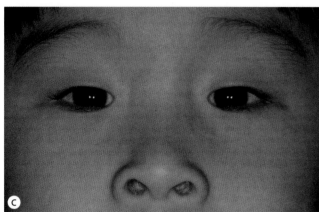

Figure 5-14 Epiblepharon repair (see Figure 5-8 for the preoperative view). (**A**) Mark and excise the redundant roll of lower eyelid skin. (Probe is in the lower canaliculus; arrows point to inferior incision line.) (**B**) The skin margins should touch slightly after resection. (**C**) Postoperative view. Note that the eyelashes are no longer against the cornea.

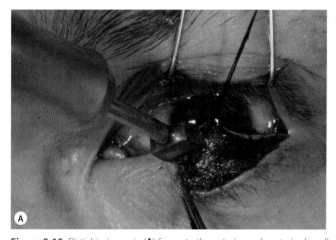

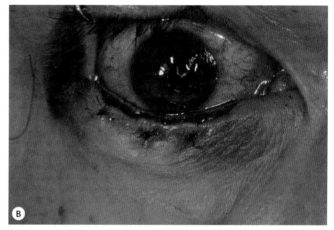

Figure 5-15 Distichiasis repair. (**A**) Separate the anterior and posterior lamella. Apply cryotherapy to the posterior lamella. (**B**) Recess the anterior lamella.

Treatment of distichiasis

The indications for treatment of distichiasis are the same as those for epiblepharon. The treatment depends on how many lashes are present. If only a few localized lashes are present, the principles outlined in the section "Treatment of Traumatic Causes of Eyelash Misdirection" can be applied. More commonly, an incomplete row, involving most of the eyelid, is seen. In these patients, *the lid margin is split into the anterior and posterior lamella along the gray line. Cryotherapy is applied to the posterior lamella*. The lamellae are reconstructed with the *anterior lamella in a recessed position* (Figure 5-15).

Distichiasis is rare and the treatment is somewhat involved. Referral to an oculoplastic surgeon is appropriate for most patients with distichiasis.

Checkpoint

- What is the most common symptom of trichiasis? What symptom in children is a good indicator of more than mild corneal exposure?
- What are the landmarks for the normal eyelid margin?
- Draw the lid margin and orientation of the eyelashes for each type of trichiasis.
- Review in your mind the treatment for:
  1. One or two misdirected lashes
  2. A 5- to 10-mm segment of misdirected lashes after trauma
  3. The entire length of the lower lid with marginal entropion
  4. The entire length of the upper lid with marginal entropion
  5. A child with epiblepharon and photophobia
  6. A child with distichiasis and moderate to severe corneal staining

Answers
1. Consider hyfrecation of involved eyelash follicles
2. Consider wedge resection of the involved lid margin
3. Tarsal fracture operation
4. First choice—tarsal fracture or terminal tarsal rotation operation. Second choice—anterior lamellar eyelash excision. Third choice—cryotherapy
5. Lower lid blepharoplasty
6. Lid splitting with posterior lamellar cryotherapy

Cicatricial and involutional entropion also cause the lashes to rub against the eye but are considered specific entities, rather than causes of trichiasis.

Major points

The normal landmarks on the lid margin include:

- The mucocutaneous junction
- The meibomian gland orifices
- The gray line
- The eyelashes

Any misdirection of the eyelashes is known as *trichiasis*.
The most common cause of trichiasis in adults is *marginal entropion*.

The signs of marginal entropion include:

- Parallel misdirected eyelashes
- Rounding of the posterior lid margin
- Anterior migration of the mucocutaneous junction

Trauma may cause trichiasis with or without lid margin irregularities.

- The misdirected eyelashes are frequently not parallel

The treatment options for trichiasis include:

- Tarsal fracture procedure
- Hyfrecation
- Pentagonal wedge resection of the eyelid with reconstruction
- Cryotherapy

Two childhood conditions cause the eyelashes to rub the cornea:

- Epiblepharon—treated with lower blepharoplasty
- Distichiasis—treated with lid margin splitting and posterior lamellar cryotherapy

Suggested reading

1. American Academy of Ophthalmology: *Basic and clinical science course: orbit, eyelids, and lacrimal system*, sect. 7, pp. 207–208, San Francisco, The American Academy of Ophthalmology, 2006/2007.
2. Anderson RL, Harvey JT: Lid splitting and posterior lamella cryosurgery for congenital and acquired distichiasis. *Arch Ophthalmol* 99:631–633, 1981.
3. Anderson RL, Wood JR: Complications of cryosurgery. *Arch Ophthalmol* 90:460–463, 1981.
4. Barber K, Dabbs T: Morphologic observations on patients with presumed trichiasis. *Br J Ophthalmol* 72:17–22, 1988.
5. Bartley GB, Lowry JC: Argon laser treatment of trichiasis. *Am J Ophthalmol* 113(1):71–74, 1992.
6. Boynton R, Naugle T: Trichiasis and distichiasis. In Levine MR, ed., *Manual of oculoplastic surgery*, 3rd edn, pp. 181–189, Boston: Butterworth-Heinemann, 2003.
7. Collin JRO: Entropion and trichiasis. In *A manual of systemic eyelid surgery*, 3rd edn, pp. 29–56 and 139–148, Edinburgh: Churchill Livingstone, 1989.
8. Kersten RC, Kleiner FP, Kulwin DR: Tarsotomy for the treatment of cicatricial entropion with trichiasis. *Arch Ophthalmol* 110:714, 1992.
9. Martin RT, Nunery WR, Tanenbaum M: Entropion, trichiasis and distichiasis. In McCord CD, Tanenbaum M, Nunery WR, eds, *Oculoplastic surgery*, 3rd edn, ch. 8, pp. 230–248, New York: Raven Press, 1995.
10. McCord CD, ed.: *Eyelid surgery, principles and techniques*, ch. 5, pp. 57–79, Philadelphia: Lippincott-Raven, 1995.
11. Nerad J: The diagnosis and treatment of misdirected eyelashes. In *The requisites—Oculoplastic surgery*, pp. 104–119, St Louis: Mosby, 2001.
12. Nerad JA, Carter KD, Alford MA: Trichiasis: marginal entropion and other causes. In *Rapid diagnosis in ophthalmology—oculoplastic and reconstructive surgery*, pp. 96–99, Philadelphia: Mosby Elsevier, 2008.
13. Sullivan JH, Beard C, Bullock JD: Cryosurgery for treatment of trichiasis. *Am J Ophthalmol* 82(1):117–121, 1976.

Involutional Periorbital Changes: Dermatochalasis and Brow Ptosis

Introduction

With time, the tissues in the periorbital area and face tend to sag. The periocular changes include a drooping of the brow known as *brow ptosis*, excessive accumulation of skin in the upper lid known as *dermatochalasis*, and a *prolapse of orbital fat* in the upper and lower lids caused by weakening of the fibrous orbital septum and orbital connective tissues. Characteristic changes in the midface, lower face, and neck occur as well. These anatomic changes occur in all patients to some degree as they age. In some patients, family traits may cause an exaggerated aging process. In others, earlier trauma or facial nerve palsy may add to the involutional process.

In each case, *you must understand the patient's complaint regarding these changes*. Many patients you see will complain about *decreased vision* due to the sagging tissues around the eye. Other patients may be more concerned about their *appearance*. One of the most important parts of the history-taking process is to understand the patient's complaint so that the appropriate concerns are addressed during surgery. In this chapter, we will discuss the functional changes of the periocular region—those changes that affect the vision. In the next chapter, "Aesthetic Surgery of the Face," we will discuss the aesthetic changes of the lower eyelids and face. There is a big overlap between the two approaches. Patients with functional changes have aesthetic issues and vice versa but, for the most part, your patients will be coming to you with complaints about *how they see versus how they look*. Part of your job is to sort out the relative importance of these complaints. In general, your aesthetic patients will be more

demanding and require more time. Your reimbursement for treatment to improve "how the patient looks" will be much higher than for treatment to improve "how the patient sees." In many cases, the operation will be the same or very similar. This can be a tricky area. Over time, you will develop your own ideas and learn to apply them on an individual basis.

A detailed examination will identify specific anatomic abnormalities that need to be addressed during surgery. These abnormalities include (1) low brow position; (2) abnormal brow contour, especially temporal droop; (3) redundant eyelid skin and muscle; (4) prolapsing orbital fat; (5) upper eyelid ptosis; (6) lower lid retraction; (7) lower eyelid laxity; and (8) abnormal orbital bony architecture. Midface, lower face, and neck changes should be identified as well. Once these individual factors are identified, their specific relationship to one another needs to be determined (**Figure 6-1**).

An operation is planned to correct the functional or aesthetic anatomic abnormality identified. Functional operations include *browplasty* and *upper blepharoplasty*, and will be discussed in this chapter. A variety of other procedures are available to complete the rejuvenation of the entire face, including lower blepharoplasty, forehead, midface, face, and neck lifts. Additional aesthetic operations including wrinkle reduction using laser resurfacing or chemical peels are available for patients seeking treatment in these areas. We will describe these procedures in the next chapter.

We will cover procedures that make your patient "see better" first. These include functional browplasty and upper blepharoplasty. We will discuss the principles of upper blepharoplasty from a reconstructive point of view. Although

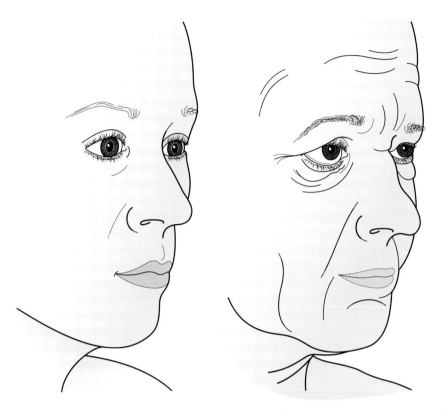

Figure 6-1 The aging face. Note typical involutional changes of the face, including descent of tissues, loss of subcutaneous fat, and deepening of skin wrinkles. Aging creates predictable "sags and bags": temporal brow droop, dermatochalasis, fat prolapse in the eyelids, lower eyelid laxity, malar mounds, deepening of the nasojugal fold (tear trough) and melolabial fold, marionette lines, jowling, loss the sharp angle between the neck and chin, and cervical banding.

this procedure is essentially the same for reconstructive and aesthetic purposes, there may be individual differences, depending upon the patient's goals. We will point out some of these nuances. Procedures that make your patient "look better" will be covered in the next chapter. As usual, in every operation, you should make an attempt to avoid complications of surgery including asymmetry, dry eye, lower lid retraction, and postoperative hemorrhage.

Anatomic considerations

The eyebrow

Parts of the eyebrow

The eyebrow has three parts, the *head*, *body*, and *tail*. The direction of the brow hairs varies from upward in the head of the brow to horizontal and slightly downward in the tail of the brow. The eyebrow is part of the forehead with similar thick skin and abundant sebaceous glands. The thick skin of the brow blends in with the thinner upper eyelid skin of the skin fold (Figure 6-2). You will be able to see and feel this transition.

Male and female eyebrows

The male and female brows differ considerably in position and shape. The *male brow is lower than the female brow*, resting at the edge of the superior orbital rim. The female brow is higher, especially in its temporal aspect, and sits above the orbital rim. The *female brow tends to be somewhat thinner* and is frequently manicured to emphasize a temporal arch with

the highest point generally occurring at the junction of the body and tail of the brow (see Figure 2-4).

Although we take these gender differences for granted, they are part of our culture in which looking young is emphasized. Like other secondary sexual characteristics, the brow position and contour send subtle clues regarding youth and reproductive ability. The thick low male brow is considered a sign of virility. The high arched brow of a woman is a sign of youth and vitality, which diminishes over time, seen as a temporal brow ptosis.

Movement of the eyebrow

The normal eyebrow *moves independently* of the upper lid. Extreme elevation of the eyebrow, as seen with severe upper lid ptosis, causes only slight elevation of the eyelid. The elevator of the eyebrow is the *frontalis muscle* (Figure 6-3), which extends from the brow over the forehead to merge with the broad fibrous tissue of the galea aponeurotica. Elevation of the frontalis muscle causes the *horizontal furrows* frequently seen in the forehead. Innervation of the frontalis, like that of other muscles of facial expression, comes from a branch of the *facial nerve*, the *frontal branch*. This single nerve provides innervation to the brow on the same side. The approximate position of the frontal nerve can be estimated by drawing a line from the tragus of the ear to 1 cm above the tail of the brow (see Figure 2-27).

Surgery in the path of the frontal branch of the facial nerve should be undertaken with caution to avoid damage to this nerve. Because this single nerve causes elevation of the brow, inadvertent injury to the brow may cause a prolonged paresis or permanent paralysis of the eyebrow.

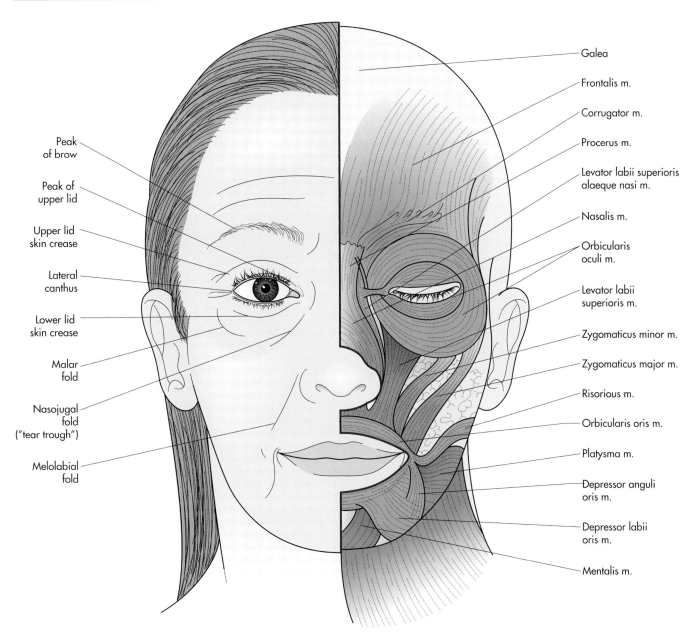

Peak
of brow

Peak of
upper lid

Upper lid
skin crease

Lateral
canthus

Lower lid
skin crease

Malar
fold

Nasojugal
fold
("tear trough")

Melolabial
fold

Galea

Frontalis m.

Corrugator m.

Procerus m.

Levator labii superioris
alaeque nasi m.

Nasalis m.

Orbicularis
oculi m.

Levator labii
superioris m.

Zygomaticus minor m.

Zygomaticus major m.

Risorious m.

Orbicularis oris m.

Platysma m.

Depressor anguli
oris m.

Depressor labii
oris m.

Mentalis m.

Figure 6-2 Surface landmarks of the face and brow.

Temporal brow droop

You will notice that the width of the frontalis muscle stops short of the tail of the brow. Consequently, elevation of the temporal brow often becomes deficient with aging, causing a temporal brow droop (Figure 6-4). As the brow droops, the upper lid skin fold is pushed down, accentuating the upper lid fold, often misinterpreted as redundant skin. Look for this problem in your older patients. It is so common that you may be ignoring it.

The glabellar folds

The *protractors*, or *depressors*, of the eyebrow are the orbital orbicularis, the procerus, and the corrugator muscles (Figure 6-5). Contraction of the *orbicularis muscle* closes the eye and pulls the eyebrow down. The vertical fibers of the *procerus muscle* at the head of the brow are responsible for the hori-

zontal furrows in the glabella. The *C-shaped corrugator muscle* pulls the head of the eyebrow medially and downward, causing the *vertical glabellar wrinkles*. Wrinkles in the area of the glabella are a common cosmetic concern among women. In many cases, these wrinkles may give an anguished or angry look to the face (see Figure 2-16).

The muscles of the eyebrows are among the most important muscles of facial expression. They are strong indicators of mood and feeling. This is best demonstrated by a simple diagram of the familiar *happy face* (Figure 6-6). A downward slope to the medial aspect of the eyebrows with associated glabellar wrinkles tends to convey *anger*. A drooping of the temporal brow suggests *melancholy*. Arched normally contoured eyebrows indicate happiness. Elevation of the arched brow with associated forehead furrows tends to indicate surprise. You may have seen this diagram in other texts. It is a very useful concept.

There are many operations that raise the eyebrows. Compare the extremes—a temporal direct brow lift and a coronal forehead lift—the former lifting the lateral part of the eyebrow and the latter lifting the eyebrows and entire forehead. You will see that the temporal lift uses a short incision placed at the lateral third of the brow hairs. It corrects the temporal sag and helps to clear the field of vision. It does nothing for the medial brow or the glabella. The coronal forehead lift is performed through an incision across the top of the head from "ear to ear." The entire forehead and eye-brows are raised. In addition, the glabellar folds, forehead furrows, and the redundancy of the eyelid skin under the medial brow are all improved. The overall result of the coronal lift is more aesthetically pleasing. Most forehead lifts are done for the "cosmetic" improvement and are "self-pay" procedures. You can guess that the recovery time and operating time for the two procedures are much different. Despite a long scar in the hairline for a coronal lift, it is less visible than the shorter scar over the eyebrow. However, the top of the head is left with some degree of numbness. You will learn which procedure is the best choice for your patient. I have

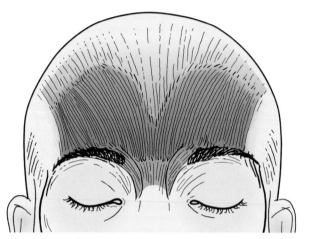

Figure 6-3 The frontalis muscle. Note that the frontalis muscle ends lateral to the body of the brow. Note the presence of the corrugator superciliaris and procerus muscles.

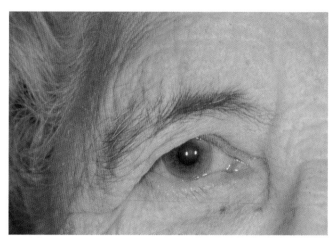

Figure 6-4 Temporal brow droop is one of the most common, yet unappreciated, causes of visual loss.

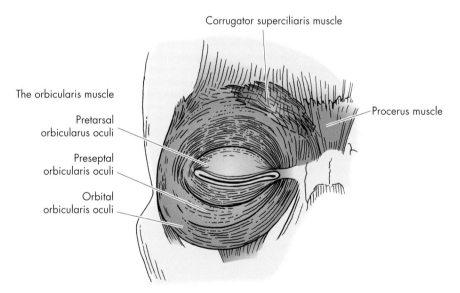

Figure 6-5 Muscles that close the eyes: the orbicularis muscle, pretarsal, preseptal, and orbital; corrugator muscle; and procerus muscle.

Corrugator superciliaris muscle

The orbicularis muscle

Pretarsal orbicularus oculi

Preseptal orbicularis oculi

Orbital orbicularis oculi

Procerus muscle

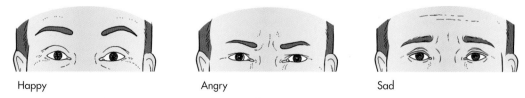

Happy

Angry

Sad

Figure 6-6 Position of brows as an expression of mood. *Left*, Happy. *Center*, Angry, mean. *Right*, Sad, melancholic (modified from Ellenbogen, 1983).

somewhat arbitrarily divided these procedures as "functional eyebrow lifting procedures" and "cosmetic forehead lifting procedures" and will discuss them in separate chapters.

Facial proportions

The proportions of the "normal" face are *divided into thirds*: the upper third from the hairline to the pupil; the middle third from the pupil to the alae of the nose (the 'mid' face), and the lower third from the nose to the chin. These thirds occur in roughly equal portions in a well-balanced face. Changes in the position of the eyebrows and the hairline may change the facial proportions. In a general sense, people with a higher forehead are thought to be somewhat more intellectual; hence the term "high brow." Changes in the male forehead associated with aging and male pattern baldness affect the proportions of the face. In general, a high forehead is considered to less aesthetically pleasing. The length of the forehead is influenced by browplasty. Incisions placed between the eyebrow and the hairline tend to shorten the forehead, and incisions placed in the hair tend to elevate the hairline, increasing the length of the forehead. These factors may contribute to the choice of incision placement in the patient's forehead. We will talk more about rejuvenation operations that lift the upper, lower and 'mid' face.

The upper eyelid

The skin fold, superior sulcus, and skin crease

The upper eyelid consists of three parts:

- The upper lid skin fold
- The upper lid sulcus
- The pretarsal eyelid

The skin and muscle between the eyebrow and the lid crease form the *upper lid skin fold* (see Figure 6-2). To have normal movement of the eyelid, there needs to be some redundancy in the eyelid tissues. This movement is provided by the skin fold. The skin fold is bounded by the eyebrow above and the skin crease below.

The *upper lid skin crease* is formed by attachments of the levator aponeurosis extending through the orbicularis into the skin. As the levator contracts, the skin crease is pulled upward, accentuating the *superior sulcus*. The upper lid skin crease is slightly higher in women than in men. A man's skin crease is usually at 6–8 mm whereas a woman's skin crease is usually between 8 and 10 mm above the lid margin. As the patient ages, the pretarsal skin sags somewhat, and the upper lid skin crease may change. The natural skin crease position can be estimated in a simple procedure performed before marking for blepharoplasty. Elevate the eyebrow and give the patient a target. As you elevate the target, you will see the upper eyelid skin tuck into place. This is the line of the original skin crease. In general, this position corresponds to the height of the upper eyelid tarsus.

A complex interaction of anatomic factors affects the fullness of the skin fold and the depth of the sulcus. *Younger patients tend to have a minimal skin fold. The brow is well supported, and there is little prolapse of orbital fat* (key factors for a young skin fold). The levator muscle pulls the pretarsal portion of the lid into the orbit. In children, the skin fold appears to be more a part of the eyebrow than of the eyelid. As the bony forehead develops in children and young adults, the fold lifts and remains tight against the brow, and a superior sulcus develops. With age, the brow descends and orbital fat prolapses, tending to fill in the sulcus and to increase the fullness of the skin fold of the older adult (Figure 6-7). You may want to reread this. It is an important concept if you want to attain any level of sophistication in performing blepharoplasty.

Individual facial proportions and bony features greatly influence the size of the skin fold. Some patients with a high or prominent brow will always have a minimal skin fold with a deep superior sulcus. Other patients with a flat brow have a full skin fold and shallow sulcus even as children. It is important to recognize these anatomic features because browplasty and blepharoplasty will not give the same results for each patient.

The upper eyelid skin and the orbicularis muscle

The upper eyelid skin is the thinnest skin of the body, allowing free movement of the eyelid. You will notice that the eyelid skin is much thinner than the eyebrow skin above.

The muscle underlying the eyelid skin is the orbicularis muscle. You are familiar with the three portions of the orbicularis muscle: the orbital, the preseptal, and the pretarsal portions. The orbital orbicularis muscle interdigitates with the procerus, corrugator, and frontalis muscles at the glabellar region (see Figure 6-5).

Relaxation of the frontalis muscle causes the brow (and underlying orbital orbicularis muscle) to fall. Correction of brow ptosis repositions the brow and orbital orbicularis muscle at the rim. Upper lid blepharoplasty removes a portion of the preseptal orbicularis and tightens the pretarsal orbicularis and skin.

The wrinkle lines in the lateral canthus, or "crow's feet," arise from contraction of the orbital orbicularis muscle.

The orbital septum

The orbital septum lies directly beneath the orbicularis muscle. It is a fibrous layer arising from the periosteum of the orbital rims. The septum functions as an anatomic boundary of the lids, separating the eyelids from the orbit (Figure 6-8). Although this fibrous tissue is quite tough, it also allows for vertical movement of the eyelid. With aging, weakening of the orbital septum allows fat to prolapse in the eyelid. When no fat prolapse is present, the orbital septum is not opened during upper lid blepharoplasty. When orbital fat prolapse is present, the orbital septum may be opened and fat is excised or repositioned. Fat prolapse is the main indication for blepharoplasty in the lower eyelid. Because the septum is not elastic, it should never be sewn closed as this may contribute to lagophthalmos. With aging, the smooth transition from the lower eyelid to the cheek is lost. Fat prolapse and associated cheek descent transforms the single convex surface of the eyelid and cheek to the so-called "double convexity" that is part of the aging midface. We will learn about this more later.

The preaponeurotic fat

The upper eyelid preaponeurotic fat is divided into two compartments containing the *preaponeurotic* or *central fat* and the *nasal* or *medial fat*. The lacrimal gland fills in the temporal aspect of the preaponeurotic space in the upper lid (Figure 6-9). The lacrimal gland is distinguished from the fat by its whitish color and lobulated surface. A branch of the palpe-

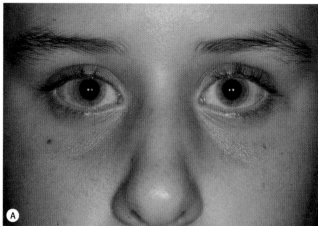

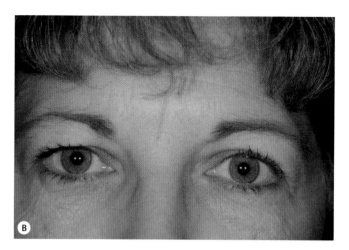

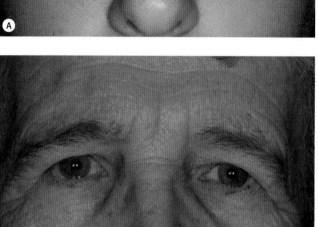

Figure 6-7 The typical superior sulcus by age. Note progression of brow ptosis crowding the sulcus. (**A**) Teenager: the brow is well supported and independent of the eyelid. (**B**) Middle-aged woman: mild generalized brow ptosis contributing to the fullness of the sulcus. (**C**) Older woman: note the prominent temporal brow ptosis.

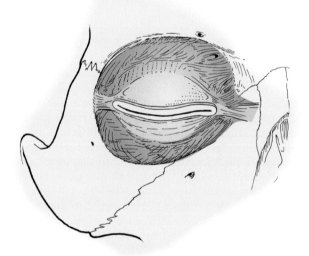

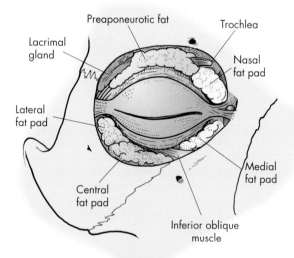

Figure 6-8 The orbital septum.

Figure 6-9 The preaponeurotic fat. Note central and nasal fat pads. Lacrimal gland is temporal to the central fat pad.

bral artery runs posterior to the nasal fat pad. You should be careful not to inadvertently cut this artery because brisk bleeding will occur. The nasal fat pad is whiter in color than the central fat pad.

The amount and position of the fat prolapse varies from patient to patient. No fat prolapse is seen in many patients.

These patients may have dermatochalasis only and do well with only skin and muscle being removed during upper lid blepharoplasty. Nasal fat prolapse is especially common, but patients may have fat prolapse in any combination of locations (Figure 6-10).

The lower eyelid

The lower eyelid position and contour

The normal lower eyelid *rests at the limbus*. The lateral canthus is slightly higher than the medial canthus in most patients. The lowest point of the lower lid is inferior to the lateral limbus (see Figure 6-2).

The position of the lower eyelid is dependent on several factors including:

- The inferior rim bony prominence
- The horizontal tension of the lower eyelid
- The length of the anterior or posterior lamellae of the eyelid

We saw in our discussion of ectropion (see Chapter 3) that patients with less prominent inferior orbital rims (maxillary hypoplasia or "hemiproptosis") are more susceptible to lid retraction and ectropion. Another way to evaluate this is to view the patient from the side and draw a line from the cornea to the inferior orbital rim. If the line slopes toward the cheek, the patient is said to have a *negative vector* (the same as what we have termed hemiproptosis). Shortening of the skin, muscle, or conjunctiva from sun, disease, trauma, or surgery can cause lower lid retraction. You will learn to respect the forces that hold the lower eyelid in position. It does not take much to alter the balance of these forces to cause lower lid retraction, the most common complication of lower lid blepharoplasty.

The lower eyelid skin and muscle

The *lower eyelid skin is thin* like the upper eyelid skin. Because there is less movement of the lower eyelid than of the upper eyelid, the lower eyelid anterior lamella has less redundancy than the upper lid skin fold provides. Similarly, the less well-developed lower lid retractors do not create the same pull as the levator muscle, making the lower lid skin crease not apparent in most adults.

Briefly, let's consider the general aging changes of the face:

- Sagging ("descent") of facial features
- Deepening of facial wrinkles
- Loss of subcutaneous tissue ("deflation")

You have seen this in your patients, but may be unaware of the process. Changes in the connective tissue occur. Loss of strength allows the face to sag, seen as descent of the malar fat pad, deepening of the nasolabial fold, and the creation of cheek jowling. Orbital fat prolapses forward because of a weakened orbital septum. The skin loses elasticity, creating fine wrinkling on the skin surface and the deep dynamic lines in the face that form as a result of the movement of the underlying muscles. The subcutaneous tissue, primarily fat, tends to atrophy. The face can appear as an "empty sac." The orbit appears hollow with deepening of the superior sulcus, often masked by a brow ptosis.

The parts of the orbicularis muscle in the lower eyelid have the same names as those in the upper eyelid. The orbital portion extends on the cheek. In young patients, there is a smooth transition from the eyelid margin to the cheek. With aging, the lower eyelid preaponeurotic fat prolapses forward, and a convexity to the surface of the lower eyelid is created. The descent of the cheek, once cushioning the inferior orbital rim, causes the orbital rim to be palpable and appear depressed. The smooth transition from the eyelid to the cheek is lost and a "double convexity" (Figure 6-11)

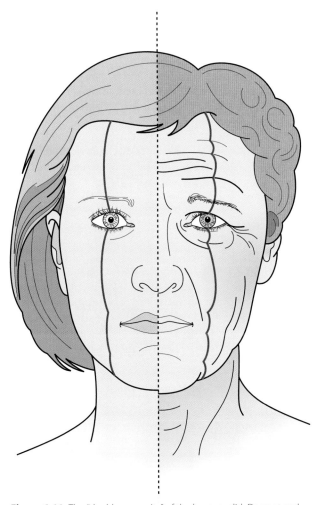

Figure 6-11 The "double convexity" of the lower eyelid. Descent and deflation aging changes transform the youthful smooth facial contours into a series of "sags and bags." As the cheek descends and the eyelid fat prolapses forward, the normal smooth contour of the lower eyelid is lost and the "double convexity" forms (based on McCord, Ch. 2, Fig. 2.14).

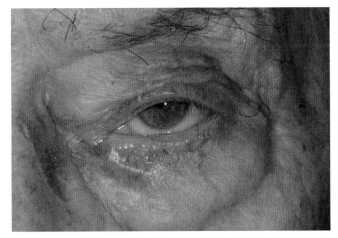

Figure 6-10 Lower eyelid fat prolapse and prominent upper nasal fat prolapse. Brow ptosis, blepharoptosis, and punctal ectropion are also present—all examples of involutional changes.

is created in profile. Lifting the cheek (midface) in combination with lower eyelid blepharoplasty can restore the youthful smooth profile to the eyelid and cheek. As you become more aware of facial aesthetics, you will notice how the aging process affects all your patients. We will talk more about the anatomy that applies to aesthetic procedures in the next chapter.

The lower eyelid fat

The lower lid fat includes *nasal, central,* and temporal fat pads (see Figure 6-9). The nasal fat pads in both upper and lower lids are somewhat whiter than the other fat pads.

Checkpoint

At this point, you should understand the changes that occur in the aging of the face:

- Most changes can be described as "descent and deflation"
  - Generalized increased laxity of tissues
  - Loss of soft tissue volume
- Brow ptosis, especially temporal
- Descent of the midface
- Redundant skin and muscle of the upper lid skin fold (made worse by brow ptosis)
- Weakening of the orbital septum causing fat prolapse
- Remind yourself of these points:
  - The differences in the male and female brow
  - How the brow position and contour reflect mood
  - The muscles responsible for the horizontal and vertical glabellar furrows
  - How to mark the upper lid skin crease
  - The number of fat pads in the upper and lower lids

History

Introduction

Taking the history and doing the physical examination tend to occur simultaneously. Before the patient even speaks, you will be formulating an opinion about the patient's structural abnormalities and the potential for correcting each abnormality. But beware, what you see and what the patient sees may be different. Resist the temptation to skip the history taking. Let the patient tell you what is bothering him or her. You may be surprised.

The patient's complaint

The most important part of the patient interview is the *patient's complaint*. You must have a complete understanding of the patient's concerns and expectations for the outcome of the operation. Is your patient concerned about the loss of visual field? Or is your patient interested in changing the appearance of the eyes? Both are valid reasons for seeking your help, but each goal may require a different approach to meet your patient's expectations. At some point during your discussion, you should ask your patient about the primary purpose of the operation, "Do you want to look better, or do you want to see better?"

Even functional goals involve a change in the patient's appearance. Often it is helpful to have the patient show you the problem in a mirror. Remember, what you see may not be what the patient sees. When you think that you understand the patient's problem, explain your perception, again using the mirror, to confirm that both you and the patient have the same understanding of the problem. The ultimate success of the blepharoplasty and browplasty has as much to do with understanding the patient's concerns and goals as it has to do with your surgical technique.

Here is a warning: remember that, even though your patient may be having a blepharoplasty for functional reasons, he or she may anticipate a certain "cosmetic" result. If the main complaint is related to loss of vision, both you and your patient should have a common understanding about what would be a "reasonable" cosmetic outcome related to the proposed operation. This avoids postoperative complaints after functional blepharoplasty such as, "What about this wrinkle here?" or "I thought my eyelids would look more open." If the patient's primary concern is the aesthetic outcome, the patient is more likely to be pleased if the procedure is not billed to medical insurance even if there is a visual function component to the problem. When the goal of the operation is to restore visual function, this should be noted in the medical record as part of the documentation of the necessity for surgery.

General medical and ocular history

You will need to review the patient's general medical condition and medications. Most patients will be healthy enough to tolerate the surgery you plan. Make sure hypertension is controlled. Remind the patient to stop all aspirin-containing medications and platelet inhibitors 10 days before surgery. All nonsteroidal anti-inflammatory drugs should be stopped 5 days before surgery.

How about the feared "dry eye." It is best to ask about a burning or foreign body sensation in the eyes and the use of artificial tears. A sensitivity to moving air, from ceiling fans, air vents, or windshield defrosters, may indicate a "dry eye." Asking if the patient has been told if he or she has a dry eye is not helpful. Many patients have been given this diagnosis incorrectly, and it will not likely complicate your blepharoplasty result. A patient who benefits from using artificial tears once a day does not really have a "dry eye." We will talk about this topic more in Chapter 10.

Is helpful to know if the patient has had any previous blepharoplasty. If so, any drooping upper lid skin is usually the result of untreated brow ptosis. During your interview, you may notice a sign of facial asymmetry and want to ask about any pre-existing facial nerve palsy.

Physical examination

Questions to be answered

In the physical examination, you will be answering these questions:

- What is the normal anatomy and function?
- What is the structural abnormality? How does the patient's anatomy differ from normal? How are functions altered?

- What is the patient's complaint? What are the patient's goals? (functional or cosmetic) What is the patient's desired outcome? (specific postoperative appearance) What is the potential for meeting these goals?
- What are the options for attaining the patient's goals? What is the best surgical plan?
- Are there contraindications for getting the desired result?

Don't memorize these questions. You are already answering these questions about your patients without knowing it. Many of the problems that we are addressing in this chapter are really not "abnormalities;" rather, they are normal anatomic consequences of aging. For most patients, you will be comparing their current anatomy with what was probably present many years before. We will look at the examination with these thoughts in mind.

Examine each portion of the periorbital anatomy including the eyebrow, the upper lid, and the lower lid. It is a good idea to perform an anterior segment examination to identify any coexisting eye abnormalities, especially factors related to maintaining a healthy precorneal tear film.

During the examination, you will be comparing the patient's periocular anatomy to the stylized "normal" or "desirable" anatomy for the patient's gender. As you gain experience, you will be able to visualize the patient's potential for that "perfect" look or normal function.

Examination of the eyebrow

The height and contour of the brow

The examination should always begin at the eyebrow. The *height and contour of the eyebrow* should be noted. You will recall that the normal male brow is at the rim and relatively flat. The normal female brow is above the rim and arched temporally. Remember to look at some young adults to help you understand where the normal brow position is. A good way to judge the height of the brow is to palpate the brow between your index finger and thumb relative to the orbital rim. Is there a generalized ptosis of the brow or is there more of a mild temporal droop? Brow furrows indicate that the patient is trying to see by using the brows to elevate the lids. One of those furrows may be a good place to hide a browplasty scar.

The supraorbital ridge

Is the supraorbital ridge prominent or flat? Lifting the brow with your finger can give you an estimate of the potential depth of the superior sulcus. A flat supraorbital ridge with relatively prominent eyes does not offer much potential for a deep superior sulcus. Remember, the majority of cosmetic surgery is soft tissue surgery, not bone surgery. A browplasty redrapes the tissues over the skeleton. It is like reupholstering a sofa. If the frame does not have the correct proportions, adding new fabric may not meet the customer's goal. As you get experience, you will learn to see the potential effect of a browplasty or blepharoplasty on the appearance of a particular patient. You will see an older patient with very ptotic brows and drooping upper lids, but you will also recognize the patient's handsome or beautiful bone structure, which will make your surgery look good.

The position of the eyebrow must be considered before any decision regarding upper lid blepharoplasty can be made. *Aging causes changes throughout the whole face.* Removing only skin in the area of the skin fold, blepharoplasty, is generally not the complete answer. It can be the best compromise, however. If the eyebrow is markedly drooped, consideration should be given to a browplasty. Commonly, the temporal aspect of the eyebrow droops the most, and a small temporal direct browplasty can be used to lift the eyelid. When a more complete brow ptosis exists, elevation of the entire brow should be considered. If the patient is interested in removing the forehead and glabellar furrows or "cleaning up" the sagging skin above the medial canthus, the best treatment is one of the cosmetic forehead procedures that provide lift across the entire forehead. Blepharoplasty can be performed on a patient with a drooping brow, but remember that the eyebrow and the eyelid should function independently. You must leave enough skin between the skin crease and the eyebrow, at least 10–15 mm, to allow independent action to occur.

Examination of the upper eyelid

The examination of the upper eyelid in preparation for blepharoplasty is focused on the extra tissues in the skin fold and the position of the eyelid.

Skin fold

Your examination of the skin fold has already started. The biggest factor in the fullness of the skin fold is the eyebrow position. Look at your younger patients (or young television personalities). You will see that, if the brow is in a good position, there really is not much skin fold to deal with. You can estimate the amount of redundant skin and muscle in the skin fold if you lift the brow into the normal position at or above the rim. If you lift the brow higher, you can see any fullness of sulcus if there is prolapsed orbital fat present. You should note the amount and position of the fat (central or nasal fat). It is especially common to see prolapsed nasal fat. In older patients, you may see sagging pretarsal skin that should be tightened during the blepharoplasty.

Upper eyelid height

As you lift the upper lid skin fold up, note the position of the upper eyelid. Frequently, upper eyelid ptosis coexists with dermatochalasis. The combination of upper eyelid blepharoplasty and ptosis repair is quite common.

In general, *redundant upper eyelid skin does not change the eyelid position (margin reflex distance; MRD)*. To determine the MRD_1, simply elevate the upper skin fold slightly to check the position of the upper lid margin (recall that the MRD_1 is the distance from the corneal light reflex to the upper eyelid margin). Levator function can be recorded, but it is not necessary if ptosis repair is not being considered.

If you and your patient feel that the problem interferes with vision, you should record this in the medical record. Typically, a *ptotic brow hanging over the superior orbital rim or dermatochalasis with upper lid skin resting on the eyelashes is considered to affect vision significantly.* Visual field measurements with the eyelid skin or ptotic brow in resting position can be used to demonstrate a field defect that improves when the brow and skin fold are lifted. These visual field measurements may be required for reimbursement from Medicare or private insurance. You may need to take photographs to document the necessity for surgery.

Examination of the lower eyelid

Prolapsing orbital fat

Lower eyelid blepharoplasty is a cosmetic procedure except in rare patients. *In contrast to the upper lid blepharoplasty, in which the emphasis of the operation is removing skin and muscle with variable amounts of fat, the lower lid blepharoplasty involves primarily the removal or repositioning of fat and a minimal removal of skin.* Evaluate the amount of fat in each compartment. This will help you intraoperatively. If you know that there is no prolapse of the lateral fat pad, you won't have to look there during surgery.

Redundant skin and muscle

Next look to see how much redundant skin and muscle are present. Younger patients often have fat prolapse without redundant lower lid skin. Older patients have both fat prolapse and redundant skin and muscle present (Figure 6-12). You should note whether any *lower eyelid malar bags* or *festoons* are present (Figure 6-13).

Lower eyelid position

The most common complication seen with lower lid blepharoplasty is lid retraction, so it is important to note the preoperative position of the lower eyelid and any predisposing factors that could contribute to lower eyelid retraction postoperatively. The normal lower lid rests at the limbus. The position of the lower eyelid, the MRD_2, is measured in millimeters from the corneal light reflex to the lower eyelid margin. Lower lid retraction can occur naturally or may be

the result of previous blepharoplasty or any trauma where anterior lamellar shortening has pulled the lid inferiorly.

The lateral canthus is usually 1–2 mm higher than the medial canthus. The contour of the lower eyelid normally has a gentle curve up toward the lateral canthus. The lowest point of the lower eyelid is inferior to the lateral limbus. The position of the lower lid is related to both lower lid laxity and eyelid bony architecture.

Lower eyelid laxity

Lower lid laxity should be estimated during the lower eyelid examination. Two tests are useful. The *lid distraction test* measures the distance that the lower eyelid can be pulled directly off the eye. The normal eyelid should not pull more than 6 mm away from the eyeball. The *snap test* determines the ability of the eyelid to return to normal position after it

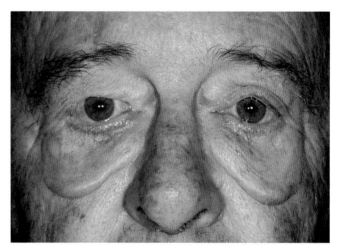

Figure 6-13 Lower eyelid festoons. Note the patient has had previous upper eyelid reconstruction procedures on both upper eyelids.

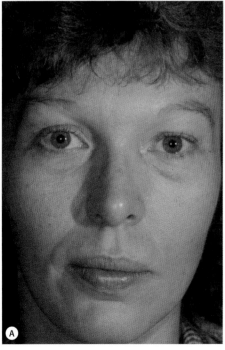
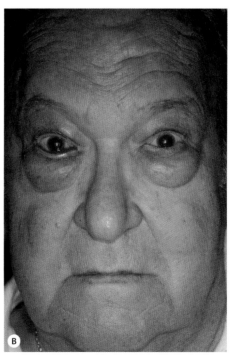

Figure 6-12 Lower eyelid examination. (**A**) Fat prolapse without redundancy of skin and muscle. (**B**) Fat prolapse with redundant skin and muscle. Note left lower eyelid retraction and bilateral upper eyelid retraction suggesting thyroid eye disease.

has been pulled away from the globe. The lower eyelid is pulled down and released. The position of the eyelids is evaluated without the patient blinking. As the patient blinks, the eyelid will return to normal position. A healthy lower lid should return to normal position without a blink or with one blink. If several blinks are required for the lid to return to normal position, the lid is lax. These tests were discussed in more detail in Chapter 3 (see Figures 3-6 and 3-7). Lower lid laxity should be corrected at the time of lower lid blepharoplasty to avoid lid retraction or ectropion.

The inferior orbital rim

A significant, often overlooked, factor related to the lower eyelid position is the anterior projection of the inferior orbital rim. If the midface is somewhat hypoplastic, the lower lid is relatively poorly supported and tends to be retracted in the resting position. As we discussed earlier, patients with this midfacial hypoplasia are said to be "hemiproptotic" or have "shallow orbits." The term *orbito-ocular disparity* is also used, emphasizing that the cornea is more anterior than the inferior orbital rim. In aesthetic surgery, as we discussed above, the term used is *negative vector orbit*. These patients are at risk for lid retraction after any lower eyelid operation.

The relationship between the inferior orbital rim and the position of the eye varies among individuals, but also tends to vary among races. Asian patients tend to have high cheekbones and a low predisposition for lid retraction. African American patients tend to have the opposite facial characteristics, with maxillary hypoplasia causing prominent eyes and inferior scleral show. Caucasian patients tend to have bony architecture intermediate between African American and Asians. It is important for you to recognize lid retraction or the potential for it to occur after blepharoplasty, because it changes the patient's appearance and can contribute to corneal exposure.

Keep in mind that lower blepharoplasty is primarily an operation designed to remove excess fat. As your experience in cosmetic surgery increases, you may learn techniques to reposition the fat to create a more youthful and graceful contour over the inferior orbital rim. In older patients, you will usually remove a small amount of skin and muscle in addition to the prolapsing orbital fat.

Lid retraction is the most common complication, so look for preoperative lid retraction, lid laxity, or hemiproptosis to help you plan the lower lid blepharoplasty. The *transconjunctival approach* for fat excision is a good solution for removing excess fat without affecting the lower lid position (more on this surgical approach later). When you need to excise skin and muscle to reduce lower eyelid skin redundancy, you will probably tighten the lower eyelid to avoid retraction.

General skin condition

As you perform more periocular operations, you will quickly recognize the signs of damaged skin. Changes related to *sun damage* and *smoking* should be noted. *Deep facial wrinkles, blotchy pigmentary changes, loss of skin elasticity, and thinning of the dermis that allows the deeper vessels to be visible* are signs of actinic damage. Smoking causes *premature aging and deep furrowing of the skin*. Small vessel damage predisposes patients to poor healing and potential flap necrosis.

Explain to your patient that blepharoplasty will not change the condition of the skin. Upper and lower lid blepharoplasty restores the structure to the periocular tissues, but cannot remove all the periocular wrinkles, even in normal skin. In many patients, *laser resurfacing* or chemical peels will improve the rhytids and pigment changes related to aging or sun damage. We will talk about how to make and keep the skin looking young in the next chapter.

Checkpoint

- What is the most important part of the history taking?
- Review the points of the physical examination (Box 6-1). You should be able to write these points down from memory
- What are the factors related to the depth of the superior sulcus? Consider brow height, supraorbital ridge prominence, and the components of the skin fold
- What do the MRD_1 and MRD_2 represent? What are normal measurements?
- Describe the lid snap and lid distraction tests for evaluating lower lid laxity

Contraindications to surgery

Inability to meet the patient's goals

The main contraindication to proceeding with surgery is the inability to meet the patient's goals for surgery. The patient may not have realistic expectations. You and the patient may not be a good personality match. A technically perfect operation will not be satisfactory to the patient if you don't meet his or her goals.

During your interview, watch how the patient blinks and moves the face. Is the *blink rate* normal? Does the patient blink infrequently (Parkinsonism) or blink excessively (reflex irritation or essential blepharospasm). Does the eye close

---

Box 6-1

The Periocular Physical Examination

The eyebrow
- Brow position
- Brow contour
- The supraorbital ridge

The upper eyelid
- The eyebrow
- The superior sulcus
- The skin fold
  - Redundant skin and muscle
  - Prolapsing orbital fat
- The upper eyelid position: MRD_1

The lower eyelid
- Prolapsing orbital fat
- Redundant skin and muscle
- Lower lid retraction: MRD_2
- Lower lid laxity
- The inferior orbital rim

completely with a blink. An *incomplete blink* is associated with facial nerve weakness or a cicatricial process of the eyelids. *Lagophthalmos* means that the eye does not close completely at rest. If the *Bell's phenomenon* is normal, sleeping with the eyes open a small amount does not cause corneal drying. *Lower eyelid retraction* will exacerbate any tendency for corneal irritation postoperatively.

We already talked about the diagnosis of *dry eyes* and the usefulness of questions about eye irritation associated with air circulating across the eyes. During slit lamp examination, look at the size of the tear lake, the thickness of the conjunctiva, and any corneal staining. The Schirmer's test with a topical anaesthetic is not an extremely reliable test, but a result of less than 5 mm of wetting suggests caution. If you are not familiar with these tests, ask a colleague to do an examination to identify risk factors that will increase the chance of corneal exposure after surgery.

"Dry eyes" or blinking abnormalities should be considered relative contraindications for blepharoplasty procedures. You should always tell your patient that eye irritation is always a possibility. In most patients, the irritation can be managed with lubricants and tincture of time. The more aggressive the blepharoplasty or ptosis surgery, the more likely that dry eye will develop. If you think your patient is at risk, remove somewhat less skin and muscle. Some surgeons do only skin resection in these patients. If you follow these guidelines, very few, if any, of your patients will have long-term problems with irritation.

Browplasty

Planning the browplasty and upper eyelid blepharoplasty

If your patient is young and has no evidence of brow ptosis, an upper lid blepharoplasty is the obvious choice for saggy skin in the upper eyelid. If the brow is ptotic, you have three choices:

- Elevate the entire brow (+/– blepharoplasty)
- Lift the temporal brow (+/– blepharoplasty)
- Do blepharoplasty alone

Your decision will depend largely on the patient's expectations. As we discussed above, if the brow is low and the patient wants a "cosmetic result," the best choice is an endoscopic forehead lift or other type of forehead lift. Besides lifting the eyebrow, the entire forehead is raised with an improvement in forehead furrows, glabellar folds, and the "multicontoured" areas of the medial canthus. All this can be accomplished with minimal visible scarring. These operations are relatively time consuming and are usually reserved for cosmetic indications. The technique for these operations will be discussed later in this chapter.

If the patient is purely interested in lifting the brow for visual function reasons, a direct browplasty is best. Forehead tissue directly above the brow is removed. This provides a strong lift of the brow. A scar directly above the brow is produced. Exchanging the preoperative melancholic sleepy look of the patient with temporal brow ptosis for the alert "happy face" of the arched brow can have a dramatic effect on the appearance of a patient, especially an older patient

(Figure 6-14). An alternative for men with deep forehead furrows is the indirect or midforehead lift. This operation removes a horizontal strip, or two ellipses, of forehead tissue halfway up the forehead with the incision hidden in a forehead furrow (Figure 6-15).

Most patients older than age 50 have an element of *temporal brow ptosis*. This can be addressed simply with a *temporal direct browplasty*. This procedure is a useful adjunct to an upper lid blepharoplasty when there is a temporal ptosis. This operation is simple and leaves an acceptable scar for most patients except those who are most concerned about a cosmetic result. If you plan to do blepharoplasty operations in older adults, you should learn this operation.

An alternative to the temporal direct browplasty is the *transblepharoplasty* (or *transeyelid*) *browplasty*. In this procedure, the *temporal half of the brow is tacked to the periosteum or attached to the bone with a "carpet tack" device*. The browplasty is performed through the blepharoplasty skin crease incision so there is no *additional scar*. This procedure is less powerful than the lateral direct browplasty and does not lift the medial brow. Transblepharoplasty browplasty is most commonly used as an adjunct to a blepharoplasty when there is mild brow ptosis or temporal brow ptosis and the patient does not want a full forehead lift. You will want to learn this procedure for patients having blepharoplasty who have mild sagging of the temporal eyebrow that will interfere with a good blepharoplasty result.

As you can see from Box 6-2, there are many types of browplasty operations. As is the usual case, this means that none is perfect. Each has its pros and cons. So learn the procedures that suit your patient population and skill level. Consider the following order of learning browplasty operations. For the beginning surgeon, the direct temporal approach is a good way to get rid of the temporal hooding in an aging patient where a blepharoplasty alone is not enough. As you get more experience, try more difficult procedures. Combining an upper blepharoplasty with a transblepharoplasty brow lift is the next step and not much more difficult. It is useful for the same problem as the temporal direct browplasty, but does not leave a scar because you use the blepharoplasty incision to get to the brow. You should consider learning these procedures.

As you master simpler operations, you can move to more difficult procedures. The aesthetic "endoscopic" forehead techniques that I use most often use the same initial approach as the transblepharoplasty browplasty and, when performed this way, is not a huge step further. The midforehead operation we describe is useful in only a few patients, mainly men with deep forehead furrows. It does have the advantage of not creating arched brows, but it is not an easy dissection plane. It seems less "scary" than the bigger forehead procedures, but it is not easier. Often the scar, even though hidden in a furrow, is deeper than I like. The pretrichial lift is not difficult as you get more experience with larger flaps and has the big advantage of lowering the hairline, which is a real bonus for many women. For both the coronal and the pretrichial forehead lifts, numbness of the forehead and crown of the head is pronounced, so make sure that your patient is ready for that. The traditional coronal flap is a powerful procedure and not much more difficult than the pretrichial lift but, for most patients with a normal hairline wanting an aesthetic lift, I prefer the modified endoscopic lift. The endo-

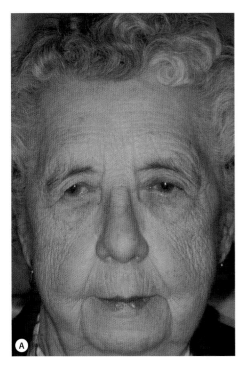

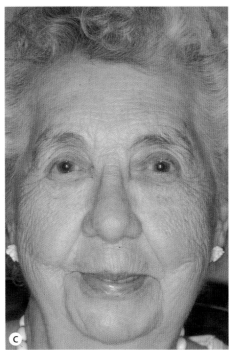

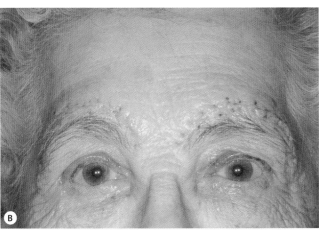

Figure 6-14 Direct browplasty. (**A**) Preoperative melancholic look resulting from the temporal brow ptosis. (**B**) One week after direct browplasty, upper lid blepharoplasty, and ptosis repair. (**C**) Postoperative alert and "happy face" look with brow elevated and natural contour restored.

scopic lift is not easy but, like all procedures, as your skill level and experience increase, you will get good results and your operating time will reduce to a reasonable time. If you move onto aesthetic facial procedures, the pretrichial, coronal, and endoscopic lifts are often combined with midface and lower face lifts.

Direct browplasty

The direct forehead lift provides a good functional eyebrow lift. It lifts the entire brow from the head to the tail of the brow. The contour of the brow can be influenced to a large degree, depending on the amount of tissue excised over a region of the brow. The direct browplasty is best suited for women who desire a functional improvement of their eyebrow position. The familiar temporal arch preferred by most women can be recreated by excising more tissue temporally than medially. The complete direct browplasty is not recommended for the patient desiring true cosmetic surgery.

You can use the complete direct browplasty in men, but you should try to minimize the feminization of the eyebrow. The ellipse of skin excision should be drawn to avoid a typically female temporal arch. You will not be able to avoid the smooth superior edge of the eyebrow where brow hairs are always lost to some degree, tending to give the upper eyebrow a manicured look, rather than the typical male feathered look.

Before any browplasty, you should discuss the possibility of *scarring*, *asymmetry*, and *numbness*. Scarring will be present in all patients, but is acceptable to older patients. Asymmetry can occur, but should be modest. Some degree of hyperesthesia in the area immediately above the incision is common. Direct incision of the supraorbital nerve at the head of the brow should be avoided to prevent permanent numbness of the entire forehead and scalp on the same side.

The complete direct browplasty is a relatively easy operation. Many of your patients with functional brow ptosis will be good candidates for this operation.

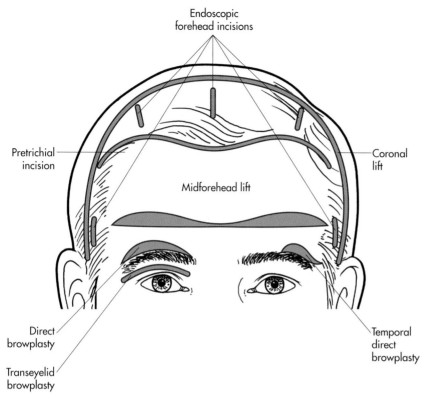

Figure 6-15 Browplasty operations: coronal, endoscopic, midforehead, direct, temporal direct, and transblepharoplasty.

Box 6-2

Comparison of Browplasty Procedures

Procedure	Advantages	Disadvantages
Direct temporal	Easy Minimal visible scar Corrects the commonly seen temporal hooding	Does not lift central brow
Direct	Easy Elevates central brow Good for facial nerve paralysis	Visible scar Some temporary hyperesthesia
Transblepharoplasty	Lifts temporal brow No scar Good adjunct to blepharoplasty	Not a powerful lift Moderate difficulty Some forehead tenderness Visible mound in some
Midforehead	Lifts entire brow Avoids arched brow of direct approach Avoids bigger flap Minimal hyperesthesia	Selected patients Deepens forehead furrows Visible scar Not easy dissection plane
Pretrichial	Powerful lift Minimal hairline scar Lowers hairline Smoothes forehead and glabella	Numb above hairline Moderate difficulty Risk to frontal branch
Coronal	Powerful lift, the "gold standard" Scar hidden in hair Smoothes forehead and glabella	Numb above incision Moderate difficulty Raises hairline Risk to frontal branch Large flap
Endoscopic	Good lift Scars hidden in hair Minimal numbness Can smooth forehead and glabella	Not as powerful as coronal Difficult Some extra equipment ? duration of lift

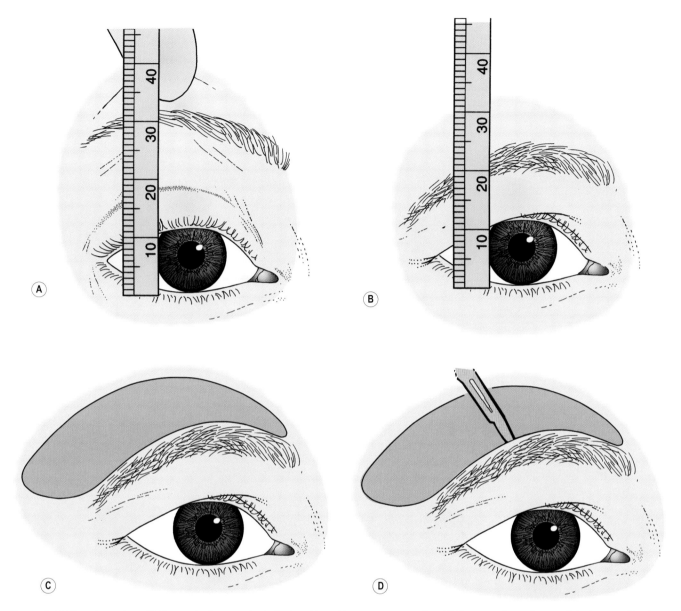

Figure 6-16 Direct browplasty. (**A**) Elevate the brow to the desired position with some overcorrection. (**B**) Place a marker at the top of the brow and let the brow drop. (**C**) Mark an ellipse of tissue to be removed (the normal range of excision is 10–15 mm). (**D**) Make a skin incision through the subcutaneous tissue to the frontalis and orbicularis muscles. (**E**) Excise the skin and muscle to the periosteum. Do not excise muscle over the head of the brow to avoid anesthesia of the forehead. (**F**) Layered closure. In patients with brow paralysis, suture the muscle to the periosteum. In other patients, close the subcutaneous layer with interrupted sutures and the skin with a running suture. Note that the position of the brow is overcorrected more for patients with brow paralysis.

The direct browplasty includes:

- Skin marking
- Anesthesia
- Skin and muscle excision
- Closure

The steps of the complete direct browplasty are:

1. Mark the skin
   A. Mark the amount of resection preoperatively. Hold the eyebrow in the desired position at (men) or above (women) the rim. Place a ruler next to the inferior brow hairs. Allow the brow to drop to the relaxed position. Record the distance that the eyebrow drops. Multiply this number by a factor of 1–1.5 times to give the final height of the planned excision. Measure at least two points above the eyebrow. Draw an ellipse from the eyebrow hairs to the marks placed above the brow (Figure 6-16, A–C).
   B. The shape of the ellipse should correspond to the change in contour anticipated. Usually 8–15 mm of tissue is excised with the greater measurements being temporal.
   C. Do not extend the temporal incision more than 1 cm lateral to the tail of the brow to avoid inadvertent damage to the frontal nerve.
2. Administer anesthesia
   A. Instill topical anaesthetic drops.

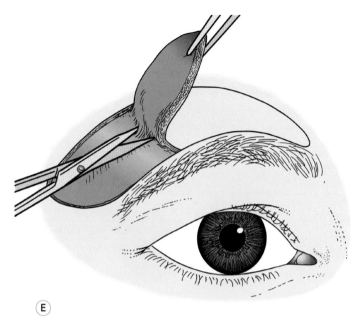

(E)

Figure 6-16 Continued.

(F)

B. Inject local anaesthetic into the skin down to the periosteum. Avoid injection into the supraorbital vein.

3. Excise skin and muscle in one layer
   A. Use a no. 15 blade to incise the skin. Make a deeper incision using the blade, CO_2 laser, or Colorado needle to deepen the incision *to the subcutaneous fat. You must keep the excision superficial at the head of the brow to avoid damage to the supraorbital nerve* (Figure 6-16, D).
   B. Some surgeons prefer to bevel the blade during the skin incision with the thought that fewer brow hair follicles will be cut. In my experience, this has not made much difference and, in almost all patients, some superior brow hairs are lost independent of the skin incision technique.
   C. Use a Stevens scissors, Colorado needle, or CO_2 laser *to excise the skin and muscle layer*. You will be dissecting in the loose areolar layer anterior to the periosteum (Figure 6-16, E). Stay superficial to the frontalis near the tail of the brow.
   D. You will need to use some *cautery* at this point. Cauterize the biggest vessels and cover the wound with a wet sponge and go on to the other eyebrow. Most of the smaller vessels will stop bleeding without cautery.

4. Close the wounds with a layered closure
   A. Use a 4-0 PDS suture (P-3 needle Z494G) to close the deep tissues with a few interrupted sutures and a 5-0 Prolene suture (Ethicon 8698 P-3 needle) for a continuous skin closure (the blue Prolene suture is easier to see than a black suture against dark brow hairs) (Figure 6-16, F).
   B. Place topical antibiotic on the wounds.
   C. Remove the skin sutures in 7–10 days.

The postoperative care of the patient and side-effects of this procedure are minimal. Scars take 6 months, or longer, to

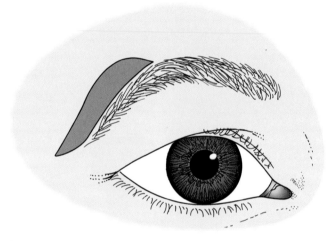

Figure 6-17 Temporal direct browplasty.

fade well. Numbness resolves slowly over the same time period, as long as you have not cut the supraorbital nerve. Your patients will be much more tolerant of any scarring and numbness if they know what to expect from your preoperative discussions.

Temporal direct browplasty

This procedure is anatomically the same as the complete direct browplasty, but is performed only in the *lateral one half or one third of the eyebrow* (Figure 6-17). Remember to avoid the path of the frontal branch of the facial nerve to prevent the possibility of a complete brow paralysis. This procedure is an excellent choice for repair of functional brow ptosis. It is very useful as an adjunct to upper lid blepharoplasty. It is equally helpful in both men and women because the high arch of a complete direct browplasty can be avoided. The temporal aspect of the eyebrow scars less than the medial aspect. There is less risk of hyperesthesia as well. The technique of the temporal direct browplasty is the same as that of the direct browplasty with only the lateral portion of the brow being elevated.

The temporal direct browplasty does not correct a complete brow ptosis. A small amount of scarring is always present temporally; however, this is generally well tolerated. This scarring may be unacceptable for a patient who wants the ultimate procedure.

Midforehead lift

The midforehead lift uses incisions placed in forehead furrows to lift the entire eyebrow and lower forehead (see Figure 6-15). Staggered incisions across the forehead brow can provide lift for the glabellar area as well.

The midforehead lift tends to be *more useful in men* than in women because men frequently have deeper forehead wrinkles. There is less feminization with the midforehead lift than with the direct lift, because the brow is lifted evenly across its entire length without creating a great deal of arch. The hairs on the superior edge of the eyebrow are not violated, so the typical male feathered edge to the superior brow is not altered. The midforehead lift can be used in women, but the benefits, compared with those for a direct browplasty, are greater for men. The scar from a midforehead lift is better hidden than that from a direct browplasty if there are deep forehead furrows present. Like all brow incisions placed below the hairline, the forehead is shortened a small amount. The midforehead lift is not ideally suited for patients with a completely smooth forehead.

Two types of midforehead lift operations are possible. The first type includes skin and subcutaneous tissue excision only. The second type includes brow suspension with sutures.

In the first technique, an ellipse of tissue is drawn in a forehead furrow to correct the height and contour abnormality. The vertical height of the proposed excision should be 1–1.5 times the measured brow droop. The brow incision may extend across the forehead or it may be staggered in alternate wrinkle lines for better camouflage. The ellipses can be drawn above or below the forehead wrinkle. Skin and subcutaneous tissue only are excised. The frontalis muscle should not be excised because this may cause some forehead weakness above the incision. In older patients, it can be difficult to identify the frontalis muscle. Frequently, all you will see is a faint pink layer of tissue within the subcutaneous tissue of the forehead and brow. After the skin excision, close the wounds in a layered closure similar to that for the direct browplasty.

The suture suspension midforehead lift involves the formation of a skin flap and suture suspension of the eyebrows.

The suture suspension midforehead lift includes:

- Marking the skin
- Injecting local anaesthetic
- Making the skin incision
- Dissecting in the subcutaneous plane
- Suspending the brow with sutures
- Excising the redundant skin
- Closing the wound

The steps of the suture suspension midforehead lift (suture suspension) are:

1. Mark the skin
   A. Mark a horizontal forehead furrow 2–4 cm above each brow (Figure 6-18, A). No measurements are made.
2. Administer anesthesia
   A. Instill topical anaesthetic drops.
   B. Inject local anaesthetic into the tissue down to the periosteum.
3. Make a skin incision
   A. Make an incision into the skin to the *subcutaneous level*.
   B. If you cut more deeply through the subcutaneous fat, you will see the faint pink layer of the frontalis muscle. Try to avoid this.
4. Dissect a plane within the subcutaneous tissue
   A. In the subcutaneous plane, anterior to the frontalis muscle, dissect inferiorly to the brow hairs. This is a *difficult step* because there is no true tissue plane. All the dissection is sharp. Make sure that you do not make the forehead flap so thin that a part of it will die (Figure 6-18, B and C).
5. Perform suture suspension
   A. Place two 3-0 Gore-Tex sutures (Gore 3N10 PH-24 CV-3 needle) at the junction of the thirds of the eyebrow.
   B. Pass each needle deep into the periosteum at the level of the skin incision.
   C. Tie each suture temporarily in a "hang back" fashion, estimating the proper height and contour (Figure 6-18, D).
   D. With the patient in the sitting position, check the height and contour.
   E. Make adjustments as necessary until height and contour are acceptable. A second suture may be used at the junction of the medial and central thirds of the brow if there is a residual medial brow ptosis. Overcorrect the brow height moderately.
   F. Tie the sutures.
6. Make a skin excision
   A. Drape the excess skin over the incision and mark the excess.
   B. Excise the excess skin sharply with the scalpel (Figure 6-18, E).
7. Close the wound
   A. Close the skin in a layered fashion as explained above (Figure 6-18, F).

In this operation, the *amount of lift is determined by the tightness of the sutures* rather than the amount of skin excision alone. Consequently, the skin excision is not measured or marked at the beginning of the procedure. *Intraoperative suture placement and adjustment are the critical parts of this operation*. This technique offers the ability to get a slightly better contour and perhaps a more long-lasting result because of the suture placement. In theory, there is less numbness of the forehead than with the skin flap midforehead lift. This procedure is more difficult than the skin excision midfore-

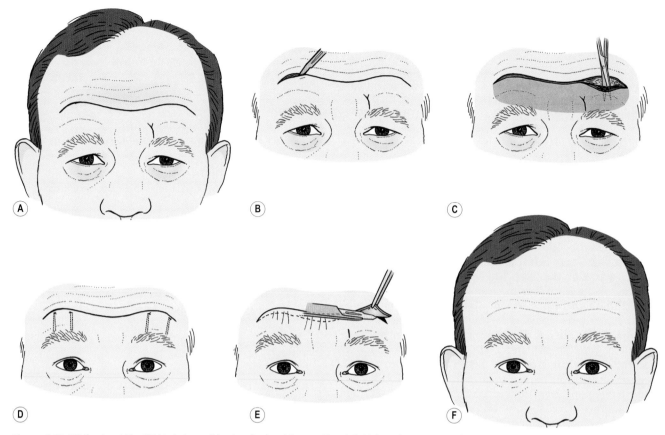

Figure 6-18 Midforehead lifts. (**A**) Mark the excision in a forehead furrow. (**B** and **C**) Make a skin incision with a no. 15 blade. Dissect a skin flap with Stevens scissors or a Colorado needle within the subcutaneous layer (sharp dissection required). (**D**) Place brow suspension sutures using 3-0 Gore-Tex. (**E**) Mark and excise the excess skin. (**F**) Close the subcutaneous layer and the skin.

head lift flap or direct brow lift. Skin flap elevation requires attention so that the skin flap will remain viable.

Few complications occur with the midforehead lift. Asymmetry is possible and, if marked, it can be corrected with a reoperation. Scarring is always present to some degree, and it takes months for the scars to disappear. There is generally some numbness above the skin incision, which improves with time. This is not the ultimate cosmetic procedure, but it works well for many patients, especially those with deep forehead furrows (Box 6-3).

Transblepharoplasty browplasty

The transblepharoplasty or transeyelid browplasty is performed through the upper lid skin crease incision in conjunction with an upper lid blepharoplasty. This operation is useful for the patient with a *mild brow ptosis* who would benefit from a slight brow elevation in conjunction with blepharoplasty, but who does not want the scar of a direct temporal browplasty or a full brow lift using an endoscopic or coronal forehead lift.

The transeyelid browplasty operation includes:

- Marking the skin and injecting anesthesia
- Making the blepharoplasty incision
- Performing the brow dissection
- Elevating the brow
- Closing the blepharoplasty incision

Box 6-3

Suture Suspension: Midforehead Lift

Skin marking

- Horizontal furrow only

Anesthesia

- Local anesthetic down to the periosteum

Skin incision

- Into the subcutaneous layer anterior to the frontalis muscle

Dissection of skin plane

- Sharp dissection in the same plane anterior to the frontalis muscle inferiorly to the brow

Suture suspension

- 3-0 Gore-Tex sutures (Gore 3N10 PH-24 CV-3 needle) from brow to the periosteum
- Careful adjustment for height and contour

Skin excision

- Excess skin draped over the wound and excised

Closure

- 4-0 PDS interrupted sutures in the subcutaneous layer (Ethicon P-3 needle Z494G)
- 5-0 Prolene or nylon running skin suture (Ethicon 8698G or 698G P-3 needle)

The steps of the transeyelid blepharoplasty are:

1. Mark the skin and administer anesthesia
   A. Mark the excess skin for upper lid blepharoplasty.
   B. Inject local anaesthetic as you would normally for blepharoplasty.
   C. Inject additional local anaesthetic at the superior orbital rim and under the eyebrow.
2. Make the skin incision and perform the standard blepharoplasty excision of skin and muscle (Figure 6-19, A)
3. Dissect under the brow
   A. Dissect superiorly toward the brow, *beginning at the superior edge* of the blepharoplasty incision.
   B. Extend the dissection superiorly in the *preseptal plane to the orbital rim at the arcus marginalis.*
   C. *Extend the dissection above the rim, anterior to the periosteum for approximately 1.5 cm* for the lateral half of the eyebrow (Figure 6-19, B).
      (1) You can *remove* or *sculpt brow fat* at this point. If the brow is particularly heavy, your patient may benefit from removal of the brow fat pad. This should be necessary only in very full eyebrows. Dissect in the subcutaneous fat posterior to the eyebrow hairs to meet the previous dissection anterior to the periosteum.
      (2) Elevate and fixate the brow
         a) Suture technique
            i) Extend the dissection above the rim, anterior to the periosteum for approximately 1.5 cm for the lateral half of the eyebrow (Figure 6-19, B).
            ii) You can remove or sculpt brow fat at this point. If the brow is particularly heavy, your patient may benefit from removal of the brow fat pad. This should be necessary only in very full eyebrows. Dissect in the subcutaneous fat posterior to the eyebrow hairs to meet the previous dissection anterior to the periosteum.
            iii) Elevate the brow, pass a 4-0 PDS (Ethicon P-3 needle Z494G) suture through the soft tissues under the inferior edge of the eyebrow hairs. Place the suture at the junction of the body and tail of the brow.
            iv) Next pass the same suture through the periosteum 1 cm above the supraorbital rim and make a temporary tie (Figure 6-19, C and D).
            v) Repeat the browplasty on the other side and inspect to ensure symmetry. Check the final height and contour with the patient in the sitting position. Additional sutures can be passed if necessary to improve the brow contour.
            vi) A superficial pass of the needle under the eyebrow will create dimpling of the brow. In some cases, you will lose some motility of the eyebrow.
            vii) You will not be able to elevate the head of the eyebrow because of the position of the supraorbital nerve.
         b) Endotine forehead fixation technique
            i) The Endotine forehead fixation technique is an easy and clever way to fixate the eyebrow to the scalp. An Endotine device or "carpet tacks" is used to attach the elevated brow to the skull (Figure 6-20, http://www.coaptsystems.com). This is currently my favored technique for fixation using the transblepharoplasty approach.
            ii) Following blepharoplasty, you will perform the same approach to the rim. At the rim, use the microdissector needle to elevate the periosteum and dissect superiorly on the frontal bone for 2–3 cm. This is a subperiosteal dissection, not a preperiosteal dissection as above. As you are subperiosteal, there is no brow fat pad sculpting. Do this from the lateral canthus to the supraorbital neurovascular bundle.
            iii) Using the hand drill, make a bone hole about 12 mm superior to the p 60 rim, about 12 mm medial to the temporal line. Clean the bone fragments from the hole. A flat end of a Senn retractor (Storz N4780) is useful to give exposure to the bone.
            iv) Push the Endotine into place. "Hang" the periosteum of the frontal bone over the tines using a Freer elevator. Examine the position of the brow. You can unhook it and push the brow higher if necessary. Once you have a reasonable position, check for contour, height, and symmetry with your patient in the sitting position.
            v) This is a much more satisfying procedure than the suture fixation technique. Both these techniques "push" the eyebrow into position and are less powerful than procedures that "pull" the eyebrow up from above. The long-term effectiveness has not been proven.
            vi) When you are comfortable with this technique, learn to do the broader elevation that I describe in the section on endoscopic brow lifting technique in the next chapter. With more knowledge of the temporal anatomy and a little practice, you can release a significant amount of the forehead and temple, including the release of the conjoined tendon, through the eyelid.
      (3) After either fixation technique, close the wound. Open the septum and remove fat, if necessary, after fixing the brow. Then use your usual closure.

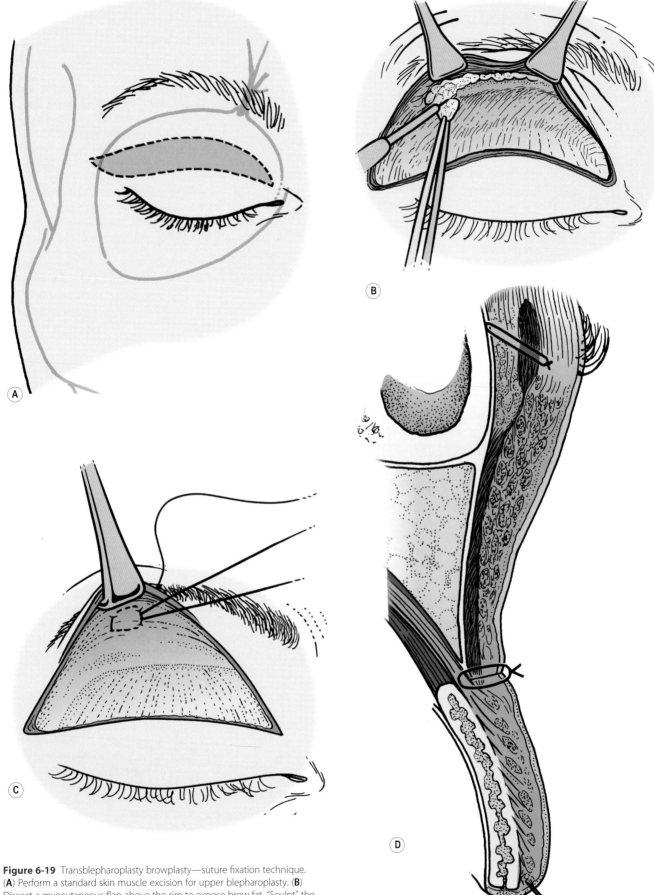

Figure 6-19 Transblepharoplasty browplasty—suture fixation technique.
(**A**) Perform a standard skin muscle excision for upper blepharoplasty. (**B**)
Dissect a myocutaneous flap above the rim to expose brow fat. "Sculpt" the
brow fat as needed. (**C**) Elevate the brow with sutures. (**D**) Sagittal view with
brow fixation and skin sutures in place.

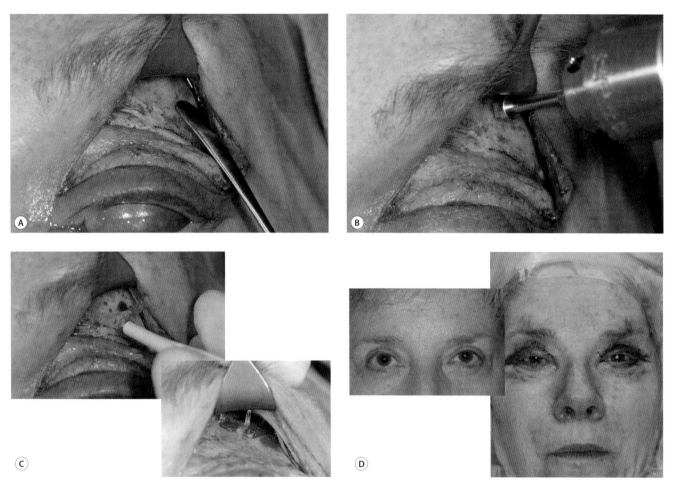

Figure 6-20 Transblepharoplasty browplasty—Endotine forehead fixation technique. (**A**) Dissect a myocutaneous flap superiorly from the standard blepharoplasty excision to the superior orbital rim. Incise the periosteum from the supraorbital notch to the lateral canthus. Elevate the brow in the subperiosteal plane (shown). (**B**) Drill a hole 12 mm above the rim, 12 mm medial to the temporal line. (**C**) Push the Endotine into the drill hole. Set height of brow by pushing tissues onto the tines. (**D**) Intra op and post op views.

Remember that you excise less skin and muscle for blepharoplasty when performing a browplasty. The transeyelid browplasty should be considered as an addition to upper lid blepharoplasty in younger patients looking for a deeper superior sulcus. The elevation provided is not enough for a complete brow ptosis or more than mild to moderate amounts of temporal brow ptosis. As you might expect, some temporary numbness will occur above the brow. Despite these limitations, this browplasty can be useful for patients undergoing simultaneous blepharoplasty (Box 6-4).

Upper eyelid blepharoplasty

Preoperative considerations

Blepharoplasty is a commonly performed procedure in both men and women. The upper lid blepharoplasty *removes redundant skin and muscle from the upper skin fold. Variable amounts of fat are excised,* depending on the amount of fat prolapse and the goals of the operation.

Upper lid blepharoplasty can be considered to be either functional or cosmetic. When the patient complains that vision is blocked by the redundant skin fold and the examination supports this complaint, upper lid blepharoplasty is considered to be a reconstructive procedure reimbursed by insurance. Each insurance carrier has slightly different requirements for payment, but they usually include:

- A visual complaint
- An upper lid skin fold that hangs over the lashes on physical examination
- Superior visual field loss of 15 degrees or more (sometimes described as a 20% loss)
- Photographs that document the condition

Visual field loss can be demonstrated by performing visual field examination with the lids and brow in a resting position compared with the lids and brow taped in an elevated position. A large isopter is chosen to map the peripheral field using either an automated or a Goldmann field technique. Tangent screen or confrontation fields may be used if other techniques are not available. The difference in the degrees of

Transblepharoplasty Browplasty—Endotine Fixation

Skin marking and anesthesia
- Administer intravenous sedation
- Mark an upper eyelid skin crease and blepharoplasty incision
- Mark the high point of the eyebrow (usually at the lateral one third)
- Inject local anesthetic and administer topical drops

Skin incision
- Perform a standard upper lid blepharoplasty operation (see below)

Brow dissection
- Dissect anterior to the septum to the arcus marginalis
- Cut periosteum. Subperiosteal dissection for 3 cm
- Consider temple and conjoined tendon release

Brow fixation
- Drill hole 12 mm superior and 12 mm medial to temporal line
- Position 3.5 mm Endotine forehead device
- Suspend brow tissues onto tines
- Inspect for height, contour, and symmetry

Closure
- Use a standard blepharoplasty closure

peripheral field in the untaped and taped screening test represents the amount of visual field loss caused by the dermatochalasis. The exact amount of field loss that defines a "functional" condition varies among insurance carriers.

Although all upper lid blepharoplasty procedures are similar, an individual patient's goals, expectations, and demands can be quite different. Patients who are interested in visual field improvement are generally tolerant of minor amounts of asymmetry postoperatively. These patients view their operation as a necessary procedure that will improve their vision. Patients who are interested in a cosmetic improvement have often given the operation a great deal of consideration and have specific results in mind. For the most part, these expectations are reasonable, although the demands on the surgeon's time and expertise are usually greater.

Brow ptosis, dermatochalasis, and upper lid ptosis frequently occur together and combine to cause visual field loss in patients undergoing blepharoplasty. Blepharoplasty, browplasty, and ptosis repair are considered separate operations and should be reimbursed independently if the specific contributions to visual loss are documented. In many cases, insurance payers fail to realize the importance of these independent procedures, and reimbursement for each may be difficult to obtain. Operations designed primarily to offer an improvement in appearance should be considered cosmetic surgery with payment provided by the patient, not through insurance reimbursement.

As with any type of operation, the *ultimate success of the procedure depends on meeting the expectations of the patient.* Sometimes, the patient may claim to be interested in obtaining an improvement in visual function from the blepharoplasty, but he or she really wants a cosmetic result that the insurance company will pay for. Every patient undergoing blepharoplasty derives some cosmetic benefit, independent of the main purpose of the procedure. Although functional

and cosmetic blepharoplasty are the same procedure, less skin removal and, in most cases, no fat removal are required to lift the skin fold off the lashes and restore the visual field. Cosmetic surgery requires great attention to symmetry and generally attempts to recreate a deep sulcus. The surgeon and the patient must agree on the goals of the surgery to avoid patient disappointment and surgeon frustration when good visual improvement is obtained that does not meet the cosmetic concerns of the patient. If the patient's main concern is to alter appearance, then the procedure is classified as cosmetic. Recall our earlier discussion of "how the patient looks" versus "how the patient sees."

Upper eyelid blepharoplasty technique

Review the indications for browplasty in association with blepharoplasty before you decide to do a blepharoplasty alone. Remember that patients who have a redundant upper lid skin fold commonly have an element of temporal brow ptosis or complete brow ptosis. The steps of the upper lid blepharoplasty are the same whether or not you do a browplasty. In most patients, blepharoplasty accompanying browplasty will require less skin removal.

The steps for functional and cosmetic blepharoplasty are the same and are considered in this section together. In general, more skin and fat are removed for cosmetic indications. Some surgeons do not consider fat removal a part of a functional blepharoplasty. Lower blepharoplasty is always considered to be a cosmetic procedure and will be discussed in the next chapter with other aesthetic facial procedures.

The upper lid blepharoplasty includes:
- Skin marking
- Anesthesia
- Skin incision
- Skin and muscle excision
- Fat excision
- Closure

The steps of the upper lid blepharoplasty are:

1. Mark the skin
   A. The most important part of the upper lid blepharoplasty operation is marking the appropriate amount and location of the skin and muscle to be removed. Perhaps a better way to think of this is *marking a symmetric amount of skin that will remain between the eyebrow and the skin crease on each side.*
   B. There are two parts to blepharoplasty marking: *the skin crease* and *the upper limit of the skin excision.* The procedure for marking the skin crease has been discussed previously. With the patient in a supine position, manually elevate the eyebrows just to the level at which the eyelashes start to lift. Ask the patient to slowly look from downgaze to upgaze and you can identify the patient's natural skin crease where the skin tucks in. As the patient moves the eye, make a few small marks in the crease. With the patient's eyes resting closed, connect the marks and extend the skin crease from the punctum to the lateral canthus. Extend the curved skin crease incision laterally to the lateral orbit rim or slightly beyond.

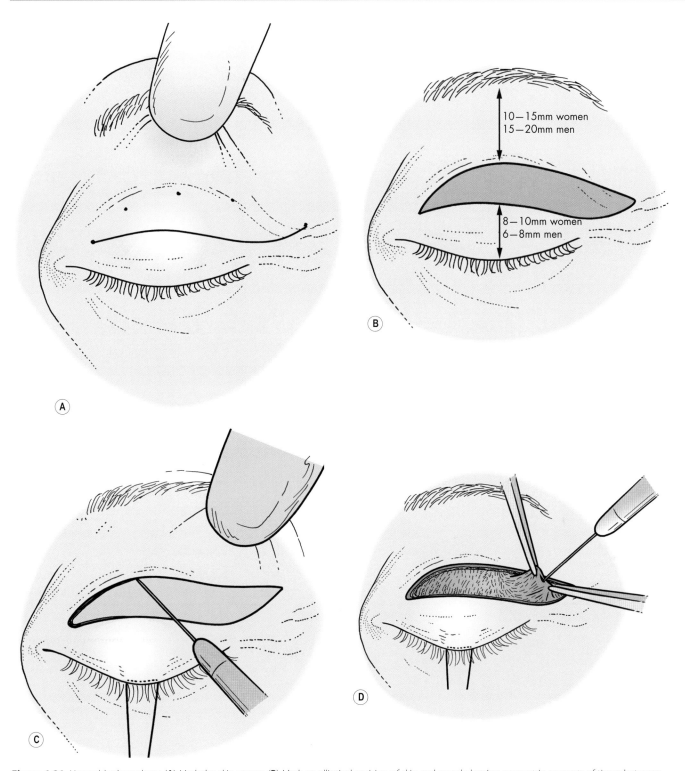

Figure 6-21 Upper blepharoplasty. (**A**) Mark the skin crease. (**B**) Mark an elliptical excision of skin and muscle leaving symmetric amounts of tissue between creases and brows. (**C**) Excise a skin and muscle flap using the Colorado needle. (**D**) Open the entire orbital septum. (**E** and **F**) Excise fat using scissors or a thermal cautery. (**G**) Pass two interrupted skin crease-forming sutures to the aponeurosis. Excise any "dog-ear" at the medial canthus. (**H**) Close the skin with an interrupted dog-ear suture and a running skin crease suture.

C. The upper line of the skin incision should *leave between 10 and 15 mm of skin between the eyebrow hairs and the skin crease.* Remember that you must leave symmetric amounts of skin on each side (Figure 6-21, A).

D. Use a caliper to measure 10–15 mm down from the base of the eyebrow hairs to the eyelid skin and

place a mark. Do this in several locations across the eyelid, marking the upper limit of skin and muscle removal. *Some judgment and experience are necessary to know how much skin to leave.* To be on the safe side, *15 mm of skin is appropriate for all patients.* When a more cosmetic result is necessary, the remaining skin can be left at 10 mm. If a browplasty or blepharo-

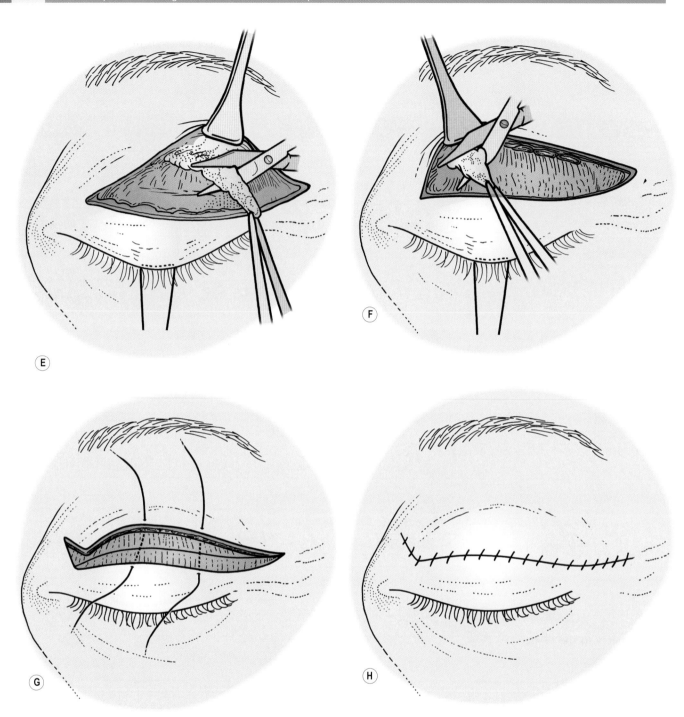

Figure 6-21 Continued.

plasty is undertaken at the same time, you will want to leave slightly more skin between the brow hairs and the skin crease. Your patient is unlikely to have problems with lagophthalmos or cornea exposure if you leave 15 mm of skin. *You should reconsider your marking if you find that you are leaving 10 mm or less skin between the skin crease and the brow hairs.* You must preserve the *independent movement of the eyebrow and eyelid.* If you cut off too much skin, you will pull the brow down, which distorts the normal anatomy and interferes with closure of the eyelids.

E. Have the patient sit up to observe the position and shape of your marks. The skin crease should fit in naturally with the patient's crease. The lateral extension should fall into a "laugh line." The upper incision marking should be visible hanging over the tarsus following the contour of the lid. There is usually some space between the upper and lower incisions laterally to correct temporal hooding. Watch the patient open and close the eyes, and you can see how symmetric the planned skin excisions will be.

2. Administer anesthesia
   A. Upper lid blepharoplasty is usually performed under local anesthesia. Your patient will probably benefit from some intravenous sedation as well.
   B. You might like the following injection technique because it causes very little discomfort. Inject 0.1 ml of local anaesthetic with epinephrine in two or three spots within the area of planned excision. Remember that the needle should be placed just underneath the skin and not in the muscle to avoid a hematoma. After 30 seconds, inject an additional 1–1.5 ml in each upper lid. Injection of this additional local anaesthetic will not cause pain. Hold gentle pressure on the injection sites with a gauze pad to prevent any bleeding.
   C. The patient can be prepped and draped while you scrub. Leave the entire face in the surgical field.
3. Incise the skin
   A. Sit at the patient's head with your assistant at the side on which you are operating. Stabilize the lid margin with a 4-0 silk suture passed through the meibomian gland orifices of the upper lid margin. As you get more comfortable with eyelid surgery, you may decide that the traction suture is not necessary.
   B. I prefer to do upper blepharoplasty using a CO₂ laser or Colorado microdissection needle. I rarely, if ever, use scissors any longer. Some surgeons prefer to use a blade for the initial skin incision, which makes a very smooth clean wound. Next, using either the laser or the needle, extend the skin incision through the orbicularis muscle to the septum. With the microdissector needle, use light long "paintbrush-like" strokes across the muscle with only the tip of the needle just touching the tissue. Any tissue build-up on the needle (or excess smoke) suggests that you are moving too quickly or are placing the needle too deeply, "pushing the tissue" rather than vaporizing it. The painting laser technique is similar, but there is no tissue contact. If you linger with either tool, you will deliver excess energy to the tissue and cause thermal damage. Learn to use the microdissection needle before using the laser. There is nothing wrong with scissors alone, but you will be spoiled with the hemostasis of the laser or needle.
   C. As you pass through the thin orbicularis muscle to the orbital septum, you will notice that the *color changes from pink to white*. If you observe closely, you may see a few *small vessels and nerves running perpendicular to the direction of the orbicularis fibers* in the preseptal plane (Figure 6-21, B).
4. Excise skin and muscle
   A. After you have made the skin incision, *excise the skin and muscle as one layer*. It is a good exercise to try to preserve the orbital septum.
   B. Dissect inferiorly from the superior incision toward the skin crease *in the preseptal plane*. This dissection is facilitated by your grasp of the septum with your nondominant hand as your assistant pulls the orbicularis muscle away from you. *You will see the*

fibrous bands of the orbital septum spread as they are pulled apart (make sure you understand this technique of "pulling" the tissue planes apart—very important). This is an avascular plane that is easy to work in. Continue the dissection inferiorly to the upper lid skin crease and then excise the skin and muscle flap, cutting it off at the crease (Figure 6-21, C). By not opening the septum, you will be sure that the levator has not been violated. If you do cut a bit of the levator, there is usually no need to reattach it.
   C. If there is no prolapse of orbital fat or you are not planning fat excision, you can close the skin at this point.
5. Remove fat
   A. Fat removal is a common part of upper lid blepharoplasty especially when the goal is to provide a deep superior sulcus.
   B. Open the septum at the superior edge of the ellipse. Your patient may not tolerate dissection posterior to the septum with the microdissector needle. If so, you will need to switch to Westcott scissors or use a disposable thermal cautery. Dissection posterior to the septum is possible with the CO₂ laser also.
   C. Open the septum widely over the pad or pads that you plan to excise. In many cases, the only excision necessary is the medial pad (Figure 6-21, D).
   D. Tease the septum off the fat moving inferiorly to the reflection of the septum on the levator aponeurosis. Now dissect the septum off the fat superiorly toward the superior orbital rim. As you pull the septum away from the orbital fat, you will see fibrous strands that are easily identified and cut. At this point, the preaponeurotic fat should be clearly visible.
   E. Now dissect the preaponeurotic fat off the levator toward the superior orbital rim. The fat most easily seen is the *preaponeurotic, or central, fat pad.*
   F. You will see a *thin fibrous capsule with small vessels covering the fat*. Open the capsule. You will see the free-flowing *yellow fat* of the central or preaponeurotic fat pad.
   G. If you want to remove the medial (nasal) fat, you may need to open the septum more medially. Dissect more posteriorly until you see the *white nasal fat pad*. At this point, it is reasonable to inject some additional local anaesthetic into the fat pads. If you are combining a blepharoplasty with a ptosis repair, finalize the aponeurosis advancement before injecting additional local anaesthetic.
   H. Open the medial fat pad capsule and dissect posteriorly. Take care not to *cut the medial palpebral artery*. If you cut this artery, brisk bleeding follows. If you cause bleeding, quickly place pressure on the area. Identify the source of the bleeding and use bipolar cautery to coagulate the vessel. Because you have already injected the additional local anaesthetic into the fat, you can cauterize the artery without creating excess pain.
   I. Once the excess fat pad or pads are exposed, you can trim the redundant fat anterior to the superior rim.

Trim away slightly more fat in women than in men and *never take fat posterior to the superior orbital rim*. As with the skin and muscle excision, the most important point is to leave symmetric amounts of fat behind rather than to remove symmetric amounts of fat (Figure 6-21, E and F). The current trend is to remove less fat. Excessive fat removal, especially medially, gives a characteristic "operated on" deep unnatural look. Remember, loss of fat is a characteristic of aging, in general, so be conservative.

J. Your fat excision will generally proceed without bleeding because there are very few vessels within the fat itself. If you are concerned about causing bleeding, you can cauterize the fat before cutting. Bipolar cautery can be used to melt away some fat to make perfect symmetry between the two sides.

6. Close the skin

A. *Reform the skin crease* with two interrupted sutures. Use one or two interrupted sutures passed from the skin edge to the aponeurosis at the level of the skin crease (top of tarsus). Pass one suture at the peak of the lid and an additional suture medial to the lateral canthus. Crease formation is not necessary in younger patients with less lax skin.

B. Make a *small dog-ear excision* of any redundant skin and muscle at the medial canthus (Figure 6-21, G) using the *Burrow's triangle technique*.

C. The reformed skin crease should be measured to be symmetric. This is a good time to place the patient in a sitting position to make a final check for symmetry in the skin fold, crease height, and contour. When you are satisfied, close the skin. There are several options for skin closure. I prefer a 5-0 fast absorbing gut suture for the interrupted and deep sutures for most patients (Figure 6-21, H). This is not a perfect suture as it unties easily so you want to use four or more ties. The sutures last more than a week, but usually fall out on their own. Patients like not having sutures out. Good alternatives are continuous 6-0 nylon or Prolene sutures. For younger, more "cosmetic" patients, I use a continuous or running "subcuticular" suture with Prolene that can easily be slid out at the first postoperative visit. I no longer use 7-0 Vicryl suture for skin closure, as this suture material lasts too long and may leave suture tracks.

D. Place some topical antibiotic ointment on the wound and in the conjunctival cul de sac. As usual, ask your patient to use cold compresses placed over the eyes for the first 24–48 hours. Let your patient know what to expect for a normal recovery period and give the patient a number to call if any concerns come up (Box 6-5).

Postoperative complications

Complications are rare, but include:

- Asymmetry
- Reoperation
- Scarring
- Corneal exposure

Box 6-5

Upper Eyelid Blepharoplasty

Skin marking

- Mark symmetric skin crease incisions (6–8 mm for men; 8–10 mm for women)
- Mark the upper limit of skin and muscle resection, leaving 10–15 mm between the brow and the mark

Anesthesia

- Administer intravenous sedation
- Administer topical drops and inject local anesthetic

Skin incision

- Use a 4-0 silk traction suture
- Cut through skin only

Skin and muscle excision

- Dissect skin and muscle off the orbital septum
- Remember to pull the layers apart and cut the bands on stretch

Fat excision

- Open the septum at the upper skin incision
- Dissect the septum off the anterior surface of the fat
- Dissect the fat off the aponeurosis
- Inject additional local anesthetic
- Open the medial fat pad
- Excise fat, leaving symmetric amounts.
- Be conservative
- Don't excise posterior to the superior orbital rim

Closure

- You many choose to reform the skin crease with sutures
- Use a continuous suture to close the skin

- Lagophthalmos
- Blindness
- Death

The most common complication is *asymmetry*. The best tactic to avoid asymmetry is careful marking preoperatively. If asymmetric brow ptosis is present, this may lead to asymmetric skin folds as well. Reoperation is rarely necessary, but occasionally some skin fold or skin crease asymmetry may need to be addressed. Scarring or wound infections are rare. Inferior corneal exposure occurs to a mild degree in many patients in the early postoperative course. As the orbicularis function returns, the exposure resolves. Corneal exposure can be managed with topical lubricants and massage. If exposure persists beyond 4–6 months postoperatively, consider exploration of the surgical wound to lyse any scars contributing to incomplete closure or lagophthalmos. In patients with extreme corneal exposure, skin grafting may be necessary, but generally leaves a less than ideal cosmetic appearance. Blindness secondary to postoperative hemorrhage occurs rarely after any blepharoplasty operation. If your patient has more than mild discomfort or severe lid swelling in the first 24 hours, you should be called immediately. You should let your patient know what to expect postoperatively—"*Sore and swollen is normal, your vision will be blurry from the ointment. If your eye hurts badly, swells closed or you can't see at all, call us right away, that's not normal.*" In many patients with orbital hemorrhage, opening the surgical wound and evacuating the hemorrhage can restore lost vision. Death is an extremely unlikely event after eyelid surgery.

- Upper lid blepharoplasty reduces the skin fold by removing redundant skin and muscle. Fat removal and eyebrow elevation will reduce the skin fold further and deepen the superior sulcus.
- Remember to consider browplasty for any patient undergoing blepharoplasty. Browplasty may not be practical for every patient. Remember to preserve the independent function of the brow and lid by leaving 10–15 mm of skin between the upper lid skin crease and the brow hairs whether or not browplasty is performed.
- Review the skin marking procedure and steps of the upper lid blepharoplasty in Box 6-5.

At this point, you should be able to treat the majority of your patients with "functional" or "restorative" periocular problems. As always, you need to appreciate the normal anatomy and how it is altered by time or disease. You should develop an interest in how your instruments and your hands—your "tools of the trade"—work to give you the desired result. We have looked primarily at the upper face—the forehead, and upper eyelids and some procedures to improve eyebrow position and remove the extra skin on the eyelid. In the next chapter, "Aesthetic Surgery of the Face," we will reinforce the concepts that you have already learned with regard to the upper face. We'll look at the mid and lower face. At the same time, we'll put the *sags, bags and wrinkles* that we see into the framework of the *descent and deflation* process that begins and continues through adulthood. There will be a great deal of overlap in this chapter and the next, but we will shift our emphasis to *how the patient looks, rather than how the patient sees*. The next chapter was a fun chapter for me to write. I hope that you find it interesting and useful for you and your patients.

Major points

- Laxity of the periorbital tissues is responsible for the brow ptosis, dermatochalasis, and fat prolapse seen with aging.
- There are three fat pads in the lower eyelid and two fat pads in the upper eyelid. Weakness of the orbital septum and intraorbital fibrous tissues allows the fat to prolapse forward.
- The typical woman's eyebrow sits above the superior orbital rim and is arched upward. The typical man's eyebrow sits at the superior orbital rim and is thicker and flatter than the female eyebrow.
- The height and contour of the eyebrow should be noted on examination. Temporal brow ptosis is common because of the normal anatomy of the frontalis muscle, which ends medial to the tail of the brow.
- The brow is an important muscle of facial expression. The height and contour of the brow suggest mood.
- Browplasty elevates the drooping eyebrow into anatomic position at or above the superior orbital rim, which improves the patient's vision and appearance.
- The type of browplasty in your practice will depend largely on the patient's goals with regard to "reconstructive" or "cosmetic" results. Common types of browplasty in use in oculoplastic surgery include:
  - Direct or temporal direct browplasty
  - Midforehead lift
  - Endoscopic forehead lift
  - Pretrichial or coronal lift
- Understanding the patient's complaint and goal is critical for achieving success in browplasty and blepharoplasty operations.
- Brow ptosis is a contributing factor to dermatochalasis in most patients. Some consideration to browplasty should be given for all patients undergoing blepharoplasty. Practical considerations prevent the use of browplasty in many patients.
- Upper eyelid blepharoplasty reduces the upper lid skin fold by removing mainly redundant skin and muscle.
- The depth of the superior sulcus depends on:
  - The position of the eyebrow
  - The prominence of the superior orbital rim
  - Redundant skin and muscle of the upper lid skin fold
  - The presence of prolapsing orbital fat
- Symmetry of the skin folds is achieved by leaving equal amounts of skin between the brow and the upper lid skin crease. Leave at least 10–15 mm of skin, depending on your goals. Brow height and remaining orbital fat should be made symmetric as well.

Suggested reading

1. Aiache AE, Ramirez OH: The suborbicularis oculi fat pads: an anatomic and clinical study. *Plast Reconstr Surg* 95:37–42, 1995.

2. Albert DM., Lucarelli MJ: Aesthetic and functional surgery of the eyebrow and forehead ptosis. In *Clinical atlas of procedures in ophthalmic surgery*, pp. 263–283, Chicago: AMA Press, 2004.

3. American Academy of Ophthalmology: *Basic and clinical science course: orbit, eyelids and lacrimal system*, sect. 7, pp. 135–145, 228–248, San Francisco, The American Academy of Ophthalmology, 2006/2007.

4. Biesman BS: *Lasers in facial aesthetic and reconstructive surgery*, Baltimore: Williams & Wilkins, 1999.

5. Brown BZ: Blepharoplasty. In Levine MR, ed., Manual of oculoplastic surgery, 3rd edn, pp. 77–87, Boston: Butterworth-Heinemann, 2003.

6. Chen WPD, Khan JA, McCord CD, eds: *The color atlas of cosmetic oculofacial surgery*, Elsevier, 2004.

7. Ellenbogen R: Transcoronal eyebrow lift with concomitant upper blepharoplasty. *Plast Reconstr Surg* 71(4):490–499, 1983.

8. Fagien S, ed.: Chapters II-6 through II-12. In *Putterman's cosmetic oculoplastic surgery*, 4th edn, pp. 67–145, Philadelphia: Elsevier, 2008.

9. Johnson CM Jr, Waldman SR: Midforehead lift. *Arch Otolaryngol* 109(3):155–159, 1983.

10. Moses JL, Tanenbaum M: Blepharoplasty cosmetic and functional. In McCord CD, Tanenbaum M, Nunery WR, eds, *Oculoplastic surgery*, 3rd edn, ch. 11, pp. 285–317, New York: Raven Press, 1995.

11. Nerad J: The involutional periorbital changes: dermatochalasis and brow ptosis. In *The requisites—Oculoplastic surgery*, pp. 120–156, St Louis: Mosby, 2001.

12. Nerad JA, Carter KD, Alford MA: Upper eyelid dermatochalasis. In *Rapid diagnosis in ophthalmology—oculoplastic and reconstructive surgery*, pp. 72–75, Philadelphia: Mosby Elsevier, 2008.

13. Nerad JA, Carter KD, Alford MA: Brow ptosis. In *Rapid diagnosis in ophthalmology—oculoplastic and reconstructive surgery*, pp. 68–69, Philadelphia: Mosby Elsevier, 2008.

14. Shorr N, Hoenig JA, Cook T: Brow lift. In Levine MR, ed., *Manual of oculoplastic surgery*, 3rd edn, pp. 61–75, Boston: Butterworth-Heinemann, 2003.

15. Wobig, JL, Dailey RA, Surgery of the upper eyelid and brow. In Wobig JL, Dailey RA, eds, *Oculofacial plastic surgery: face, lacrimal system, and orbit*, pp. 34–53, New York: Thieme, 2004.

CHAPTER 7

Aesthetic Surgery of the Face

Chapter contents

Introduction

This chapter has lots of new material not contained in my original book, *Oculoplastic Surgery—the Requisites*. Aesthetic surgery is a booming area that used to be on the periphery of "traditional" oculoplastic surgery. All across surgical specialties, interest in facial rejuvenation has increased dramatically in the last 10 years. Based on the material in the last chapter, you should be able to treat the majority of your patients with "functional" or "restorative" periocular problems. Facial rejuvenation is another area where your expertise as a reconstructive surgeon can be put to good use. All reconstructive procedures have an aesthetic element in addition to the primary goal of restoring function. And vice versa, all aesthetic procedures depend on reconstructive concepts that form the basis of a successful rejuvenation procedure. In this chapter, we will emphasize those concepts.

In Chapter 6, we looked at aging changes around the eyes from the point of view of restoring the function of the eyes lost with the common aging changes. We have looked primarily at the upper face, the forehead, and upper eyelids and some procedures to improve eyebrow position and remove the extra skin on the eyelid. In this chapter, we will reinforce the concepts that you have already learned with regard to the upper face. We'll look at the mid and lower face. At the same time, we'll put the *sags, bags and wrinkles* that we see in the framework of the *"descent and deflation"* process that begins and continues through adulthood.

You may already be familiar with many of the procedures discussed here. For the advanced surgeon already incorporating these techniques in his or her practice, this will serve as a review. For the resident or surgeon interested in learning these procedures, my hope is to provide a general scheme of options for rejuvenation. We will start with the anatomic and pathologic basis of skin changes, followed by their prevention and the medical and surgical options for treatment. The "nonsurgical" treatments include exfoliants, Botox® and filler injections, laser resurfacing, and chemical peeling. The surgical options include forehead lift, midface lift and lower face and neck lift.

As always keep the big picture in mind. Skim over the material initially and go back over it in a more detailed fashion. Pick out areas that you and your patients are interested in. Start with easy skin care options and proceed to the next level when your skills permit it. For more advanced operations, you will need extra reading, observation, and mentoring before you take them on. At the end of this chapter, no matter what your personal goals are in the area of facial rejuvenation, you should have a good base to build on.

Evaluation and treatment of aging

What happens in aging? The conceptual approach of *"descent and deflation"* is a good way to organize your thoughts. As we age, supporting tissues stretch causing the familiar "sags and bags" of aging. Accompanying this laxity is a general loss of soft tissue thickness. In the current jargon, this is referred to as a loss of facial *"volume."* A combination of thinning of the subcutaneous layer and facial fat pads combines with generalized tissue laxity to give a characteristic aged facial profile. Temporal brow drooping and the formation of the melolabial fold are familiar examples. Thinning of the skin, primarily the dermis, causes the skin to *"wrinkle"* and develop other surface changes (Figure 7-1).

There is a complex interplay of *internal* and *external* causes of aging. Forgive this simplification, but I think you will find that this scheme will provide a basis for evaluating your patient's aging changes. You will also see that these concepts will help you organize and present a treatment plan to your patient (Boxes 7-1, 7-2 and 7-3).

Anatomic considerations

The skin

In Chapter 2, we discussed the facial anatomy in some detail. Here, we will review features that you can easily apply to the

---

Box 7-1

Concepts of Facial Aging
- "Descent and deflation"
  - Supporting tissue laxity
  - Loss of facial volume
- Evaluate your patient in terms of
  - "Sags and bags"
  - "Wrinkles" and other skin changes

Box 7-2

Causes of Aging
- Internal
  - Genetics
    - — "I am starting to look like my mother"
  - Disease
    - — Diabetes, thyroid, menopause
- External
  - Sun damage
  - Tobacco

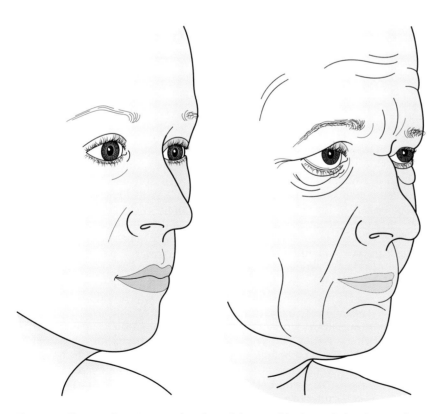

Figure 7-1 The aging face. Note typical involutional changes of the face, including descent of tissues, loss of subcutaneous fat, and deepening of skin wrinkles. Aging creates predictable "sags and bags": temporal brow droop, dermatochalasis, fat prolapse in the eyelids, lower eyelid laxity, malar mounds, deepening of the nasojugal fold (tear trough) and melolabial fold, marionette lines, jowling, loss of the sharp angle between the neck and chin, and cervical banding.

sags, bags and wrinkles approach to the evaluation and treatment of your patients. We will start at the surface and work our way inward.

The *skin* has two layers, the epidermis and the dermis. You will recall that the *epidermis* is rapidly turning over with young cells originating at the deep basal layer and maturing as the cells migrate toward the surface. As the cells move upward, they lose their nuclei, flatten, and eventually become keratinized. Pigment cells are scattered in the deep layers of the epidermis. With aging, the epidermis thins. A *generalized loss of pigment* occurs but, at the same time, focal areas of pigmentation, *dyschromias*, occur. *Premalignant and malignant changes* include actinic keratosis, basal cell carcinoma, and squamous cell carcinoma. Laser resurfacing (the ablative type) and chemical peeling remove the epidermis, which removes abnormal surface cells and improves color changes. The real improvement that results from these procedures comes in improvements in the underlying dermis, however.

The *dermis* is a connective tissue layer made of *collagen and elastin fibers* surrounded by a watery mixture known as the *ground substance*. The dermis also contains fibrous cells and the *skin adnexae—the hair follicles, oil and sweat glands*. We will discuss a variety of lesions related to the adnexae in Chapter 11. Blood vessels, lymphatics, and nerves also travel within the dermis.

There are two layers of the dermis: the more superficial *papillary* and the deeper *reticular dermis*. Aging changes damage the collagen and elastin fibers of the dermis, resulting in a loss of dermal thickness and elasticity. Loss of the dermal thickness allows normal and telangiectactic vessels to become apparent.

The loss of skin elasticity causes *wrinkles* or *rhytids* to form. Wrinkles that form while the underlying muscle contracts are called *dynamic wrinkles*. Over time, as the skin loses its elasticity, the repeated folding of the skin creates lines that remain without any underlying muscle contraction known as *adynamic wrinkles*. Resurfacing and peeling procedures remove the epidermis and cause thermal damage to the dermis. Repair of the damage results in thickening of the dermis and the return of some elastin fibers resulting in a more elastic skin—and fewer wrinkles. A new layer of epidermis grows back from regenerative cells derived from the

underlying adnexae. The new epidermis is lighter in color with fewer patchy dyschromias and premalignant changes. Botulinum injections relax the underlying muscles resulting in improvement of dynamic wrinkling. When adynamic wrinkles remain, injectable filler agents "plump up" the dermis and "fill in" the creases.

A part of facial "deflation" is a loss of subcutaneous fat in aging. The cherubic look of the youthful face is lost, especially in patients who are normal weight or tending to be slim. In heavier patients, some of the typical deflation features may not be obvious and the patient may have a more youthful facial appearance. Injection of filler materials or autologous harvested fat can mask the loss of facial fat giving a more rounded youthful look.

Superficial musculoaponeurotic system (SMAS)

In Chapter 2, we spent a great deal of energy talking about the muscles of facial expression and the investing fibrous layer known as the SMAS (superficial musculoaponeurotic system). If this is sounding pretty hazy to you, it might be worth going back and rereading the last sections in Chapter 2 before you move on. Hopefully, you will recall that the SMAS layer coordinates facial movements by physically linking the mimetic muscles together. Strong fibers attach the SMAS to the underlying bone and in turn attach to the skin itself (osseo-cutaneous retaining ligaments). These ligaments are strongest along the inferior and lateral orbital rim extending onto the zygoma, as well as along the mandible. Lax tissues "hang" over the sturdy attachment points. Combined with the loss of associated fatty tissues, this process is responsible for the characteristic "sags and bags" of the face—*deepening of the melolabial fold, jowling, and marionette lines*. The anatomic extensions of the SMAS—the temporoparietal fascia (TPF), the galea, and platysma—develop laxity as well. *Temporal brow drooping and platysmal banding* are the manifestations of this process.

Tightening of the SMAS layer and its counterparts is the basis of modern face, neck, brow, and temple lifting procedures.

As the SMAS stretches, its associated fat pads fall, contributing to the sags and bags we have just discussed. A deep plane of fat exists behind the orbicularis muscle overlying the inferior rim (the suborbicularis oculi fat pad; SOOF) and extends superiorly over the lateral rim to overlie the superior orbital rim (the retroorbicularis fat pad; ROOF). The fullness of the lateral portion of the eyebrow and the tissues over the superior orbital rim seen in youth are due to a full and well-supported ROOF. Drooping of the ROOF is a cause of temporal eyebrow ptosis and is corrected with the browplasty or forehead lift operations. The *malar fat pad* is a collection of fat on and within the anterior surface of the SMAS over the malar eminence (Figure 7-2). A full normally positioned malar fat pad contributes to the high full cheek in children and young adults. We will see below that the descent of the SOOF and the malar fat pad is a characteristic feature of facial aging, the formation of the so-called *double convexity* deformity.

In the child, the facial profile from the lower eyelid to the cheek extends inferiorly in a smooth convexity (Figure 7-2). Over time, this single curve changes into a double curve. Here is what happens. Let's look at the development of the

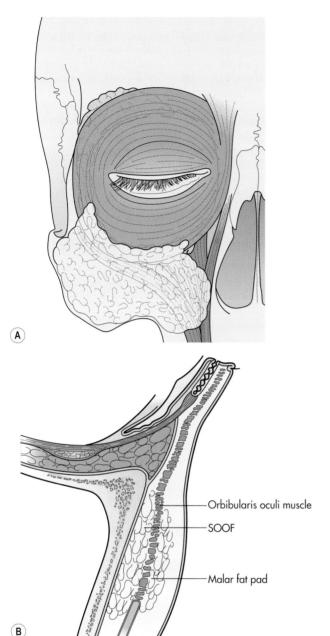

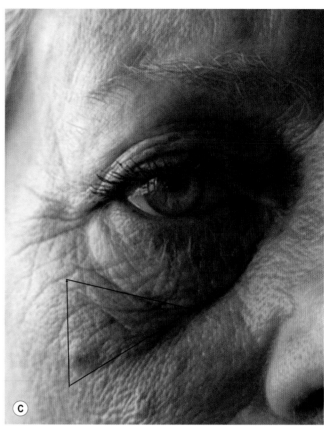

Orbibularis oculi muscle

SOOF

Malar fat pad

Figure 7-2 ABC. ROOF, SOOF, and malar fat pads. (**A**) The orbicularis muscle separates the RO/SOOF from the malar pad. (**B**) Side view of retro-orbicularis fat from malar fat. (**C**) Lower eyelid landmarks—malar triangle (mound), nasojugal sulcus (dark curved line), palpebral malar sulcus (lighter curved line).

cheek convexity first. As the SMAS stretches in the lateral midface, the malar and the suborbicularis fat pads fall ("descend") in a characteristic manner creating the "malar mound" laterally. Medially, the cheek descent causes the inferior orbital rim to lose its soft tissue padding (part of the "deflation" look). This used to be referred to as a "long lower eyelid." Now the term "skeletonization" of the lower orbital rim is in vogue, emphasizing the loss of tissue over the inferior orbital rim. The feature most commonly emphasized is deepening of the nasojugal fold (so-called "tear trough" deformity). As the cheek tissues descend inferiorly and medially, the melolabial fold deepens. The *eyelid convexity* develops as the orbital septum thins and fat prolapses forward. The aging adult develops a bulge of fat prolapse in the lower eyelid, a hollow at the rim, and a bulge of drooping cheek, the double convexity.

What can be done to improve this—essentially "rejuvenate" the midface? There are some options for restoring the smooth single curve of youth. Lifting the cheek (midface lift) improves the melolabial fold and lifts some tissue over the rim. Trimming some fat from the lower eyelid with a blepharoplasty reduces the lower eyelid convexity. Maybe even repositioning the eyelid fat over the inferior rim—"flipping the fat"—will help to fill in the hollow at the rim. A less invasive way to camouflage the double convexity is to fill in the "tear trough" with an injectable filler or autogenous fat transfer. You can see this can be a complicated issue.

My hope is that by now you are starting to understand the normal anatomy and what happens to that anatomy with aging. The options for rejuvenation are numerous and complex. So how do you decide what can or should be done? Let's look at the options from simplest to more com-

Table 7-1 Options for rejuvenation

	Prevention	
Wrinkles	Sunscreen and stop smoking	All ages
Dynamic wrinkles	Botulinum injection	30–40+ years
Adynamic wrinkles	Fillers	40+ years
Surface texture and color changes	Laser resurfacing or chemical peels	40+ years
Sags and bags		
Dermatochalasis	Blepharoplasty	35+ years
Lower eyelid fat prolapse	Blepharoplasty	35+ years
Brow ptosis	Browplasty or forehead lift	40–50+ years
Deepening of melolabial fold	Midface lift	40–50+ years
Jowling and marionette lines	Facelift	50+ years
Platysmal banding	Liposuction and platysmaplasty	50+ years

plicated. As you might imagine, this algorithm follows a chronological progression of patient age (Table 7-1).

Look this over a few times. It is important because it summarizes the facial aging scheme and gives you some direction in what procedures that you might consider offering your patient interested in facial rejuvenation.

Checkpoint

- What do we mean by intrinsic and extrinsic causes of aging?
- What are the two main extrinsic causes of aging?
- What is the difference between dynamic and adynamic wrinkles?
- What is the SMAS?
- Do you understand the concept of "descent and deflation"?
- Starting with the forehead, describe some characteristic "sags and bags"

Philosophy toward aesthetic surgery

As you add cosmetic procedures to your reconstruction practice, I suggest you consider your own, as well as your patient's, philosophy regarding aesthetic surgery. *All your patients age…* now consider:

- Mind set 1
  - Many of your patients would like to look younger
  - Most of your patients will not be interested in any rejuvenation
  - Few will be able to pay for these procedures

- Mind set 2
  - All your patients would like to look younger
  - Many of your patients will be interested in rejuvenation
  - Many are able to pay for these procedures
  - And are happy to enter a discussion about options for rejuvenation

Over the last several years, my philosophy has changed from the former to the latter. If you are interested in doing aesthetic surgery, you will want to adopt a version of mind set 2. Make your services known. Likely, you will see that many of the patients in your practice have a similar philosophy. And many new patients will be interested in coming to your practice. That being said, your job is to educate your patients and help them decide what is best for them. "Talking your patient in to a procedure" that they don't really want, or can't afford, is a fast way to a slow aesthetic practice.

Making a decision: the "cost"–benefit ratio

The menu

There are many reasons for the increasing interest in cosmetic surgery. Youth remains a priority in our society. We are all "hard wired" to be attracted to youthful features. Patients are living longer. The "baby boomer" population is aging and remaining active. Most patients who look younger feel younger. The introduction of less invasive procedures, especially Botox injections, has made the opportunities for rejuvenation more available to patients, often serving as an introduction to other aesthetic procedures. Society is accepting these procedures more readily. More men are having procedures done. And no doubt a constant barrage of marketing makes the option of rejuvenation procedures appear attractive to the general public.

In the next sections, we will deal with the "menu" of aesthetic procedures available that your patients might choose from. Your job is to offer them procedures that suit their needs and are safe. I like the scheme of evaluating your patient in terms of:

- Wrinkles
- Sags and bags
- Contributing factors
  - Intrinsic: age, genetics, skin type, diabetes, cardiovascular condition
  - Extrinsic: sun exposure, smoking

This system lends itself well to selecting the right menu choices, depending on your patient's desire for a "snack" or a full "seven course meal."

All patients over 40 years have some degree of all these aging changes. So how do you and your patient make a decision about which of many choices for rejuvenation is appropriate? It all comes down to the perceived *cost–benefit ratio*. You are going to offer only procedures within your skill set that you think will address the patient concern and offer a benefit to the patient with a minimal risk. As we said, your job is to educate the patient with regard to the benefit and risk of a particular procedure. As cosmetic procedures are completely elective, the decision to proceed really comes down to the patient's perception of the cost–benefit ratio. If the patient perceives no benefit, even "no risk" does not make the patient want to have the procedure (mind set 1). If the patient perceives a benefit and the risks appear minimal, he or she will elect to proceed with surgery.

The medical risks of all these procedures are very low, but you must factor in cost and "down time" (swelling, bruising, pain, and time out of the public eye) on the risk side of the ratio. Patients prefer low-cost procedures with little down time. You will find that many patients are interested in trying that "appetizer" from the long "menu of rejuvenation" options. This is where Botox and fillers have received widespread acceptance. Later, the patient may come back for a second or third course. A few patients are "hungry" and will order "full meal" on the first visit. You might want to remind your patients that more "involved" treatments with longer recovery almost always have more effect and longevity than procedures with less down time. Ultimately, it is the patient's choice with your wise counsel.

Where do you start?

With regard to your level of expertise, Botox and filler injection technique skills are acquired easily with some practice, so that is a good place to start. You may already know how to do a functional upper blepharoplasty and direct browplasty. An aesthetic blepharoplasty in a younger patient is not any more difficult. In some ways, it is easier because there is usually much less redundant tissue. It goes without saying that your technique must be meticulous and your bedside manner very accommodating. Next, you might want to offer laser resurfacing or chemical peels. Then think about lower blepharoplasty, generally considered more difficult and risky than upper blepharoplasty. As your skills increase, you can learn pretrichial or coronal forehead lifting. With the brow and temple anatomy well understood and perhaps your familiarity with the endoscope for retrieving stents and doing endoscopic dacryocystorhinostomy (DCR), you might want to do endoscopic forehead lifting with your upper blepharoplasty (the technique that I have outlined below is not a big jump). Taking courses, viewing DVDs, mentoring with an experienced colleague, and trips to the anatomy lab will help you tremendously.

At this point, you are well on your way to a full "aesthetic menu" for your patients. Each of us has different interests and practice situations. Very few surgeons do only "cosmetic" surgery. The market is very competitive for these higher reimbursement cases. You can choose to limit your expertise to periocular procedures, or move further into midface, face, and neck lifting.

In the next sections, we will consider the first of these procedures in some detail. I would like you to have an understanding of midface, lower face, and neck lifting procedures, but have not given you details. There are many other procedures that you should at least be aware of, such as cheek and chin implants, rhinoplasty, and hair replacement, that are not covered in this text. There are many texts available that you can use when you want more specifics. Some of these are listed in the Suggested Reading. Before we head toward the procedures, we should talk about *prevention of facial aging*, an important topic for all our patients for both functional and aesthetic reasons (Box 7-4).

Box 7-4

Scheme for Aesthetic Evaluation

- Wrinkles
  - Dynamic wrinkles
  - Adynamic wrinkles
  - Surface texture, fine wrinkles, and color changes
- Sags and bags
  - Brow ptosis
  - Dermatochalasis
  - Lower eyelid fat prolapse
  - Deepening of melolabial fold
  - Jowling and marionette lines
  - Loss of cervicomental angle
  - Platysmal banding
- Contributing factors
  - Intrinsic–age, skin type, diabetes, cardiovascular condition
  - Extrinsic—sun exposure, smoking

Prevention and medical treatment of the skin

We talked about intrinsic and extrinsic factors that play a role in aging. We cannot change our genetic predisposition to specific *intrinsic* aging changes. No better example of the aging patient is the person who sees his or her genetic future and presents with the complaint, "I am starting to look like my mother." In other cases, an inherited less desirable feature may have been present for years: "I have been self conscious of these bags under my eyes since high school." As the saying goes, we cannot pick our parents, but we can maintain a healthy diet and keep active. Both are important factors in preventing vascular disease and diabetes. *Extrinsic* causes of aging can be modified. Smoking accelerates aging significantly. As you will see in your practice, there is an obvious difference in the appearance of the 45-year-old patient who has been a long-standing smoker compared with a patient of similar age who has never been a smoker. You are familiar with the term *smoker's lips*, the fine vertical creases at the vermillion border of the lips. *Sun exposure* is the other major cause of facial aging. I have to credit a dermatology lecturer, whose name I have long since forgotten, with this example: "If you want to know the effects of sun on your own skin, compare your cheeks. That is, the cheeks on your face compared with the 'cheeks' on your bottom. They both have the same number of birthdays and the same parents." Most of us no longer have that "baby bottom skin" on our faces largely due to actinic damage. Lightly pigmented skin ages more easily than darker skin. Skin that tans, rather than burns, is less easily damaged by the sun. You will find it more difficult to judge the age of a darkly pigmented patient compared with a lightly pigmented patient. So the message to our patients is to *apply a sunscreen* every morning as part of a daily hygiene regimen. Some actinic damage can be reversed by a daily application of *tretinoin crème* (0.25– 0.50% bid or qhs, Retin-A, Renova, Avita). These keratolytic agents remove a thin layer of the epidermis and promote remodeling of the dermis to a small degree. Some patients will have trouble with skin irritation and erythema and will require holidays from treatment.

Keep in mind our scheme for evaluation and treatment. Is your patient concerned about *wrinkles* or *sags and bags*? We will talk about how to improve the wrinkles with Botox injection, injectable fillers, and skin resurfacing in the next sections. Later in the chapter, we will discuss some of the surgical procedures for rejuvenating your patient who complains of sags and bags (Box 7-5).

Botulinum (Botox®) injection

Principles

Botulinum toxin was introduced to the medical community in the late 1970s by Alan Scott as an investigative treatment for strabismus. The pharmaceutical industry picked up Botox as an "orphan drug" for treatment of facial dystonias, primarily essential blepharospasm, in the mid-1980s. Since that time, the indications for this powerful neurotoxin have exploded. The Federal Drug Administration (FDA) approval for Botox as a treatment for glabellar wrinkling was granted in 2002. The muscle weakening effect of Botox is due to inhibition of the release of acetylcholine from the presynaptic neuron at the neuromuscular junction, causing a chemodenervation lasting 3–6 months.

Wrinkles in the skin are caused by contraction of the underlying muscles. As we have shown earlier, the wrinkling is directed 90 degrees from the pull of the underlying muscles. Think of the horizontal forehead rhytids resulting from the contraction of the underlying vertically oriented frontalis muscle or the radially oriented crow's feet at the lateral canthus resulting from circular orientation of the underlying

orbicularis muscle. In Chapter 2, we talked about the glabellar wrinkling causing contraction of the underlying procerus and corrugator muscles (Figure 7-3). In youth, the plump skin barely shows a wrinkle with facial movement. As the skin thins, facial movements are accompanied by "dynamic wrinkles." With further aging and loss of the elastic nature of the skin, wrinkles present without muscle contraction develop, known as "adynamic wrinkles." As Botox blocks the underlying muscle contraction, it is most useful for the treatment of dynamic wrinkles. The primary regions where Botox is used are in the forehead, glabella, and crow's feet.

Technique

Botox is available in a powder form with 100 u of Botox in each bottle. The powder is typically dissolved with 2 cc of sterile saline (resulting in a dilution of 5 u/0.1 cc of fluid). You should avoid vigorous shaking of the bottle as the Botox is easily degraded. Typically 2.5–5.0 units are injected in each site. (0.05–0.10 cc of solution). Some surgeons change the concentration depending on the site. Typical injection sites and dosage are chosen as shown in Figure 7-4. You might want to review the sites for Botox injection in cases of

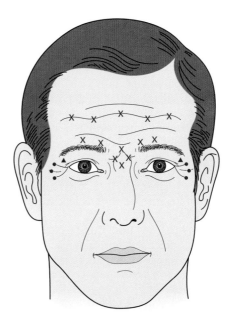

x = 5 units
• = 2.5 units for crows feet
▲ = 2.5–5 units for brow ptosis

Figure 7-4 Botox injection sites for forehead furrows, glabellar lines, and crow's feet.

Box 7-5

Evaluation and Treatment Simplified

Is your patient concerned about:
- Wrinkles?
- Sags and bags?

Are the wrinkles:
- Seen only with facial movements? Dynamic wrinkles
  - Treat with Botox
- Seen at rest? Adynamic wrinkles
  - Treat with fillers
- Generalized
  - Treat with resurfacing or peels
  - May need Botox and fillers

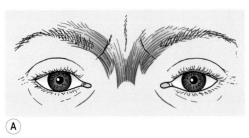

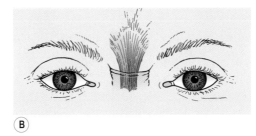

Figure 7-3 The glabellar furrows. (**A**) Corrugator muscle action causing vertical furrows in the glabella. (**B**) Procerus muscle causing horizontal furrows in the glabella.

essential blepharospasm and hemifacial spasm shown in Chapter 9 (Figures 9-8 and 9-9).

The glabella or midway up the forehead are good places to start treatment with Botox. Use lower doses and fewer sites until you have experience. Injection technique is straightforward. Use a short 30-gauge needle and inject just under the skin. You should not be intradermal. Injection into the muscle can cause hemorrhage. Around the eyes, stay peripheral to the orbital rim to avoid an upper eyelid ptosis. It's a good idea to always point the needle away from the eye.

Undertreatment is more desirable than the total paralysis of overtreatment. Even worse is the occasional upper eyelid ptosis that will persist for several weeks once it occurs. Iopidine™ (apraclonidine 0.5%) eye drops have been recommended to treat Botox-induced ptosis. This α2-adrenergic agonist causes Müller's muscle to contract, elevating the upper eyelid 1–3 mm. I have no experience with this, however. Few patients will experience dry eye symptoms after treatment, but a lubrication regiment of artificial tears three or four times a day is reasonable. You should avoid treatment of the lower face, at least until you get experience. Unsightly abnormalities in movements of the mouth are tell-tale signs of overtreatment with Botox.

A good rule of thumb is—Botox is best for the upper face. Fillers are best for the lower face.

With some experience, you can use Botox in conjunction with fillers. Botox eliminates the tissue elevation (smooth the "hills") caused by the underlying muscle contraction. Fillers eliminate any remaining depression (fill the "valleys"). Botox has been advocated prior to a surgical forehead lift, hoping to facilitate the release and maintain forehead elevation while postoperative adhesions form. Botox injection in the neck can be used to improve platysmal banding in the neck. Injection of 5 units per site in several sites along the bands can give temporary improvement. A good time to "practice" is on your functional patients with facial dystonias or facial nerve synkinesis.

Remember, the best aesthetic result occurs when a new "refreshed look" is not attributed to any treatment at all. You want your aesthetic outcomes to look natural. Consider the example of hairpieces—have you ever seen a good toupee? No, you only see the bad ones. Similarly, it does not matter if you are doing Botox injections or a facelift, your patient should not have an unnatural "operated on look."

Injectable fillers

Principles

Botox works well for dynamic wrinkles but does not completely eliminate adynamic wrinkles. These "wrinkles at rest," like a depressed scar, are most visible with a light directed from the side casting a shadow over the valley, making the depression visible. When you eliminate or "fill" the depression with injection of a filler product, the shadowing is gone. Typically, this is most useful in the area of the adynamic wrinkles at the lateral canthus, on the sides of the mouth (vertical jowl lines and the marionette lines), at the margins of the lips, and in the glabella (with caution because necrosis has been seen).

Fillers can also be used as a "volumizing agent" to replace facial deflation. You can restore the fullness of the youthful face with injection of filler products into the melolabial fold, the nasojugal fold, the ROOF, and in the lip itself. The most common use is to fill in the valley (the crease) of the melolabial fold. In many cases, more advanced uses of fillers, often in significant amounts, can be used to "reshape" or "volumize the face". These techniques include filling the fat pads in the malar region and jowls and depression overlying the temporalis muscle.

Fillers can be divided into products that have a *temporary* or a *permanent* effect. The safest and simplest fillers to use are the temporary products, all of which contain a variation of hyaluronic acid (HA). As you recall, HA is a main component of the ground substance of skin and is very hydrophilic, pulling water into the dermis. HA products have replaced the collagen-based products popular in the past. They last twice as long and have no tendency to create allergic reaction, so no skin testing is required. These products vary in terms of thickness. Thinner HA materials can be used to improve fine wrinkles, whereas thicker materials are used for more prominent lines and for providing volume. In practice, it is easiest to stock and use one type of HA filler that will work in all regions of the face for most patients. I would suggest that you use only HA products until both you and your patients get experience with the effect of the filler. Some patients will want more volume than others (related to personal preference or expense), so don't overtreat initially. You can add more filler later if needed.

HA products are injected in the mid-dermis. With experience, you may vary the depth depending on the area and the filler, but you should not inject very superficially or into the underlying fat. Your careful injection technique and massage will give a uniform distribution of the material. The result is immediate. Swelling and bruising are minimized by ice application after injection. The effect lasts from 6 to 12 months. If any filler material is left over after the initial injection, you should keep it on hand in case your patient requests a bit more volume in the subsequent week after treatment. Although rarely, if ever, necessary, the injection can be reversed by injection of hyaluronidase (Wydase).

Injection into the crow's feet or the melolabial folds is the easiest. When you get more experience, you can inject the nasojugal fold and the lips. Small depressed scars can be improved somewhat. If adynamic wrinkles remain after Botox injection into the forehead and glabella, you can add a small amount of filler (especially in men with deep wrinkles). Check out the tips for injection of HA fillers in Box 7-6.

Most "permanent filler" products contain particulate matter and derive their long-lasting effect by stimulating new collagen production in the dermis. The effect is delayed and cumulative over many injections. These fillers should be delivered deeper in the dermis. There is no current consensus on the safest and most effective type of long duration filler product at this time. None are FDA approved for cosmetic use except for human immunodeficiency virus (HIV) lipodystrophy patients. The benefit of a "permanent" effect is attractive to patients, but there is no good way to reverse an unwanted outcome. Rare, but reported, side-effects, such as granuloma formation, are difficult to deal with. I would suggest that you do not use these materials

Box 7-6

Tips for HA Filler Injection

Injection technique

- 27–30 gauge needle
- Consider topical anesthetic crème
- Local anesthesia for lips
- Use linear threading or serial puncture
- Aim for injection into dermis
- Fill completely, but no overfill
- Avoid lumps
- Smooth with massage
- Stop if skin blanches

Wrinkles

- Thin products for fine wrinkles
- Inject into superficial dermis
- Areas
    - Smoker's lips
    - Crow's feet
    - Glabella*
    - Forehead

Volume replacement

- Thicker products
- Inject into deeper dermis
- Areas
    - Melolabial fold
    - Nasojugal fold
    - Brow fat pad
    - Lips

Postinjection care

- Massage
- Ice
- Touch up in 1–2 weeks if necessary

*Glabellar injections have been associated with skin necrosis.

Box 7-7

Choice of Fillers*

Temporary 6–12 months

- Hyaluronic acid based
    - Restylane/Perlane
    - Juvéderm Ultra/Ultra Plus
    - Hyalaform
    - Captique

Longer acting—permanent

- Calcium hydroxyapatite beads—Radiesse, Radiance, Radiance FN
- Polymethylmethacrylate (PMMA) microspheres—Artefill
- Silicone oil—Silikon 1000, Adato Sil-ol 500
- Poly-L-lactic acid—Sculptra

Autogenous fat injection

*Many of the fillers above are not FDA approved for cosmetic use.

so check the literature and talk with your colleagues to find out the latest information on the effectiveness, duration, and safety of new products as they become available (http://www.juvedermusa.com, http://www.restylaneusa.com).

Technique

In the United States, Botox was introduced before fillers and, at this time, Botox is used much more commonly. With the introduction of fillers in the United States and heavy marketing, many patients are requesting fillers with or without Botox. Keep in mind that some of your patients will have generalized wrinkling as well. This is where laser resurfacing or chemical peeling can improve skin texture, tone, and color over the periocular region or the whole face. Once you have experience with treating all three types of wrinkles—dynamic, adynamic, and generalized—you can tailor your treatment to the wrinkles that bother your patient most.

until you are very comfortable with your techniques using HA products.

A final option for "reinflating the deflated face" is using autogenous fat injections. Using liposuction technique, you can harvest fat either from the neck during a facelift procedure or from another site on the body. Prior to injection, the fat cells are separated out via a centrifugation technique. Small or, in some cases, large amounts of fat can be injected into the face to re-establish the smooth contours of youth. The results and longevity are variable but, in some cases, the improvement is spectacular. For most surgeons, this is a technique that is added to a "mature" aesthetic practice.

My goal in this section is to have you remember the principles of Botox and injectable filler use. Botox and fillers are a good place to start your aesthetic practice. Patients with less aged skin may have only dynamic wrinkles and respond well to Botox alone. Patients with more aged skin will have both dynamic and adynamic wrinkles. If Botox alone does not do enough, you can add an HA-based filler. The currently available products are listed in Box 7-7. Start with one or two HA products and get confident using them. As you get more experience, you might want to learn to use longer lasting fillers. Keep in mind that this field is changing rapidly,

Checkpoint

- Think about your personal philosophy regarding "cosmetic surgery" for your patients. Start thinking about the menu of aesthetic treatments you may want to offer
- Name two types of skin products that help prevent aging changes—are you using them?
- What is the difference between dynamic and adynamic wrinkles?
- Remember, Botox for upper face, fillers for the lower face. As you get more experience, you can "bend" the rules
- Sketch out potential sites for Botox
- Sketch out the potential sites for filler injection
    - Wrinkles
    - Volume (clue: eyelids and cheek)
- Why should you use fillers with caution in the glabella?
- When are Botox and fillers helpful together?

Skin resurfacing and chemical peeling

Introduction

Some patients develop generalized wrinkling, texture changes, and areas of pigmentation that are not easily treated with the localized injection techniques we have talked about. In these patients, laser resurfacing or chemical peeling tightens the skin and gives a fresh layer of epithelium. Although the treatments are different in application, the effect is the same. The surface epithelium is removed and the dermis is damaged. Re-epithelialization brings about a thicker layer of new cells (less atypia) with more even pigmentation. Over a few months following treatment, the dermis undergoes a "remodeling" process, increasing in thickness and containing more collagen, elastin, and ground substance. The overall result is a smoother thicker skin with fewer wrinkles.

Fitzpatrick classification system of skin type

The Fitzpatrick Classification (Table 7-2) is useful for selecting which of your patients are good candidates for treatment. This classification is based on a patient's tendency to tan rather than burn when exposed to sunlight. Your patients with lighter skin color will respond best to resurfacing and peeling procedures with less risk of post-treatment hyperpigmentation, the most common side-effect. When you are learning these treatments, pick patients with mild to moderate aging changes with skin types I–III. You will get a reasonable effect and will avoid unwelcome post-treatment pigmentary changes.

Treatment principles

Mastering the "art" of laser resurfacing and chemical peeling is to understand and then match the severity of the sun damage (depth of damage) with the penetration of the laser or peeling agent (depth of the treatment). The treatment and healing process leaves a healthier skin.

We talked in some detail about the intrinsic and extrinsic causes of skin damage. As you will need to match the degree of damage with the severity of treatment, let's look at how to recognize the amount of damage present. Mild sun damage is seen as abnormalities in the skin *texture and pigmentation*. The damage is seen mostly within the epidermis. As *wrinkling* develops, the damage is first within the superficial part of the dermis, the papillary dermis. These patients

have surface and pigment changes as well as dynamic and early adynamic wrinkles. As the sun damage progresses, the deeper reticular dermis is affected. These patients have *many wrinkles at rest*. The skin starts to appear leathery and can take on a yellow discoloration.

Before you embark on these treatments, you should prepare the skin medically. After treatment, you should recommend a long-term skin maintenance plan. For most of your patients, retreatment over the years will be required to maintain optimal skin condition.

Pretreatment

You should start pretreatment care at least 6 weeks prior to resurfacing or peeling. *Tretinoin* (0.025–0.05%) should be applied qhs or bid. For patients with moderate amounts of pigmentary changes, a bleaching agent such as topical *hydroquinone 4%* should be applied bid. This will even out the dyschromias and minimize the possibility of post-treatment hyperpigmentation. It's a good idea to avoid treating patients with easily tanning, olive or darker skin (types IV–VI) until you have considerable experience. *Sun blocks* containing zinc oxide or titanium oxide, rather than chemical sunscreens, are best and should be applied each morning. *Valacyclovir* (Valtrex) 500 mg po bid and *Cephalexin* (Keflex) 500 qid should be started the day before treatment and continued until the skin is re-epithelialized (usually 7–14 days depending on the treatment).

In the next two sections, we will discuss the principles of laser resurfacing and chemical peeling techniques with the idea of matching the depth of treatment to the depth of the damage. As you already know, the deeper the damage, the greater the effect. However, with deeper treatments, healing is prolonged and the risk of complications, including infection, scarring, and hyperpigmentation, is increased. With moderate treatment, you will get an improvement with low risk of complications.

Laser resurfacing

Laser energy can be used to improve skin texture, pigmentation, and wrinkling. Many types of lasers and techniques have been described in recent years to improve facial skin health. In my opinion, the gold standard remains the CO_2 laser ablative resurfacing technique*. The chromophore for the CO_2 laser is water (10,600 nm wavelength). As human tissues contain a large amount of water, high laser energy levels will instantly vaporize the tissue. When lower energy is absorbed, the tissues will absorb heat. *Ablative* resurfacing techniques (either CO_2 or Erbium YAG) vaporize the epithelium and deliver heat into the dermis. As the new epithelium regenerates, the result is a smooth healthy layer of cells without blotchy pigmentation. During the recovery process, the underlying dermis goes through a remodeling process that promotes collagen production resulting in a more plump skin with fewer wrinkles. Recently, *nonablative* lasers have been developed that deliver energy to the deeper layers without removing the surface epithelium. The intended result is improvement of wrinkles without the crusty healing

Table 7-2 Fitzpatrick Classification System

Skin type	Skin color	Characteristic
I	Very white or freckled	Always burns, never tans
II	White	Usually burns, tans less than average
III	White to olive	Sometimes mild burn, tans about average
IV	Brown	Rarely burns, tans more than average
V	Dark brown	Rarely burns, tans profusely
VI	Black	Never burns, deeply pigmented

*With a CO_2 laser on hand for resurfacing, you will also have a great incisional laser with excellent hemostatic properties. Erbium YAG wavelength lasers do not provide the same hemostasis.

phase of epithelialization. As you might expect, the result is faster healing, but a less dramatic reduction in wrinkling. More recently, laser techniques have developed known as fractional resurfacing. Using this technology, microscopic "holes" are burned through the epithelium with most of the energy delivered deeply. The consensus opinion regarding the results of this technique is not in yet. No doubt there will be continued efforts to achieve the most improvement with the least "down time" and possible side-effects. There is no "right" technique or laser.

As you will see with peeling, in your early treatment experience, it is best to pick one laser technique and get familiar with delivering a fixed amount, or a narrow range, of energy to mild to moderately damaged skin. As we said already, it is best to pick lighter skinned patients with skin types I–III. Once you are confident with your technique and happy with your results, you can treat patients with deeper damage using higher energies. Treating darker skinned patients is more unpredictable so be wary of moving to darker skin types. Always keep in mind that higher energy means more improvement, but will prolong recovery and increase the risks of postoperative problems such as scarring, prolonged erythema, hyperpigmentation, hypopigmentation, and infection.

As we discussed above, pretreatment with tretinoin (Retin-A, Avita, Renova) and sunscreen is mandatory. Some physicians will pretreat with bleaches, but this is not usually necessary. Cells for re-epithelialization migrate to the surface from the underlying dermal glands so patients should have not used Accutane (isotretinoin) for 6–12 months prior to resurfacing (remember this medication reduces sebaceous gland function). There is a paucity of these glandular structures in the neck so you should not resurface below the mandibular line.

Periocular treatment is a very effective adjunct to upper and lower blepharoplasty. As you know, upper blepharoplasty is primarily a skin- and muscle-removing operation. Lower blepharoplasty is primarily a fat-removing operation. Neither should be used for removing fine wrinkles in the eyelid skin. Resurfacing works well in this regard and can be performed at the same time. As the healing process is accompanied by a period of erythema often lasting weeks, you should warn your patients about demarcation lines separating treated and untreated areas. Similarly, occasionally, noticeable alterations in skin pigmentation (hypo- or hyper-) can result. You can minimize these problems by "feathering" the treatment edges so that more heavily treated areas blend with normal skin using intermediate treatment intensity. After epithelialization, 7–10 days, your patients can wear make up to hide any color changes.

Treatment may be directed at the periocular area alone or the full face. Full face resurfacing will avoid the "transition" zones around the eyes and can greatly improve the superficial and deep wrinkles around the mouth and in the vertical pleated folds that occur at the sides of the mouth and jowls. Similarly, "smoker's" lips respond well. As you will not be resurfacing the neck skin, you must stop at the mandibular margin and do some feathering to minimize the transition from treated to untreated areas.

Infiltrative local anesthesia with mild sedation works well for eyelid resurfacing. For full face treatment, infiltrative and regional blocks (infraorbital, mental, and supraorbital nerve blocks) are necessary. Most of your face patients will do best with monitored anesthesia care (MAC) sedation or general anesthesia. Safety precautions should be followed to avoid accidental laser injury. Staff should all wear goggles and the patient should wear metal corneal shields. The surgical field should be surrounded with wet drapes and a smoke evacuator is necessary. Supplemental oxygen should be turned off during treatment.

You can change the depth of treatment by adjusting the laser power or density of the laser energy delivery. You can also change the depth of treatment with an additional one or two more passes of the laser. Remember that matching the depth of the burn to the depth of the damage is the key to "art" of resurfacing. Initially pick patients with mild to moderate damage and use the suggested settings below. Watch how the color changes on the treated skin—pink is light treatment, yellow is heavy treatment. The ideal treatment color is described as "chamois" color.

With experience, you will learn how to modify the settings or add treatment passes. When preparing to treat your patient, select the appropriate settings, get a comfortable grip on the hand piece, and fire a test against a tongue blade to see that the laser is working correctly. Depress the foot pedal for each laser burst. As you get experience, you can use repeated timed firings by holding the pedal down. Position the hand piece with the laser aimed perpendicular to the skin surface. Most lasers have a collimated hand piece that does not require an exact focal distance, making your hand positioning more flexible. Put the laser pattern bursts next to each other on the skin, with about a 10% overlap. When you complete one pass of the entire treatment area, you should remove the charred epithelium with a soaking wet gauze pad. Dry the skin to remove all water before another pass (Figure 7-5).

Do your second pass with the laser moving in a slightly different direction to insure even coverage. In general, the cheeks and forehead tolerate two or three passes. The eyelid skin and lips are thinner and tolerate only one or two passes. Use only one pass when feathering into the neck at the mandibular line and on the pretarsal skin. If a patient has especially deep vertical pleated wrinkles or smoker's wrinkles of the lips (or elsewhere), mark these areas before you start. You can laser along your marks before swelling occurs, then add the two passes you planned for an additional effect.

A general protocol is presented in Box 7-8.

Post treatment

Your post-treatment care starts on the initial visit. Part of your "benefit and risk" discussion includes an explanation of the "down time" of healing. No matter how you explain the immediate postoperative appearance, most patients will be alarmed by how they look. Photos are helpful. Obviously, your goal is not to scare your patient away, but to educate them—some preoperative reassurance that, despite how they look for a few days after surgery, they will do well. You will save the patient some worries and save yourself some phone calls. Erythema is the most common longer term issue, so be sure to remind your patient that this is normal and will resolve over several weeks, but can persist for 3 or more months. It is important to remind your patients that any sun exposure while the skin is still pink can result in long term pigmentation changes.

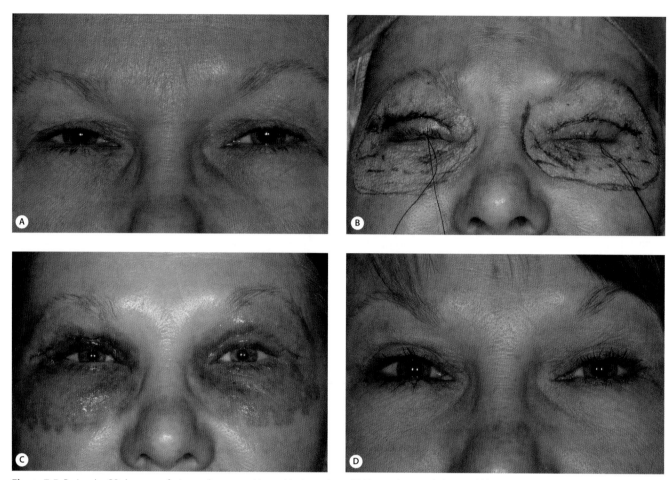

Figure 7-5 Periocular CO_2 laser resurfacing and upper and lower blepharoplasty. (**A**) Upper dermatochalasis, mild lower eyelid fat prolapse. (**B**) Light CO_2 resurfacing and 4 lid blepharoplasty—markings to show rims and feathering. (**C**) Re-epithelialization nearly complete after 8 days. (**D**) Improved upper skin fold and no lower fat prolapse. Improvement of lower lid fine wrinkles.

Serious complications are unlikely and reduced by appropriate skin pretreatments, antibiotics, and antiviral agents. Hyperpigmentation should be treated aggressively with bleaching agents (hydroquinone 4% cream; Eldoquin Forte) if a tendency becomes apparent after a few weeks of healing. Pruritis is common and can be helped with Benadryl, cool compresses, and Domeboro soaks. Scarring is uncommon and is best avoided by conservative treatment. Over-the-counter pain medications such as Tylenol or Celebrex are recommended. You should consider anti-anxiety agents, such as Xanax, in all your patients. It is worth giving a prescription for narcotic pain medication in case the other medications do not provide enough relief. After the first 2 days, the pain should reduce each day. Increasing pain over the first week or two should be an alarm for the possibility of bacterial or viral infection. Diagnostic help with cultures and sensitivities for bacterial and KOH scrapings should be performed.

Chemical peeling

Peels can be classified by depth and peeling agent. *Superficial peels* extend through the epidermis to the papillary dermis. *Medium depth peels* extend from the papillary dermis to the upper reticular dermis. *Deep peels* extend into the mid-reticular dermis. In general terms, the common peeling agents that you should know about can be classified as:

- Superficial agents
  — Retinoic acid (Retin A)
  — Alpha hydroxy acid (AHA)
  — Jessner's solution
- Medium depth agents
  — Trichloroacetic acid (TCA)
- Deep agents
  — Phenol in Baker's formula

You will see that it is a bit more complicated than this because many agents are available in different concentrations and are often applied together or sequentially. The depth of penetration is also affected by skin pretreatment protocols, rubbing during application, and varies according to skin type.

Your patient should already be on *retinoic acid* (not to be confused with tretinoin, Accutane) as a pretreatment. When used for months, this product will have a mild peeling effect. *Alpha hydroxy acid (AHA) products* (glycolic acid, most commonly) are used as the familiar "lunch time" peels. These agents give a superficial peel, improving mild wrinkling and pigmentation. They require repeated treatments to give much effect. *Jessner's solution* is considered a superficial peeling agent when used alone, but is most commonly used as a "primer" applied immediately prior to a stronger agent (commonly TCA). The primer application increases the penetration of the second agent. Like pretreatment and primer applications, degreasing the skin with acetone immediately prior to treatment will also affect the depth of penetration.

Trichloroacetic acid (TCA) is a good choice to start your peeling practice. The percentage of TCA applied affects the penetration, ranging from superficial depth (10–30% TCA) to medium depth (35–50% TCA). A user-friendly TCA product is the Obagi Blue Peel. Color is added to this product to help give an even application. *Phenol* 89% used alone is a medium depth peel. Phenol is used most commonly as the active ingredient in the Baker–Gordon formula. Septisol soap, croton oil, and water are added to create a deeply penetrating mixture and should not be used without considerable experience with other weaker agents. Aside from the danger of an excessively deep peel, cardiac toxicity can be seen.

You can see that there are many factors that affect the depth of the peel. It is good to use one type of peel (TCA) and pretreatment (retinoic acid) so that you can get familiar with its effect. Pick mild to moderate damage in lighter patients. Once you are familiar with the effect, you can modify your "standard" treatment based on the depth of damage and the skin type. A suggested protocol is outlined in Box 7-9. The procedure may be applied to the entire face or just the periocular region. Your post-treatment care is the same as we described above for laser resurfacing.

Checkpoint

- Do you have a general idea of the Fitzpatrick Classification of skin types?
- What effects do resurfacing treatments and chemical peels have on the epidermis? And the dermis?
- What are some of the risks of these procedures? Most common? Most serious?
- Remember the key to these procedures is matching the depth of the treatment to the depth of the damage. Try to get an idea of what mild, moderate, and severe skin damage looks like
- Avoid any deep peels until you have considerable experience with more superficial peels

---

Box 7-8

CO$_2$ Laser Resurfacing for Mild to Moderate Sun Damage

Pretreatment

6 weeks before—Tretinoin 0.05% bid for 6 weeks

2 days before—and continued until epithelialized

- Valacyclovir 500 mg po bid
- Keflex 500 mg po qid

Treatment

Safety precautions—eye glasses for staff, wet drapes around field and over any endotracheal tube, metal contact lenses for patient, wet gauze over teeth CO$_2$ laser* settings with computer pattern generator hand piece

- Power
- Density
- Pattern
- Size

Periorbital region

- First pass
  - Settings: power 250 mJ, density 4, pattern 5, size 5
  - Upper eyelid: eyebrow to skin crease
  - Lower eyelid: 2–3 mm below lashes down to slightly below rim
  - Remove char with wet gauze
- Second pass
  - Settings: power 200–250 mJ, density 4, pattern 5, size 5
  - Same as above plus
    — Upper pretarsal skin (2 mm above lashes)
    — One pass inferior to rim to feather
  - Remove char with wet gauze

Face

- Deep wrinkles
  - Consider marking and treating with one pass before general treatment, using settings below

- First pass
  - Settings: power 300 mJ, density 4, pattern 3, size 8
  - Hairline to mandible (treat just into hairs)
  - Remove char with wet gauze
- Second pass
  - Settings: power 300 mJ, density 4, pattern 3, size 8
  - Same as above plus one row inferior to mandible—feather
  - Remove char with wet gauze

Post treatment

First 48 hours post treatment

- Dressing options
  - Biomembrane occlusive dressing for 48 hours, change and use an additional 48 hours if necessary (Silon TSR, http://www.silon.com) or
  - Aquaphor or Vaseline ointment
    — Cool compresses or rinses (or shower) every 30 minutes
    — Reapply ointment after each soaking or rinse
- Oral pain meds—Celebrex, Percocet
- Sedation—Xanax

After 48 hours every 2–4 hours

- If using dressing, remove in office on pod 2
- Switch compresses to warm when tolerated
- Dilute vinegar (1 tsp per cup of water) or Domebrero astringent soaks q30 minutes
- Apply Aquaphor or Vaseline ointment after each soaking or rinse ointment q2 hours
- Benadryl prn itching

*Using Coherent 5000 c CO$_2$ laser. Current model is Ultrapulse Lumenis, http://www.lumenis.com.

Box 7-9

Medium Depth Peeling Protocol

Patient selection: skin types I–III

- Mild to moderate damage
- Epidermal texture and pigment changes
- Dynamic wrinkles and superficial wrinkles at rest

Pretreatment

- 6 weeks before—Tretinoin 0.05% bid for 6 weeks
- 2 days before—and continued until epithelialized
  - Valacyclovir 500 mg po bid
  - Keflex 500 mg po qid

Treatment

- Agents
  - Jensen's solution to face and extending to the inferior border of the mandible and neck
  - 35% TCA solution to face ending at mandible
- Application
  - Patient supine with head elevated 45 degrees
  - Degrease the skin with alcohol or acetone
  - Wet, not saturated, folded 2 × 2 gauze
  - Stretch skin during application
  - Avoid overlapping passes
  - "Frost" will develop and show you how deep the penetration is
    - Ideal—white frost with pink showing through, indicating a medium depth treatment

- — Light white frost—superficial treatment
- — Heavy all-white frost—deep treatment
- Periocular region
  - — Apply from eyebrow to superior orbital rim
  - — No upper eyelid application
  - — Treat lower eyelid from 2–3 mm below margin and down
- Face
  - — Treat from just within hairline to mandible
  - — Feather with Jensen's or more dilute TCA inferior to mandible 1 cm below mandible
- Neck and chest
  - — With experience, you can extend treatment

Post treatment

- Initial—Rinse skin with water
- First 48 hours post treatment
  - Biomembrane dressing (Silon TSR, http://www.silon.com), change and use an additional 48 hours if necessary
  - Oral pain meds—Celebrex, Percocet
  - Sedation—Xanax
- After 48 hours every 2–4 hours
  - Cool water rinses or compresses
  - Dilute vinegar (1 tsp per cup of water) or Domeboro astringent soaks q30 minutes
  - Aquaphor ointment
  - Benadryl prn itching

Lower eyelid blepharoplasty

Preoperative considerations

Lower lid blepharoplasty is frequently done *in combination with upper lid blepharoplasty*. The majority of complications from lower lid blepharoplasty are associated with *lower lid retraction*. As already discussed, the extent of skin and muscle excision, if necessary at all, should be conservative in all patients. When an element of lid laxity is present, lid tightening should be done if any skin and muscle resection is planned. Lower lid blepharoplasty can be combined with a midface lift or other facelift procedures, which may be done under general anesthesia.

There are two lower eyelid blepharoplasty procedures. The *transcutaneous lower eyelid blepharoplasty* is used to remove skin, muscle, and fat. The *transconjunctival lower eyelid blepharoplasty* is used for patients who require fat removal only. (As you will see, many surgeons combine a transconjunctival fat removal with a small "pinch" skin-only blepharoplasty.)

Transcutaneous lower blepharoplasty

Transcutaneous lower blepharoplasty includes:

- Marking the skin
- Instilling local anesthesia
- Making a skin incision
- Dissecting a skin and muscle flap
- Opening the orbital septum, dissecting, and excising prolapsing orbital fat
- Consideration of a lateral canthoplasty

- Conservative skin and muscle excision
- Closing the skin

The steps of the transcutaneous lower eyelid blepharoplasty are:

1. Mark the skin
   A. Mark a subciliary incision 2–3 mm below the lower lashes. Extend the mark from the punctum to the lateral canthus and bring it approximately 5 mm lateral to the lateral canthus in a wrinkle line (**Figure 7-6, A**).

2. Administer anesthesia
   A. Consider intravenous sedation.
   B. Inject the lower eyelid anteriorly with a 30-gauge needle passing just beneath the skin (1.5–2 ml). Take care not to cause a hematoma.
   C. Prep and drape the patient, leaving the entire face in the operating field.

3. Make a skin incision
   A. Use a Colorado needle to cut along the subciliary incision (**Figure 7-6, B**). A no. 15 blade or CO_2 laser may be used.

4. Dissect a skin and muscle flap
   A. Dissect a *skin and muscle flap* inferiorly to the orbital rim (**Figure 7-6, C**).
   B. As with upper lid blepharoplasty, "pull apart" the orbicularis and septum and you will see *small fibers stretching from the posterior surface of the orbicularis to the septum* that can be cut. In many patients, you will see one or two neurovascular bundles in the post-orbicular fascia running perpendicular to the muscle

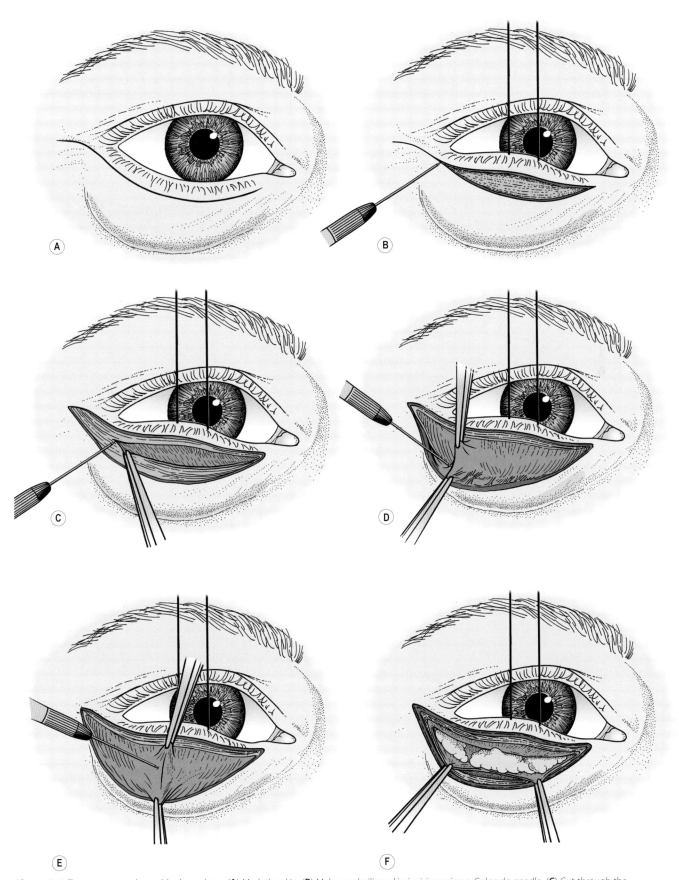

Figure 7-6 Transcutaneous lower blepharoplasty. (**A**) Mark the skin. (**B**) Make a subciliary skin incision using a Colorado needle. (**C**) Cut through the orbicularis muscle to the orbital septum. (**D**) Dissect a skin and muscle flap. (**E**) and (**F**) Open the orbital septum and identify the three lower lid fat pads. (**G**) Dissect and excise the prolapsing orbital fat with Westcott scissors. (**H**) Consider a lateral canthoplasty. (**I**) Perform a conservative skin and muscle excision. (**J**) Consider using a deep fixation suture temporally into the periosteum (a version of the preperiosteal midface lift). Close the skin with a running suture.

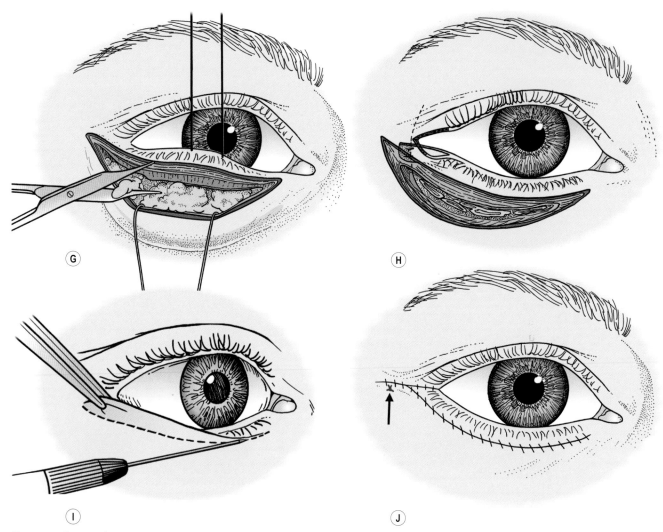

Figure 7-6 Continued.

fibers (as in the upper eyelid). These nerves are a subtle, but helpful, surgical landmark, indicating the depth of the septal plane.

5. Open the orbital septum and dissect the orbital fat
   A. You will identify the orbital septum as a thin fibrous layer covering the orbital fat. The septum has many thin layers to it. In older adults, the septum may be quite thin (which allows the orbital fat to prolapse).
   B. Open the septum with Westcott scissors. Cut the septum overlying the fat to protect the underlying lower lid retractors (Figure 7-6, D).
   C. The three fat compartments in the lower lid are the *nasal*, *central*, and *lateral fat pads*. Generally, the nasal and central fat pads are easy to see. You have already opened the orbital septum so the individual fat compartments should be visualized. Open the thin fibrous fat capsule over each pad. There are small vessels in the capsule that may require some cautery. Dissect the capsule posteriorly to the white band of tissue, *the lower lid retractors* (Figure 7-6, E and F). As you continue to elevate the fat off the retractors inferiorly, you will see a thicker horizontal band of

fibrous tissue, Lockwood's ligament. Just posterior to *Lockwood's ligament*, within the retractors, lies the inferior oblique muscle.

D. Before fat excision, *inject some additional local anesthetic* into the fat. Use bipolar cautery at the base of the fat pads and *excise the fat at or just anterior to the inferior orbital rim*. It is much better to be conservative with fat excision than to be overaggressive. *Fat excision posterior to the inferior orbital rim will result in the patient having a hollow gaunt look, which is difficult to correct.* For your first few operations, be conservative and have the patient sit up after the fat excision to estimate if further excision is necessary. Generally, little bleeding results with fat excision. You should look at the amount of fat in all three compartments.

E. Generally, the nasal and central fat pads are not difficult to identify, *but the lateral fat pad may be somewhat more hidden.* Remember, it is not the amount of excision that needs to be symmetric, but rather that you *leave symmetric amounts of fat* in each orbit. Using the inferior orbital rim as a landmark is helpful. In general, you should not remove any fat posterior to the inferior orbital margin.

(1) Your preoperative evaluation should give you the location and relative amount of fat that is prolapsing (during the exam, position a directional light over the patient and ask them to look up. Note in the chart something like 4+ fat prolapse medial pad, 2+ central pad, 0-1+ lateral pad, moderate nasojugal fold centrally).

F. There is a trend toward smaller amounts of fat excision in both upper and lower eyelids. Some patients benefit from *"repositioning"* of the orbital fat over the inferior rim to mask the descent of the malar fat that occurs with aging. In these cases, dissect the nasal and central fat pads free. Excise any fat that you feel is excessive, but be conservative. "Flip" the remaining fat over the rim (where you have noted a hollow preoperatively) and suture in place with a running 6-0 Vicryl suture. You will be filling the "tear trough" so only the nasal and central pads are rotated over the rim.

6. Consider a lateral canthoplasty

A. Before skin and muscle excision, consider a lateral canthoplasty or lower lid tightening. I use a *lateral tarsal strip* type procedure (see Chapter 3). Make a canthotomy incision extending into the previously marked wrinkle line using Westcott scissors or a Colorado needle.

B. Perform a cantholysis. Make a strip of bare tarsus by dissecting the anterior lamella off the tarsus and denuding the lid margin and posterior aspect of the tarsus of the epithelium. Suture the strip onto the inner aspect of the lateral orbital rim with a double-armed 4-0 Mersilene suture on a P-2 half-circle needle (see lateral tarsal strip procedure in Chapter). Use moderate tightness and slight superior placement of the lateral canthal angle (Figure 7-6, G). Remember the precautions about the patient with hemiproptosis (or "negative vector"), in whom lid tightening can exacerbate lid retraction.

C. *There are several variations of the lateral canthoplasty procedure.* Some surgeons plicate the tendon. When performing an upper lid blepharoplasty at the same time, you might try to pull the lateral canthal tendon superiorly through the upper lid incision and anchor it to the lateral orbital rim periosteum. This works well in younger patients who do not require much lid tightening. For the vast majority of patients who need lower eyelid tightening, I use a lateral tarsal strip type procedure.

7. Excise skin and muscle

A. With the lateral canthus sutured into position, drape the skin and muscle over the edge of the lid margin. A conservative amount of skin and muscle should be excised (usually 2–3 mm). I use a marking pen to outline the excess skin at the lid margin. *Avoid the tendency to remove much more skin laterally than medially.* This is a common cause for the temporal droop of the lower lid, or scleral show, seen in patients postoperatively. Again, remove a conservative amount of skin and muscle (Figure 7-6, H). Your

skin excision can be slightly less conservative if you have tightened the lid. Once the skin and muscle have been removed, the skin should lie nicely in position. Some surgeons choose to have the patient sit up at this point to check if enough skin has been removed. This is a reasonable step to perform in your early experience.

8. Close the skin

A. I usually place a *deep fixation suture* at the lateral canthus, giving further lift and support of the lateral lid tissue. I use a 4-0 PDS suture (Ethicon Z504G P-2 needle, 8 mm reverse cutting, clear) to place a stitch through the orbital orbicularis muscle flap 1 cm below the lateral canthus and pull this tissue up, attaching the muscle to the periosteum of the lateral orbital rim. Try not to dimple the skin. In some cases, you may want to perform a bit of a preperiosteal midface lift to give extra elevation of the cheek. You will learn how to do this later in the chapter. These fixation sutures are helpful in preventing the temporal lower eyelid droop that is a tell-tale sign of an aggressive lower eyelid blepharoplasty.

B. Next, place an interrupted 6-0 Prolene or nylon suture into the edge of the skin and muscle flap directly to the most lateral edge of the tarsal strip to nicely reform the canthal angle. Use one or two more to close the canthotomy. I use a running closure with the same suture (or sometimes a 5-0 fast absorbing gut suture) to close the skin from the punctum to the lateral canthus (Figure 7-6, I).

C. Place some topical antibiotic ointment on the wound and in the conjunctival cul de sac. As usual, ask your patient to use cold compresses placed over the eyes for the first 24–48 hours. No oral antibiotics are used. It can be worthwhile to use 5 days of oral steroids (60 mg prednisone per day) (Box 7-10).

Transconjunctival lower eyelid blepharoplasty

This approach is *useful in younger patients with no excess skin and muscle.* The fat can be removed through a transconjunctival incision without placing any scars on the skin. In patients in whom lower eyelid laxity exists, a lateral canthoplasty can be performed, but it generally is not necessary as the majority of these procedures are performed on younger patients.

The transconjunctival lower blepharoplasty includes:

- Marking
- Anesthesia
- Conjunctival incision
- Orbital fat exposure
- Excision of prolapsing fat
- Elective lower lid tightening
- Conjunctiva closure

The steps of the transconjunctival lower blepharoplasty are:

1. Mark the skin

A. No formal marking is done on the conjunctiva. However, you may find it helpful to mark the bulging fat pads on the skin surface as a reminder to you.

Box 7-10

Transcutaneous Lower Eyelid Blepharoplasty

Skin marking

- Mark a subciliary incision 2–3 mm inferior to the eyelashes
- Extend the mark from the punctum to 5 mm lateral to the lateral canthus

Anesthesia

- Administer topical anesthetic drops
- Inject 1–2 ml of local anesthetic under the skin

Skin incision

- Make a subciliary incision with a Colorado needle

Skin and muscle flap dissection

- Dissect a skin and muscle flap to the inferior orbital rim
- Remember to "pull" the orbicularis muscle and the septum apart

Fat excision

- Open the septum
- Expose the three fat pads: lateral, central, and nasal
- Inject additional local anesthetic
- Excise the fat anterior to the orbital rim, leaving symmetric amounts of skin
- Consider fat repositioning over the inferior rim

Canthoplasty

- Consider a lateral canthoplasty type procedure to tighten the lid in any patient undergoing skin and muscle excision (usually lid laxity is present)

Skin and muscle excision

- Remove a minimal amount of skin and muscle (usually less than 3 mm)
- Avoid excessive skin removal temporally

Closure

- Consider a deep fixation suture laterally
- Use interrupted sutures for the canthotomy
- Use a running skin closure for the subciliary incision
- Do not close the septum

2. Administer anesthesia
   A. Consider intravenous sedation.
   B. Place topical anesthetic drops in the conjunctival cul de sacs.
   C. Inject local anesthetic under the palpebral conjunctiva and again under the skin anteriorly.
3. Make a conjunctival incision
   A. Use two *4-0 silk sutures* through the lid margin as traction sutures. If lid tightening is not anticipated, evert the lower lid over a retractor ("shoehorn"— Jaeger retractor or a small Desmarres retractor). As you get more experience, you will not need the traction sutures.
   B. Use a no. 15 blade or a Colorado needle to make an incision at the inferior edge of the tarsus. Be extremely careful using the Colorado needle, especially if you are not using a corneal protector. This incision is through the conjunctiva and lower lid retractors to the level of orbicularis muscle (Figure 7-7, A).
   C. If lid tightening is anticipated, the conjunctival incision is preceded by a small lateral canthotomy

and cantholysis. The inferior conjunctival incision is then performed and extended into cantholysis (Figure 7-7, B and C). You will find that using the canthotomy/cantholysis approach makes it easier to see the fat, especially in the lateral compartment. I find that it is very difficult to "flip the fat" without a canthotomy.

4. Dissect a skin and muscle flap
   A. If you are used to doing only anterior approach lower lid surgery, these steps will seem somewhat unfamiliar initially. The goal of your dissection is to now elevate the orbicularis off the orbital septum and extend the dissection inferiorly to the orbital rim (Figure 7-7, D and E). Once dissection in this plane is started, it will become familiar to surgeons used to the anterior approach because the remainder of the dissection is essentially the same.
   B. Pull the edges of the conjunctival wound apart, separating the orbital septum from the orbicularis muscle. Follow this plane inferiorly to the inferior orbital rim. You will see the preaponeurotic fat posterior to the orbital septum.
5. Expose the orbital fat
   A. The same technique of orbital fat dissection and removal is carried out through this incision. I find it helpful to place another suture at the edge of the conjunctival wound to retract this tissue superiorly. A Desmarres lid retractor or a Jaffe lid speculum is useful to retract the lid margin and tarsus away from the fat. If a lateral canthotomy and cantholysis have not been performed, it is somewhat difficult to get to the lateral fat pad, but your persistence and experience will allow this to be done.
   B. Open the septum and elevate the fat off the retractors (Figure 7-7, F).
   C. Inject additional local anesthetic into the fat. Open the fat capsules, exposing all three fat pads. Use bipolar cautery if necessary.
6. Excise the redundant orbital fat
   A. Trim the fat off just anterior to the inferior orbital rim (Figure 7-7, G). This is the time for repositioning the fat to "soften" the inferior rim.
7. Close the conjunctiva
   A. When no lid tightening procedure has been used, suture the conjunctiva with either interrupted or running sutures. I usually close the wound with two or three 5-0 or 6-0 fast absorbing gut sutures (Figure 7-7, H).
   B. If lid tightening is necessary, close the medial two thirds of the wound and perform a tarsal strip type of canthoplasty. Place the canthus slightly high with appropriate lid tightening.
   C. When only fat removal is anticipated, some surgeons will make the initial incision in the fornix through the conjunctiva and lower lid retractors going directly into the fat in the preaponeurotic area. In theory, this approach is less likely to cause lower lid retraction, because the orbital septum is not opened at all. All fat excision is carried out from behind the intact orbital septum. This approach is used when there is a

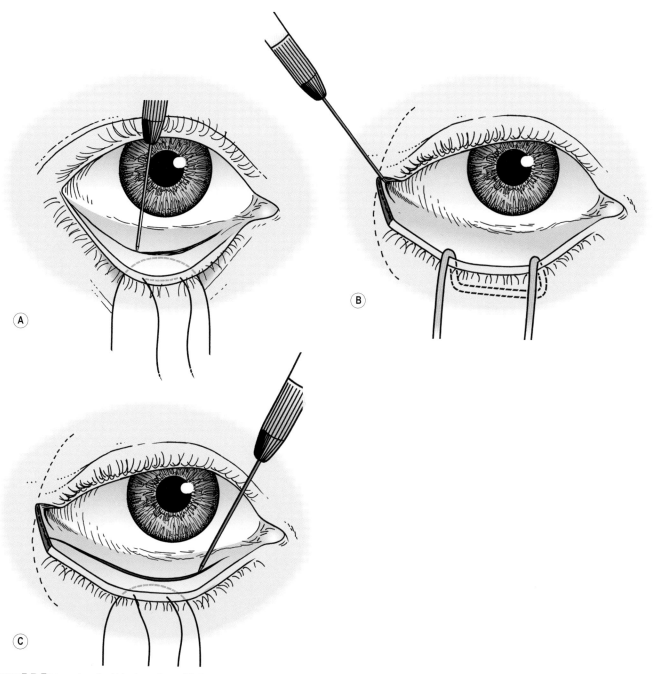

Figure 7-7 Transconjunctival blepharoplasty. (**A**) Conjunctival incision at the inferior tarsal margin (no lid tightening anticipated). (**B**) and (**C**) Canthotomy/cantholysis and conjunctival incision (when lid tightening is anticipated). (**D**) Dissect a skin and muscle flap to the inferior rim (remain anterior to the septum). (**E**) Lateral view of preseptal dissection. (**F**) Use Westcott scissors to open the orbital septum and expose the orbital fat. (**G**) Excise (or reposition) prolapsing orbital fat. (**H**) Close the conjunctiva with interrupted sutures and canthoplasty closure to rim. (**I**) Canthoplasty closure with interrupted sutures.

mild to moderate amount of fat to excise and minimal eyelid laxity. Some surgeons add a "pinch" skin-only blepharoplasty to remove fine wrinkles of the lower eyelid skin. The advantage of this combined anterior and posterior approach is that the possibility of lid retraction is minimized. This is not a procedure that I do often. Its main use is where a small amount of fine skin wrinkling persists (often in patients wanting a touch up after an earlier lower blepharoplasty). Laser resurfacing of the lower eyelids is an alternative to improve these wrinkles.

Complications of lower eyelid blepharoplasty

The most common complications of lower lid blepharoplasty include *lid retraction* and *asymmetry*. Avoiding these complications starts with an appreciation of the anatomy and anatomic factors that relate to one another and may cause problems. Remember to *offer only realistic goals* to your patient. Avoid any patient with unrealistic expectations who may cause you to be overly aggressive. *The best way to avoid lower lid retraction is to be conservative in any skin excision.*

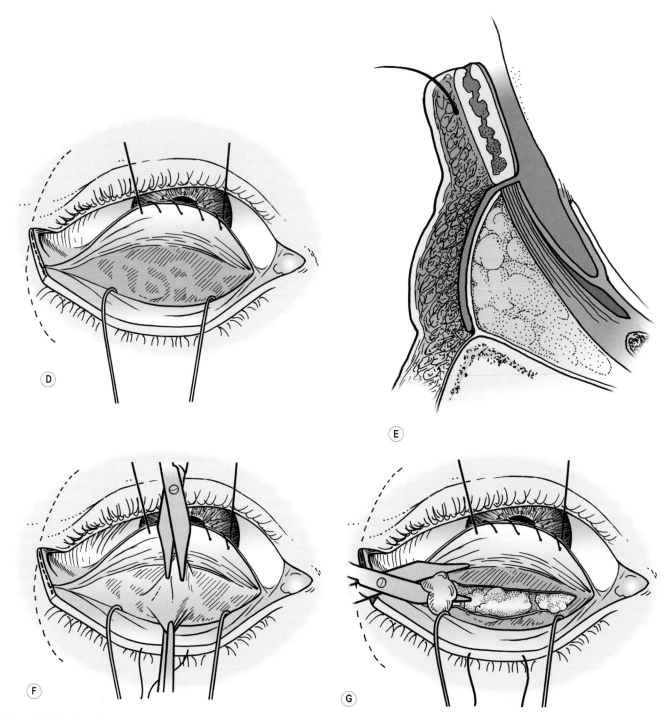

Figure 7-7 Continued.

Lower lid retraction and scleral show may be caused by excess skin and muscle excision or uncorrected lid laxity. Both these problems are exacerbated in patients with hemi-proptosis or midfacial hypoplasia. Lower lid retraction can be avoided by a transconjunctival approach in patients who do not need skin and muscle excision. In all patients in whom skin and muscle excision is performed, the excision should be conservative. Lateral canthoplasty for lid tighten-ing should be used whenever lid laxity is considered to be part of the problem. In patients with hemiproptosis, it may be necessary to support the lower lid with posterior lamellar grafts such as hard palate mucosa to correct or avoid further lid retraction.

If your patient develops lid retraction postoperatively, aggressive *massage* upward should be used for 2–3 months to correct minor abnormalities. If this does not work and retrac-tion is minimal, a lateral canthoplasty type of procedure may correct the retraction. The usual lateral tarsal strip operation can be used with extra attention being paid to *cutting the lateral portion of the lower lid retractors* to allow the lid to rise superiorly. If the retraction is more than 1–2 mm, it is best to perform a retractor reinsertion with a posterior lamellar spacer

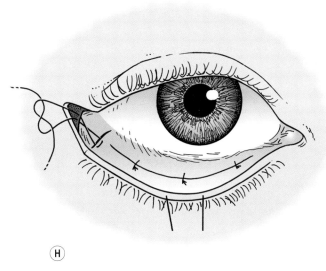

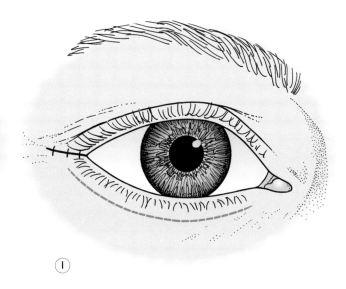

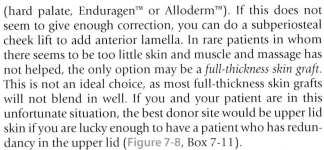

(H)

(I)

Figure 7-7 Continued.

(hard palate, Enduragen™ or Alloderm™). If this does not seem to give enough correction, you can do a subperiosteal cheek lift to add anterior lamella. In rare patients in whom there seems to be too little skin and muscle and massage has not helped, the only option may be a *full-thickness skin graft*. This is not an ideal choice, as most full-thickness skin grafts will not blend in well. If you and your patient are in this unfortunate situation, the best donor site would be upper lid skin if you are lucky enough to have a patient who has redundancy in the upper lid (Figure 7-8, Box 7-11).

Postoperative asymmetry is most easily dealt with if excess tissue is the problem. If excess skin, muscle, or fat is present, the appropriate tissue can be removed. In patients in whom unacceptable hollowness of the lower lid exists because of excess fat excision, fat grafting may be necessary to fill in the defect. If you find yourself in this situation, it may be appropriate to ask for help.

Orbital hemorrhage is a rare complication of any eyelid surgery. As is always the case, it is best to avoid complications rather than having to deal with them postoperatively. Patients should be reminded *preoperatively to discontinue aspirin, coumadin, or nonsteroidal anti-inflammatory drugs*. Vigorous pulling on the orbital fat should be avoided. The wound should be dry at the end of the procedure.

Postoperative care

At the conclusion of browplasty or blepharoplasty, patients should be given written material summarizing postoperative care. The patient should engage in little or no activity for 24–48 hours and keep cold compresses on the wound for the majority of the waking hours. If your patient develops severe pain or any proptosis, he or she should call you immediately. Ask your patients to gradually increase their activity on the second or third day postoperatively. Encourage most patients to return to work within 1 week, but remind them that bruising is common and may last for 10–14 days. In general, improvement in the patient's appearance is seen within a week or two, but mild swelling of the eyelids, especially of the pretarsal upper lid, may not resolve completely for several months.

Checkpoint

The main purpose of lower lid blepharoplasty is to remove the bulging fat in the lower eyelids. Some wrinkling will be reduced, but aggressive attempts to remove all wrinkles will create eyelid retraction. Skin resurfacing will reduce fine skin wrinkles.

- When is a transconjunctival approach to lower blepharoplasty indicated? When is a transcutaneous approach indicated?
- Avoid lower lid retraction and scleral show by:
  — Conservative skin and muscle resection
  — Lid tightening when excising skin and muscle
  — Anchoring sutures at the lateral canthus
  — Transconjunctival blepharoplasty when no redundant skin and muscle exist
- Can you explain the lower *eyelid double convexity*? You may be able to improve the nasojugal fold with "flipping the fat" over the rim, rather than excision alone
- Transconjunctival fornix fat excision and "pinch" skin removal is an alternative to transcutaneous lower blepharoplasty when there is only slight skin redundancy

With blepharoplasty, perhaps more than with any other surgery, a clear understanding of the patient's expectations is critical for success. Identification of the changes in anatomic features associated with the aging process gives a basis for choosing the correct procedure. Conservative surgery is the best way to avoid postoperative complications. If the goals of the operation are realistic and well understood, the patient and surgeon will be delighted with the postoperative result.

Forehead lifting procedures

Introduction

We have already discussed the principles of brow elevation surgery. You have seen the range of simple to more complex

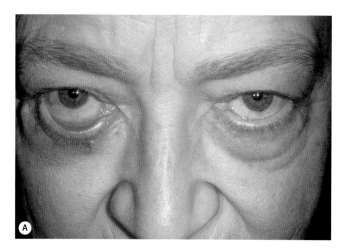

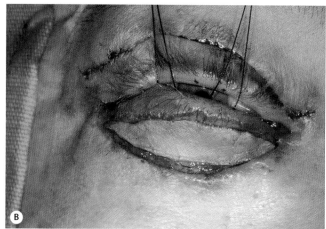

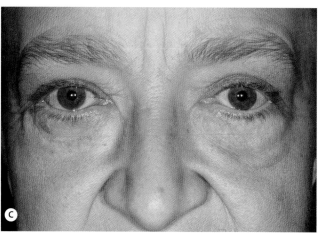

Figure 7-8 Eyelid retraction and ectropion after blepharoplasty. (**A**) Ectropion and retraction after blepharoplasty caused by excessive skin and muscle resection and lower eyelid laxity (the chin-down position of this photo does exaggerate the actual amount of eyelid retraction). (**B**) Corrected with full-thickness skin graft from upper eyelid and lower eyelid tightening. (**C**) Postoperative result.

Box 7-11

Management of Lower Eyelid Retraction after Blepharoplasty

Massage vertically, for as long as 6 months

Lateral tarsal strip

• With lysis of lateral part of lower eyelid retractors

Lateral tarsal strip and posterior lamellar spacer

• With excision of lower eyelid retractors
• Posterior lamellar spacer
  • Hard palate
  • Enduragen™ (porcine collagen sheet, http://www.porexsurgical.com)
  • Alloderm™ (human acellular dermis matrix, http://www.lifecell.com)

Add subperiosteal midface lift to above

Full-thickness skin graft as last choice

---

procedures that you can offer to restore the vision to your patient. You are already familiar with the benefits of forehead lifts in improving forehead furrows, glabellar folds, and medial eyelid fullness. If your patient is interested in "looking better" more than "seeing better,"

you will want to offer one of the forehead lifts we will be discussing. This is a good time to refer back to Box 6-2 and Figure 6-15 comparing the types of eyebrow procedures (Figure 7-9).

I will reinforce what I wrote earlier to get you ready for these procedures. You should get experience on the simpler functional browplasty operations before you move to these procedures. In some ways, they are not more difficult, but the anatomy may be less familiar and your patients may be more demanding. The "endoscopic" forehead technique that I use most often uses the same initial approach as the trans-blepharoplasty browplasty. The traditional "endoscopic" brow release is easily done through the eyelid incision. The pretrichial lift is not difficult as you get more experience with larger flaps and has the big advantage of lowering the hairline, which is a real bonus for many women. For both coronal and pretrichial forehead lifts, numbness of the forehead and crown of the head is pronounced, so make sure that your patient is ready for that. The traditional coronal flap is a powerful procedure and not much more difficult than the pretrichial lift but, for most patients with a normal hairline wanting an aesthetic lift, I prefer the endoscopic lift. The endoscopic lift is not easy but, like all procedures, as your skill level and experience increase, you will get good results and your operating time will reduce to a reasonable time. You are probably using the endoscope for some of

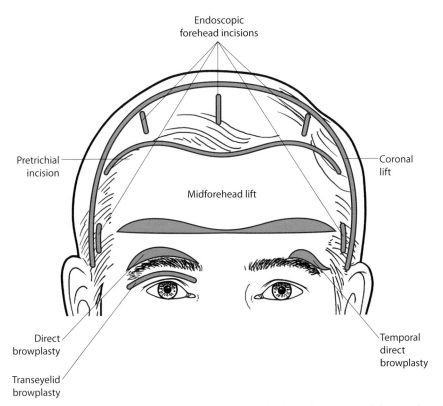

Endoscopic
forehead incisions

Pretrichial
incision

Coronal
lift

Midforehead lift

Direct
browplasty

Temporal
direct
browplasty

Transeyelid
browplasty

Figure 7-9 Browplasty operations: coronal, endoscopic, midforehead, direct, temporal direct, and transblepharoplasty.

your lacrimal procedures so you can get experience with the equipment and the technique that way. As you move toward aesthetic procedures of the face, you will combine the pretrichial, the coronal, and the endoscopic lifts with midface and lower facelifts.

The coronal forehead lift

The coronal forehead lift has been considered the gold standard of brow lifts for many years. The entire forehead is lifted through an "ear to ear" incision hidden in the hair anterior to the coronal suture. Despite the good results with coronal forehead lifts, patients complain of the long incision, which may create a "false part" in the hair when wet or blown in the wind. It takes some time for most patients to get used to the *numbness* above the incision extending to the crown of the head. Today, most patients seeking a cosmetic lift of the forehead and brow prefer the endoscopic lift. I rarely used a coronal forehead lift.

Pretrichial forehead lift

Any incision hidden in the hair used to raise the forehead will raise the hairline. A lift using an incision just anterior to, or within, the hairline will not raise the hairline. This pretrichial forehead lift is useful for your patients who have a "high forehead" as the operation *raises the eyebrow and lowers the hairline*. Essentially the same procedure performed just posterior to the hairline is known as a "trichophytic" forehead lift.

So how do you choose which forehead lift procedure to recommend? I use one of two forehead lift procedures, most commonly the endoscopic brow lift. For patients who are concerned about raising the hairline and don't mind the idea of scalp numbness, I recommend the pretrichial lift. After you get used to the size of the flap, you will find the operation relatively easy and fast. The key is to make an irregular incision at or just into the hairs and use meticulous layer closure to minimize the scar.

The procedure is an outpatient one and can be done under MAC or general anesthesia. It can be done alone, but usually it is done with a blepharoplasty or other facial procedure. *Use a fine marker to mark an irregular incision line at the hairline.* Some of the incision can include a few hairs. Extend the incision into the temporal hairline for about 4 cm with a taper. Each zig and zag is 2–3 mm. Then mark a matching "opposite" incision 1–1.5 cm anterior to the initial incision. Mark a blepharoplasty incision, if needed. *Mark the supraorbital notch and the temporal lines.* Use local injections with epinephrine superior to the hairline incision, across the eyebrows, and under the eyelid skin. Prep and drape as usual.

The steps are:

- Mark the hairline and blepharoplasty incisions
- Mark the supraorbital notch and temporal line
- Skin incision
- Develop forehead flap

The *skin incision* is made with a no. 15 blade making sharp cuts perpendicular to the skin starting at the hairline. Don't cauterize unless the bleeding does not stop with pressure. I excise the extra forehead strip next to make sure the wound is cut in an exact manner. You can excise this strip *after* you elevate the forehead, which gives you a chance to better estimate the amount of skin to excise, but it is difficult to match the "zigzags" on both sides of the wound. The cut goes through the skin fat and galea. You will elevate in the loose areolar tissue between the galea and periosteum (remember the layers of the "SCALP"—*s*kin, sub*c*utaneous fat, *a*poneurosis, *l*oose areolar tissue, *p*eriosteum). You will be raising the layers equivalent to the SMAS in the face—the *frontalis muscle* and *galea* in the forehead and the *temporoparietal fascia* in the temple.

The *forehead plane of dissection* is easy to work in. Use a Joseph skin hook in your nondominant hand to lift the flap. Use either a Freer elevator or Metzenbaum scissors to bluntly develop the plane inferiorly to about 1.5 cm above the rim. Go back to the wound lateral to the temporal line (over the temporalis muscle) and, using an Adson forceps and the same scissors, spread the temporoparietal fascia open to see the white shiny fibers of the deep layer of the temporalis fascia. Remember, if you are not certain that you are deep enough, you incise the deep layer and the muscle will be immediately visible. You should be certain that you are in the correct plane. If you are too superficial, you will damage the frontal branch of the facial nerve. As you elevate the flap, you will feel the resistance of the conjoined tendon at the temporal line.

The next steps are:

- Cut the conjoined tendon
- Expose the supraorbital nerves and vessels
- Release the corrugators
- Close the wound

Using your scissors, you can free the conjoined tendon inferiorly to the tail of the eyebrow. Remember the conjoined tendon is the fusion of the periosteum, the deep temporal fascia, and the temporoparetial fascia. You won't release the lateral canthal periosteum as you do in an endoscopic forehead lift (subperiosteal). This plane is preperiosteal.

At the lateral end of the superior orbital rim, the brow will lift freely. Elevate the forehead tissues as you move medially until you see the supraorbital vessels and nerves. Medial to the notches, lift the glabella off the bridge of the nose. The view of the corrugators is not easy, but you will be able to tear them with an elevator or using the microdissector needle.

Closure is in layers with the galeal bites holding the wound together. Use a 3-0 PDS suture (Ethicon Z398H FS-2 reverse cutting, violet suture). Next use interrupted 4-0 PDS sutures (Ethicon Z494G P-3 needle, clear suture) in the subcutaneous layer in four or five places. Finally, place a few interrupted 5-0 Prolene sutures to line up the wound. Follow with a running 5-0 Prolene closure. The dressing, wound care, and follow-up are the same as for the endoscopic forehead lift described in the next section. The "down time" for the pretrichial lift is less. Numbness persists for at least 6 months. The feeling probably never returns to normal, but does not bother most patients in the long run (see Figure 7-10).

Endoscopic brow lift

In the endoscopic brow lift operation, the brow and forehead are lifted through 2–3 cm vertical incisions in the hair. Instruments are introduced through the scalp incisions to elevate the periosteum off the frontal bone. The corrugator and procerus muscles are visualized with the endoscope and weakened to eliminate glabellar wrinkles. Fibrous attachments of the brow to the temporal and superior orbital rim are released and the forehead is lifted. Alternatively, the periosteal attachments at the brow can be released through a blepharoplasty incision (using the same approach as transblepharoplasty browplasty). The released and elevated forehead is then secured to the skull using a variety of techniques. The scalp and periosteum scar to the frontal bone in an elevated position.

The endoscopic brow lift is an attractive alternative to the coronal lift because it causes *minimal hypesthesia and the scarring is minimal*. It *lifts the entire brow and reduces forehead and glabellar wrinkles*. The long-term effectiveness of this procedure is not totally established, but surgeons, as a whole, feel that the results are long-lasting. As you might expect, new skills and instrumentation are required for this procedure. Care must be taken to avoid injury to the frontal and supraorbital nerves. The endoscopic brow lift is used as a cosmetic procedure only (Figure 7-11).

The endoscopic lift is probably the most difficult browplasty procedure to learn. Like any procedure, think about the basics before you get absorbed in the details of the procedure. In its simplest form, you are going to use a small incision in the hair to release the forehead and scalp from the attachments to the skull. You will then pull the scalp up and anchor it back to the skull in a more superior position—all this to lift the eyebrows. From the eyebrows to the top of the head, the surgical plane you will work in is the subperiosteal plane, lifting the tissues off the frontal bone. Laterally, you won't be lifting in the subperiosteal plane because the temporalis muscle is strongly attached to the periosteum. To release the scalp in this area, you will have to work in the plane anterior to the muscle. An important step, and a slightly more difficult step, is connecting the deeper plane over the forehead to the more superficial plane laterally over the temporalis muscle. To do this, you open both planes separately, creating two "pockets," and then join the two "pockets" (planes) by cutting the *conjoined tendon* at the *temporal line* to create one larger pocket. After releasing a few more attachments to the skull, the anterior scalp will be easy to lift. Let's review the anatomy of the temporal scalp.

You will remember that the anterior attachment of the temporalis muscle is the *temporal line*. You can feel this on your own skull. It is the bony ridge that separates your "temple" from your "forehead." If you are trying to learn this, I expect you are palpating your own forehead now. As you clench your teeth together, you will feel the temporalis muscle contract posterior to the temporal line. Likely, you can palpate your own temporal line as well. If you look at a human skull, you can always see this line. Remember, anterior to the temporal line, the plane of dissection is subperiosteal. If you were to stay in the subperiosteal plane as you dissect laterally beyond the temporal line, you would have to elevate the temporalis muscle off the skull. As this strong

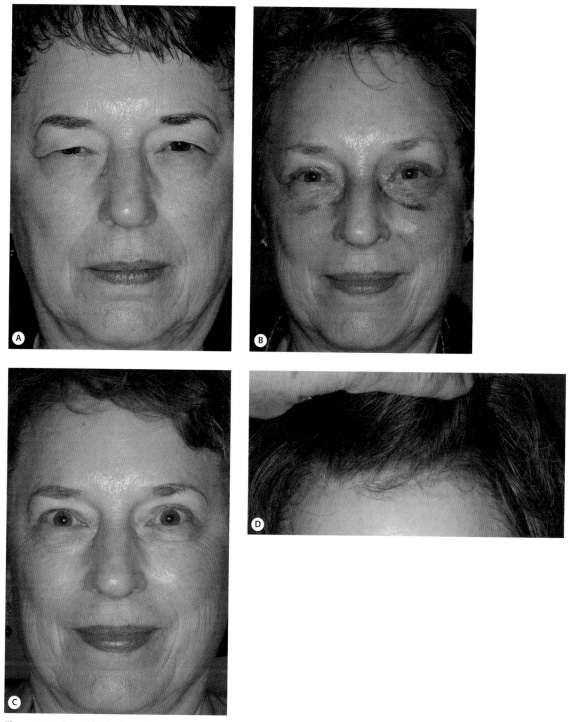

Figure 7-10 Pretrichial forehead lift. (**A**) Brow ptosis, dermatochalasis, high forehead. (**B**) Pretrichial browplasty and upper blepharoplasty (1 week). Note pretrichial incision and still moderately high forehead after 15 mm scalp excision. (**C**) and (**D**) 6 months postoperatively. Hairline incision with minimal scarring and hypesthesia after 6 months.

muscle is firmly inserted into the mandible below, elevating the muscle is not going to do anything for you in terms of releasing the scalp to allow a vertical lift. You must release the muscle from the scalp by dissecting anterior to the muscle and its fascial layer.

The periosteum of the forehead fuses with fascia overlying the temporalis muscle at the temporal line. This line of fusion, known as the *conjoined tendon*, separates the two tissue planes that you will be working in. To move from the subperiosteal plane to the plane anterior to the temporalis muscle, you will need to cut or tear the conjoined tendon. When you have done this, you have connected the "central pocket" of the forehead with the "lateral pocket" of the temple. By connecting these two pockets, you have released the forehead and scalp from the skull from ear to ear and from the top of the head down toward the eyebrows.

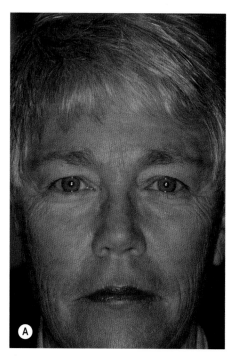
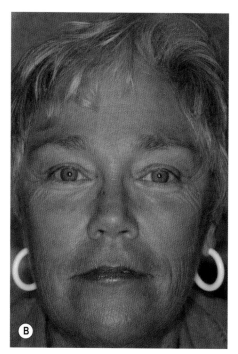

Figure 7-11 Endoscopic brow lift and upper lid blepharoplasty. (**A**) Preoperative brow ptosis and dermatochalasis. (**B**) Postoperative improvement. Lifting the eyebrows improves the cosmetic result of an upper lid blepharoplasty in most patients.

The remaining attachment of the forehead to the skull is the periosteum along the supraorbital ridges and along the lateral orbital rim. Using the traditional endoscopic brow-plasty, these attachments are released through incisions in the scalp when viewed from above with the endoscope. For the surgeon who starts his career from the "eye outward," these attachments are much easier to see directly through blepharoplasty incisions than from above using the endo-scope. For me, this modification (explained to me several years ago by one of my former fellows, Gene Howard) greatly simplified the soft tissue release portion of the operation. *A complete release of the soft tissue is the key to a successful endo-scopic forehead lift.* Remember, as in any "flap" repair, it is the release of the soft tissues, not how hard you pull them, that makes the procedure work. You may find it interesting that some surgeons do not feel that any forehead fixation is nec-essary after adequate forehead release.

Now that you have the idea of releasing the scalp and forehead from the skull, keep in mind that the frontal nerve travels in the loose connective tissue that overlies the temporalis muscle. This nerve can be easily injured and, on some occasions, will not recover leaving the patient with an eyebrow and forehead that do not move. *The key to avoiding damage to the frontal nerve is to keep your flap dissection deep in the temporal pocket, against the deep temporalis fascia.* The frontal nerve will be superficial in the scalp flap (within the temporoparietal fascia). Marking the path of the nerve on the patient ahead of time will remind you to be careful.

The remaining portion of the operation is anchoring the forehead back to the skull in a more superior position. We will talk briefly about a few of the options for incisions and anchoring later.

As always, try to get the "big picture" before focusing on the details. Keep that in mind when you read the next steps and use the hierarchal outline to "learn in layers," one easy layer at a time. The steps of the endoscopic browplasty are:

- Preoperative considerations
- Mark the incisions
- Anesthesia
- Make brow incisions
- Perform the upper blepharoplasty
- Release the forehead and scalp
    - At the rim
    - Over the forehead
    - To the crown
    - Over the lateral orbital rim
    - Over the temporalis muscle
    - Connect the pockets—cut the conjoined tendon
- Anchor the forehead flap
- Close the wounds

1. Preoperative considerations
    A. 1 day preoperatively.
        (1) Wash the hair with shampoo the night before.
        (2) Oral prednisone 60 mg 1 day preoperatively.
    B. In the operating room.
        (1) Mark the *upper blepharoplasty* (see blepharoplasty section below) *and the peak of the brow* (usually at the lateral one third of the brow).
            a) Mark before the patient goes to sleep; you will be able to watch how the eyelids move and the skin fold forms.

b) Look at the patient in the sitting position to see that the mark conforms to the natural contour of the superior rim and brow.

c) Take care to leave 10–15 mm of skin between the upper incision line and brow hairs. Be conservative with skin removal when lifting the brow.

(2) *Position the patient* on the operating table with the head slightly off the top end of the table, neck slightly extended.

a) *General anesthesia* is best for the first several cases.

b) With more experience and speed, you can do this under local anesthesia with sedation.

C. Mark, anesthetize, and prep the patient (Figure 7-12, A).

(1) When the patient is asleep, finish marking

a) The *supraorbital notches and nerves.*

b) A *horizontal line across the forehead*—2 cm above rims.

c) The *temporal line.*

d) The path of the *frontal nerve.*

e) Five *scalp incisions.*

   i) Three vertical incisions behind hairline.

      (a) At midline: 1.5–2 cm behind hairline, 2–3 cm long.

      (b) At peak of brows: 1.5–2 cm behind hairline, 2–3 cm long radically oriented.

      (c) Behind temporal hairline bilaterally.

   ii) Use a ruler to mark a line from the lateral ala to the lateral canthus to the hairline. Use this line to center the temporal marks.

      (a) 2 cm behind hairline, mark a 2–3 cm line parallel to the hairline.

(2) Inject local with epinephrine for hemostasis.

a) 2% lidocaine (Xylocaine) with 1:100,000 epinephrine in combination with 0.5% bupivicaine (Marcaine).

b) Inject about 1 cc at all incision lines.

c) Infiltrate in a "tourniquet" from lateral canthus, across brows, across scalp from ear to ear—about 20 cc.

d) An option for hemostasis and anesthesia is the injection of Klein solution diffusely throughout the flap ("tumescent anesthesia"—more on this technique later).

(3) Prep and drape the patient.

a) Wash the hair with prep solution.

   i) "Twist" the hair away from incisions and secure with small rubber bands. The easiest way is to put the band over hemostat blades and use the hemostat to twist the hair and then slip the band over the tuft of hair.

b) Prep the entire face.

c) Drape using a head drape with a plastic "pocket" to catch any drainage of blood or irrigation during the operation.

2. Incisions

A. Make the central scalp incisions.

(1) Using a no. 15 blade, open the central skin incision to the periosteum.

(2) Make a small drill hole at the superior end of the central wounds. This will be used to help estimate the lift at the conclusion of the operation.

(3) Elevate the periosteum with a Freer elevator.

(4) Elevate the periorbita laterally to the adjacent incisions at the eyebrow peaks.

   (a) Again using a no. 15 blade, open the temporal brow incisions.

(5) Cut or spread until you find the deep temporalis fascia.

   (a) You will see a white layer with crossing fibers.

   (b) If you are uncertain whether you are at the correct layer, knick it with the blade and you will see the underlying temporalis muscle.

   (c) You can start to spread in the plane anterior to the deep temporal fascia ("opening the temporal pocket"), but I usually save this until later.

   (d) Don't bother to coagulate these scalp wounds at this point. Most of the bleeding will stop on its own and you won't risk damaging hair follicles.

B. Perform an upper blepharoplasty.

(1) Use the standard skin muscle excision.

(2) Leave the septum closed and dissect to the superior rim.

(3) If you think fat removal is necessary, go back at the end and do a more conservative fat excision than you would do if you were doing a blepharoplasty alone.

3. Release the forehead and scalp (Figure 7-12, B)

A. At the rim. Cut the periosteum at the rim using a Freer elevator.

(1) Have your assistant elevate the eyelid skin and brow with a Desmarres retractor so you can see.

(2) Use the Frazier suction in your nondominant hand to help with visualization of the periosteum.

(3) Incise the periosteum just superior to the rim and elevate the periosteum off the frontal bone.

(4) Be aware of where the supraorbital neurovascular bundle is (you marked it preoperatively). Do not cut the bundle, but carefully elevate the periosteum around it.

(5) Extend the dissection superiorly onto the forehead for 2 cm (you marked this horizontal line preoperatively).

B. Over the forehead. Now move back to the central incisions. Lift the central incision and enter the subperiosteal space with the malleable elevators (Daniel endoforehead elevators, http://www.snowdenpencer.com).

(1) Elevate the forehead flap inferiorly to the horizontal line you have drawn.

(2) Elevate the forehead laterally to the temporal line (you are now completing the "central pocket").

   a) You may want to use the other central incisions to help with this.

(3) Pass the elevator through the central incision to elevate the glabella over the nasal bridge.

(4) In a few minutes, you will connect the central pocket with the "temporal pocket" by cutting the "conjoined tendon."

C. To the crown.

(1) Using the same incisions, elevate the scalp to the crown of the head.

(2) This will allow the entire scalp to lift superiorly when you elevate the brow.

D. Over the lateral orbital rim.

(1) Go back to the eyelid incision and extend the periosteal incision at the superior rim along the lateral orbital rim. You will need to wear a headlight for the rest of this flap elevation (if you are not already wearing one).

(2) Gradually elevate the periosteum laterally off the rim to the lateral canthal tendon. You will see later that this tissue can be tough to elevate. The area is part of the suspensory system of the SMAS known as the *orbital retaining ligament*.

   (a) Start to dissect more deeply. You are looking for the fascia that overlies the temporalis muscle (remember this is the deep temporalis fascia).

   (b) When you find this fascia (white vertical bands), start to elevate superiorly and laterally over the temporalis muscle (you are creating the "temporal pocket").

   (c) Be careful how far inferiorly you extend this dissection. The inferior extent of this elevation is the *sentinel vein* that you may see in the fat overlying the fascia at this level. You are very close to the frontal branch of the facial nerve, so you should stop.

E. Over the temporalis muscle.

(1) Go back to the temporal incisions and use an elevator to lift the scalp off the temporalis.

   (a) Posteriorly to the ear.

   (b) Inferiorly to the lateral incision.

(2) Medially to the temporal line.

F. Connect the pockets—cut the conjoined tendon.

(1) Now you will connect the temporal pocket with the central pocket by cutting the conjoined tendon.

   (a) The easiest way to do this is with Metzenbaum scissors put into the temporal pocket through the lateral canthus where you have just dissected.

(2) Remember that, in the traditional endoscopic brow operation, the "pockets" were dissected using the endoscope from above.

G. Release the forehead around the nerves (Figure 7-12, C)

(1) This is the only portion of the procedure that I do using the scope. From the central forehead incision, pass the endoscope into the central pocket and visualize the nerves as they exit the bone.

(2) Carefully elevate the periosteum off the notch or a foramen if it exists.

   (a) If you are having trouble locating the nerves, pass a 20-gauge needle through the forehead into the pocket adjacent to the nerve and visualize the needle point with the scope. You can also palpate the notch.

(3) If you want to avulse the corrugators, you can do so at this point with endoscopic forceps visualizing from above with the scope. You can also do this through the blepharoplasty incision with some practice. Be conservative as this can leave depressions and allow the heads of the brows to separate a bit. A better description than avulsing the corrugator might be to "tear them up." Sometimes a nerve hook is helpful to separate the muscle from the nerve.

H. Anchor the scalp (Figure 7-12, D).

(1) There are several ways to anchor the central scalp to the skull in the new higher position (Figure 7-12, E).

   (a) Endotine forehead fixation devices. I think these proprietary "carpet tacks" are the easiest of the techniques. Using the drill mark in the skull you made at the beginning of the operation, drill the fixation hole for placement of the Endotine in the two temporal "peak" incisions. Snap the Endotine into position in the bone. Use a Joseph skin hook to pull the scalp superiorly and then push the scalp onto the hook. Place the other Endotine and check for height and symmetry. You are aiming for a 1.5–2 cm lift of the scalp wounds in most cases. The eyebrows should be superior to the rim at this point.

   (b) Bone tunnels. This technique uses drill holes you make in the outer table of the frontal bone to anchor the scalp directly to the skull with sutures. This is slightly more involved than the Endotine technique, but is less expensive as there is no expense for the fixation devices.

   (c) Bone screws. 14 mm long and 1.5 mm in diameter. This is the technique originally described to anchor the scalp. The pilot drill holes are redrilled to accommodate a 1.5 by 14 mm screw. The screw is screwed into position such that the head of the screw will protrude from the scalp when the wounds are closed. The scalp is elevated and staples are placed posterior to the screw giving a lift roughly the length of the incision. This is a good technique, but it requires that the screws be removed in 1 week. In the meantime, the screws protrude from the scalp. There can be some hair loss around the screw.

(2) Elevate the temple by excising a 1–1.5 cm ellipse of scalp from the posterior edge of the wound.

You will anchor and elevate the temple by sewing the subcutaneous layer to the temporalis fascia. I use 3-0 PDS (Ethicon Z398H FS-2 needle) suture passes to anchor the anterior edge of the scalp wound to the temporalis fascia at the posterior edge of the wound.

4. Close the wounds
   A. Close the blepharoplasty incisions with 5-0 fast absorbing gut or 6-0 nylon. Remember to be conservative with any fat excision.
   B. Use staples to close the scalp wounds (35 N or W). I do not use drains, but some surgeons do. Generally this makes the procedure an overnight stay.

5. Postoperative care
   A. Wash the hair, dry with a towel. Dress the wounds with antibiotic ointment, Kling wrap, and Elastoplast bandage.
   B. Give an intravenous dose of 6–10 mg of dexamethasone (Decadron) in the operating room. Give oral prednisone 60 mg per day for 5 postoperative days. Give an oral antibiotic of your choice for 7 days. For pain and anxiety, give Celebrex, alprazolam (Xanax). If pain is not relieved, you can give a narcotic.

Postoperatively, your patient will be uncomfortable with a headache and tightness of the scalp. Give the same advice and instructions as you would for a blepharoplasty: "Discomfort, swelling, and blurry vision are expected. Severe pain, eyes swelling closed, or no vision are not normal, so call us if you have these problems." Ask your patient to keep the Kling on for 24–48 hours (often it will fall off sooner). I see these patients 1 week postoperatively, but you might want to see your more demanding patients in 24–48 hours.

Some comments with regard to dissection technique and fixation. I like the transblepharoplasty approach. It simplifies the forehead and conjoined tendon release, but does require a blepharoplasty incision. You can try the entire release with the endoscope at some point and decide for yourself.

If you like a "traditional" endoscopic approach, an alternative set of forehead incisions that you might prefer are vertical incisions just medial to the temporal lines (3 cm) and a *horizontal* incision (4 cm) placed centrally 1–2 cm behind the hairline. The longer horizontal incision still avoids cutting the supraorbital nerves and allows good mobility of the endoscope, so that you do not need to put the scope into any of the other openings. I recently learned this technique from my colleague, Jeff Carithers, and am using it for our more recent cases. It also makes sense to have your assistant hold the endoscope so you can use a bimanual scalp elevation technique, one hand with the elevator and the other palpating the skin over the elevator. A good assistant should "swivel" the endoscope to visualize your elevator, without advancing the scope into the wound. The bimanual endoscope technique is used in skull base endoscopic procedures and frees a hand to palpate the elevators through the scalp. Your movements will be much more coordinated. With the central horizontal incision technique, you do not need to move the scope out to the lateral scalp incisions. These incisions permit your elevator to enter the central pocket, the temporal pocket, and to cut the conjoined tendon. There are no scalp incisions over the temporalis muscle. Fixation at the temporal incisions gives a great vertical lift and helps to avoid spreading the heads of the eyebrows apart—something that can occur with aggressive corrugator excision and a temporal pull.

Another interesting variation combines the best of both the pretrichial lift (no raised hairline) and the endoscopic technique. In this variation, the central horizontal incision between the supraorbital nerves is made 5–10 mm behind the hairline—a "trichophytic" incision. The incision is made with a long bevelled incision about 5 mm long, cutting the hair shafts, but preserving the follicles. The forehead lift is performed through this central incision and the lateral incisions as described above. The forehead central lift is created by excising an appropriate amount of forehead inferior to the central incision. This scalp incision is cut with an opposite bevel of the adjacent wound. The hair follicles grow through this flap and the scar is well hidden. The hairline is not raised centrally. Standard fixation is done laterally. There is minimal numbness of the scalp. As you can imagine, there are many variations that make sense and will work for your patient. It is best to use one technique first, get a general familiarity with it, and modify it to what works effectively and efficiently for you.

As we discussed above, there are many fixation techniques. The original technique used a mini screw protruding through the temporal wounds. This technique is a good starting place, as you already have drills and plating systems available. It is awkward for the patient to have hardware sticking out that requires removal in the clinic. The Endotine forehead system (Coapt, http://www.coaptsystems.com) allows you to bury the fixation device. This technique is simple, effective, and has replaced the screw technique. The cost of the device has to be passed on to your patient making your operation either more expensive or less profitable. The bone tunnel jig invented by Jonathan Sykes (Medtronics/Xomed Brow Lift Bone Bridge SSK #37-47100 and #37-47105, http://www.xomcat.com) is clever, inexpensive, and works well. It allows suture fixation of the forehead to the bone. It pays for itself quickly, and you can vary the tunnel position and number to provide a multivector pull depending on how you want to contour the brow.

Checkpoint

- Do you remember the types of browplasty we discussed in the last chapter (direct, direct temporal, midforehead and transblepharoplasty)?
- What is the main advantage of a pretrichial or trichophytic brow lift over an endoscopic forehead lift? What are the disadvantages?
- Review in your mind:
  — Layers of the soft tissue over the frontal bone (SCALP)
  — Layers of the scalp over the temple
  — What layers fuse at the conjoined tendon?
- What are the SMAS equivalent layers:
  — Over the temple
  — Across the skull
  — In the neck

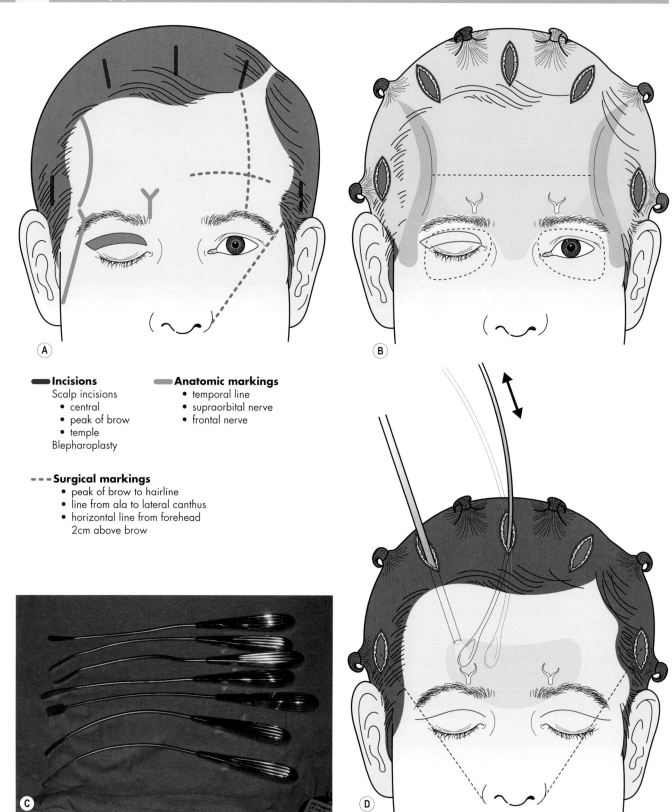

Incisions
Scalp incisions
 • central
 • peak of brow
 • temple
Blepharoplasty

Anatomic markings
 • temporal line
 • supraorbital nerve
 • frontal nerve

Surgical markings
 • peak of brow to hairline
 • line from ala to lateral canthus
 • horizontal line from forehead 2cm above brow

Figure 7-12 (**A**) Endoscopic browplasty landmarks. (**B**) Areas of forehead and superior orbital rim release: Yellow area is a subperiosteal release of the rim and conjoined tendon through the eyelid incision. Blue area superior to the dotted line is a non-endoscopic subperiosteal dissection though the scalp wounds above. Blue area inferior to dotted line is an endoscopic release of the rim, nerves and glabella. Green area is an endoscopic dissection deep to the superficial temporal parietal fascia, superficial to the deep temporalis fascia. Note that areas of dissection overlap one another. (**C**) Endoscopic forehead elevators. (**D**) Endoscopic release of supraorbital nerves. (**E**) Endoscopic view of supraorbital nerve branches. (**F**) Brow fixation. a) Endotine brow fixation devices in place with scalp elevated. Scalp closure with staples. b) Original "mini screw" fixation—prior to stapling scalp in position on left side and after scalp stapling on right side. Blepharoplasty wounds are closed with running suture. (**G**) Endotine device—described as a "carpet tack" to hold scalp in position. (**H**) Brow lift bone bridge tunnel fixation (current favorite technique). a) Bone tunnels drill through outer table of skull with suture in tunnel. b) Bone tunnel "jig" used to drill skull.

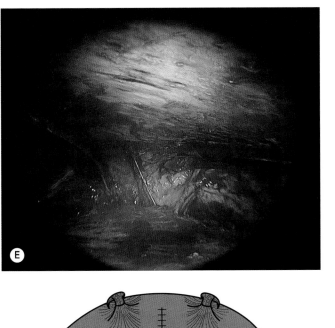

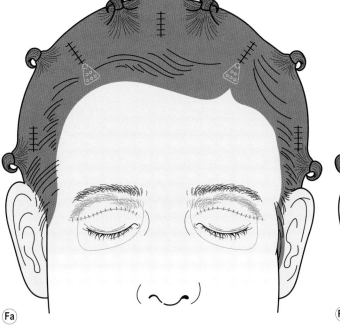

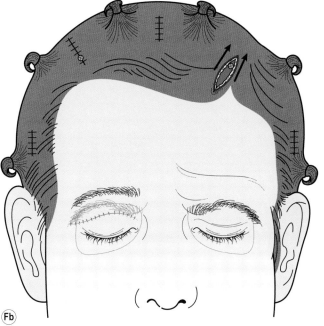

Figure 7-12 Continued.

Facelift operations

Introduction

Facelift technique is a huge topic—way too big for us to cover with detail—so my goal is to leave you with some principles that will give you an overview and provide a basis for more detailed study. Let's review what we have discussed so far. We suggested an approach to facial rejuvenation using the "descent and deflation" approach to evaluation and treatment. Treatment is directed at the patient's complaint— "wrinkles" or "sags and bags." Wrinkles occur due to the loss

of tissue plumpness resulting from age and the sun-related damage to collagen, elastin, and the ground substance. Wrinkles are improved with Botox, fillers, resurfacing, and peels. Meanwhile, as part of the same processes, the facial tissues become lax and develop the characteristic "sags and bags" that we have been discussing (see Box 7-12). Sags and bags are improved with face "lifting" operations. Many of your patients will want help with both "wrinkles" and "sags and bags."

Years ago, face lifting procedures were limited to celebrity figures who had "skin tightening only" operations. The results were faces that were pulled tightly, resulting in a

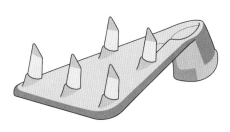

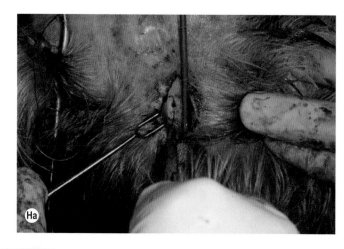

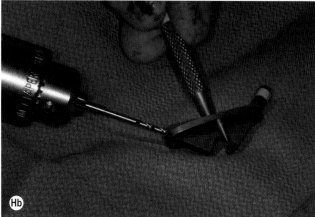

Figure 7-12 Continued.

Box 7-12

"Sags and Bags" of Facial Aging

Upper face
- Forehead furrows
- Brow ptosis
- Upper eyelid dermatochalasis

Midface
- Lower eyelid and cheek double convexity
  - Cheek descent
  - Tear trough formation (nasojugal fold deepening)
  - Lower eyelid fat prolapse
- Malar mound formation
- Deepening of the melolabial fold
- Lower face
- Jowling
- Marionette lines
- Prejowl sulcus

Neck
- Loss of cervicomental angle
- Platysmal bands

"windswept" appearance. A subcutaneous dissection plane was created and the skin was pulled tight, with a predominantly posterior, not vertical, pull. Excess skin was excised and the wounds were closed with the tension on the skin closure. With all the lift due to tightening, the skin results

were temporary, scarring was poor, and second operations were common.

We have already seen the "face lifting" procedures for the upper face—the forehead lift, various browplasties, and the upper blepharoplasty. We have stressed the anatomic extension and equivalence of the temporoparietal fascia (TPF), the frontalis and galea, the SMAS, and the platysma. And we have just seen how the forehead procedures tighten or lift the TPF and galeal layers. Contemporary face lifting procedures of the midface, lower face, and neck involve tightening the SMAS and platysma. Facelift operations are divided into:

- Upper facelift—elevation of frontalis, galea, and TPF
  — Lifts eyebrow
  — Improves forehead and glabellar lines
- Midface lift—vertical elevation of SOOF portion of SMAS
  — Raises cheek
  — Improves melolabial fold
- Lower face lift—superior (and lateral) elevation of SMAS
  — Improves melolabial fold
  — Improves jowls
- Neck lift
  — Includes superior and lateral lift of platysma
- Neck liposuction and/or fat excision
- Platysmal plication
  — Improves mandibular line (jowling), sharpens cervicomental angle, removes platysmal bands, and improves "turkey gobble"

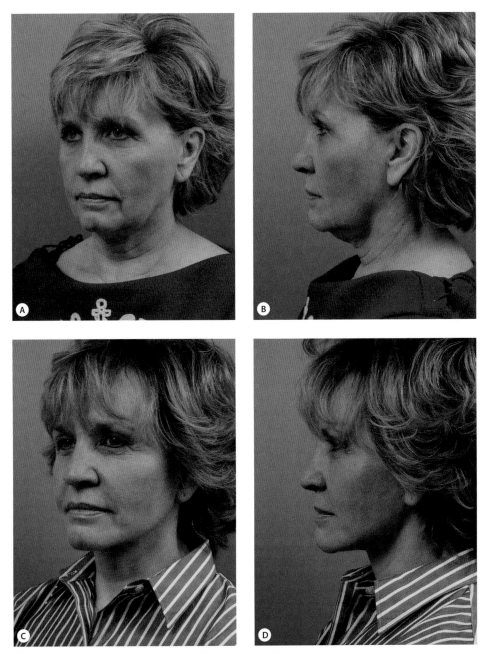

Figure 7-13 Pre- and postoperative face, midface, and neck lift. Preoperative oblique and lateral views—note deep melolabial fold, jowling, marionette lines, and loss of cervicomental angle. Postoperative oblique and lateral views—melolabial fold, jowling, and marionette lines are reduced. Malar fat pad is elevated. Cervicomental angle is sharpened (courtesy of Jeffrey Carithers, MD).

The improvement that follows a lower face and neck lift is the result of a predominantly superior (and somewhat lateral) elevation of the strong SMAS layer and platysma. These layers are anchored to periosteum over the mastoid bone and the parotid fascia and perichondrium anterior to the ear. The excess skin is draped over the incision line, excised, and closed with little tension. The result is more natural, longer lasting lift.*

The standard "facelift" gives its main improvement at the mandibular border (jowling) and neck. Although the exact

manner in which the SMAS is tightened varies with the technique, all improve jowling and marionette lines. Further improvement in the neck comes from a combination of liposuction and platysmal plication (repair of the any central dehiscence between the heads of the platysma). The result is a smooth mandibular line and a sharp cervicomental angle (see Figure 7-13). The melolabial fold is lessened with this lift but can be helped more with a midface lift. The midface lift gives a more vertical elevation of the SMAS and the associated fat pads (malar fat pad and suborbicularis oculi fat) restoring fullness to the cheek over the zygoma, at the same time lessening the fold.

One last point—these procedures "reupholster the old furniture." If the "frame" is good, the "new fabric" will look great. Defects in the underlying facial skeleton will not be

*Some of the "mini" facelifts today still use this skin tightening technique. These procedures can be used on younger patients with or without surgery on the neck. Lesser effectiveness and longevity is the trade-off for somewhat less "down time."

helped by rhytidectomy procedures. A low hyoid bone will never give a sharp cervicomental angle. A retruded chin or shallow cheekbones may require implants to repair the frame in order to make your upholstery job the masterpiece you and your patient are expecting. We will save these topics for your more advanced study.

In the next two sections, we will cover the basic concepts of the lower face and neck lift procedure and the midface lift. You will be ready for some more in-depth reading, cadaver dissection, and mentoring with a colleague so that you can do these procedures on your patients.

Lower face and neck lift

Modern facelift techniques vary in terms of which layer is tightened and how the tightening is accomplished. Most experienced facelift surgeons use SMAS tightening procedures. The common variations of SMAS tightening techniques are:

- SMAS plication
- SMAS imbrication ("SMAS" ectomy)
- Deep plane SMAS lift

Imagine an analogy with eyelid ptosis correction, the levator aponeurosis advancement operation. In this procedure, which you will learn about in the next chapter, you will tighten, or shorten, the levator muscle in much the same way as you tighten the SMAS. The eyelid ptosis correction starts with an inconspicuously placed incision (in the skin crease). Next you will dissect down to the levator and shorten it to raise the eyelid. Before you close (or more likely earlier in the case), you will remove extra skin (blepharoplasty). So your ptosis surgery is very similar in concept to a facelifting procedure. The levator muscle complex can be compared to the fibromuscular SMAS—each is shortened to lift the tissue.

Let's go back to the exposed levator aponeurosis. To shorten the aponeurosis, one option might be to place a suture in the aponeurosis some number of millimeters superiorly, shortening the aponeurosis by pulling it down and suturing it to the tarsus (no dissection required, just folding or "plication" of the aponeurosis on itself). A second option would be to excise a strip of aponeurosis and suture the cut edge down to the tarsus (excision of a piece of aponeurosis, but no dissection to mobilize it, "imbrication"). The third option, advancement, is what is most commonly done. The aponeurosis is detached from the tarsus and a plane of dissection is performed posterior to the aponeurosis freeing the aponeurosis from the underlying tissue. The aponeurosis is then sewn back to the tarsus and excess tissue is excised. This is the same concept as the deep plane facelift.

Plication and imbrication techniques may be well suited for a particular patient of yours. These are less invasive and lower risk than the deep plane technique. As versions of the deep plane facelift are generally considered the most effective, natural, and long-lasting facelift, I have chosen to discuss this technique. To do so, we will have to consider the neck as well because the face and neck are usually done together in patients undergoing deep plane facelifting. These are considered advanced techniques.

The lower facelift steps are often performed at the same time as a forehead lift, upper and lower blepharoplasty, and

midface lift. We will discuss the principles of midface lifting in the last section.

The facelift procedure can be done under general anesthesia or with deep sedation (or a combination). Surgeon's preferences for the choice of local anesthetic agent vary widely. Often a combination of a short- and long-acting local anesthetic with dilute epinephrine (1 : 200,000 or less) is used. In 1987, Jeffrey Klein described a technique known as tumescent anesthesia. This technique is widely used to facilitate body liposuction procedures and is used by some surgeons for facial surgery as well. Preoperatively, a solution containing dilute lidocaine and epinephrine (Klein's solution) is injected into the subcutaneous fat in quantities large enough to swell the tissue (tumescent means swollen and firm). The infiltration minimizes bleeding and bruising, facilitates subcutaneous dissection, and eliminates the need for general anesthesia. You might try this for your forehead lift procedures and any lower face procedures. Injection of local with epinephrine and tumescent anesthesia are both well-accepted techniques. At the other end of the spectrum, some facial surgeons prefer that any local anesthetic contain no epinephrine at all. They would argue that they want to see any bleeding at the time of surgery and control it in the operating room. One complication of facelift surgery that you will want to avoid is postoperative hemorrhage or hematoma formation under the facial flap. My preference is for a combination of short- and long-acting agents with dilute epinephrine added.

The steps of the deep plane facelift include:

- Skin making
- Pre- and retroauricular skin incisions
- Subcutaneous skin flap elevation of the face and neck
- Liposuction of the neck
- Platysmaplasty
- Superior and lateral suspension of the platysma muscle
- Dissection posterior to the SMAS (deep plane)
- Superior suspension of platysma and SMAS
- Redraping, trimming, and closing the skin
- Skin marking and incisions

Prior to the operation, markings are made to remind us of important landmarks (Figure 7-14):

- The mandibular line and angle
- The zygomatic arch
- The path of the frontal branch of the facial nerve (from the tragus to a point 1 cm lateral to the brow)
- A line drawn from the angle of the mandible to the malar eminence denotes the limit of the subcutaneous dissection and the start of the deep dissection of the SMAS
- Erb's point, 6.5 cm inferior to the auditory canal, is marked denoting the approximate location of the greater auricular nerve
- A transverse submental incision is marked
- The facial incisions are marked anterior to the ear extending superiorly to the temporal hairline. The incision is extended inferiorly and around the ear in a position just anterior to the ear crease so that, when the ear relaxes, the incision falls in the crease. About two thirds of the way up the ear (at the ear canal), the incision is extended posteriorly into the hairline at a slight inferior angle (Figure 7-14)

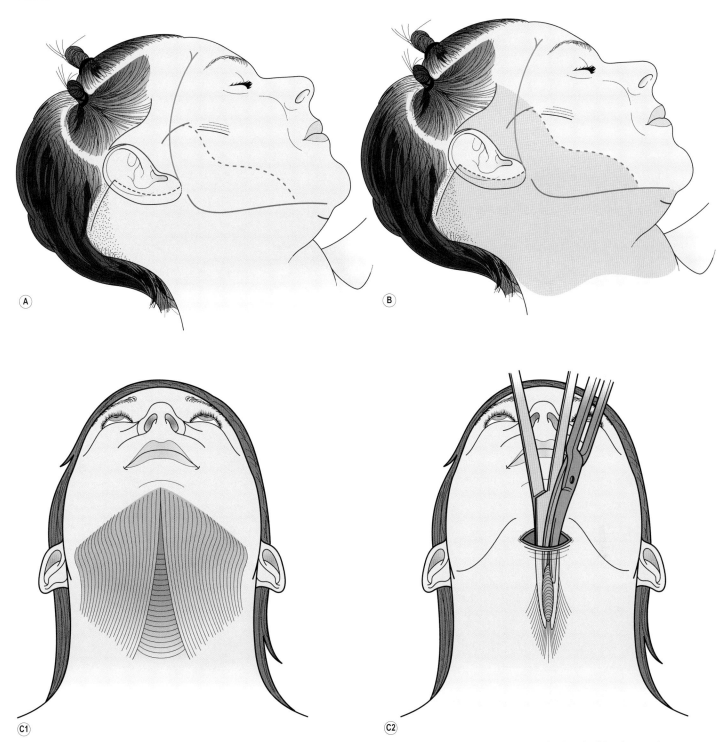

Figure 7-14 Modified deep plane face lift operation. (**A**) (i) Anatomic landmarks. 1) zygomatic arch. 2) zygomaticus major muscle. 3) path of facial nerve. 4) angle of mandible. (ii) Incisions. 1) anterior hairline alternative incision of Brennan. 2) preauricular incision onto tragus. 3) retroauricular incision onto bowl. 4) posterior hairline incision. 5) submental incision. (iii) Skin flap elevation extending to 3 points. a) to McGregor's patch. b) one third distance from tragus to melolabial fold. c) mandibular retaining ligaments, dotted line showing extent of facial subcutaneous dissection. (**B**) Subcutaneous dissection area. (**C**) 1) Platysmal banding due to central dehiscence of the muscle heads. 2) Clamping and cutting of platysmal heads following subcutaneous fat excision through a submental incision. 3) Vertical suturing of platysmal heads. (**D**) Skin flap reflected. SMAS incision marked. (**E**) SMAS incision beginning over parotid and extending toward melolabial fold. (**F**) Suspension and suturing of SMAS in primarily a vertical direction. (**G**) Excision of excess skin. Take care to excise only half of the redundant tissue at the ear lobule to avoid a "pixie ear". (**H**) Interrupted and running sutures with no tension on wound. Often a drain is placed.

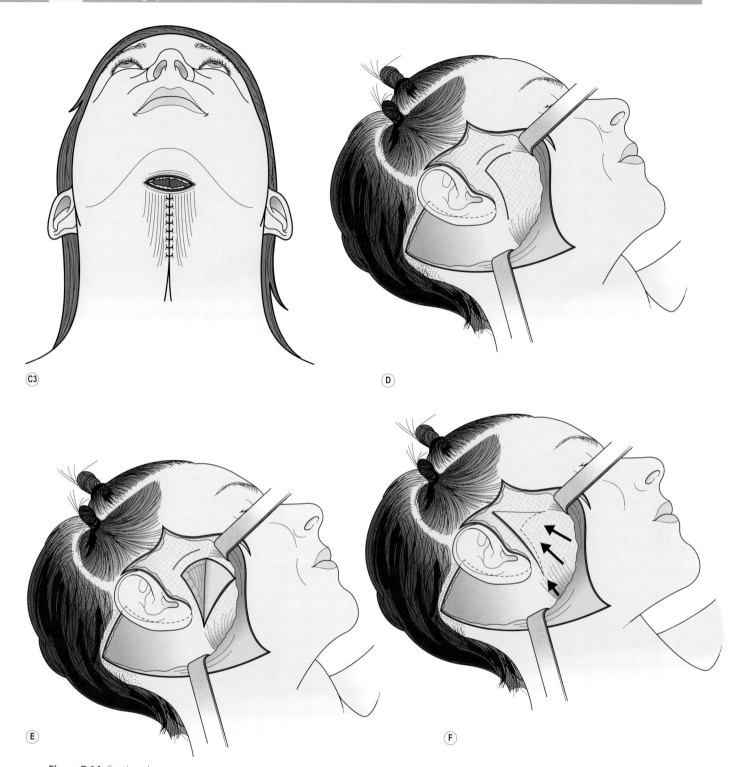

Figure 7-14 Continued.

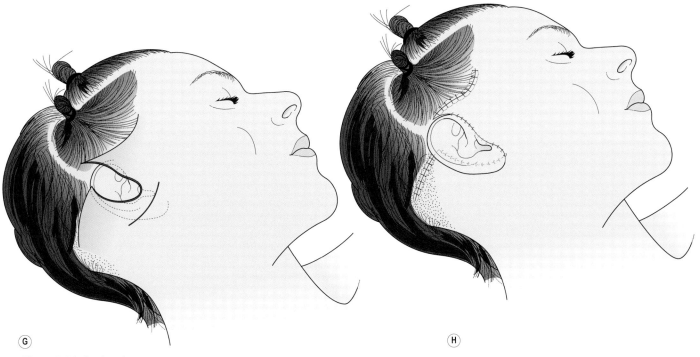

G   H

Figure 7-14 Continued.

Subcutaneous skin flap elevation of the face to the mandible (Figure 7-14, B)

From the preauricular incision, a subcutaneous dissection plane is developed extending beyond the anterior edge of the parotid gland (about 4.5 cm) and to the superior border of the zygomatic arch. Remember to be superficial over the arch as the frontal branch is most superficial at this point. A safe dissection is facilitated by stretching the skin tightly with aid of a multivectorial pull with the help of your assistant. Watch the outline of the tips of your curved facelift scissors moving under the flap. You will extend the flap toward the melolabial fold until the cheek frees up.

From the posterior incision, you will complete the subcutaneous dissection into the hairline posteriorly and inferiorly down to the angle of the mandible. As the postauricular flap develops inferiorly over the sternocleidomastoid muscle, be careful not to injure the posterior auricular nerve. This nerve is most commonly seen where the sternocleidomastoid and platysmus muscles cross (the *Erb's point* we just marked), but can be injured anywhere along its course to the ear lobe. You will recall that this nerve provides sensory innervation to the ear. You will eventually continue the subcutaneous plane of dissection over the platysma medially into the neck but, before loosening up the neck tissue, will do liposuction and any necessary platysmal plication in the neck.

Liposuction of the neck

Liposuction is performed along the mandibular border to reduce the jowl fat and anteriorly in the neck to reduce the "gobble" of preplatysmal subcutaneous fat. Using a standard microcannula (3 or 4 mm), passes are made in crossing directions to remove the subcutaneous fat. As you move over

the mandible with the liposuction cannula, you will have to stay superficial to avoid damage to the *ramus mandibularis* (causing lip depressor paralysis). Pinching the skin between your fingers helps to stay superficial and is a good way to judge the amount of fat present.

Platysmaplasty

If platysmal banding is present you will open the transverse submental incision next and dissect through the fat to find the medial edges of the platysma. Any midline fat anterior to the platysma can be excised directly with scissors at this point (some prefer using a cannula, but the scissors leave a bit more fat, which is not a bad thing in many patients with thin skin in this area). The central dehiscence between the two platysma bellies responsible for the banding is identified. Fat posterior to the platysma can be excised, but only with extreme care as you will be close to the jugular vein. Any redundancy in the muscle bellies can be clamped and excised, which will help to sharpen the neck. Notched incisions of the platysma at the cervicomental angle will sharpen the neck, but are usually not necessary. You will repair the platysmal dehiscence with six or eight passes of 3-0 PDS suture starting at the hyoid bone and extending to the mandible (Figure 7-14, C).

As you get more experience, you may want extra platysmal tightening at the angle using opposing interlocking crossed 2-0 Prolene sutures (going from the left medial platysmal edge to the right mastoid fascia, and opposite for the other side).

With the fat removed from the neck and the platysmal dehiscence repaired, you are ready to free up the remaining layers that will be lifted. First, you will free the platysma from the lateral side and then go back to the face for the sub-SMAS dissection. After you develop the deep plane dissection under the SMAS, you will come back to secure the platysma superiorly and laterally.

Dissection posterior to the SMAS (deep plane)

The SMAS is tightly adherent to the underlying parotid fascia. Anterior to the parotid gland, you will incise the SMAS and begin a careful sub-SMAS dissection (Figure 7-14, D). This is about at the point of our diagonal line drawn at the beginning of the case. If you were doing an SMAS excision procedure, you stop here, excise a strip of SMAS, and sew the edges together for the lift.

The deep plane dissection extends anteriorly in the sub-SMAS plane toward the melolabial fold. This is a dangerous zone as the facial nerve branches are no longer protected by the parotid tissue and have emerged from the anterior edge of the gland. Your sharp dissection plane will be deep to the SMAS, but superficial to the zygomaticus major muscle. You can feel the origin of this muscle under the body of the zygoma, especially if you pull the corner of the lip down. This is close to the superior limit of the sub-SMAS dissection— 1 cm inferior to the arch. You will want to curve the SMAS incision slightly anteriorly to make sure that you avoid the frontal branch of the facial nerve. At this point, you will be releasing the *zygomatic* and some of the *orbitomalar retaining ligaments*. This release will free up the SMAS (Figure 7-14, E).

As you continue your sub-SMAS dissection toward the melolabial fold, the facial nerve branches are deep to you in the parotidomasseteric fascia bound down to the masseter muscle. With vertical spreading of the scissor blades, you will be able to release the thin *buccal retaining ligaments* (that extend from the masseter to the melolabial fold), further releasing the SMAS (see Figure 7-14, E). At the inferior aspect of the deep plane, you will see the platysmal fibers superficial to your dissection continuous with the SMAS flap. Now go back to the posterior subcutaneous dissection plane and find the lateral edge of the platysma inferior to the mandible and free up a few millimeters deep to the platysma.

Suspension of platysma and SMAS

The final steps are to anchor the lateral platysmal flap and the SMAS flap laterally and superiorly. As much vertical elevation as possible is desirable, as opposed to a more lateral pull, which gives an "operated on" look. Use 2-0 PDS sutures to anchor the SMAS and platysma flap at key points from the periosteum over the mastoid to the parotid fascia and the temporalis fascia anterior to the ear. You can place some additional 3-0 PDS sutures anchoring the platysma to the sternocleidomastoid muscle fascia (Figure 7-14, F). Before anchoring the skin flap, place a Jackson Pratt (JP) or similar drain in the neck extending from the cervicomental angle to retroauricular incision out a stab wound.

Redraping, trimming, and closing the skin

The last steps are to anchor, trim, and close the skin flap. A good anchor is at the junction of the vertical and horizontal retroauricular incisions using a skin staple. Place deep strong anchoring sutures at the temporal hairline, the ear lobule, and periosteum behind the ear to give a superior vector to pull the skin flap (Figure 7-14, G). There should not be excessive tension on the skin. Remember the SMAS is supporting the tension. Excise excess skin at the ear and trim the "dog-ears" that you form at the hairline and behind the ear. Use staples to close the skin at the temporal hairline. Use a 5-0 fast absorbing running gut suture behind the ear. Lastly, trim the preauricular skin. Leave plenty of skin inferior to the lobule in order to avoid the pulled "pixie ear" deformity. In fact, you may want to push the lobule up a bit with extra skin. This wound will always retract. A pixie ear is difficult to fix. Run the preauricular skin with a 5-0 fast absorbing gut suture (Figure 7-14, H).

Apply antibiotic ointment on the wounds and a pressure dressing around the head and neck. It is reasonable to use steroids and oral antibiotics for the first 5–7 days postoperatively for most patients.

There are many variations of the technique depending on the surgeon's preference and the patient's needs. The principles are the same, however. You can see that this is an involved operation. You will need to start with more basic techniques. Some suggestions are presented in Box 7-13. There are many good texts available (some listed in the Suggested Readings). Courses are helpful. There is no substitute for cadaver dissections and mentoring with an experienced colleague.

Midface lift procedures

Introduction

The midface lift procedure raises the position and increases the projection of the cheek using a strong vertical pull that is not obtained with the standard lower facelift. Both the melolabial fold and the tear trough are lessened. With more pull, you can create a slight elevation of the corner of the mouth. A number of techniques have been described. It's best to consider the lifts in terms of *minimal, moderate,* and *maximal lift*. These descriptions fit the surgical approach used as well: the *preperiosteal, subperiosteal,* and *endoscopic* approaches (see Box 7-14).

Preperiosteal approach

You will use this approach at the time of a lower blepharoplasty to prevent lower eyelid retraction. The improvement

---

Box 7-13

Steps to Learning Deep Plane Facelift

- Full-thickness preauricular skin graft harvest
  - Preauricular incision, +/− post-tragal incision
  - Undermining in subcutaneous plane
  - Layered closure
- Retroauricular skin graft harvest
  - Incision placement
  - Undermining and closure
- Mustarde cheek flap
  - Developing a large subcutaneous plane
- Intumescent technique
  - Large reconstructive facial flaps
  - Forehead lifts
- Subcutaneous flap dissection and SMAS plication
- Subcutaneous flap dissection and SMAS imbrication
- Neck liposuction

in cheek projection is minimal, but the vertical height of the lower eyelid is shortened. You will raise a myocutaneous flap to the inferior rim. The flap can be either myocutaneous or transconjunctival. At the rim, use a Freer elevator to tease open the fat posterior to the orbicularis (the SOOF) off the bone. Elevate in this *"preperiosteal plane"* inferior and lateral to the orbital rim for 2–3 cm (you are deep to the orbicularis, so this is not really the subcutaneous plane). Once the cheek (which includes the malar fat, the orbicularis, and SOOF) is released, make a small flap of orbicularis and subcutaneous (malar) fat hinged inferiorly. Pass a 4-0 Vicryl or PDS suture though this flap and suture it to the fascia at the lateral orbital rim. One or two sutures will suffice. The lift gives mild cheek elevation.

You will find this type of "mini midface" lift is useful when you do a lower transcutaneous blepharoplasty with skin removal. Adding a lateral tarsal strip canthoplasty to correct lower eyelid laxity is a good way to prevent lower eyelid retraction or abnormal contouring ("round eye"). You can cause some temporary numbness in the distribution of the zygomatic temporal nerve. There is not much improvement medially in the tear trough with this technique. This is a relatively easy technique. You should learn to do this if you will be performing lower eyelid cosmetic blepharoplasties. The cheek lift procedures that we will describe below are advanced topics. At this point, get the big picture. We won't go into detail.

Subperiosteal midface—eyelid approach

Using the same blepharoplasty approach, you can get a greater and a more medial lift by elevating the cheek medial and lateral to the infraorbital nerve in the *subperiosteal* plane (Figure 7-15, A). As you enter the subperiosteal plane 2–3 mm inferior to the rim, try to leave some periosteum intact. Elevate inferiorly. You will be on the surface of the maxilla deep to the facial muscles (Figures 7-15, B and C).

Try not to stretch or injure the nerve, as many patients will have some temporary numbness of the face. As you approach the gingival sulcus, you will need to stretch or tear the periosteum to get a release of the cheek (you can feel the most inferior dissection limit by putting your index finger in the mouth). Now anchor the free superior edge of the periosteum to the tuft of remaining periosteum along the rim with four or five 4-0 Vicryl or PDS sutures (Figure 7-15, D).

Coapt makes a midface suspension device, the Endotine Midface B, that makes suspension easy. These procedures provide a moderate lift of the cheek and reduction of the melolabial fold. They are very good techniques to recruit excess skin into the eyelid as required in repairing lower eyelid retraction after blepharoplasty, often combined with hard palate or other posterior lamellar spacer grafts (Figure 7-16).

Subperiosteal midface lift with forehead lift

A stronger lift can be achieved by anchoring the released midface up to the temporalis fascia. You can easily connect the temporal pocket of your forehead lift to the subperiosteal space of the cheek. The deep temporal fascia is accessed using endoscopic or open forehead lifting procedures. You can do an open subperiosteal cheek release from above, as described, or from below through the gingival sulcus. Another alternative, but technically demanding, is an endoscopic release of the cheek, starting from the deep temporal fascia in the brow and dissecting inferiorly to the lateral canthus. The path from the temporal pocket to the cheek is anterior and deep to the frontal branch of the facial nerve. Further subperiosteal dissection will get you into the subperiosteal plane of the cheek.

Fixation sutures, usually 2-0 PDS, can be passed transcutaneously or transgingivally through the cheek tissue at the melolabial fold at about the level of the ala. Alternatively, but more challenging, you can pass a suture through the cheek tissue endoscopically. The suture is then passed back through the previous tunnel and secured to the temporalis fascia or to tunnels made in the skull near the temporal line. Similar fixation can be obtained with the Coapt Endotine Midface ST device. These procedures improve the position and prominence of the cheek (Figure 7-16, F). You will see considerable improvement in the melolabial fold, the tear trough, and the corner of the mouth not easily appreciated with less powerful midface lifts.

Aside from access to the temporal pocket, lifting the forehead at the same time allows the redundant cheek tissue that forms at the lateral canthus to redistribute itself superiorly. These midface lifts are a nice complement to other facial rejuvenating procedures, as we'll see below.

Midface lift with deep plane facelift

With experience, you will see that the procedures that you do on one part of the face have to "match," "blend in," or *harmonize* with the rest of the face to maintain a natural look. You can do an upper blepharoplasty alone and get a nice natural look but, as your facility with forehead lifting improves, you will start to see that many of your patients would look "better"—more natural—if you also lifted the forehead. Soon, your lower blepharoplasty procedures look better if you lift the cheek some. Similarly, if you do a lower

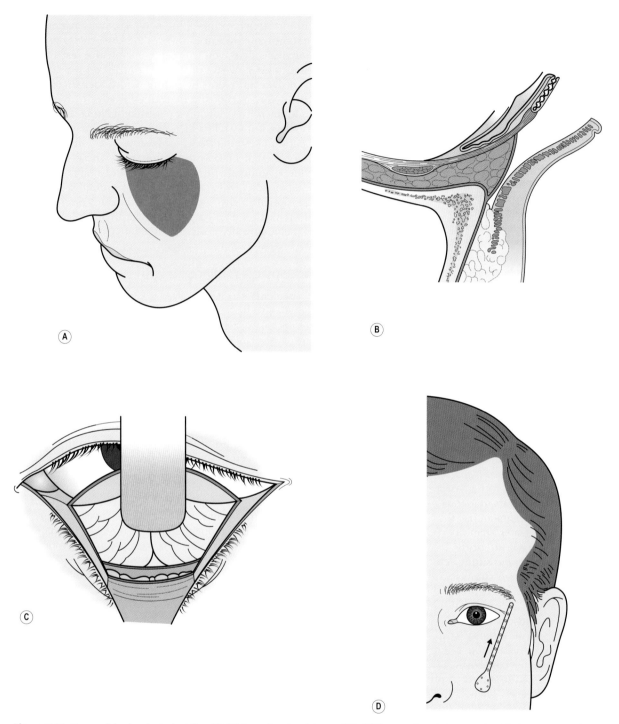

Figure 7-15 Transeyelid subperiosteal midface lift. (**A**) Area of undermining and lift. (**B**) Transconjunctival approach with dissection in subperiosteal plane over maxilla. (**C**) Transcutaneous or transconjunctival approach used to elevate periorbita at rim. Transoral route using a gingival buccal incision can also be used. (**D**) Elevation and fixation with sutures or Endotine "midface" device.

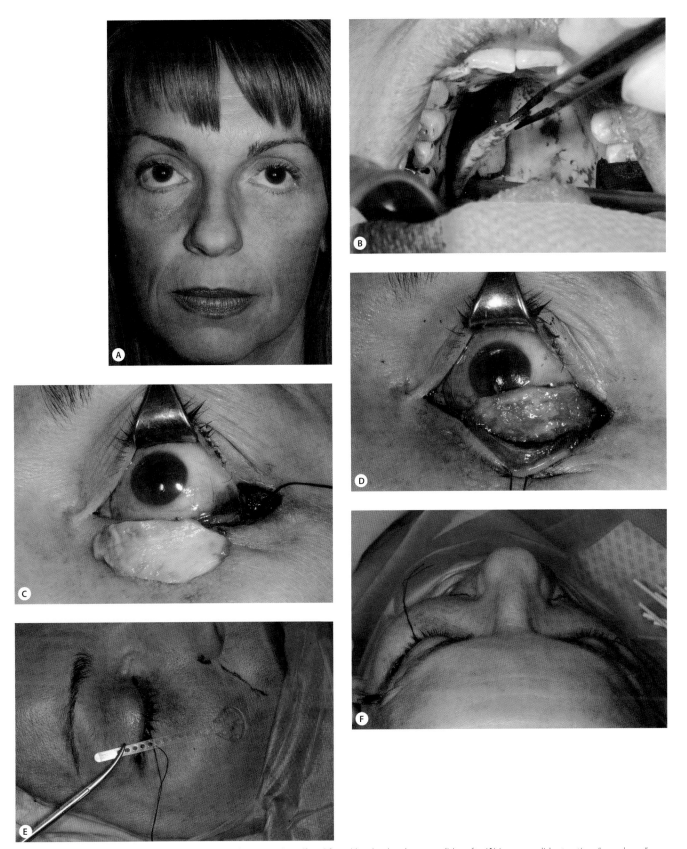

Figure 7-16 Lower eyelid retraction repaired with subperiosteal midface lift and hard palate lower eyelid grafts. (**A**) Lower eyelid retraction, "round eye," a complication of lower blepharoplasty. (**B**) Intraoperative view of hard palate harvest. (**C**) Hard palate—mucosal side shown. (**D**) Lower eyelid retractors disinserted and hard palate graft placed. No conjunctival covering is necessary. (**E**) Endotine midface device. (**F**) View from above showing prominence of left malar eminence after first side is elevated. (**G**) Postoperative appearance after 6 weeks. Slight swelling and asymmetry are still present. The lower eyelid position is improved. (**H**) Healing hard palate harvest sites.

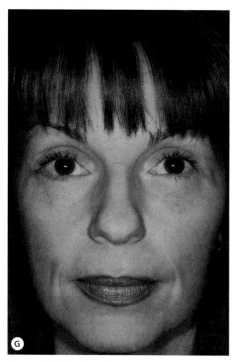

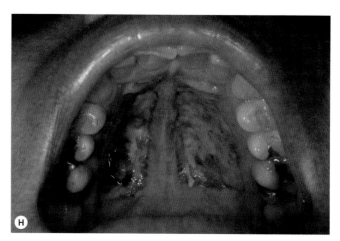

Figure 7-16 Continued.

facelift without giving enough cheek elevation, you may not get the natural look that you and your patient are looking for. For this reason, many surgeons routinely combine midface procedures with lower facelifts. In fact, the best result is often obtained when the patient has upper, mid, and lower face procedures at the same setting.

The standard order (with some individual surgeon and patient variation) is upper and lower blepharoplasty, forehead, lower face and neck, midface. You may be doing Botox and filler injections at the beginning of the case and finishing with some resurfacing or peeling. It makes for a long day in the operating room, but the result gives a nice balance to the "new" facial features. Experienced surgeons can spend 8 or more hours doing these cases, so choose combinations carefully until you can proceed safely and quickly.

This ends our primer of aesthetic surgery of the face. There is a lot to learn here. Remember to get the "big picture." The anatomy is complex and best learned by reviewing this material a few times, then going on to other texts (some in the Suggested Readings), then to the cadaver lab, and finally watching or assisting other colleagues. Aesthetic procedures are not the type of cases that are easy to "practice on" with your patients, so start with some of the simple, more functional procedures that we have discussed. Videos are great for getting familiar with more complex operations. But nothing is better than a good teacher with you in the operating room. Do your homework and prepare ahead so you don't waste any precious operating room experience (Box 7-13).

Checkpoint

- What are the temporoparietal fascia equivalent layers:
  — On the face
  — Across the skull
  — In the neck
- Three ways to tighten the SMAS are:
  — Plication
  — Imbrication—"SMAS" ectomy
  — Advancement—Deep plane SMAS lift
- Review the basic steps of the neck and facelift (not in detail)
  — Face—skin flap, neck liposuction, retroauricular and neck flap, platysmaplasty, SMAS dissection, SMAS and neck suspension, skin draping and excision, closure
- Neck, face, and forehead lifts can be combined for a "full facelift"
- Blepharoplasty, laser resurfacing, peeling, and Botox can be performed at the same time
- The midface lift elevates the cheek vertically, reducing the depth of the melolabial and nasojugal folds. The malar projection increases

Major points

- Lower eyelid blepharoplasty reduces lower eyelid fullness by removing mainly lower eyelid fat. Minimal skin and muscle are removed.
- Lower eyelid retraction is the most common complication after lower lid blepharoplasty. The position of the lower eyelid is influenced by:
  - Prominence of the inferior orbital rim relative to the eye
  - Tension of the lower eyelid
  - Length of the anterior and posterior lamellae
- Transconjunctival lower blepharoplasty is useful to remove fat while minimizing the risk of lower lid retraction.
- There are intrinsic and extrinsic causes of aging:
  - Intrinsic causes include genetics and disease
  - The two main extrinsic causes of aging are smoking and sun exposure
- It is useful to describe aging based on the concepts of "descent and deflation". This describes the typical stretching of tissues with loss of facial volume.
- It is useful to describe treatments based on the concepts of improving "sags, bags, and wrinkles".
  - Examples of sags and bags are temporal hooding of the upper eyelid, deepening of the melolabial fold, and jowling
  - Wrinkles result from loss of volume and skin elasticity
- Sags and bags are treated with "lifting procedures." Wrinkles are improved with Botox and fillers, resurfacing, and peels. There are overlapping areas of improvement with each type of treatment
- Wrinkles are described as:
  - Dynamic—occurring with underlying muscle action, treated with Botox
  - Adynamic—present at rest, treated with fillers
- The muscles of facial expression are innervated by the facial nerve, with almost all the muscles being innervated from under the surface.
- The facial muscles are interconnected by a fibrous layer known as the superficial musculoaponeurotic system (SMAS). Extensions of the SMAS include the:
  - Temporoparietal fascia (TPF) onto the temple:
  - Galea across the skull
  - Platysma in the neck
- The SMAS is supported by the osseo-cutaneous retaining ligaments. Tightening the SMAS is the basis of modern facelifting procedures.
- A layer of fat is found behind the orbicularis muscle:
  - The SOOF — suborbicularis oculi fat inferiorly
  - The ROOF — retroorbicularis oculi fat superiorly
- A fat pad overlies the orbicularis at the malar eminence known as the malar fat pad.
- The lower eyelid double convexity forms from:
  - An "eyelid convexity" as the orbital septum thins allowing orbital fat to prolapse forward
  - An "orbital rim hollow" as the cheek descends and the bony rim becomes visible (the tear trough)

- A "cheek convexity" as the melolabial fold forms
- The malar fat pad and cheek drop exposing the inferior orbital rim (tear trough)
- When performing periocular aesthetic or functional surgery, make sure that the goals are well established. Is the operation to "make you see better" or "make you look better".
- All patients who would like to minimize aging changes should wear a sunscreen an apply tretinoin crème (Retin-A).
- Botox is used to reduce dynamic wrinkles. Fillers are used to improve adynamic wrinkles. Botox should be used primarily in the upper face. Fillers should be used primarily in the lower face.
- The most commonly used fillers are hyaluronic acid based, which draw water into the tissue to rehydrate the skin ground substance. The effect lasts 6–12 months.
- Laser resurfacing and chemical peels improve:
  - Wrinkles
  - Dyschromias
  - Premalignant skin changes

Hyperpigmentation is the most common undesired effect. Avoid all sun exposure while the skin in pink in the healing phase. The safest patients to treat have light skin tones (Fitzpatrick skin types I–III).

- Understanding the patient's complaint and goal is critical for achieving success in aesthetic procedures.
- Set realistic expectations—"Under promise, over deliver".
- Upper eyelid blepharoplasty reduces the upper lid skin fold by removing mainly redundant skin and muscle. Lower eyelid blepharoplasty reduces lower eyelid fullness by removing mainly lower eyelid fat. Minimal skin and muscle are removed.
- Lower eyelid retraction is the most common complication after lower lid blepharoplasty.
- Transconjunctival lower blepharoplasty is useful to remove fat while minimizing the risk of lower lid retraction.
- The type of browplasty in your practice will depend largely on the patient's goals with regard to "reconstructive" or "cosmetic" results. Common types of browplasty in use in oculoplastic surgery include:
  - Direct or temporal direct browplasty
  - Midforehead lift
  - Endoscopic forehead lift
  - Pretrichial, trichophytic or coronal lift
- Full facelift includes brow, face, neck, and midface.
  - Brow—elevates brows, improves forehead and glabellar rhytids, and reduces upper eyelid hooding
  - Face—reduces jowling and melolabial fold
  - Neck—reduces jowling, sharpens cervicomental angle, eliminates "turkey gobble" and platysmal bands
  - Midface—reduces melolabial fold, raises height of malar eminence, and reduces nasojugal fold

Suggested reading

1. Aiache AE, Ramirez OH: The suborbicularis oculi fat pads: an anatomic and clinical study. *Plast Reconstr Surg* 95:37–42, 1995.

2. Albert DM, Lucarelli MJ: Aesthetic and functional surgery of the eyebrow and forehead ptosis. In *Clinical atlas of procedures in ophthalmic surgery*, pp. 263–283, Chicago: AMA Press, 2004.

3. American Academy of Ophthalmology: *Basic and clinical science course: orbit, eyelids and lacrimal system*, sect. 7, pp. 135–145, 228–248, San Francisco: The American Academy of Ophthalmology, 2006/2007.

4. Biesman BS: *Lasers in facial aesthetic and reconstructive surgery*. Baltimore: Williams & Wilkins, 1999.

5. Chen WPD, Khan JA, McCord CD, eds: *The color atlas of cosmetic oculofacial surgery*. Philadelphia: Butterworth and Heinemann, 2004.

6. Ellenbogen R: Transcoronal eyebrow lift with concomitant upper blepharoplasty. *Plast Reconstr Surg* 71(4):490–499, 1983.

7. Ellis E III, Zide MF: *Surgical approaches to the facial skeleton*, ch. 1–6, pp. 3–93, Philadelphia: Williams & Wilkins, 1995.

8. Fagien S, ed.: *Putterman's cosmetic oculoplastic surgery*, 4th edn. Philadelphia: Elsevier, 2008.

9. Foster JA, Huang W, Perry JD, Holck DL, Wulc AE: Cosmetic uses of Botulinum toxin. In Levine MR, ed., *Manual of oculoplastic surgery*, 3rd edn, pp. 93–97, Boston: Butterworth-Heinemann, 2003.

10. Goldberg RA et al: Surgery of the lower eyelid. In Wobig JL, Dailey RA, eds, *Oculofacial plastic surgery: face, lacrimal system, and orbit*, pp. 83–102, New York: Thieme, 2004.

11. Johnson CM Jr, Alsarraf R: *The aging face: a systematic approach*. Philadelphia: Saunders, 2002.

12. Knize DM, ed.: *The forehead and temporal fossa: anatomy and technique*. Philadelphia: Williams & Wilkins, 2001.

13. Lucarelli MJ., Khwarg SI, Lemke BN, Kozel JS, Dortzbach RK: The anatomy of midfacial ptosis. *Ophthal Plast Reconstr Surg* 16:7–22, 2000.

14. McCord CD, Nahai F, Codner MA, Nahai F, Hester TR: Use of porcine dermal matrix (Enduragen) grafts as an adjunct to reconstructive procedures in eyelids: a review of 69 patients, 129 eyelids. *Plast Reconstr Surg* 122:1206-1213, 2008.

15. Moses JL, Tanenbaum M: Blepharoplasty cosmetic and functional. In McCord CD, Tanenbaum M, Nunery WR, eds, *Oculoplastic surgery*, 3rd edn, ch. 11, pp. 285–317. New York: Raven Press, 1995.

16. Nerad J: The involutional periorbital changes: dermatochalasis and brow ptosis. In *The requisites—Oculoplastic surgery*, pp. 120–156. St Louis: Mosby, 2001.

17. Nerad JA, Carter KD, Alford MA: Lower eyelid involutional changes. In *Rapid diagnosis in ophthalmology—oculoplastic and reconstructive surgery*, pp. 76–79, Philadelphia: Mosby Elsevier, 2008.

18. Nerad JA, Carter KD, Alford MA: Brow ptosis. In *Rapid diagnosis in ophthalmology—oculoplastic and reconstructive surgery*, pp. 68–69, Philadelphia: Mosby Elsevier, 2008.

19. Pessa JE, Garza JR: The malar septum: the anatomic basis of malar mounds and malar edema. *Aesth Surg* 17:11, 1997.

20. Shorr N, Hoenig JA, Cook T: Brow lift. In Levine MR, ed., *Manual of oculoplastic surgery*, 3rd edn, pp. 61–75, Boston: Butterworth-Heinemann, 2003.

21. Rubin M: *Manual of chemical peels*. Philadelphia: JB Lippincott Co., 1995.

22. Wobig JL, Dailey RA: Surgery of the upper eyelid and brow. In Wobig, JL, Dailey RA, eds, *Oculofacial plastic surgery: face, lacrimal system, and orbit*, pp. 34–53, New York: Thieme, 2004.

23. Wobig JL, Dailey RA: Surgery of the midface, lower face and neck. In Wobig JL, Dailey RA, eds, *Oculofacial plastic surgery: face, lacrimal system, and orbit*, pp. 103–125, New York: Thieme, 2004.

CHAPTER 8

Evaluation and Treatment of the Patient with Ptosis

Chapter contents

Introduction

Ptosis is one of the most common oculoplastic problems that you will see in your office. The concepts are simple. The symptoms relate to loss of peripheral visual field and, in severe cases, a loss of central vision. In most patients, the levator muscle and aponeurosis are responsible for the ptosis. The majority of patients with ptosis have either *congenital ptosis* caused by a dystrophy of the levator muscle or *involutional ptosis* related to aging changes in the levator aponeurosis or muscle. You can assume that your patient with ptosis has one of these two types unless a finding in the history or physical examination points to an *unusual type of ptosis*. We will approach the chapter from that perspective.

The *severity* of the ptosis and the best *treatment* are easy to determine by measurement of the *eyelid vital signs*. The treatment is almost always surgical, and most patients appreciate the improvement in their vision. Complications of ptosis repair are rare. With experience, you will find that it becomes easy to get a "good" result in most patients, but you will continue to be challenged throughout your career to get a "perfect" result in all patients.

This chapter begins with a discussion of the *normal eyelid anatomy and function*. The two common forms of ptosis, *simple congenital ptosis* and *involutional ptosis*, are discussed next. You will learn the *importance of the levator function* in

recognizing the type of ptosis and choosing the appropriate treatment. In the sections on the *history and physical examination*, you will learn the findings that identify the type of ptosis, appropriate surgical treatment, and factors that lead you to alter your usual surgical plan. The details of the *levator aponeurosis advancement and frontalis sling operations* follow. Finally, you will be introduced to the numerous *unusual types of ptosis*.

As I have emphasized before, it is important to appreciate the "normal" before moving on to the "abnormal." Spend some extra time learning the concepts related to the two common types of ptosis. By doing so, you won't miss spotting the unusual type that you are much less likely to see.

Anatomy and function

Normal eyelid position

The upper lid rests at or just below the upper limbus. The lower lid normally sits at the lower limbus. The *palpebral aperture* is the distance between the upper lid margin and the lower lid margin. The normal measurement is approximately 9 mm. The position of the upper lid is best quantified as the *upper lid margin reflex distance* (MRD_1). This measurement extends from the central corneal light reflex to the upper lid margin and is normally *4–5 mm* (Figure 8-1).

The upper eyelid retractors

The retractors open the upper eyelid. The retractors are:

- The levator muscle
- Müller's muscle
- The frontalis muscle

Functional or anatomic abnormalities in the levator muscle complex are the cause of most ptosis.

The levator muscle

The *levator muscle* is the primary retractor of the upper eyelid. This skeletal muscle is responsible for voluntary elevation of the upper eyelid. Innervation to the levator muscle is via the superior division of the third cranial nerve (the oculomotor

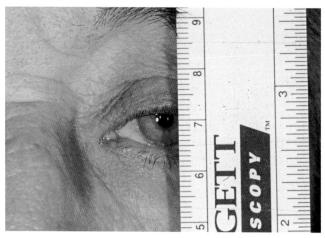

Figure 8-1 Measurement of the margin reflex distance (MRD) and the palpebral fissure. The MRD$_1$ is 1 mm. Often an estimate will suffice, 1–2 mm, in this case. The MRD$_2$ is 5 mm. The palpebral fissure is the sum of the MRD$_1$ and the MRD$_2$.

nerve). The levator muscle originates at the orbital apex and extends forward inferior to the bone of the orbital roof (Figure 8-2). At the orbital aperture, the levator is supported by *Whitnall's ligament* (see Figure 2-22). As the levator muscle travels anteriorly, it becomes a fibrous *aponeurosis* that extends inferiorly into the eyelid to insert on the anterior aspect of the tarsal plate. Fibrous extensions of the aponeurosis pass through the orbicularis muscle to create the *upper eyelid skin crease* (Figure 8-3).

Whitnall's ligament is an important anatomic landmark. The ligament extends from the fascia surrounding the lacrimal gland temporally to the trochlea medially. Whitnall's ligament is usually easy to see intraoperatively as a strong white band of fibrous tissue. Generally the tissue superior to the ligament is muscle and the tissue inferior to the ligament is aponeurosis, although variation exists among individuals. It has been suggested that Whitnall's ligament serves as a "pulley" for the levator muscle. Although the levator muscle complex does not slide through the ligament, the concept of the ligament allowing the muscle to change direction is a helpful one.

As the levator aponeurosis travels from Whitnall's ligament to the tarsus, it "fans" out to form the *horns of the levator aponeurosis*. The horns are the medial and lateral flared extensions of the aponeurosis inserting into the medial and lateral canthal regions. During operations on the levator, you will see that the lateral horn of the aponeurosis is much thicker and stronger than the medial horn. The lateral horn is cut, or released from the lateral orbital rim, to improve the typical temporal flare of Graves disease upper eyelid retraction.

Müller's muscle

Müller's muscle is responsible for the involuntary upper eyelid elevation seen in the sympathetically innervated "fight or

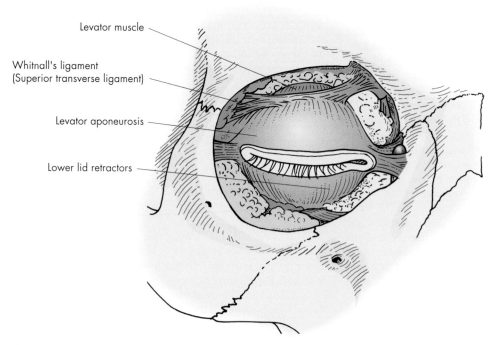

Figure 8-2 The levator complex: levator aponeurosis, Whitnall's ligament, and levator muscle.

Levator muscle

Whitnall's ligament
(Superior transverse ligament)

Levator aponeurosis

Lower lid retractors

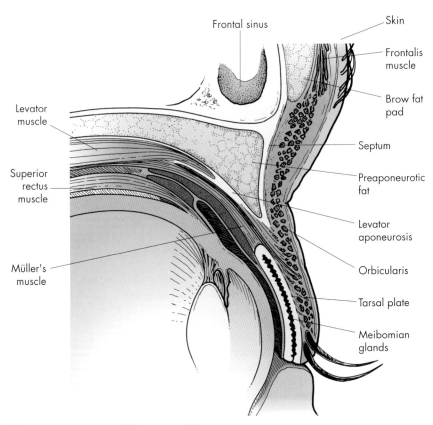

Figure 8-3 Cross-section of the upper eyelid.

Labels on figure:
- Frontal sinus
- Skin
- Frontalis muscle
- Brow fat pad
- Septum
- Preaponeurotic fat
- Levator aponeurosis
- Orbicularis
- Tarsal plate
- Meibomian glands
- Levator muscle
- Superior rectus muscle
- Müller's muscle

flight" phenomenon. Müller's muscle is "sandwiched" between the conjunctiva posteriorly and the levator aponeurosis anteriorly. Müller's muscle extends from the superior margin of the upper tarsal plate to the level of Whitnall's ligament (Figure 8-3). A prominent surgical landmark on the surface of Müller's muscle is the *peripheral arcade*, a vascular arcade extending across the muscle a few millimeters above the tarsal plate (Figure 8-4; see also Figure 2-23). You will recall that the loss of innervation to Müller's muscle results in the mild ptosis associated with *Horner's syndrome*.

The frontalis muscle

No doubt you have patients with drooping upper lids who lift their eyebrows to provide a tiny bit more upper eyelid elevation. The *frontalis muscle* lifts the brows and is a weak retractor of the upper eyelids (Figure 8-5). The frontalis muscle is part of the galea aponeurotica of the scalp. The fibrous aponeurosis extending from the occiput becomes the frontalis muscle inferior to the hairline. Like the other muscles of facial expression, the frontalis muscle is innervated by a branch of the facial nerve, *the frontal nerve* (see Figure 2-27). *Elevation of the eyebrows* and *prominent forehead furrows* seen in a patient with ptosis tell you that the drooping lids are interfering with the patient's vision. In some patients, a brow ache will occur with extended brow activity. The action of the frontalis muscle should be "blocked" with your thumb when making measurements of the eyelids.

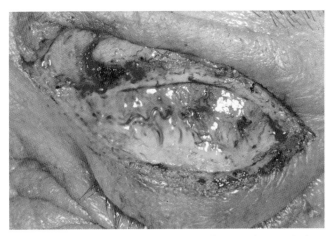

Figure 8-4 The peripheral vascular arcade in Müller's muscle. Note the line of the surgically disinserted levator aponeurosis.

The "eyelid vital signs"

The condition or "health" of the eyelid can be identified by measuring the *eyelid vital signs*:

- Margin reflex distance (MRD)
- Levator function
- Skin crease height and strength

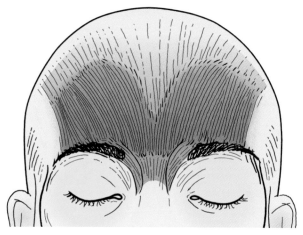

Figure 8-5 The frontalis muscle is a weak elevator of the eyelid.

We have already mentioned the MRD as a simple way to measure the height of the upper lid. The most practical measure of the strength of the levator muscle is the levator function. The *levator function* is defined as the excursion of the upper lid from extreme downgaze to extreme upgaze measured in millimeters. This movement is normally 15 mm. You will recall that the upper eyelid skin crease is created by the pull of the levator aponeurosis on the skin. The *skin crease height* is the distance from the lid margin to the crease. This height varies among individuals, but averages 6–8 mm for men and 8–10 mm for women at the highest point. The crease slopes both medially and laterally. A weak levator muscle creates less pull on the skin so the crease is less distinct or "weak." *Read this paragraph again.*

The vital signs will give you the information that you need to know to classify and treat ptosis. You will see the following concepts repeated several times in this chapter:

- Simple congenital ptosis is associated with decreased levator function
- Involutional ptosis is associated with normal levator function
- If levator function is normal, a shortening of the aponeurosis works well to lift the upper lid (a levator aponeurosis advancement operation)
- If the levator function is poor, the eyelid is surgically "connected" to the brow (a frontalis sling operation). The action of the frontalis muscle lifts the upper eyelid

Notice how important the levator function is. As you become experienced in taking care of patients with ptosis, you will see that asking "What is the levator function?" becomes the critical question (Box 8-1). We will discuss this further in the next section.

Checkpoint

- Name the retractors of the upper eyelid
- What are the "eyelid vital signs"? What are the normal measurements? Remember these findings indicate the "health" of the upper eyelid
- What are the two most common types of ptosis?
- Which of the vital signs determines the treatment of ptosis?

Box 8-1

The "Eyelid Vital Signs"

The status and health of the upper lid are measured by the "eyelid vital signs:"

- Margin reflex distance (MRD)
- Levator function
- Skin crease height and strength

The MRD describes the eyelid position:

- The MRD_1 measures the distance from the central light reflex to the upper lid margin
- The normal value is 4–5 mm

Levator function is an indicator of the strength of the levator muscle:

- The levator function is the amount of movement of the upper eyelid from downgaze to upgaze
- The normal value is 15 mm

The upper lid skin crease is formed by the pulling of the levator aponeurosis from beneath skin:

- The position and strength of the upper lid skin crease help in recognizing the amount of levator function present and the type of ptosis
- In involutional ptosis, the crease is high and pulls diffusely
- In simple congenital ptosis, the crease is not well defined and there is reduced pull
- Proper placement of the crease during surgery is important for symmetry and an optimal surgical result

---

Box 8-2

Types of Ptosis: A Simplified System

- Simple congenital ptosis
- Involutional ptosis
- "Unusual" ptosis

Classification of ptosis

A simplified system

There are many types of ptosis and many systems that classify the types (Box 8-2). From a practical point of view, most patients you will see have either *simple congenital ptosis* or *involutional ptosis*. Most of the children you will see have simple congenital ptosis. Most of the older adults you will see have an involutional ptosis. I group the other less common types into the category *unusual ptosis*. This is an oversimplification, but it works well.

The levator function: the relationship to classification

For this approach to work, you must learn the common types of ptosis well. Most of our medical training is spent learning the details of diseases that we will rarely see, an example being ptosis secondary to myasthenia gravis. For now, I will be emphasizing the two common types of ptosis. After you know all about these two types, you will be able to easily identify an unusual type of ptosis when you see something that doesn't fit with the two common types.

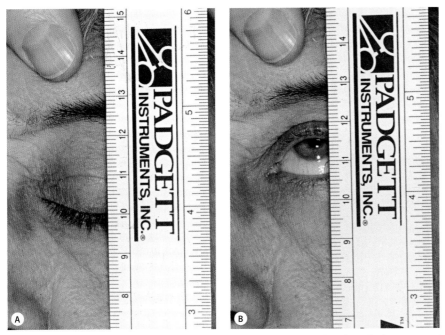

Figure 8-6 Measurement of the levator function. Note the position of the thumb on the brow, preventing any eyelid elevation by the frontalis muscle. (**A**) Eyelid in extreme downgaze. (**B**) Eyelid in extreme upgaze. The excursion of the eyelid, or levator function, is 15 mm in this case.

Box 8-3

Levator Function

Levator function is the basis of both classification and treatment of ptosis. The extremes are:
- Normal levator function
  - Seen in involutional ptosis
  - The levator aponeurosis advancement operation is the treatment
- Reduced levator function
  - Seen in simple congenital ptosis
  - The frontalis sling operation (for patients with poor levator function) is the treatment

---

Levator function is the key concept in ptosis classification and treatment. We have already stated that levator function is defined as the movement, or excursion, of the eyelid from extreme downgaze to extreme upgaze. It is measured in millimeters with 15 mm being the average normal adult measurement (Figure 8-6). The levator function is the most clinically useful indicator of the health of the levator muscle. Normal movement suggests that the levator muscle has normal strength (Box 8-3). As we have said, the levator function forms the basis of both classification and treatment of ptosis. Does the patient have "normal" levator function? Is the levator function reduced? Is it poor or absent?

Simple congenital ptosis is always associated with reduced levator function. If you see a child with ptosis and normal levator function, something doesn't make sense, and you should consider another diagnosis. *Involutional ptosis is associated with normal (or near normal function).* If you see an adult with ptosis and reduced levator function, something doesn't make sense, and you should consider another diagnosis. Are you getting the idea? So far, we know that:

- *Simple congenital ptosis* is associated with reduced levator function
- *Involutional ptosis* is associated with normal or near normal levator function
- *Unusual types of ptosis* are usually associated with reduced levator function, but levator function also can be normal

When I see a patient with ptosis, I classify the ptosis into one of these three categories. Most patients will have involutional or simple congenital ptosis. Congenital ptosis is much less common than the acquired forms of ptosis; consequently, the majority of patients will have involutional ptosis.

Tips for measuring the levator function

As you measure the levator function, you must *immobilize the eyebrow* so that the action of the frontalis muscle is eliminated completely. The amount of movement is measured with a millimeter ruler placed next to the patient's eye. The measurement is straightforward with adults, but may be difficult with children who will often elevate the chin as well as the eyes. It is sometimes helpful to practice a few times with the child before actually measuring the function. I will often demonstrate on myself to give the child the idea. Using the example of a "rocket ship" blasting off will help to hold the child's attention. Several measurements should be made until a reliable number can be obtained.

Watching *how the lid crease develops* with lid elevation will give a good idea of the function as well. As you get experience with measuring levator excursion, you will notice that the *speed of elevation* also varies among individuals. Later in the chapter, we will talk more about how levator function plays a role in treatment choice. At this point, we will discuss simple congenital ptosis and involutional ptosis in detail.

Simple congenital ptosis

Let's start with some comments on *nomenclature*. Some classification systems include congenital and acquired ptosis as the major categories. This is appropriate in some ways. Obviously congenital ptosis means that the patient was born with a drooping lid, and acquired ptosis means that the ptosis developed after birth. Unfortunately, so many varied types of ptosis fit into these two categories that you are not given any direction for a treatment plan using this classification. To avoid confusion with the inclusive term *congenital ptosis*, I like to use the term *simple congenital ptosis* to describe a specific form of ptosis present at birth. For the most common form of acquired ptosis that occurs late in life, I like to use the term *involutional ptosis* (Box 8-4).

In *simple congenital ptosis*, the eyelid is ptotic because of a *dystrophy of the levator muscle* itself. I use the term *simple* to specify that the only problem is the dystrophic levator muscle. When you perform ptosis surgery on a patient with simple congenital ptosis, you will see that the dystrophic muscle is infiltrated with fatty tissue. The muscle is no longer a healthy red color, but yellowish to a variable degree (Figure 8-7). This weak muscle cannot move well so the levator function is reduced. Usually the degree of ptosis is related to the levator function, that is the lower the levator function, the more ptosis present. In patients with

---

Box 8-4

Characteristics of the Common Types of Ptosis

Simple congenital ptosis
- Almost always bilateral, often asymmetric
- Ranges from mild to severe
- Reduced levator function
- Weak or absent skin crease
- Lid lag on downgaze

Involutional ptosis
- Often bilateral
- Ranges from mild to severe
- Normal levator function
- High skin crease
- Lid drop on downgaze

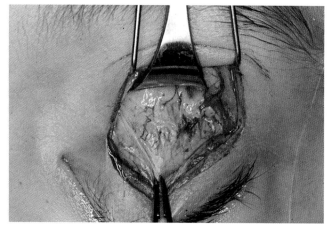

Figure 8-7 Fatty infiltration into the levator muscle seen in simple congenital ptosis.

severe ptosis, the levator function may be totally absent. In patients with mild ptosis, the levator function may be minimally reduced.

As alluded to above, *reduced levator function is associated with a weak or absent skin crease*. Remember that the skin crease is formed by attachments of the levator aponeurosis extending through the orbicularis to the skin at or near the top of the tarsal plate. If the levator is not pulling well, the skin crease will likewise not be as well defined.

Although we usually think of the upper lid not moving up well, it is probably *more accurate to think of the weak and fibrotic muscle not moving well in either upgaze or downgaze*. A characteristic of congenital ptosis demonstrating this is known as *lid lag on downgaze* (Figure 8-8).

Simple congenital ptosis *ranges from mild to severe*. In essentially all patients with congenital ptosis, the problem is *bilateral*. Sometimes, the amount of ptosis is quite *asymmetric*, and parents will only recognize that one side droops (see Figure 8-8). It is worth pointing out the bilaterality because it will probably affect some of the subtleties of the treatment.

Typically, simple congenital ptosis is associated with:

- Reduced levator function
- A weak or absent skin crease
- Lid lag on downgaze

We have stressed that levator function is the key to both classification and treatment of ptosis. For simple ptosis with levator function greater than 4 mm, a *levator aponeurosis advancement* (tightening the levator) is the correct treatment. Greater amounts of advancement are necessary for diminishing amounts of function. If the levator function is less than 3 mm, a *frontalis sling* is appropriate. For levator function between 3 and 4 mm, a generous advancement is usual, with the resection extending high above Whitnall's ligament into the muscle itself (Box 8-5).

Involutional ptosis

In contrast to simple congenital ptosis, involutional ptosis is associated with *normal, or near normal, levator function*. The traditional teaching says that the muscle is normal. The droop of the lid is suggested to be caused by the aponeurosis separating from the tarsal plate; hence, the commonly used name, *aponeurotic ptosis*. The term *disinsertion* is used, implying a slipping of the aponeurosis (disinsertion) off the tarsal plate or a thinning of the aponeurosis (dehiscence or rarefaction) itself. This pathophysiologic concept is helpful to differentiate this form of ptosis from the simple congenital form in which the muscle is weakened and much less easy to tighten surgically.

From a conceptual point of view, these features are helpful. Remember the suggested pathogenesis is that the aponeurosis is disinserted or stretched. The muscle is normal. It then makes sense that the *levator function is normal*. A *high skin crease* is the result of the levator fibers to the skin being dragged upward with the disinserted aponeurosis. The lid margin remains low throughout downgaze: *lid drop on downgaze*. This is caused by the eyelid being "longer" because of the aponeurosis disinsertion or stretching. Contrast this with the lid lag on downgaze in congenital ptosis caused by the fibrotic levator muscle.

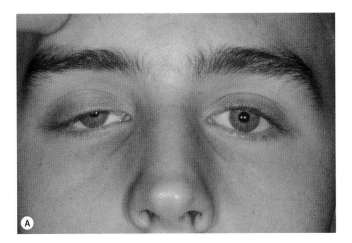

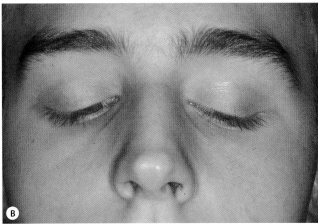

Figure 8-8 Characteristics of simple congenital ptosis, in this case bilateral and asymmetric. (**A**) Ptotic right upper eyelid with a weak skin crease. (**B**) The upper eyelid does not drop as far on the less ptotic side (lid lag on downgaze) because of the fibrosis in the weak levator muscle. (**C**) The upper eyelid does not elevate well (reduced levator function).

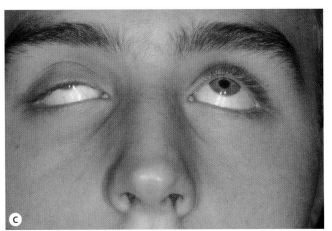

Box 8-5
Treatment of Ptosis
• Normal levator function—Aponeurosis advancement
• Poor levator function—Frontalis sling

Involutional ptosis *ranges from mild to severe*. It may be *bilateral* or *unilateral*. Usually there is an element of bilaterality to the ptosis if you look for it, although the patient often only complains about the more ptotic side.

Typically, involutional ptosis is associated with:

- Good levator function
- A high skin crease
- Lid drop on downgaze

Compare the photos of the patients with simple congenital and involutional ptosis to get these points clear in your mind (Figure 8-9). Although not all patients show these features on examination, the concept is valuable. However, as we will discuss later, the etiology of involutional ptosis as being entirely "aponeurotic" is likely not accurate.

Because patients with involutional ptosis have normal levator function, tightening the levator aponeurosis is the procedure of choice. You should notice that, as long as the levator function is good, levator aponeurosis advancement is the procedure of choice for both of the common types of ptosis.

Checkpoint

- Using our simplified classification system, what are the three types of ptosis?
- What are the characteristics of the two most common types of ptosis in terms of the "eyelid vital signs"? Describe the physical characteristics of the levator muscle and aponeurosis that account for the "eyelid vital signs" associated with each ptosis type
- What is the treatment for each type of ptosis?

History

Introduction

Your goal for the history taking and physical examination is to obtain three important pieces of information:

- Identify the type of ptosis
- Formulate a treatment plan
- Identify factors that modify treatment

With the background you have so far, you know that most children will have simple congenital ptosis, and most adults will have an involutional type of ptosis. During the history taking and physical examination, you will look for findings

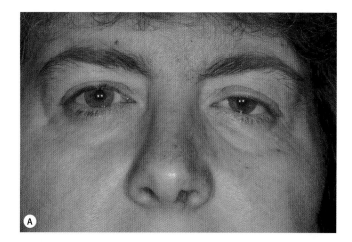

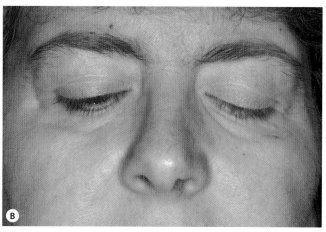

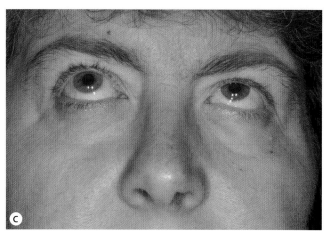

Figure 8-9 Characteristics of involutional ptosis. (**A**) Ptotic left upper eyelid with a high skin crease. (**B**) The upper eyelid shows lid drop on downgaze. (**C**) The levator function is normal.

that confirm the diagnosis. At the same time, you will be looking for factors that point away from the common diagnosis.

Once you have convinced yourself of the diagnosis, you will look for the factors that allow you to devise a treatment plan. You already know that the most important part of this is the levator function. Other factors may cause you to modify or individualize the treatment plan. Does the patient have a dry eye? Is closure incomplete? Does the normal lid have an unusual contour that you may need to match? Is the patient too frail to have an operation in the usual outpatient setting? There are many of these factors, and looking for them becomes second nature with experience.

Taking a history in children with ptosis

Is the diagnosis simple congenital ptosis? There are a few questions that you can ask to see if the child with ptosis has simple congenital ptosis. Remember that simple congenital ptosis involves only a ptotic upper lid in an otherwise healthy child with no other abnormal eye findings.

Is the ptosis congenital? When a ptosis is seen in a child, it is almost always congenital. Any onset after birth suggests a different diagnosis.

Is the ptosis unilateral or bilateral? Remember that congenital ptosis is usually bilateral, but often asymmetric. The parents may not have recognized this.

Does the lid change position? Is the lid ever open all the way? Does the lid position change with chewing or sucking?

- Any ptosis will be slightly worse when the patient is tired. Wide variations in the day are not typical of simple congenital ptosis.
- Extreme variation of the lid position from moment to moment suggests a *synkinetic form* of ptosis. As the name suggests (*syn*, same; *kinesis*, movement), these disorders include abnormal simultaneous movements of the lid and another muscle. Ptosis associated with abnormal lid movements caused by chewing, sucking, or other changes in jaw position is known as Marcus Gunn jaw winking. Ptosis associated with abnormal lid movements caused by changes in eye position is seen in third nerve palsy with aberrant regeneration.

Is there a family history of ptosis?

- Strict inheritance of simple congenital ptosis is rare.
- Occasionally a family will have several family members with ptosis without any other associated abnormality.
- More likely, a family history suggests the presence of *blepharophimosis syndrome*. The epicanthal folds and telecanthus are usually easy to recognize. The facies are usually a well-recognized "family trait" because of the autosomal dominant inheritance pattern. Often the parent bringing the child will have the syndrome. Sporadic cases are not uncommon, however.
- Congenital ptosis is not commonly associated with any ocular or systemic abnormalities. The dystrophy of the levator muscle is the only abnormality present. Rarely,

a congenital ptosis may occur as part of a syndrome. Usually the presence of a syndrome is obvious, based upon physical or neurologic development, but questions about the child's medical history are appropriate.

Formulating a treatment plan

The treatment plan for a simple congenital ptosis is based mainly on diagnosis and the levator function. Your questions in the history taking will help you confirm the diagnosis of simple congenital ptosis. More information about levator function appears later under "Physical Examination."

Identifying factors that modify the treatment plan

Now you have a good idea that the ptosis is the simple congenital type. You are planning to repair the ptosis sometime in the future. What factors should you consider that might affect the timing or the operation that you are planning?

Is the lid open above the pupil? During what part of the day?

- Surgical repair of simple congenital ptosis is usually done before the child starts school (at age 4). Features in the history suggesting the possibility of *amblyopia* should alter the timing of treatment.
- Amblyopia caused by congenital ptosis is rare. *Severe unilateral ptosis* is the most likely type to cause amblyopia. Associated astigmatism may also cause amblyopia.
- You should ask the parents to call you if the child stops trying to see out from under the drooping eyelid.
- A history of previous ptosis surgery makes your operation more difficult. Previous ptosis repair, especially levator aponeurosis advancement (tightening) procedures, puts the patient at risk for corneal exposure after more advancement.

By the end of the history taking, you should have an idea whether the ptosis is the simple congenital type. You should also have some idea of what operation the child will need and factors that might influence the timing of the operation. In the physical examination, you will confirm your impressions (Box 8-6).

Taking a history in adults with ptosis

The goals of the history taking for an adult are the same as those for a child but are somewhat more involved because there are more unusual types of ptosis in adults. The goals are:

- Determine the etiology of the ptosis
- Identify any characteristics suggesting an unusual type of ptosis
- Identify factors that modify the planned operation
- In the adult, an additional piece of information to obtain is documentation of the effect of the ptosis on the patient's vision

Is the diagnosis involutional ptosis? The first part of the history taking will help you determine if the ptosis is the usual involutional type of ptosis seen as the most common acquired ptosis in adults.

Is the ptosis acquired or has it been present since birth? When was the onset? What is the rate of progression?

Box 8-6

Children with Ptosis: History Taking

Goals
- Confirm diagnosis and etiology
- Identify any characteristics of unusual types of ptosis
- Identify factors that modify the operation

Simple congenital ptosis
- Unilateral or bilateral ptosis since birth
- No other associated eye or systemic problems
- Could amblyopia be present?
  - How severe is the ptosis?
  - Is the ptosis unilateral or bilateral?
  - How much time is the lid above the pupil?

Factors suggesting an unusual type of childhood ptosis
- Associated strabismus
- Family history
  - Blepharophimosis syndrome
- Developmental delay
  - Many syndromes associated with ptosis
- Extreme variation of ptosis from minute to minute or throughout the day
  - Lid movement associated with chewing or sucking
  - Lid movement associated with eye movements

- Most adults will have an acquired form of ptosis, usually the common involutional type. The *onset* is difficult to identify as the *progression* is usually so gradual over several years that no particular time can be identified as the exact onset.
- An acute onset suggests a diagnosis other than involutional ptosis.
- An exception to this is the onset of involutional ptosis *after cataract surgery.* This is uncommon today, but occurred often when a superior rectus fixation suture was used in cataract surgery.
- Occasionally an adult will have *pre-existing congenital ptosis* that has slowly gotten worse over time or may have asymmetric congenital ptosis that can no longer be ignored because the "normal" side has progressively drooped more. A review of old photos is rarely necessary because the physical examination will probably confirm the reduced levator function of congenital ptosis.
- Remember that any cause of ptosis in a child persists into adulthood.

Identifying factors that modify the treatment plan

The remaining portion of the history taking will help you identify factors that may cause you to modify the usual levator aponeurosis advancement procedure performed on patients with involutional ptosis. One of the main goals is to identify the patient who may develop corneal exposure if the eyelid is elevated.

Is there a history of previous ptosis operations? A history of previous lid operations may be a warning sign that the levator aponeurosis has already been shortened so that further tightening may cause lagophthalmos. Second operations tend to be more painful for the patient and technically more demanding for the surgeon.

Does the patient have symptoms of "dry" eye? Symptoms such as burning or eye irritation with air movement across the eye may suggest an undiagnosed dry eye condition. The frequent use of eye drops or ointment may mean that the patient has a known dry eye problem (Box 8-7).

Is there a history of facial nerve palsy? A history of facial nerve palsy signals the potential for poor blinking and lagophthalmos after surgery.

What is the patient's general health?

- Is the patient taking a long list of medications? This may suggest to you that the ptosis repair should be done in an operating room with more supervision than in an office or an outpatient operating room.
- Is the patient particularly nervous during the examination, suggesting to you that you would like an anesthesiologist present to help with sedation?

By the end of the history taking, you will have obtained a large amount of information. You have a good idea whether the ptosis is typical of simple congenital ptosis or an involutional type. You have looked for unusual features that might suggest that this is not the usual congenital or acquired ptosis. You have started to make a treatment plan. You know

---

Box 8-7

Adult with Ptosis: History Taking

Goals
- Confirm diagnosis and etiology
- Identify any characteristics of unusual types of ptosis
- Identify factors that modify the operation

Involutional adult ptosis
- Indefinite onset, gradual progression
- No other associated eye or systemic problems
- What is the patient's complaint?
  - Most commonly, visual loss
    - Peripheral vision: mild to moderate cases
    - Central vision: severe cases
  - Brow ache or headache may be present
  - Occasionally, difficulty with reading
- Ptosis usually about the same severity throughout the day

Factors suggesting an unusual type of adult ptosis
- Positive family history
- Associated diplopia
- Variation in degree of ptosis
  - Minute to minute
  - With eye movements
  - Better after naps
- Associated facial movement problems
  - History of facial nerve palsy
  - History of facial spasms

Factors that modify the operation
- Possible corneal exposure
- Dry eye symptoms
- Use of eye drops or ointment
- Previous eye or lid operations
- History of facial nerve weakness
- Patient's general health
- Patient preference for a particular outcome

---

how the patient's vision is affected and the goals of treatment. You have begun to identify factors that would make you want to modify the usual surgery. With this information in hand, you are ready to do the physical examination. You know what points you need to emphasize during the physical examination to confirm or deny your findings in the history taking.

Physical examination

Introduction

As we have seen above, a good history prepares you to do a directed physical examination. As in all fields of medicine, the history and physical examination are highly complementary. The goals of the physical examination are:

- Classify the type of ptosis based on levator function
- Identify findings suggesting that an unusual ptosis is present
- Document the degree of ptosis
- Look for factors that might modify the usual ptosis operation

The *eyelid vital signs* give an assessment of the overall condition of the eyelids. Remember the eyelid vital signs:

- Margin reflex distance (MRD)
  - MRD_1 and MRD_2
- Levator function
  - Excursion from downgaze to upgaze
  - Speed of excursion
- Skin crease height and strength

You should measure the eyelid vital signs in every patient with ptosis.

The margin reflex distance

We used the term, *margin reflex distance* (MRD) earlier. The MRD is a useful measurement for describing the position of the eyelids. Before the introduction of the MRD, the *palpebral fissure* measurement was used. This distance is the millimeters measured between the upper and lower lids. A normal palpebral fissure is 9–10 mm. For the palpebral fissure measurement to be meaningful in describing the upper lid position, the lower lid must be in the normal position. A fissure of 9 mm could mean that the upper lid is crossing the pupil and that the lower lid is 4 mm below the lower limbus. For this reason, the palpebral fissure, or aperture, measurement has largely been replaced by the MRD measurement.

Useful refinements of the MRD measurement are the MRD_1 and MRD_2. MRD_1 designates the distance of the upper lid from the corneal light reflex. MRD_2 designates the distance of the lower lid from the corneal light reflex. These measurements give a good mental picture and accurately define the position of the upper and lower lids.

The MRD_1 measures the degree of ptosis. It should be measured using a penlight and a millimeter rule. With the patient at your eye level, ask him or her to look straight ahead at a distant target. Shine the penlight at the patient's eye. The distance from the corneal light reflex to the upper lid margin, measured with the millimeter rule, is the MRD_1. With some experience, it is easy to estimate the MRD_1, if you assume that the corneal diameter is 10 mm and that the normal upper lid resting position is just below the upper limbus. The normal MRD_1 is between 4 and 5 mm. If the lid margin crosses the pupil, the MRD_1 is 0 mm. If the lid margin is about halfway down from the limbus to the corneal light reflex, the MRD_1 is 2.5 mm (a good number to remember because this is the MRD_1 often considered to indicate that a visual impairment exists) (Figure 8-10).

It is important to remember that the patient should be relaxed during this measurement. The frontalis muscle should not be contributing to the lid opening. As we stated earlier, it is best to stabilize the brow during this measurement. Take care not to push the lid down. I usually ask the patient to close the eyes and then open them in a comfortable position. Often the patient will be somewhat anxious during the initial part of the examination, and the eyes will be open more than usual. It is important to recognize this and help the patient relax during this measurement.

With experience, it is easy to accurately estimate the MRD just by watching the patient while obtaining the history. Although for the sake of organizing this textbook, I have separated history taking and physical examination, as you probably already know, many observational measurements are made while obtaining the history. As you have probably heard before in your training, the physical examination starts when the patient walks into the examination room.

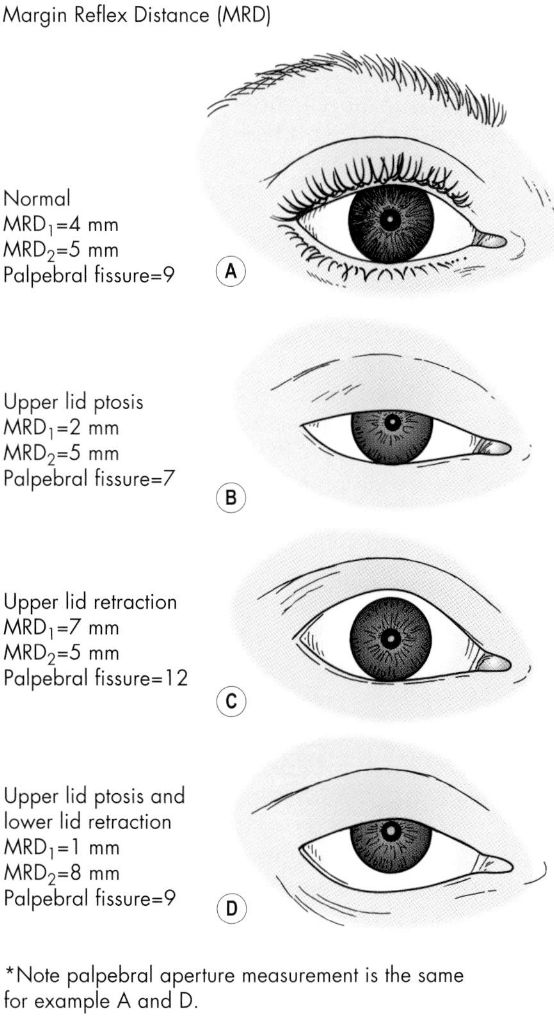

The levator function

We have stressed the importance of the levator function in determining the "health" or "strength" of the levator muscle. Practice measuring levator function in adults before you try to get accurate measurements in children. Remember to block the action of the brow with your thumb and don't allow the head to tip up with eye elevation.

The conventional levator function is a measurement of *distance* (*levator excursion*). I believe that it is worth considering a refinement in the measurement of levator function, an estimate of the *speed of the excursion*. As your measurements get more accurate, you will notice that the excursion of the upper lid is much slower in patients with some of the unusual types of ptosis. You will realize that many "involutional" ptosis patients have normal or near normal excursion, but very slow rates of eyelid elevation. This explains, in part at least, why ptosis repair is not always straightforward.

The skin crease height and strength

The distance from the upper lid margin to the skin crease is the skin crease height. As we stated earlier, in adult women, the measurement is 8–10 mm and in adult men the measurement is 6–8 mm. In children, the height is somewhat less.

The skin crease is important for three reasons:

- It tells you about the type of ptosis
- It gives you an estimate of the levator function
- It provides the standard incision line for opening the eyelid in most ptosis operations

You will see a weak, or indistinct, skin crease in simple congenital ptosis. The weaker the levator muscle is, the weaker the crease. Any patient with reduced levator function will have a weakened skin crease. You will see a formed crease in most patients with involutional ptosis. In many patients, the lid crease will be higher on the more ptotic side. The standard ptosis operations begin with an incision in the skin crease. This incision gives you access to the levator aponeurosis and muscle. The wounds heal with minimal scarring.

The physical examination of the child with ptosis

Is the diagnosis simple congenital ptosis? The levator function will be reduced in simple congenital ptosis. There should be no other anatomic abnormalities present.

Measure the eyelid vital signs.

- You will probably see a bilateral, often asymmetric, ptosis. It is likely that you will have to estimate the MRD_1.

Margin Reflex Distance (MRD)

Normal
MRD_1=4 mm
MRD_2=5 mm
Palpebral fissure=9   (A)

Upper lid ptosis
MRD_1=2 mm
MRD_2=5 mm
Palpebral fissure=7   (B)

Upper lid retraction
MRD_1=7 mm
MRD_2=5 mm
Palpebral fissure=12   (C)

Upper lid ptosis and
lower lid retraction
MRD_1=1 mm
MRD_2=8 mm
Palpebral fissure=9   (D)

*Note palpebral aperture measurement is the same for example A and D.

Figure 8-10 MRD and palpebral fissure measurements. Note that the palpebral fissures measure the same in examples (**A** and **D**) although each represents a different clinical condition. (**A**) Normal: MRD_1 of 4 mm, MRD_2 of 5 mm, and palpebral fissure of 9 mm. (**B**) Upper lid ptosis: MRD_1 of 2 mm, MRD_2 of 5 mm, and palpebral fissure of 7 mm. (**C**) Upper lid retraction: MRD_1 of 7 mm, MRD_2 of 5 mm, and palpebral fissure of 12 mm. (**D**) Upper lid ptosis and lower lid retraction: MRD_1 of 2 mm, MRD_2 of 7 mm and palpebral fissure of 9 mm.

- The levator function will be reduced to some degree. The reduction in levator function is usually an indication of the amount of ptosis.
- The skin crease will be weakened, depending on the amount of levator function. If a child is difficult to examine, your best estimate of the levator function may be the depth of the crease.

Measure the visual acuity. The vision may not be possible to measure, but fixation should be steady and maintained. Any associated ocular abnormalities suggest the possibility of a syndrome.

Is the external appearance of the child normal?

- The appearance should be normal in simple congenital ptosis
- The most common abnormal facies is seen in blepharophimosis syndrome
- Remember that many other syndromes can have ptosis as one of the associated findings

Measure the motility.

- Normal motility is associated with simple congenital ptosis
- The most common motility disturbance seen in children with ptosis is a localized weakness of the superior rectus muscle (said to occur in about 5% of patients born with ptosis)
- Any bizarre movement of the upper lid associated with eye movement should suggest aberrant regeneration of the third nerve

Ask the child to open and close the mouth and move the jaw around. No movement of the eyelid should occur with simple congenital ptosis. Any lid movement will diagnose a Marcus Gunn jaw winking ptosis.

Formulating a treatment plan

The measurement of the levator function is the main factor in choosing an advancement or a frontalis sling operation.

What is the levator function?

- Ptosis with poor levator function (1–3 mm) requires a frontalis sling operation
- Ptosis with medium to good levator function (>4 mm) can be corrected with a levator tightening (levator advancement) operation

Identifying factors that modify the treatment plan

Look for problems that would cause you to do the surgery earlier than usual or lift the lid less than near the anatomic normal.

Check for amblyopia. If amblyopia, due to deprivation or astigmatism, is present, plans for surgery should be made.

Look for risk factors that increase the chance of corneal exposure (rare in children):

- Facial nerve palsy
- Poor Bell's phenomenon
- Lagophthalmos (possibly caused by previous ptosis surgery)
- Poor tear film (rare) seen on slit lamp examination

- Corneal exposure. This is almost never a problem in children. However, if corneal exposure is already present, it will be worse after the lid is elevated

The physical examination of the adult with ptosis

Is the diagnosis involutional ptosis? After the history taking in an adult, you have the idea that this slowly progressive ptosis is the involutional type. During the physical examination, you will confirm that the levator function is normal and that there are no other anatomic abnormalities present.

Measure the eyelid vital signs.

- You will probably see a bilateral, often asymmetric, ptosis. Accurately measure the MRD_1 and MRD_2.
- The levator function will be normal. Levator function should not be less than 12–13 mm. Watch the speed of the lid excursion. Slight reduction in lid speed should suggest a myogenic type of unusual ptosis.
- The skin crease may be higher than normal.

Does the patient have normal facial expression?

- Weakness of the facial muscles is associated with the myogenic types of unusual ptosis.
- Is there hyperkinetic movement of the face suggesting hemifacial spasm or aberrant regeneration of the facial nerve?

Measure the motility.

- The eye movements should be normal for the patient's age in involutional ptosis.
- Any reduction in motility or symptoms of diplopia should suggest a diagnosis other than involutional ptosis. Conditions associated with types of unusual ptosis with decreased motility include myasthenia gravis, third nerve palsy, and chronic progressive external ophthalmoplegia (CPEO).
- Any bizarre association of the upper lid position (ptosis or lid retraction) with eye movements should suggest aberrant regeneration of the third nerve.

Is the pupil normal? Are there signs of Horner's syndrome? Do you see any *miosis* or *lower lid elevation* to suggest that a loss of sympathetic tone is responsible for the patient's *mild ptosis* (*Horner's syndrome—upper lid ptosis, lower lid elevation, miosis,* and *anhidrosis of the ipsilateral side of the face*)?

Formulating a treatment plan

By definition, patients with involutional ptosis have normal levator function. You have confirmed the levator function as discussed earlier. All instances of involutional ptosis can be repaired with a levator aponeurosis advancement operation.

Identifying factors that modify the treatment plan

You are planning a levator aponeurosis advancement operation. You are now looking for findings that will individualize the operation for the patient. If the patient had symptoms of dry eye elicited in the history, you should be especially diligent in looking for findings suggesting that opening the eyelid to the normal anatomic height would cause corneal exposure.

Decide if additional procedures such as a blepharoplasty or browplasty are necessary. Older patients often have dermatochalasis and brow ptosis accompanying involutional ptosis.

Look for risk factors that increase the chance of corneal exposure.

- Have the patient close the eyes forcefully. The eyelashes should be *buried* (turned inward and not visible).
- Have the patient close the eyes gently and lift the lid to evaluate the *Bell's phenomenon*. A poor Bell's phenomenon is only a relative contraindication for ptosis repair.
- Look for *lagophthalmos* (possibly caused by previous ptosis surgery).
- Look for *lower eyelid retraction* from any cause.
- Do a slit lamp examination to *evaluate the tear film*. If the tear film is minimal, do a *Schirmer's test*. If corneal exposure is present preoperatively, it will be worse after elevating the lid.
- Use the maximal treatment for any corneal exposure before proceeding with ptosis repair. Consider punctal plugs. If you cannot eliminate the symptoms and signs of corneal exposure, you should re-evaluate the need for eyelid elevation. If the benefits outweigh the risks, plan a conservative elevation (Box 8-8).

Do you plan unilateral or bilateral operations? As we said earlier, most involutional ptosis is bilateral, but often asymmetric. Commonly, the patient complains only about the worse side. You should point out any bilateral ptosis. Occasionally, when the more ptotic eyelid is raised, the less ptotic eyelid will drop. Based on the principles of *Hering's law* (simultaneous innervation), the less ptotic eyelid receives the same innervation as the more ptotic eyelid. When the more ptotic eyelid is raised, any "extra" innervation to the less ptotic eyelid disappears, leaving the patient with a ptosis on the unoperated side. Explain this to the patient preoperatively to avoid an "unexpected" operation on the "good" side.

Make sure you address your patient's concerns.

- Most patients complain of *decreased peripheral vision*. If the patient complains of *loss of central vision*, I usually lift the lid with my finger to make sure that lifting the lid improves the vision. Don't proceed with ptosis repair if your patient doesn't see an improvement. There are many causes of decreased central vision in elderly patients that are more common than upper lid ptosis.
- The same thing is true for *complaints about reading*. You should be able to confirm that lifting the lid with your patient trying to read actually improves the reading.

Box 8-8

Ptosis: Physical Examination

Goals
- Identify the type of ptosis
- Formulate a treatment plan
- Identify factors that might modify the treatment

Characteristics of simple congenital ptosis seen on examination
- Moderate to severe ptosis, sometimes mild
- Usually bilateral, often asymmetric
- Triad
  - Weak or absent skin crease
  - Reduced levator function (0–10 mm)
  - Lid lag on downgaze
- "Chin-up" position is common
- Vision, motility, and remainder of eye examination otherwise normal
- Amblyopia occurs rarely

Characteristics of involutional ptosis in adults seen on examination
- Mild to moderate ptosis, but sometimes severe
- May be unilateral or bilateral
- Triad
  - Normal levator function (13–17 mm)
  - High skin crease
  - Lid drop on downgaze
- Brow elevation, deep forehead wrinkles often seen
- Vision, motility, and remainder of eye examination otherwise normal
- Other associated periocular aging changes

Physical findings suggesting an unusual type of ptosis
- Decreased vision or relative afferent pupillary defect, especially with other cranial neuropathies
  - Tumor or inflammation at the junction of orbit and brain

- Anisocoria
  - Horner's syndrome
- Motility problem
  - Paralytic: third nerve palsy
  - Restrictive: infiltrative orbital tumor, i.e., metastatic disease
- Proptosis
  - Infiltrative orbital tumor, i.e., metastatic disease
  - Graves' disease associated with myasthenia gravis
- Variation of severity of ptosis and during examination
  - Myasthenia gravis, especially if fatigability is present
  - Third nerve palsy with aberrant regeneration
  - Facial nerve palsy with aberrant regeneration
  - Hemifacial spasm (pseudoptosis)
  - Essential blepharospasm (pseudoptosis)
- Abnormal facial movements
  - Facial nerve palsy with aberrant regeneration
  - Hemifacial spasm (pseudoptosis)
  - Essential blepharospasm (pseudoptosis)

Make a treatment plan based on the levator function. The following factors might modify the usual repair:
- Risk of corneal exposure
  - Facial nerve weakness
  - Scarring of the eyelid
  - Poor Bell's phenomenon
  - Decreased tear lake
  - Corneal staining
- Associated periocular problems
  - Unusual lid contour
  - Brow ptosis
  - Dermatochalasis

- It is important to discuss the *issues of appearance* with all patients. Although your patient may complain about a drooping upper lid, an equal, but sometimes unspoken, concern may be about some baggy upper lid skin. Setting clear goals for the ptosis operation (or for any operation) ensures a happy outcome. Remember our comments about "seeing better" versus "looking better."

Surgical correction of eyelid ptosis

Documentation of the need for ptosis repair

In most patients, ptosis repair is undertaken to improve the visual function. To be eligible for insurance reimbursement, documentation of the medical necessity for repair is necessary. Each insurance carrier has different requirements for documentation, including one or more of the following items:

- Patient complaint
- Physical findings
- Visual field testing, demonstrating an improvement with eyelid elevation
- Photographs

You have already noted the patient's complaint regarding the drooping lids in the history. Common complaints are *decreased vision* (usually peripheral, sometimes central vision), *heaviness of the eyelids, brow ache or headache, difficulty reading,* and *neck ache* (from lifting the chin).

The examination should document the upper eyelid height, the MRD_1. Supporting information includes *elevated or arched eyebrows, prominent forehead furrows,* and a *chin-up position.*

Visual field testing should be done with the eyelids in the relaxed ptotic position and with the eyelids taped open. An improvement in the superior visual field of at least *12 degrees* is required (this amount varies among insurers).

Photographs demonstrating the position of the ptotic lid are sometimes required.

Preoperative and postoperative considerations

As with any operation, the goals and risks should be discussed with the patient. For most patients, an improvement in the visual field is the expected goal. Complications are rare, but include asymmetry, corneal exposure, hemorrhage, blindness, or death. Remember to be inclusive for medical legal reasons, but put risks into perspective for the patient. Hemorrhage leading to blindness is rare. Death would be an extremely unlikely event during or after ptosis repair. Reoperations are not common.

Ask your patients to stop all medications with any anticoagulant effect before operation. These products include aspirin or products containing aspirin, platelet inhibitors (10 days), nonsteroidal anti-inflammatory agents (3–4 days), and some herbal remedies and supplements (three Gs—garlic, ginkgo, ginseng, and high doses of vitamin E). Remember that most patients do not consider aspirin or other over-the-counter medicines to be "real" medicines, so ask specifically about aspirin, "baby aspirin," or "arthritis pills." Warfarin (Coumadin) should be stopped with the internist's consent (usually 4–5 days ahead of the operation). It seems likely that eyelid operations while on Coumadin increase the likelihood of serious bleeding; however, there are no studies regarding this. Many patients have undergone eyelid operations while anticoagulated, without suffering serious complications. As you know, the indications for anticoagulation are highly varied. In most cases, stopping anticoagulation is the best choice. As always, you should consider the risks versus the benefits of discontinuing anticoagulation. If there is any question, it is best to consult with the patient's internist.

Give your patients reasonable postoperative expectations. This will decrease the number of phone calls to you and give the patient some peace of mind postoperatively. You might say, "Some discomfort is expected for 24–48 hours. A small amount of bloody tears or light-colored drainage from the wound is normal. Let me know if the bleeding doesn't stop with light pressure. You should call if pain in or behind your eye is severe. Bruising and swelling are common for 2 weeks." The patient should plan to rest with ice bags on the eye for 1 or 2 days. After 48 hours, warm wet compresses are helpful. Give your patients an emergency number to call.

Relationship of levator function to treatment

We already know that the levator function is the most important factor in choosing the type of ptosis operation. If levator function is good, the lid will lift well if the levator aponeurosis is "tightened" or "shortened" surgically. This is like a rubber band: the shorter band is stronger and capable of lifting more.

Aponeurosis advancement or shortening procedure works less and less well as the levator function decreases. Two problems occur with a weak muscle that is tightened, as in a patient with congenital ptosis with poor levator function. The first problem is that the muscle can eventually stretch out and the lid becomes low again. Remember that the normal muscle fibers have been replaced with fat and fibrous tissue. With very poor levator function (1–2 mm), the muscle is totally replaced with fat and often won't even hold a suture. The second problem relates to the inability to close the eye postoperatively. The normal lid opens and closes because the individual levator muscle fibers contract to open the upper eyelid and relax to allow the orbicularis muscle to close the eyelid. *A weak muscle doesn't have as much contraction or relaxation. In fact, the weak lid is relatively static (that is what the levator function is measuring).* Consequently, when a weak muscle is tightened, it can be shortened enough to open the lid because the fibrous tissue in the muscle holds it open. Unfortunately, lacking the normal relaxation of the levator muscle, the eye will stay open to a degree (lagophthalmos). *Remember tightening the muscle doesn't improve the levator function or movement of the eyelid; it essentially only resets the lid height.*

With this in mind, you can understand that, at some point, trying to tighten a weak levator muscle will not be acceptable because of the lagophthalmos created. When you use a levator aponeurosis advancement operation in children with simple congenital ptosis, the lowest amount of levator function that will allow the eyelid to lift without creating corneal exposure is about 3 mm. Adults with reduced levator function in this range do not tolerate the lagophthalmos created by a levator aponeurosis operation.

When the levator function is poor, a frontalis sling operation is used to lift the lids. Although the lids are suspended or "tied" open, the contraction and relaxation of the frontalis muscle allow some movement of the upper eyelid that helps to keep the cornea moist.

Checkpoint

- You already know the two operations to treat ptosis: the levator aponeurosis advancement and the frontalis sling operations. You should now understand why each works and when you would choose one over the other.
- The levator aponeurosis advancement operation is used in patients in whom the levator function is good.
- The frontalis sling operation is used in patients in whom the levator function is poor.
- Children tolerate lagophthalmos better than adults. Here are some possible reasons:
  — Children seem to have a better tear film. Most adults with ptosis are older. Older patients have reduced tear production and quality.
  — Most adults with reduced levator function have an unusual type of ptosis. They often have other problems associated with ptosis such as incomplete closure of the lids (common in the myogenic type of ptosis) or reduced eye movements and a poor Bell's phenomenon.

The levator aponeurosis advancement operation

The levator aponeurosis advancement operation is one of the most common oculoplastic operations performed. *It is the procedure of choice for adults with involutional ptosis.* These patients with ptosis have normal levator function so tightening of the levator aponeurosis makes sense.

The technique is not easy, but it is within reach for most ophthalmologists interested in learning it. You must memorize each step, and then learn the technique for each step. There is an "art" to the final adjustment in height and contour that comes with experience. Even the best of ptosis surgeons are occasionally frustrated by an unpredictable result.

This operation is most easily done using local anesthesia. Injection of local anesthetic under the skin provides enough anesthesia to operate on the aponeurosis but does not paralyze the deeper levator muscle. This makes intraoperative adjustment of the lid height and contour possible. This benefit of local anesthesia is lost when this operation is performed under general anesthesia, as is required with children.

The levator aponeurosis advancement operation includes:

- Patient preparation
- Skin incision
- Identification of the levator aponeurosis
- Dissection of the levator aponeurosis off Müller's muscle
- Levator aponeurosis advancement

- Intraoperative adjustments to height and contour
- Closure

The steps of the levator aponeurosis advancement operation are:

1. Prepare the patient
   A. Use *light intravenous sedation.* Don't make the patient too sleepy or adjustment later will not be possible.
   B. Instill topical drops.
   C. Mark an upper lid skin crease incision.
      (1) Elevate the brow with your finger until the eyelashes start to lift up. Ask the patient to look up and down. Watch where the skin crease forms. Mark symmetric creases from the lateral canthus to the punctum, usually around 6–8 mm from the eyelid margin for men and 8–10 mm for women (Figure 8-11, A).
      (2) Often, you will be marking a blepharoplasty elliptical excision for an upper lid blepharoplasty at the same time.
   D. Inject local anesthetic with epinephrine just under the skin.
      (1) Inject 0.1 ml into two or three spots. Apply light pressure. Wait 10 seconds.
      (2) Inject an additional *1–1.5 ml* of local anesthetic slowly, across the proposed incision.
      (3) Avoid injecting deeply into muscle. You do not want to cause a hematoma, which will make height and contour adjustment difficult.
   E. Prep and drape the patient.
2. Make a skin incision
   A. Place a 4-0 silk suture through the meibomian glands along the lid margin for a traction suture. Use a cutting needle (Ethicon 783 P-3 cutting needle). As you get more experienced, you may decide that the traction suture is not necessary.
   B. Stretch the skin taut placing your fingers on both sides of the wound.
   C. Use a Colorado needle or a no. 15 blade to incise the skin. Try not to cut through the muscle (Figure 8-11, B).
   D. You will need cautery at this point if you use a no. 15 blade.
3. Identify the levator aponeurosis
   A. Incise the orbicularis muscle across the wound.
   B. *Dissect the orbicularis superiorly off the orbital septum* for about 5 mm. Learn to look "through" the septum to see the yellow of the preaponeurotic fat. Looking through the tissues is helpful to keep oriented. It takes a little practice (Figure 8-11, C). Sometimes light pressure on the eye will make the fat more visible.
   C. Open the septum.
      (1) Use a thermal cautery or a Westcott scissors in your dominant hand and Paufique forceps in your nondominant hand to open the septum. The unipolar current of the Colorado needle causes pain posterior to the septum for most patients. If you have dissected 5 mm superior to the skin crease, you will be high enough to avoid damage to the aponeurosis.

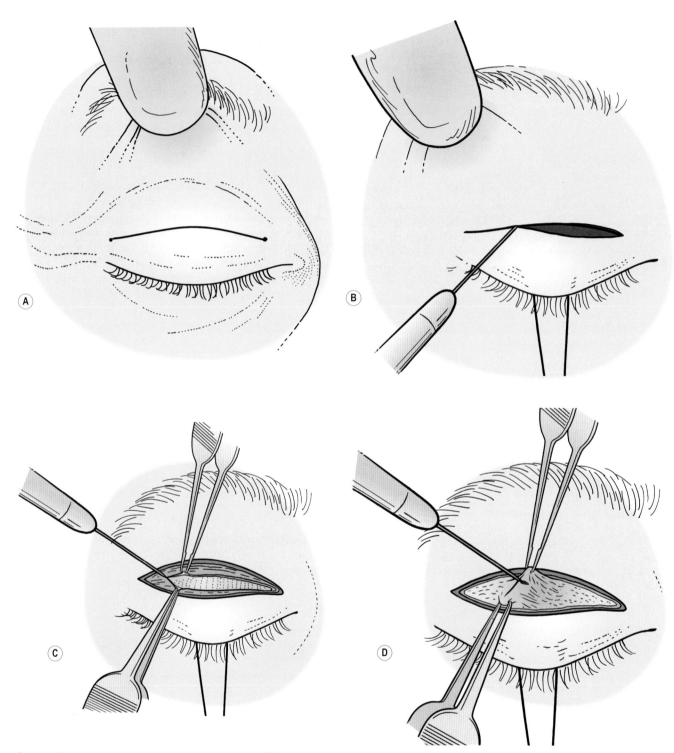

Figure 8-11 Levator aponeurosis advancement operation. (**A**) Mark an upper lid skin crease incision. (**B**) Place a 4-0 silk traction suture. Make a skin incision with the Colorado needle. (**C**) Dissect the orbicularis muscle off the septum superiorly for 5–10 mm. You should be able to see the preaponeurotic fat through the septum. (**D**) "Buttonhole" the septum with the Colorado needle, Westcott scissors, or thermal cautery. (**E**) Open the septum completely to the left and right. (**F**) Dissect the preaponeurotic fat off the aponeurosis. (**G**) Disinsert the aponeurosis from the face of the tarsal plate. Create a plane of dissection between Müller's muscle and the aponeurosis. "Pull" the tissues apart to visualize bands of tissue between the layers. Use the curve of the Westcott scissors (convex up) pushing against the undersurface of the aponeurosis to separate and cut these bands. The thermal cautery works well for this also. (**H**) Make a lamellar pass through the medial one third of the tarsus using a double-armed 5-0 nylon suture. (**I**) Pass each needle through the undersurface of the aponeurosis. (**J**) Advance the aponeurosis onto the tarsus and tie the suture with a temporary knot. Check the height and contour of the lid. Contour adjustments are made by moving the tarsal bite. Height adjustments are made by moving the aponeurotic sutures superiorly or inferiorly. (**K**) Aim for a 1 mm overcorrection. When the correct height is obtained, tie the nylon suture permanently. Trim off redundant aponeurosis using a Westcott scissors. (**L**) Rarely, a temporal droop is present. It can be corrected with an additional vertical pass of the nylon suture from the tarsus to the aponeurosis. (**M**) Form the skin crease using two interrupted skin sutures from the skin edge to the aponeurosis at the superior tarsal margin to the skin. (**N**) Close the skin crease with a running absorbable or permanent suture at a higher or lower position in the aponeurosis.

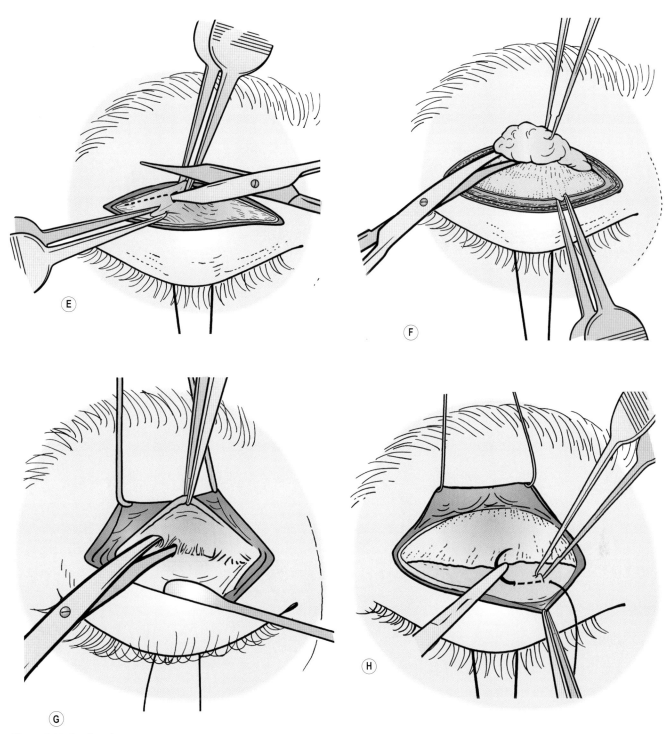

Figure 8-11 Continued.

(2) Ask your assistant to *lift the septum toward the ceiling.*

(3) While you do the same, make an opening *through the septum* to see the preaponeurotic fat. You will be lifting the septum off the aponeurosis so don't worry about cutting it (Figure 8-11, D).

(4) Open the septum to the left and then to the right (Figure 8-11, E). If you are using a scissors, you can easily slide the blades under the septum. *If you are unsure where you are, ask the patient to look up and you can see the aponeurosis move.*

D. Dissect the septum off the preaponeurotic fat.

E. Dissect the preaponeurotic fat off the aponeurosis (Figure 8-11, F).

F. For most cases, I use a thermal cautery to work posterior to the septum (two battery "hot" cautery). It works for both cutting and cautery. You will see that it is especially useful when dissecting the aponeurosis free from the underlying Müller's muscle. You have to make sure that all

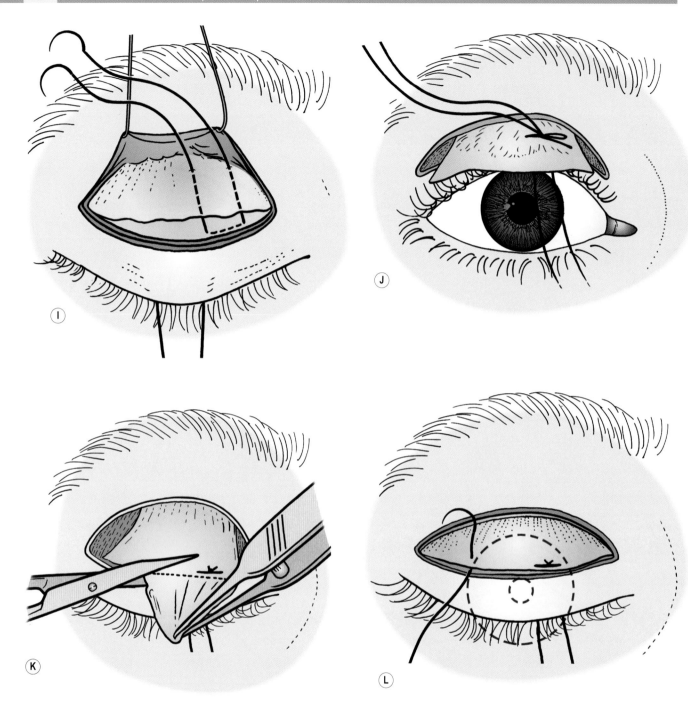

Figure 8-11 Continued.

supplemental oxygen is turned off using the hot cautery. This cautery adds a few dollars to the disposable materials costs of the operation, however.

4. Dissect the levator aponeurosis off Müller's muscle

    A. Disinsert the levator aponeurosis from the anterior surface of the tarsus using either the Colorado needle or Westcott scissors, "baring" the superior margin of the tarsus.

    B. Dissect the orbicularis muscle off the superior one third of the tarsus.

    C. Dissect the aponeurosis free from Müller's muscle.

        (1) To dissect a plane between Müller's muscle and the posterior surface of the aponeurosis, begin

by pulling the edge of the aponeurosis superiorly and the tarsus inferiorly.

(2) Slide your cutting instrument superiorly on the surface of the tarsus. As you pull the aponeurosis away from the tarsus, you will easily enter the correct plane between the two layers. This is an important step to master so that you don't get bleeding into Müller's muscle.

(3) You should see the peripheral arcade in Müller's muscle.

(4) Müller's muscle is too sensitive to grasp with forceps. The assistant should put tension on Müller's muscle with a Q-tip.

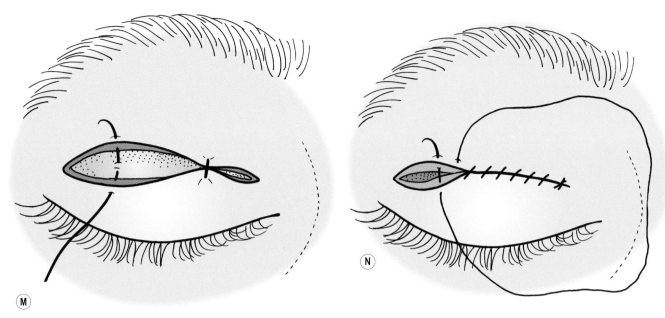

Figure 8-11 Continued.

(5) Pull the aponeurosis away from Müller's muscle. You will see *thin adhesions* stretching between Müller's muscle and the posterior surface of the aponeurosis. Carefully cut these to safely free the aponeurosis without making Müller's muscle bleed (Figure 8-11, G). The hot cautery works well for this.

(6) Continue the dissection superiorly about 10–12 mm.

5. Advance the levator aponeurosis onto the tarsus

A. Pass a double-armed 5-0 nylon suture (Ethicon 7731, S-24 spatula needle) into the tarsus. The horizontal position of the needle pass on the tarsus largely determines the contour of the eyelid.

(1) Ask the patient to open both eyes. Grasp the wound with forceps where you want to place the peak of the eyelid (just nasal to the pupil).

(2) Make the needle pass in a *lamellar fashion about 3 mm inferior* to the superior tarsal margin (Figure 8-11, H) at the point you have chosen. Make a *long needle pass* to include the *medial 5 mm of tarsus*. A long needle pass helps to give a smooth eyelid contour. A short needle pass tends to cause a sharp "peak" in the eyelid margin where the suture is placed.

(3) Pass the arms of the suture through the back of the aponeurosis about 10–15 mm superiorly, depending on how much lift you want (Figure 8-11, I).

(4) Ask your assistant to pull the aponeurosis inferiorly against the tarsus as you tie a *temporary knot* (Figure 8-11, J). Make sure that the aponeurosis is tight against the tarsus.

(5) Ask the patient to open both eyes. Check the *height and contour* with the patient in the reclining position.

6. Make intraoperative adjustments to height and contour

A. The contour should be smooth with the peak just nasal to the pupil. *Aim for a 1 mm overcorrection,* leaving the lid at or just above the limbus.

(1) First, inspect the contour. *If the lid peak is not in the correct position,* you will have to reposition the tarsal bite. If the peak is too sharp, broaden the tarsal bite.

(2) *If the lid is too high or too low,* untie the knot and back the sutures out of the aponeurosis. Reposition the sutures at a more appropriate position.

B. When you are happy with the height and shape, *have the patient sit up* and make a final inspection before you close.

(1) We use an operating table with pneumatic lifts that easily sits the patient up on the operating table—a must if you are doing many ptosis operations or blepharoplasties.

(2) If you are not perfectly satisfied with the height or contour, readjust the position of the suture in the tarsus or aponeurosis.

C. When you are pleased with the final height and contour, *tie the suture permanently* (Figure 8-11, K).

D. Trim off the extra aponeurosis.

E. If there is a small amount of temporal droop, you can place an additional suture temporally (Figure 8-11, L); usually not necessary.

(1) You will find that it is difficult to get a smooth contour in very lax upper eyelids. It is best to avoid these cases in the beginning. As you get more experience, you can add an extra tarsal bite or two to smoothen the contour, but it can be tricky.

7. Close the skin

A. Consider one or two *sutures to reform the skin crease.* Pass an absorbable suture from the skin edge to the aponeurosis at the superior margin of the tarsus to the opposite skin edge. If you are doing bilateral surgery, make sure this stitch is symmetric (Figure 8-11, M). Gut sutures have a tendency to untie, so the interrupted skin crease formation sutures give a little extra security in the wound closure.

  B. Use either 6-0 fast absorbing plain gut (Ethicon 1916, PC-1 needle) or 6-0 nylon (Ethicon 1698G, P-3 needle) (Figure 8-11, N).
8. Provide postoperative care
  A. Instill topical antibiotic ointment in the eye and on the wound three times per day.

The levator aponeurosis advancement operation in children

The levator aponeurosis advancement procedure for simple congenital ptosis is the same procedure as it is for involutional ptosis. The operation is more difficult, however, because you will have to estimate the amount of resection. This takes some experience; consequently, most ophthalmologists do not operate on children with ptosis.

There are as many techniques for estimating the amount of resection as there are surgeons. All techniques are based on one of two well-known principles for estimating the amount of resection. The *levator function technique* assumes that the eyelid height, set during general anesthesia, will elevate or drop a predictable amount after the operation based on the patient's levator function. The easiest way to remember this is to *set the intraoperative lid height where you want the lid to be when the patient wakes up if the levator function is 5–6 mm.* If the levator function is less than 5–6 mm you must advance the aponeurosis more to set the lid height higher than what you want postoperatively. For more than 5–6 mm of levator function, you must set the lid height lower, expecting that the levator will lift the lid more than the orbicularis muscle will cause it to drop (Box 8-9). *In this technique, the amount of advancement is determined intraoperatively.*

The second technique, which we will call the *MRD technique*, is based on the amount of ptosis present preoperatively. With this technique, the levator aponeurosis is advanced a certain amount, depending on the preoperative MRD. There is no adjustment based on levator function. *The amount of resection is determined preoperatively.* For mild ptosis (MRD$_1$ of 3 mm), the resection would be 10–13 mm. For severe ptosis (MRD$_1$ of 0 mm), the amount of resection would be 23 mm or more (Box 8-10).

Although these techniques seem quite different, they are similar in principle because the degree of ptosis is usually related to the amount of levator function. I rely mainly on the *levator function technique*, but combine the estimates (part of the "art" of ptosis surgery). If a patient has moderate ptosis with an MRD$_1$ of 2 mm and the levator function is 6 mm, I start with a resection of about 16 mm. If the intraoperative height is lower than where I want it postoperatively, I will resect a little more. If the intraoperative lid height is higher than where I want it to be, I will back off a few millimeters. You can see that the amount to resect is an educated guess. *A good rule to follow is that, if you don't think the lid is high enough intraoperatively, resect more. It is difficult to overcorrect congenital ptosis.*

You should notice that the least amount of resection is 10 mm. Whitnall's ligament is usually at about 13 mm in a child so

---

Box 8-9

The Levator Advancement Operation

Prepare the patient
- For local anesthesia, use light intravenous anesthesia
- Mark an upper lid skin crease incision
- Inject local anesthetic with epinephrine

Make a skin incision
- Place a 4-0 silk traction suture
- Make a skin incision
- Open the orbicularis muscle

Identify the levator aponeurosis
- Dissect the orbicularis off the orbital septum
- Open the septum
- Dissect the septum off the preaponeurotic fat
- Dissect the preaponeurotic fat off the aponeurosis

Dissect the levator aponeurosis off Müller's muscle
- Disinsert the levator aponeurosis from the anterior surface of the tarsus
- Dissect the aponeurosis free from Müller's muscle

Advance the levator aponeurosis onto the tarsus
- Pass a double-armed 5-0 nylon suture into the tarsus in a lamellar fashion
- Pass the arms of the suture through the aponeurosis
- Pull the aponeurosis inferiorly against the tarsus as you tie a temporary knot

Make intraoperative adjustments
- Aim for a 1 mm overcorrection
- Alter the horizontal position of the suture in the tarsus to change the contour
- Alter the vertical position of the suture in the aponeurosis to change the lid height
- Tie the knot permanently when satisfied with the height and contour

Close the skin
- Reform the skin crease (optional)
- Use a running suture to close the skin

Box 8-10

Estimating the Amount of Resection for Simple Congenital Ptosis

Levator function technique (based on Berke, 1959)

Levator function	Intraoperative lid height
2–3 mm (poor function)	At upper limbus
4–5 mm (poor function)	1–2 mm overlap
6–7 mm (fair function)	2 mm overlap
8–9 mm (good function)	3–4 mm overlap
10–11 mm (good function)	5 mm overlap

MRD technique (based on Beard, 1981)

Preoperative MRD1	Amount of resection
3–4 mm (mild ptosis)	10–13 mm
2–3 mm (moderate ptosis)	14–17 mm
1–2 mm (marked ptosis)	18–22 mm
0–1 mm (severe ptosis)	>23 mm

you will need to *dissect above Whitnall's ligament in all children except those with the mildest ptosis*. This operation is usually called a *levator muscle resection*.

You will almost never need to resect above Whitnall's ligament in patients with involutional ptosis. *It is best not to operate on patients with simple congenital ptosis until you are very comfortable with levator aponeurosis advancement in adults.*

The frontalis sling operation

The most common indication for the frontalis sling operation is simple congenital ptosis with poor levator function, but the operation is used for any type of ptosis with poor levator function. Any of a variety of suspension materials can be used to "sling" the lid open. The "gold standard" has been autogenous fascia lata harvested from the patient's thigh. More commonly now, tissue bank fascia is used. Many surgeons prefer using alloplastic materials. Regardless of the material, the technique is nearly the same.

The frontalis sling operation includes:

- Patient preparation
- Skin incisions
- Suturing of the fascia to tarsus
- Passing the fascia to the brow
- Skin crease closure
- Adjustment of height and contour
- Closure of forehead incisions

The steps of the frontalis sling operation are:

1. Prepare the patient
   A. The operation is usually performed under *general anesthesia in children,* but can be performed under *local anesthesia in adults.*
   B. Mark an *upper lid skin crease incision* and *2–3 mm blepharoplasty* in most children.
   C. Mark *three 4 mm incisions on the forehead.* Place an incision just above the brow hairs slightly medial to the medial canthus and slightly lateral to the lateral canthus. Mark a third incision 1–2 cm above the brow in line with the pupil (Figure 8-12, A).
   D. Inject local anesthetic with epinephrine into the proposed incision site.
   E. Prepare and drape the patient.
2. Make the skin incisions
   A. Use a 4-0 silk suture as a traction suture through the lid margin (Ethicon 783 P-3 cutting needle).
   B. Use a no. 15 blade to *open the brow incisions* down to the periosteum.
      (1) Try not to cut the supraorbital neurovascular bundle.
      (2) Spread the wound open with a hemostat. You will need to "seat" the knot of the fascia in this wound later.
      (3) You will see some bleeding that usually stops with pressure.
   C. *Incise the skin crease* with a no. 15 blade or a Colorado needle.
   D. *Identify the levato*r using the same technique as in the levator advancement procedure.
3. Suture the fascia to the tarsus

A. "Bare" the superior half of the tarsus by dissecting the orbicularis off the tarsus.
B. Suture the fascia to the tarsus (5-0 polyester, Davis and Geck 2828-23 D-1 spatula needle). You will need two strips of fascia for each eyelid (Figure 8-12, B).
   (1) Suture the middle of the length of the first strip of fascia to the upper third of the tarsus at the peak of the lid.
   (2) Suture the same piece of fascia to the tarsus at the *medial limbus.*
   (3) Repeat with the second strip of fascia, sewing it next to the first suture and then at the *lateral limbus.*
4. Pass the fascia
   A. Thread the fascia onto a *Mayo trocar* (this is a thick needle used for general surgical closures, made by Richard Allen Medical (http://www.ramedical.co.uk, available through Aspen Surgical Products, 888 364 7004, half-circle, style 216703).
   B. *You will pass the fascia through the skin crease incision under the orbital septum and out the brow wounds* using a Webster needle holder (Figure 8-12, C).
      (1) Place a *Jaeger lid plate* in the superior conjunctival fornix to protect the eye (with experience, you may find it easier not to use the lid plate).
      (2) Load the fascia through the needle eye. Pass the needle though the crease incision posterior to the septum. As you advance superiorly, *skim under the periosteum* inferior to the superior orbital rim (don't pass the needle into the periosteum directly at the rim or the fascia will not move).
      (3) Pass the *medial fascia strip ends* out the medial brow incision.
      (4) Pass the *lateral fascia strip ends* out the lateral brow incision.
      (5) This pattern makes two small triangles from the tarsus to the brow (the Crawford technique, see Figure 8-12).
   C. Inspect the lid contour.
      (1) Pull the fascia superiorly through the brow incisions. Tug on the sutures independently to make the best eyelid contour.
      (2) If the contour is good, proceed to the skin crease closure. If the contour is not reasonable, repass the tarsal sutures laterally or medially to give a natural lid contour.
5. Close the skin crease
   A. Use two or three interrupted 7-0 Vicryl sutures (Ethicon J-546) to form the skin crease (remember that poor levator function means no natural crease). Pass the suture through the skin edge to the top of the tarsus and then out the opposite skin edge. Follow with a running suture using 5-0 fast absorbing gut.
6. Adjust the height and contour
   A. Pull the fascia superiorly again to adjust the height. *Tie the fascia so that the lid margin is at the limbus* (Figure 8-12, D).

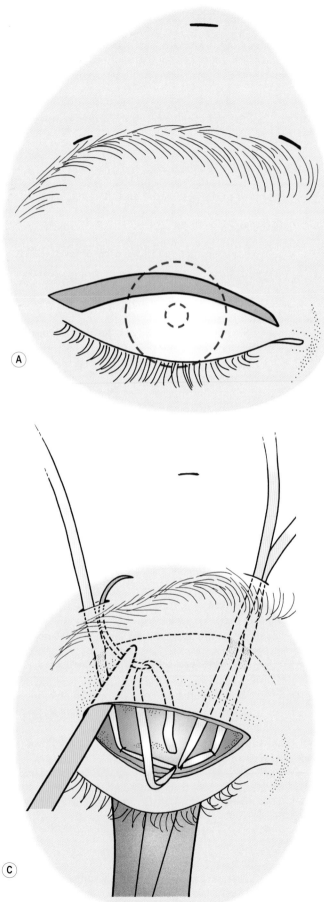

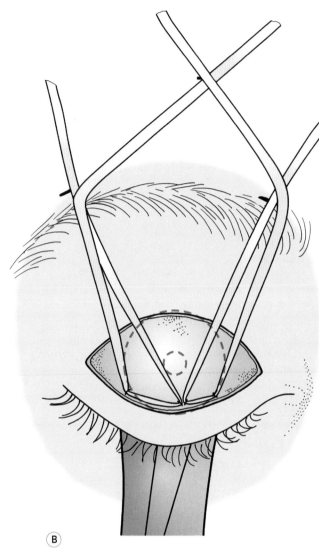

Figure 8-12 The frontalis sling operation. (**A**) Mark a 2–3-mm blepharoplasty ellipse at the skin crease. Mark brow wounds medial to the lateral canthus and lateral to the supraorbital notch. Mark a third incision 1.5 cm above the brow just nasal to the pupil. (**B**) Place a 4-0 silk traction suture. Excise the skin muscle flap and bare the anterior surface of the tarsus. Suture the fascia strips to the tarsus using a 5-0 polyester suture. (**C**) Pass the fascia under the orbital septum near the arcus marginalis and out the brow wounds using a Mayo trocar. Note the Jaeger lid plate in position protecting the eye. Close the skin crease using skin crease-forming sutures. (**D**) Tie the fascia at the brow wounds, adjusting the height and contour to rest at the upper limbus. (**E**) Pass one end of each fascia strip out the apical incision and make a final tie. Close the brow wounds with absorbable suture.

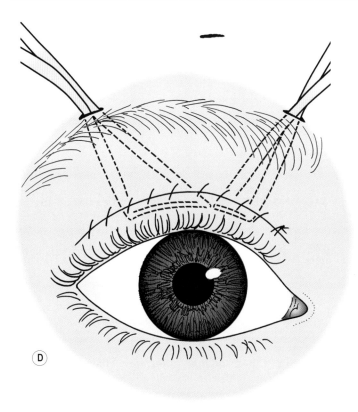

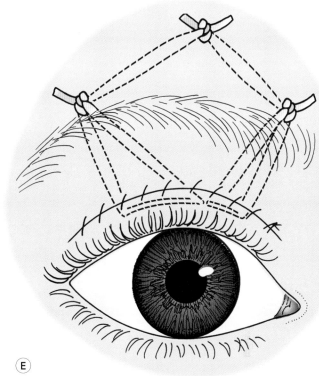

Figure 8-12 Continued.

(1) Use a square knot tied over a piece of 5-0 Vicryl suture. Tie the Vicryl suture over the square knot so it will not slip. Three throws of fascia in the knot usually makes an unacceptably large knot that can be visible through the skin.

(2) Cut one end of fascia off 1 cm past the knot.

B. Pass the long end of each piece of fascia out the central incision using the Mayo trocar.

(1) Tie the knot in the same way. Trim the ends of the fascia.

(2) Use a smooth forceps to slip the ends of the fascia under the frontalis muscle.

7. Close the forehead incisions

A. Use 5-0 fast absorbing gut suture with interrupted passes (Figure 8-12, E).

8. Provide postoperative care

A. *Place a 4-0 silk suture through the lower lid margin* and tape to the forehead (Frost suture) to avoid postoperative exposure.

B. *Remove the Frost suture* on the first postoperative day.

C. Use frequent doses of *lubricating ointment* for the first week and taper as tolerated.

D. Use *topical and oral antibiotics* for 1 week.

The frontalis sling operation is easier than the levator aponeurosis operation. The anatomic structure is simpler, and the adjustment is less subjective. Passing the fascia is somewhat intimidating initially, but it is safe if you control the needle. The results are good, but often there is some slight asymmetry. Long-term corneal exposure is rarely a problem in children.

For newborn children with a severe ptosis with poor levator function that is likely to cause amblyopia, a frontalis sling should be performed early, especially if the ptosis is unilateral. For a healthy term baby, the risk of a general anesthetic is minimal after 1 month of age. The Supramid "ski" needle and suture (3-0 Supramid Extra II 2GS-2-30, S. Jackson, Inc., http://www.supramid.com) is a convenient and effective way to suspend the eyelid open. Standard eyebrow/forehead incisions are made. No eyelid crease incision is required. Rather, two 1 mm horizontal "stab" incisions are made just above the eyelashes where the "ski" needle slides on the tarsus under the orbicularis. The sling is passed in the pentagon pattern, and the Supramid is tied at the most superior forehead wound (Figure 8-13 shows the postoperative appearance after Supramid). Although cheese wiring can occur over time, this technique usually keeps the upper eyelid elevated for a few years until a more permanent suspension material can be placed, usually at age 4–5 years. When the permanent sling material is passed, a small blepharoplasty is performed with attention to forming a deep skin crease (Box 8-11).

Dynarod frontalis sling operation

The frontalis sling operation can be performed using any number of alloplastic materials. A useful material is the silicone rod known as a Dynarod (Dynarod eyelid prosthesis, Roger Klein, Palmer, Puerto Rico, Fax: 787 888 8071). As

Box 8-11

Frontalis Sling Operation

Patient preparation

- Use general anesthesia for children or local anesthesia for adults
- Mark the upper lid skin crease incision and three forehead incisions

Skin incisions

- Make the forehead incisions and form a pocket
- Incise the lid crease
- Identify the levator
- Suture the fascia to the tarsus
- "Bare" the tarsus and secure each strip with 5-0 polyester

Pass the fascia to the forehead

- Use a Mayo trocar
- Go behind the septum and out the brow wounds
- Inspect and adjust the tarsal sutures, if necessary

Close the skin crease

- Form the skin crease with sutures
- Use a running suture for skin closure

Adjust the height and contour

- Tie the fascia at the brow
- Pass the fascia to the forehead incision and tie
- Bury the ends of the fascia
- Close the forehead wounds

this material can be adjusted or removed any time after surgery, you will find it especially useful for your patients who are at high risk for corneal exposure (patients with ptosis who have poor levator function and incomplete closure, most commonly those with myogenic ptoses). The height can be adjusted because the rod is not fibrosed into the tissues as happens with fascia strips.

The technique is similar to that described above with a few modifications. The rod is sutured to the tarsus in a similar fashion, but it is passed in a pentagon pattern (the Fox technique) using one piece of silicone rod tied at the apex of the pentagon. Two or three 3 mm segments of Watzke no. 270 sleeve are passed over the ends of the rod, securing the length of the rod (the sleeve that comes with the Dynarod seems too loose). A length of 5-0 polyester suture (the same as that used for the tarsal sutures) is tied around each sleeve to prevent slipping. A knot is tied beyond the sleeves. Should any postoperative lowering of the lid be required, the forehead wound can be opened and one or two of the inferior sleeves can be cut off, allowing the lid to drop (Figure 8-14). You will find that lowering (or raising) the sling is not necessary in most patients. Knowing that adjustments are possible gives you the confidence to raise the eyelid higher than you might otherwise. I like the option on these patients, especially when orbicularis weakness coexists.

The Dynarod silicone sling is also a useful operation for apraxia of lid opening that occurs in some patients with essential blepharospasm.

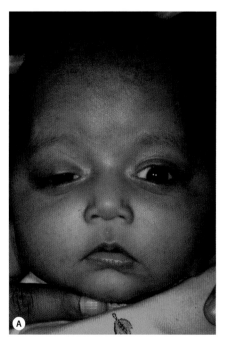 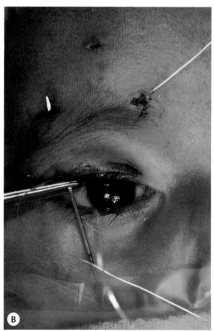 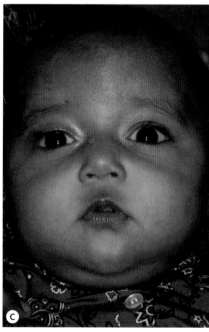

Figure 8-13 Frontalis sling with Supramid suture in newborn with severe congenital ptosis. (**A**) Right upper eyelid pupil covered most of the day. (**B**) Supramid suture on ski needle passed in pentagon pattern. (**C**) 1 week after Supramid suture frontalis sling using pentagon pattern.

Checkpoint

- At this point, you know how to treat most patients with ptosis. For patients with good levator function, do a levator aponeurosis advancement operation. For patients with poor levator function, do a frontalis sling operation.
- Children with reduced function (greater than 3–4 mm) will usually not have corneal exposure after aponeurosis advancement. It may be difficult to fully correct the lid height, however. Adults with reduced levator function (<15 mm but >10 mm) will usually do well with an aponeurosis advancement, unless there are risk factors for corneal exposure. You can see that, when you have to treat patients whose levator function is not at the extremes (totally absent or totally normal), the "rules" have to be adjusted individually for each patient.

Unusual types of ptosis

Before we proceed with this section, I want to emphasize that unusual types of ptosis are rare (by definition, but really true). Rather than spending lots of time on these now, make sure that you understand the presentations and physical findings of simple congenital and involutional ptosis, which are more commonly seen. Remember that, by learning all about the common things, you will develop a sense of when

a patient's situation does not fit a familiar pattern. With time, you will be able to identify unusual presentations quickly. Look at Box 8-12 for an overview of unusual types of ptosis. In this section, we will present each of these unusual types of ptosis with minimal detail.

Box 8-12

Unusual Types of Ptosis

Congenital ptosis

- Superior rectus weakness
- Marcus Gunn jaw winking
- Blepharophimosis syndrome

Acquired ptosis

- Neurogenic
  - Myasthenia gravis
  - Third nerve palsy
- Myogenic causes
  - Oculopharyngeal dystrophy
  - Chronic progressive external ophthalmoplegia
  - Post traumatic: Damage to the levator muscle
- Involutional ptosis
  - True "aponeurotic" disinsertion
- Post traumatic: Damage to aponeurosis
  - Lid swelling, blepharochalasis syndrome
- Pseudoptosis
  - Hemifacial spasm
  - Facial nerve palsy with aberrant regeneration
  - Contralateral lid retraction

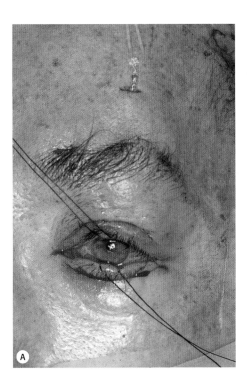
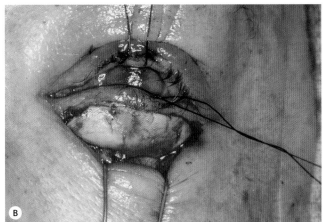

Figure 8-14 Dynarod adjustable silicone sling. (**A**) Adjustable silicone sling (Dynarod) for patients with ptosis at high risk for corneal exposure who require a frontalis sling operation. (**B**) An ear cartilage graft is placed to raise the lower eyelid. In this case, it is placed at the time of the sling procedure in a patient with a myotonic dystrophy (poor levator function, weak facial muscles, and poor Bell's phenomenon).

Unusual types of congenital ptosis

Superior rectus weakness

The typical form of congenital ptosis is said to be associated with a weak superior rectus in approximately 5% of patients. The common origin of the superior rectus and levator muscles probably explains this relation. The weakness is not easy to see because it is often difficult to examine the motility in these patients because of their age and the fact that the low upper lid obscures the view of the eye in upgaze. Weakness of the superior rectus muscle has little clinical implication. In some patients, the Bell's phenomenon may be reduced, but this rarely changes the approach to therapy in children.

Marcus Gunn jaw winking

This uncommon type of ptosis is one of the most striking. A "miswiring" of the cranial nerve V (to the pterygoid muscles) gets misdirected to cranial nerve III (to the levator muscle) causing the drooping upper eyelid to elevate with movements of the mouth (Figure 8-15). The term *synkinesis* (*same movement*) is used to describe this abnormal innervation. The parents usually note that the upper lid is ptotic and that sucking causes the upper eyelid to bob up and down. In many patients, the upper lid actually retracts above the normal position. Usually the ptosis is severe, and the movement is obvious. There is a range in presentations, however. In some patients, the ptosis will be mild and the movement almost imperceptible. You should look for Marcus Gunn jaw winking in all children with congenital ptosis by having the child eat or chew gum during the examination.

The usual patient with severe ptosis, poor levator function, and significant synkinesis will require extirpation of the levator to eliminate the abnormal movement and a frontalis sling operation to elevate the upper lid. A few patients will have minimal ptosis with good levator function and minimal synkinesis. You can use the standard levator aponeurosis advancement operation for these patients. It is said that patients may "outgrow" this condition. It seems more likely that patients learn how to control the movements of the mouth to minimize the abnormal lid movement.

Blepharophimosis syndrome

This congenital syndrome consists of *ptosis, epicanthus inversus, and blepharophimosis of the eyelids* (Figure 8-16). Blepharophimosis is inherited as an autosomal dominant disorder, so often the family is familiar with the condition. Many times, the condition is seen sporadically, so more explanation will be required in these patients. Typically, the ptosis is bilaterally symmetric and severe and is associated with poor levator function. As you would expect, there is wide range of expression. The epicanthus inversus is seen as a medial canthal fold of skin extending from the lower eyelid to the upper eyelid (remember the more common epicanthal folds originate in the upper eyelid). The horizontal aperture of the eyelid is narrowed both laterally and medially (phimosis). Telecanthus, lateral ectropion of the lower eyelids, and low-set ears with an abnormal shape are often seen. Intelligence is normal, although the facial appearance may suggest otherwise.

The ptosis is usually treated with a frontalis sling operation. Occasionally, enough levator function is present to lift the lid using the aponeurosis advancement operation. Additional procedures can be performed to improve the epicanthal folds, telecanthus, and ectropion when necessary. Considerable improvements can be made, but the final result is often less than perfect.

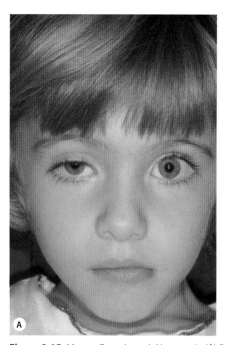
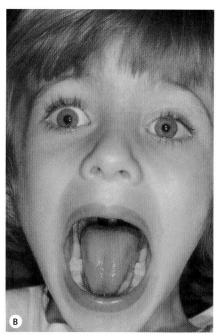

Figure 8-15 Marcus Gunn jaw winking ptosis. (**A**) Ptotic right upper eyelid at rest. (**B**) Synkinetic upper lid retraction seen with the mouth open.

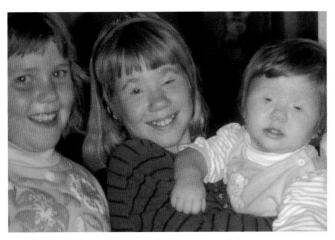

Figure 8-16 Blepharophimosis syndrome: autosomal dominant trait present in two of three siblings. Note the ptosis with poor levator function (absent skin crease), epicanthus inversus, telecanthus, and phimosis.

Unusual types of acquired ptosis

As you can see, there are many types of ptosis. Don't lose sight of what you have already learned by trying to memorize all these types. *Keep the basic concepts in mind.* Traditionally, ptosis is divided into types based on etiology:

- Neurogenic
- Myogenic
- Post-traumatic
- Pseudoptosis

We will use this classification to help organize the unusual types of ptosis. For the most part, these are self-explanatory. Patients with neurogenic ptosis have an abnormality in the innervation of the levator muscle. We already saw an example of Marcus Gunn jaw winking ptosis earlier under "Unusual Types of Congenital Ptosis." Patients with myogenic types of ptosis have normal innervation, but an abnormal muscle.

Post-traumatic ptosis usually involves scarring of the levator aponeurosis or muscle. Patients with pseudoptosis appear to have ptosis but, on close inspection, the MRD_1 is normal.

Neurogenic ptosis

Myasthenia gravis

Myasthenia gravis is an autoimmune disorder where the number of acetylcholine receptors at the neuromuscular junction is reduced. The poor conduction of the nerve results in weakness of the affected muscles. The ptosis is typically *variable*. You may see a change in the lid position from minute to minute, or changes occurring throughout the day. Remember that normal lids get slightly more droopy as the day goes on, so you shouldn't let this confuse you. Myasthenia gravis is classically associated with *diplopia*, but this has not been a helpful symptom for me to rely on. If diplopia is present, it should alert you to the possibility of myasthenia gravis, but the absence of symptoms of diplopia does not exclude the diagnosis. Systemic disease may or may not be present.

Ask your patients if the drooping remains constant during the day. If a patient tells you that the eyelid position changes dramatically, ask him or her to look up and hold the position for 30–60 seconds. If myasthenia gravis is present, the eyelid will *fatigue* and slowly drop as available neurotransmitter is used up in sustained upgaze (Figure 8-17).

Edrophonium (Tensilon) testing is the standard for the diagnosis of ptosis secondary to myasthenia gravis. Intravenous injection of Tensilon (or intramuscular injection of neostigmine, Prostigmine) will result in temporary elevation of the ptotic eyelid. The "ice test" has been suggested to diagnose myasthenia gravis. Cooling of the eyelid allows the lid to elevate temporarily.

Oral pyridostigmine (Mestinon, an acetylcholinesterase inhibitor) is the treatment of choice. Immunosuppression with steroids or other medications can be helpful. Thymectomy helps many patients, even those without a thymoma. If medical therapy is unsuccessful, surgical ptosis correction can be considered in select patients. Both levator aponeurosis advancement and frontalis sling operations have been used to improve the eyelid height, the choice depending on the levator function and the frontalis muscle activity. The variability remains, however. The presence of diplopia can preclude the possibility of successful eyelid elevation.

Third nerve palsy

Damage to the third nerve by trauma, infection, tumor, or compression causes a ptosis of the upper eyelid associated with diplopia (Figure 8-18, A). Occasionally, the palsy may be congenital. In these patients, the presence of amblyopia may preclude symptoms of diplopia. The nerve weakness may range from mild to severe. Similarly, levator function may be absent or near normal. In some patients, the palsy may be temporary.

For most patients, the main problem is not the ptosis, but the motility abnormality. The typical noncomitant strabismus makes single vision in all fields of gaze impossible. Elevation of the eyelid is possible using either a frontalis sling or a levator aponeurosis advancement operation, but surgery is usually not performed unless the motility problem can be addressed.

Many patients develop *aberrant regeneration of the third nerve*. After injury, the nerve will regenerate, but often the reinnervation is misdirected. Any branch of the third nerve may reinnervate the levator muscle. Synkinesis, in this case causing eyelid elevation, occurs when any branch of the misdirected nerve is stimulated. Typically, the ptotic upper eyelid retracts with contraction of the medial rectus or inferior rectus muscle, further complicating any repair (Figure 8-18, B). Often the pupil will show constriction with eye movements as well.

Horner's syndrome

In Chapter 2, we talked about loss of the sympathetic tone to the face causing *Horner's syndrome* (*upper lid ptosis, lower lid elevation, miosis*, and *anhidrosis of the ipsilateral side of the face*). Horner's syndrome is rare, but presents an interesting clinicoanatomic correlation (i.e., test question) that every resident needs to know. Horner's syndrome presents as a *mild ptosis with normal levator function*. It can be confused with ordinary involutional ptosis, but there are usually a few

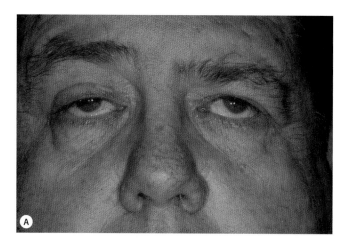

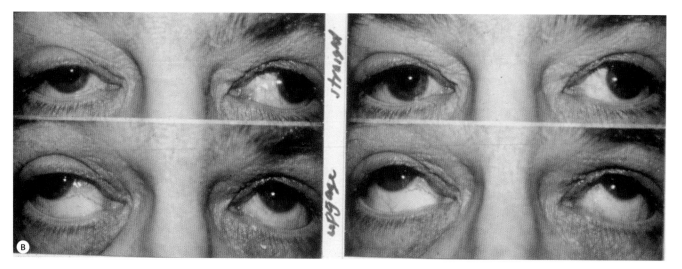

Figure 8-17 Ptosis secondary to myasthenia gravis. (**A**) Note exotropia and ptosis. Patient had variable ptosis and diplopia. (**B**) After an edrophonium (Tensilon) test (seen on lower right), the ptosis, exotropia, and elevation of the eye are improved.

clues present that will help you make the diagnosis. The associated *miosis* is usually the most obvious difference. The *lower lid elevation* may be apparent or more subtle (Figure 8-19). The anhidrosis is not visible, but many patients are aware of it if you ask. Your patient may note that the *onset* of the ptosis occurred after a chest or neck operation (in this case, you can't miss the diagnosis). Often the patient will be younger than expected for an involutional etiology. Understanding the sympathetic pathway and simple testing with eye drops will help to determine if a patient with Horner's syndrome has a *life-threatening problem or just an annoying situation.*

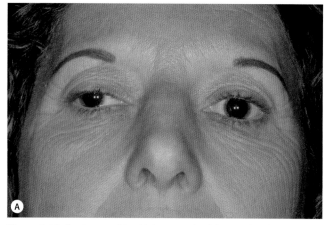

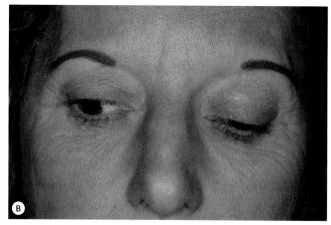

Figure 8-18 Ptosis caused by third nerve palsy. (**A**) Note that the right eye is exotropic and hypotropic. The patient has a true ptosis and a pseudoptosis secondary to the hypotropia. (**B**) Note the synkinetic elevation of the right upper eyelid with inferior rectus contraction due to aberrant regeneration of the third nerve.

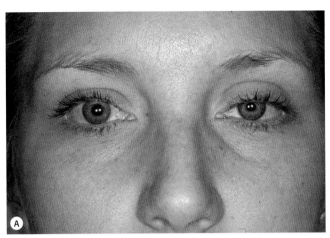 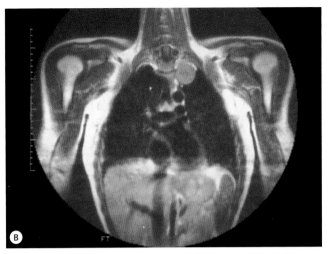

Figure 8-19 Ptosis resulting from Horner's syndrome. (**A**) Note the ptosis of the upper eyelid, the very mild "upside ptosis" of the lower eyelid, and the miosis. (**B**) This Horner's syndrome followed resection of a neurilemmoma.

Interruption of sympathetic innervation may occur at one of three anatomic areas:

- Within the central nervous system (first-order neurons)
- Between the spinal cord and superior cervical ganglion (second-order neurons)
- Between the superior cervical ganglion and the orbit (third-order neuron)

In Horner's syndrome with a *central nervous system cause*, other signs of disease are seen in the brainstem or spinal cord. *Second-order neuron damage* (so-called *preganglionic Horner's syndrome* because the interruption occurs before the superior cervical ganglion) may be caused by a chest or neck tumor (apical lung cancer, mediastinal lymphoma), cervical trauma, or congenital abnormalities ("cervical rib"). *Third-order neuron damage* (so-called *postganglionic Horner's syndrome* because the interruption occurs after the superior cervical ganglion) is usually not caused by malignancy.

Pharmacologic testing can help you determine if Horner's syndrome is present and determine a preganglionic or postganglionic etiology. *Topical cocaine drops will confirm the diagnosis of Horner's syndrome.* Cocaine prevents the reuptake of norepinephrine, causing dilation of any pupil innervated with an intact neural pathway. Interruption of the sympathetic innervation at any location will prevent dilation of the pupil with cocaine. Therefore, if the pupil of your patient with slight ptosis and miosis *does not dilate with cocaine drops,* you have confirmed the diagnosis of Horner's syndrome. Testing can also be performed using 0.5% apraclonidine (Iopidine) drops. The α_1 stimulation will cause the *hypersensitive pupil to dilate and the eyelid to rise* if there is a Horner's syndrome present.

Topical hydroxyamphetamine 1% (Paredrine) drops have been used to determine whether the block is preganglionic or postganglionic. By stimulating the release of norepinephrine at the neuromuscular junction of the third-order neuron, hydroxyamphetamine reverses the signs of preganglionic Horner's syndrome. Postganglionic Horner's syndrome will not improve with the use of hydroxyamphetamine drops because the third-order neuron is not functioning and has no neurotransmitter that can be released. Dilation with hydroxyamphetamine drops indicates a preganglionic cause (between the spinal cord and the superior cervical ganglion). Unfortunately, recently, the Federal Drug Administration (FDA) has withdrawn hydroxyamphetamine from the market. Currently, there is no other clinical test that is useful for localization of the interrupted pathway.

The ptosis of Horner's syndrome can be repaired using a slight advancement of the levator aponeurosis. Some surgeons prefer to use a resection of conjunctiva and Müller's muscle (not discussed in this text) for Horner's syndrome. Topical dilute phenylephrine (Neo-Synephrine) drops or apraclonidine 0.5% (Iopidine) can be used occasionally for temporary improvement of the upper lid ptosis (for photographs or important social occasions).

Myogenic ptosis

The common theme in this category is a primary muscle abnormality. Reduced levator function is typical so a frontalis sling operation is often required. Often the facial muscle activity and ocular motility are also reduced, complicating even a conservative frontalis sling operation. Corneal exposure is common postoperatively. In most patients with progressive myogenic ptosis, I use an adjustable and fully reversible suspension material such as the Dynarod silicone sling discussed above. As a group, these patients have the most difficult ptosis to manage.

Oculopharyngeal dystrophy

A muscular dystrophy is a progressive form of muscle wasting and atrophy of the muscle cells. Oculopharyngeal dystrophy (OPD) and myotonic dystrophy are examples of muscular dystrophies affecting the eye and periocular muscles. Oculopharyngeal dystrophy is a familial condition in which progressive bilateral ptosis develops in association with facial weakness and difficulty swallowing (Figure

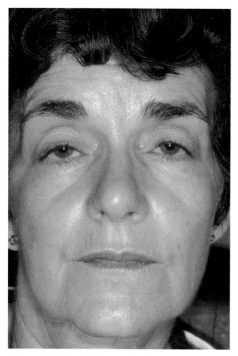

Figure 8-20 Oculopharyngeal dystrophy. Note the moderately severe ptosis with associated facial weakness in a patient with dysphagia. The patient was of French Canadian ancestry.

8-20). This dystrophy is the most common of the myogenic ptoses seen. The condition has its onset in the 40s. Probably you will recognize this condition because of the patient's flat facial expression. Swallowing problems are usually not severe at the time of initial presentation of the ptosis, but may be brought out by asking the patient to drink a glass of ice water rapidly. The classic family pedigree is of *French Canadian descent*, but many patients will not recall any French Canadian ancestry. Inheritance is autosomal dominant. Many patients will know of relatives who have ptosis and may have had some ptosis procedure in the past. Often you will see other family members after a successful ptosis repair.

Initially, the ptosis is mild with good levator function. A levator aponeurosis advancement operation is effective in these patients. Although the rate of progression is variable, most patients will require a second operation within 10 years. Because the condition is progressive, you should consider a frontalis sling operation sooner than usual in these patients in an attempt to avoid a second operation. For example, you should consider a sling in a 50- to 60-year-old OPD patient with progressive ptosis and a levator function of 8 mm. A sling performed earlier than usual for other eyelid ptosis types will save a second operation. Most patients with oculopharyngeal dystrophy do well with eyelid elevation despite the associated facial weakness.

Myotonic dystrophy

This particular type of dystrophy is associated with myotonia or a failure of muscles to relax after a sustained contraction

and is less common than oculopharyngeal dystrophy. Facial and peripheral skeletal muscle weakness is the rule (Figure 8-21). Myotonic dystrophy, unlike oculopharyngeal dystrophy, is associated with abnormalities in other organ systems. Almost any other tissue or organ can be involved including the lenses (crystalline cataract or Christmas tree cataract, see Figure 8-21, B), the hair (frontal balding), the testicles (atrophy), and the brain (weak cognitive function and personality abnormalities in some). The condition is an autosomal dominant trait.

The ptosis is slowly progressive and can be mild or severe. Motility loss is usually mild, if present. Abnormalities in almost every part of the eye have been described. Usually a conservative frontalis sling operation is required to elevate the lids. Facial weakness may complicate repair.

Chronic progressive external ophthalmoplegia

Chronic progressive external ophthalmoplegia (CPEO) is a progressive myopathy affecting the external eye muscles bilaterally. Patients develop ptosis with an extreme loss of ocular motility, often to the point of no movement (Figure 8-22, A). The pupillary muscle fibers are spared (external ophthalmoplegia). Ptosis may precede the development of the motility problem. The orbicularis is usually weak as well, often compromising closure. In most patients, the condition occurs sporadically. You will not see many patients with CPEO.

A variant of CPEO, known as *Kearns–Sayre syndrome*, is associated with other tissue changes including heart block, a pigmentary retinopathy, and sometimes peripheral muscle weakness (Figure 8-22, B). There is overlap with this syndrome and other neurologic disorders (lumped together as *CPEO plus* syndromes). Patients with ptosis and limited motility should receive a neurologic workup.

Interestingly, patients with CPEO rarely experience diplopia despite the lack of conjugate eye movements. Conservative frontalis sling procedures are useful to lift the lids. Postoperative corneal exposure is common because of poor Bell's phenomenon, incomplete blink, and lack of eye movements. Patients often require additional procedures to minimize this dryness, making the ptosis associated with CPEO one of the most difficult types to manage.

Involutional ptosis

Notice that the same involutional ptosis that we have been talking about for the whole chapter is now being discussed in this section under one of the unusual types of ptosis types, myogenic ptosis. Why?

Most surgeons consider involutional ptosis to be "aponeurotic" in origin. It has been suggested since the 1960s that a thinning or disinsertion of the levator aponeurosis is the cause of involutional ptosis. The levator muscle is said to be normal. If you study these early articles, you will see that the emphasis was on the technique of advancing the aponeurosis (rather than shortening the levator muscle) as a viable treatment of involutional ptosis. Since that time, there have been articles discussing the role of the aponeurosis as the cause of involutional ptosis. *My personal belief is that many of the cases of involutional ptosis you will see are myogenic, not aponeurotic in origin.*

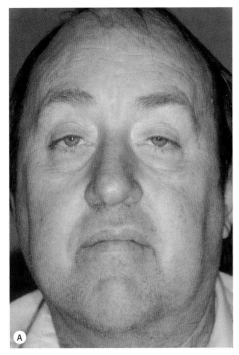

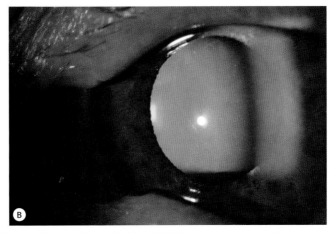

Figure 8-21 Myotonic dystrophy. (**A**) Myogenic ptosis, facial weakness, and frontal balding. (**B**) "Christmas tree" cataract of myotonic dystrophy.

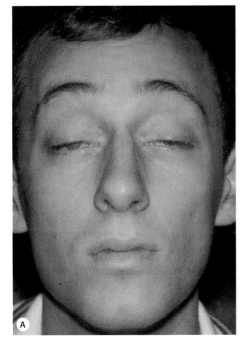

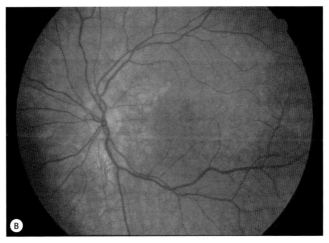

Figure 8-22 Ptosis resulting from chronic progressive external ophthalmoplegia (CPEO). (**A**) CPEO caused by defective mitochondria in the muscle cells. Note the ptosis with poor levator function and weak facial muscles. This patient had a total lack of eye movements. (**B**) Abnormalities may occur in the retina, heart, endocrine system, and central nervous system (CPEO plus). A pigmentary retinopathy is associated with the rare Kearns–Sayre syndrome (CPEO with heart block and retinopathy). This young man required a pacemaker.

Often the *levator function is reduced slightly*, in the range of 12 mm (good function when compared with congenital ptosis, but not normal). Watch the speed of the lid movement, and you will see that *excursion is slow* in many patients. Intraoperatively you will *rarely find a true disinsertion* of the aponeurosis. If you always did, it would be easy to get exactly the correct height. You will often find a *thinned aponeurosis with fatty infiltration seen in both Müller's muscle and the levator muscle*, suggesting a replacement of the normal muscle with fat, as seen elsewhere in skeletal muscles as a result of aging. We looked at 100 consecutive "involutional" ptosis patients and could demonstrate a "disinsertion" of the aponeurosis in only 5%. The majority of patients had fatty infiltration of the levator muscle and/or Müller's muscle, suggesting a myogenic, rather than an aponeurotic, cause. You will find that, in some of your involutional ptosis patients undergoing ptosis repair, an advancement of nearly the entire length of the aponeurosis will not give a normal postoperative lid height. I would consider this to be a myogenic problem. Time will tell if this theory holds true.

Post-traumatic ptosis

Any type of trauma to the levator muscle may weaken it. Any ptosis associated with a periocular laceration may be the result of damage to the levator muscle or aponeurosis. *All periocular lacerations should be inspected for the presence of orbital fat in the wound.* This means that the orbital septum has been violated and that damage to orbital structures may have occurred. If you see orbital fat, find some normal anatomic structures away from the wound that you recognize and follow the levator to ensure that no damage has occurred. You will be able to repair damage to the aponeurosis, such as an upper lid avulsion, with good results if anatomic repair can be made (Figure 8-23). If the muscle is damaged, your chance of success is reduced because of direct injury to the muscle and nerve tissue.

Scarring to adjacent structures may cause a postoperative ptosis as well.

Many surgeons believe that using *hard contact lenses* can induce an aponeurotic disinsertion as a result of the trauma of the lens rubbing on the back of the lid for many years. I personally have not seen this with any regularity, but it seems to be agreed upon by others.

Stretching of the eyelid tissues from post-traumatic swelling or rubbing of the eyes has been implicated as a cause of ptosis. Patients with recurrent bouts of idiopathic lid swelling, as seen in the *blepharochalasis syndrome*, can develop ptosis (Figure 8-24). Treatment of this type of ptosis, like that of any other, is based on the levator function. Most of these patients have normal levator function and can be treated with a levator aponeurosis advancement procedure and blepharoplasty.

Pseudoptosis

In some situations, the eyelid will appear to be low, but the levator function is not abnormal. The most common situation in my practice is patients with increased orbicularis tone who are squeezing the eyelid partially closed. This occurs in two situations: *aberrant regeneration of the facial nerve* or *hemifacial spasm*. Often the spasm is not noted or is not noted to be the actual cause of the ptosis (Figure 8-25). Beware of diagnosing ptosis in patients with facial movement abnormalities. You can reduce the spasm with botulinum toxin injections and often eliminate the "ptosis."

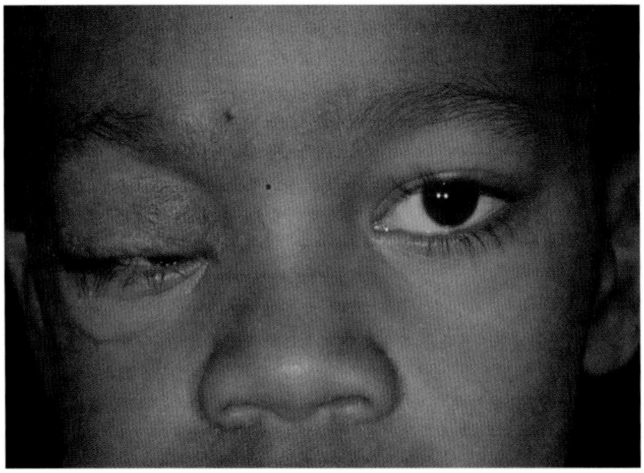

Figure 8-23 Traumatic ptosis. A 1 cm steel rod pushed through the upper eyelid and orbit into the brain of this child, leaving him with severe ptosis resulting from injury and scarring of the levator muscle.

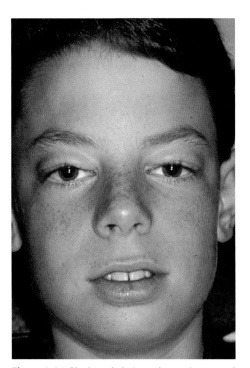

Figure 8-24 Blepharochalasis syndrome. A teenage boy with ptosis and dermatochalasis caused by recurrent episodes of eyelid swelling.

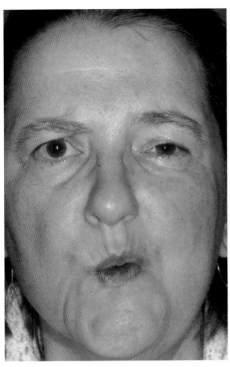

Figure 8-25 Pseudoptosis. The left upper eyelid height is low because of abnormal orbicularis contraction in this patient with aberrant regeneration of the facial nerve. This patient shows synkinesis of all the branches of the facial nerve. Note that the lower eyelid is elevated and the neck muscles are contracted.

Major points

The retractors of the upper eyelid are:

- The levator muscle
- Müller's muscle
- The frontalis muscle

Most types of ptosis are the result of a problem with the levator muscle complex.

The recognized parts of the levator muscle complex are the muscle, the aponeurosis, Whitnall's ligament, and the horns of the levator aponeurosis.

The levator muscle is innervated by the third cranial nerve and is under voluntary control.

Müller's muscle is innervated by the sympathetic nervous system.

The frontalis muscle is innervated by the facial nerve.

The condition or "health" of the eyelid can be identified by measuring the eyelid "vital signs":

- Margin reflex distance (MRD)
- Levator function
- Skin crease height and strength

The MRD is the distance from the corneal light reflex to the lid margin. The MRD_1 is the distance from the corneal light reflex to the upper lid margin (normally 4–5 mm.). The MRD_2 is the distance from the corneal light reflex to the lower lid margin (normally 5 mm).

The levator function is the excursion of the upper lid from extreme downgaze to extreme upgaze measured (normally 15 mm).

The upper eyelid skin crease is created by the pull of the levator aponeurosis on the skin. The skin crease height is the distance from the lid margin to the crease. This height varies among individuals, but averages 6–8 mm for men and 8–10 mm for women at the highest point.

A simplified classification system of ptosis includes:

- Simple congenital ptosis
- Involutional ptosis
- "Unusual" ptosis

Levator function is the key to the classification and treatment of ptosis.

Typically, simple congenital ptosis is associated with:

- Reduced levator function
- A weak or absent upper eyelid skin crease
- Lid lag on downgaze

Typically, involutional ptosis is associated with:

- Good levator function
- A high upper eyelid skin crease
- Lid drop on downgaze

The treatment of ptosis is based largely on the levator function.

- Ptosis with normal levator function is treated with a levator aponeurosis advancement operation
- Ptosis with poor levator function is treated with a frontalis sling operation

Major points Continued

Your goal for the history taking and physical examination is to obtain three important pieces of information:

- Identify the type of ptosis
- Formulate a treatment plan
- Identify factors that modify treatment

During the history taking and physical examination, you should look for information that would lead you to suspect an unusual type of ptosis:

- Any associated ocular or systemic abnormality
- A family history
- Synkinesis with the eyelids or face
- Extreme variability in lid height
- Decreased facial expression
- Anisocoria or relative afferent pupillary defect

Remember that the treatment plan for most patients with ptosis is based on confirming the diagnosis and the amount of levator function.

Factors that would modify your approach to or timing of ptosis repair include:

- Amblyopia
- Previous history of ptosis operations
- Risk factors for corneal exposure
- Patient general health concerns
- Patient preference
- Associated periocular findings

Patient concerns regarding ptosis may include:

- Loss of central vision
- Decreased peripheral vision
- Complaints regarding reading
- Heaviness of the eyes or eyebrows
- Headache, brow ache, or neck ache
- Issues of appearance

Review the steps of the levator aponeurosis advancement procedure (used for correction of ptosis in patients with greater than "poor" levator function). The better the levator function, the more easily the eyelid is lifted with an advancement procedure.

Review the steps of the frontalis sling procedure (use for patients with no or poor levator function).

Unusual types of ptosis have associated ocular or systemic abnormalities. The levator function is often reduced.

The unusual types of ptosis can be categorized as:

- Neurogenic
- Myogenic
- Post traumatic
- Pseudoptosis

Unusual types of ptosis with synkinesis include:

- Marcus Gunn jaw winking
- Third nerve palsy with aberrant regeneration
- Facial nerve paralysis with aberrant regeneration (pseudoptosis)

Unusual types of ptosis with family history include:

- Blepharophimosis syndrome
- Oculopharyngeal dystrophy
- Myotonic dystrophy

Unusual types of ptosis with facial weakness include:

- Oculopharyngeal dystrophy
- Myotonic dystrophy
- Facial nerve palsy with aberrant regeneration
- Myasthenia gravis (occasionally)

Horner's syndrome results from a loss of sympathetic tone. It includes mild ptosis, miosis, lower eyelid elevation, and anhidrosis of the ipsilateral face.

- Topical cocaine drops will confirm the diagnosis of Horner's syndrome. Topical apraclonidine 0.5% (Iopidine) will reverse the ptosis and anisocoria of Horner's syndrome.
- Traditionally, topical hydroxyamphetamine 0.5% (Paredrine) drops have been used to determine whether the block is preganglionic or postganglionic. Paredrine is currently not available, due to FDA prohibition of sales.

Suggested reading

1. Albert DM., Lucarelli MJ: Ptosis. In *Clinical atlas of procedures in ophthalmic surgery*, Chicago: AMA Press, 2004.

2. American Academy of Ophthalmology: *Basic and clinical science course: orbit, eyelids, and lacrimal system*, sect. 7, pp. 208–223, San Francisco: The American Academy of Ophthalmology, 2006/2007.

3. Anderson RL: Age of aponeurotic awareness. *Ophthal Plast Reconstr Surg* 1(1):77–79, 1985.

4. Anderson RL, Baumgartner SA: Strabismus in ptosis. *Arch Ophthalmol* 98(6):1062–1067, 1980.

5. Anderson RL, Dixon RS: Aponeurotic ptosis surgery. *Arch Ophthalmol* 97(6):1123–1128, 1979.

6. Beard C: *Ptosis*, St Louis: CV Mosby. 1981 (an older classic text).

7. Berke RN: Results of resection of the levator muscle through a skin incision in congenital ptosis. *Arch Ophthalmol* 61:177, 1959.

8. Dresner SC: Further modification of the Muller's muscle: conjunctival resection procedure for blepharoptosis. *Ophthal Plast Reconstr Surg* 7(2):114–122, 1991.

9. Jordan DR, Anderson RL: The aponeurotic approach to congenital ptosis. *Ophthal Surg* 21(4):237–244, 1990.

10. McCord C, ed.: Evaluation of the ptosis patient. In *Eyelid surgery principles and techniques*, ch. 7, pp. 99–112, Philadelphia: Lippincott-Raven, 1995.

11. McCord C, ed.: Levator surgery. In *Eyelid surgery principles and techniques*, ch. 8, pp. 113–126, Philadelphia: Lippincott-Raven, 1995.

12. McCord C, ed.: Frontalis suspension. In *Eyelid surgery principles and techniques*, ch. 9, pp. 127–137, Philadelphia: Lippincott-Raven, 1995.

13. McCord C, ed.: Decision making in ptosis surgery. In *Eyelid surgery principles and techniques*, ch. 10, pp. 138–143, Philadelphia: Lippincott- Raven, 1995.

14. McCord C, ed.: Complications of ptosis surgery and their management. In *Eyelid surgery principles and techniques*, ch. 11, pp. 144–155, Philadelphia: Lippincott-Raven, 1995.

15. Nerad J: Evaluation and treatment of the patient with ptosis. In *The requisites—Oculoplastic surgery*, pp. 157–192. St Louis: Mosby, 2001.

16. Nerad JA, Carter KD, Alford MA: Disorders of the eyelid: Blepharoptosis and eyelid retraction. In *Rapid diagnosis in ophthalmology—oculoplastic and reconstructive surgery*, pp. 102–115, Philadelphia: Mosby Elsevier, 2008.

17. Putnam JR, Nunery WR, Tanenbaum M, McCord CD: Blepharoptosis. In McCord CD, Tanenbaum M, Nunery WR, eds, *Oculoplastic surgery*, 3rd edn, ch.7, pp. 175–200, New York: Raven Press, 1995.

18. Putterman AM: Müller's muscle-conjunctiva resection. In Levine MR, ed., *Manual of oculoplastic surgery*, 3rd edn, pp. 117–123, Boston: Butterworth-Heinemann, 2003.

19. Shore JW, Bergin DJ, Garrett SN: Results of blepharoptosis surgery with early postoperative adjustment. *Ophthalmology* 97(11):1502–1511, 1990.

20. Striph GG, Miller NR: Disorders of eyelid function caused by systemic disease. In Bosniak S, ed., *Principles and practice of ophthalmic plastic and reconstructive surgery*, pp. 72–93, Philadelphia: WB Saunders, 1996.

Abnormal Movements of the Face

Introduction

Like most of our human functions, we take facial movements for granted. Quick, complete, and frequent blinks of the eyelids keep the cornea healthy. Narrowing of the eyelid fissures, or "guarding," protects an irritated eye. Reflex closure of the lids is a spontaneous reaction to avoid trauma to the eye. However, problems of both overactivity and underactivity of the facial muscles are common. Conditions related to overactivity of the facial muscles include:

- Orbicularis myokymia
- Facial tics
- Hemifacial spasm
- Essential blepharospasm

Problems of underactivity of the facial muscles are seen as well. A loss of facial expression is seen in patients with many of the myogenic ptoses that we have discussed and in patients with Parkinson's disease. *Facial nerve palsy* can occur from a number of conditions and results in typical anatomic and functional abnormalities, including incomplete eye closure and corneal exposure, ectropion, and brow ptosis.

These are situations that an oculoplastic surgeon sees daily in practice. The conditions are easily differentiated on a clinical basis and rarely require any sophisticated testing to confirm your clinical impression. Each condition of overactivity or underactivity requires a different therapeutic approach.

In this chapter, we will review the normal anatomy and function of the facial nerve and the muscles of facial expression. The pathologic conditions involving overactivity and underactivity of the facial muscles will be discussed separately. In each section, the important findings in the history and physical examination will be discussed to help you make the correct diagnosis and formulate an appropriate treatment plan. Lastly, the options for medical and surgical therapies are discussed for each disorder.

Anatomy and function

Facial nerve anatomy

The facial nerve extends from its origin in the brainstem to the innervation of the facial muscles. There are two areas of particular interest to us. The first is the point at which the facial nerve leaves the brainstem in close proximity to the fifth and eighth nerves. The second location is distal to the appearance of the facial nerve trunk in the face anterior to the tragus of the ear. From this point, the facial nerve trunk divides into five branches (Figure 9-1):

- Cervical
- Mandibular
- Buccal
- Orbital
- Frontal

These branches innervate groups of the facial muscles selectively. Depending on the cause, *facial nerve weakness* may involve the entire nerve or individual branches. Bell's palsy or injury to the nerve proximal to the branching of the facial nerve involves the entire face. Accidental or surgical trauma to the face can result in injury localized to one or more branches. All nerves have the ability to regenerate. Unfortunately, regeneration of the facial nerve after injury frequently occurs in a nonanatomic manner known as *aberrant regeneration of the facial nerve*. You may see this in a patient after a cheek laceration heals. If you look carefully, you may see

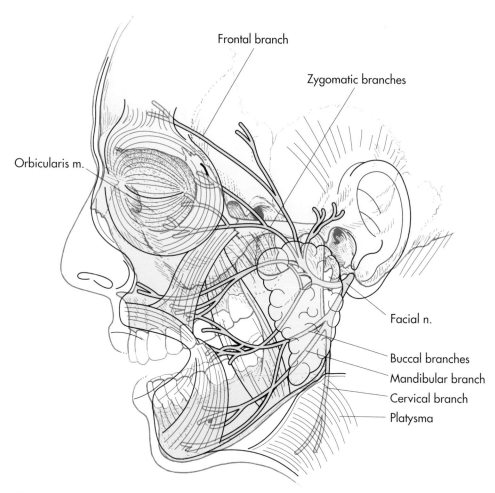

Figure 9-1 Branches of the facial nerve.

that the entire cheek moves as a whole. Similarly, after facial nerve palsy, all branches of the facial nerve will receive the same innervation. Pursing of the lips may also narrow the patient's palpebral fissure (Figure 9-2).

The facial muscles

All the muscles of the face are innervated by branches of the seventh nerve. The orbicularis muscle is responsible for eyelid closure. The orbicularis is divided into three areas. The *orbital orbicularis* causes forceful squeezing of the eye. The *preseptal* and *pretarsal* portions of the orbicularis are responsible for the quick blinks that lubricate the cornea. The orbicularis muscle receives innervation from several branches of the facial nerve such that localized trauma has to be fairly extensive to cause a significant paralysis of the orbicularis muscle. You will remember that both the corrugator and the procerus muscles are also innervated by the facial nerve (Figure 9-3). These muscles are known for the creation of the vertical and horizontal glabellar wrinkles respectively. The corrugator muscle also plays a prominent role in the forceful eyelid closure of essential blepharospasm.

The frontalis muscle lifts the eyebrows and forehead. It is innervated by a single branch of the facial nerve, the frontal branch. Injury to the frontal branch (also called the temporal branch) of the facial nerve may cause a permanent brow ptosis.

Loss of function to the lower facial muscles results in a drooping of the midface and lip as well. In patients with mild weakness, slight facial asymmetry and shallowing of the nasal labial fold will be noted. This asymmetry can be brought out by asking the patient to make a broad smile.

Overactivity of the facial muscles

Disorders

Orbicularis myokymia

Orbicularis myokymia is a common condition. It generally occurs in younger patients who note an involuntary twitching of the upper or lower eyelid. The abnormal movements are quick, lasting a second or less. The movements are easily noticed by the patient, but will require your close observation to see them. The movements result from spasm of individual bundles of muscle fibers. The muscle as a whole is not in spasm. Orbicularis myokymia is related to stress, fatigue, use of alcohol, or excessive caffeine.

Facial tics

Facial tics are voluntary movements of a group of facial muscles. In most situations, the patient is actually not aware that he or she is controlling the movements, however. The condition may be a unilateral spasm of the eye and side of

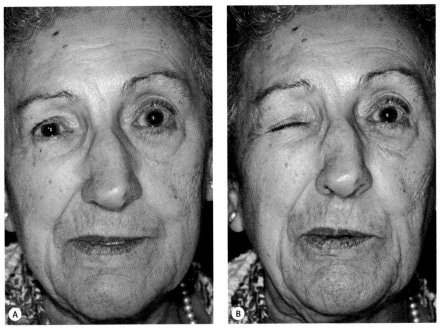

Figure 9-2 Aberrant regeneration of the facial nerve. (**A**) Right facial nerve palsy with mild tonic contracture of the right facial muscles. (**B**) Note that the palpebral fissure narrows with lip pursing.

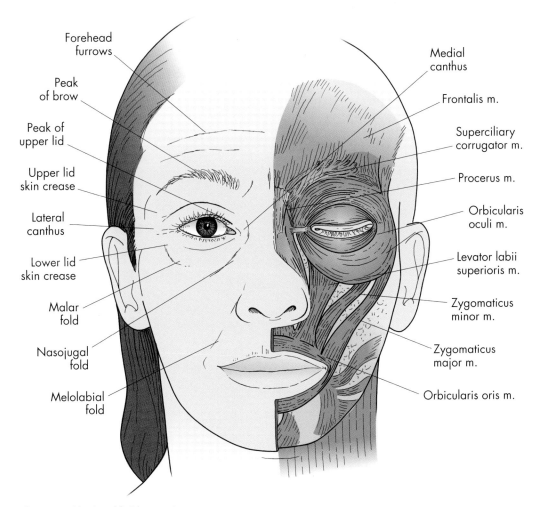

Figure 9-3 Muscles of facial expression.

the face or may be simply a bilateral increase in blinking rate. There is often some secondary gain obtained with the tic, although that is difficult to identify. Tics occur most commonly in children, but can also be seen in adults. Probably you have already seen patients with tics. We will discuss their diagnosis in more detail later.

Hemifacial spasm

Hemifacial spasm is an involuntary movement of one side of the face (Figure 9-4). The movement may be a quick apparent twitch or may be seen as a sustained spasm involving all the facial muscles on the side. The etiology of facial spasm is thought to be vascular compression of the facial nerve where the nerve leaves the brainstem. Frequently, the hemifacial spasm is accompanied by signs of mild facial weakness and aberrant regeneration.

Essential blepharospasm

Essential blepharospasm is an uncontrolled blinking or spasm of both eyes (Figure 9-5). Essential blepharospasm results from progressive degeneration of the central nervous system thought to occur in the basal ganglia. It is most commonly seen in elderly patients. Initially, the disorder may start as increased blinking, but it generally progresses to a more sustained spasm of both eyes with prominent orbital orbicularis and corrugator muscle activity. Abnormal movements of the lower face may be seen in association with essential blepharospasm, known as *Meige syndrome* (Figure 9-6).

History and physical examination of the overactive face

When diagnosing abnormal movements of the face, you will find that your history taking and physical examination

occur at the same time. You will learn to watch the patient as you take the history. As you see the type of spasms occurring, you will be able to tailor your questions to make a diagnosis.

Several factors are important in arriving at the correct diagnosis:

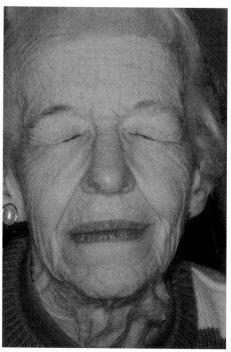

Figure 9-5 Essential blepharospasm. Bilateral involuntary closure of the eyes. Also note some lower facial movement, suggesting early Meige syndrome

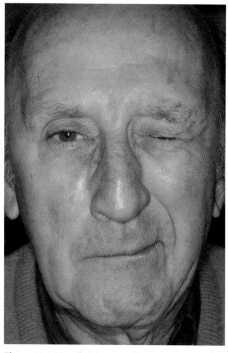

Figure 9-4 Hemifacial spasm. Note contraction of entire left side of face.

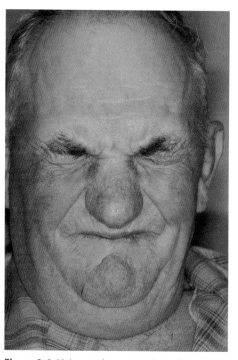

Figure 9-6 Meige syndrome: note lower facial spasm associated with blepharospasm.

- Age
- Onset
- Character of the spasm
- Quadrants of the face involved

Orbicularis myokymia and tics tend to occur in younger patients. Orbicularis myokymia and hemifacial spasm tend to occur in older adults. Orbicularis myokymia has an abrupt onset and usually lasts less than a week. The onset of facial tics may follow a particular event, and they frequently disappear spontaneously over a variable period of time. Hemifacial spasm and essential blepharospasm generally do not have a specific onset and tend to progress. As you watch the patient, you will be able to get a feel for the character of the movement problem. Is the muscle activity a quick twitch or a sustained spasm? Are you seeing an involuntary muscle activity (myokymia, hemifacial spasm, or blepharospasm), or is the abnormal facial movement the result of a voluntary coordinated movement of a group of muscles (a facial tic)? Most of all, you will want to determine which parts of the face are involved. This leads the way to determining the diagnosis (Box 9-1).

It is helpful to *divide the face into four quadrants* when evaluating patients with movement abnormalities (Figure 9-7).

First ask yourself, "Is one or are both eyes involved?"

If the answer is one eye, ask yourself, "Is the whole side of the face also involved?" If the eye alone is involved, the problem is probably myokymia. You will then know to ask about stress and fatigue. Frequently, the patient will tell you that this is a very busy time at school or work. Probably you have had an episode of orbicularis myokymia yourself.

If one eye and the whole side of the face are involved, the diagnosis is probably hemifacial spasm. In general, patients with hemifacial spasm are older than 50 years, but this condition can occur in the 40s. Beware of diagnosing hemifacial spasm in a patient younger than 40 years of age. As you initially examine the patient with hemifacial spasm, there may be no apparent abnormal movements. You may notice that, as the patient talks, the spasm starts. This is typical of hemifacial

spasm where so-called "cross-talk" of nerve fibers initiates the facial spasm. This phenomenon is bothersome to patients because the spasm often starts when they are talking to friends or business acquaintances. If you suspect hemifacial spasm, but don't see movements elsewhere on the face, look closely at the chin for dimpling of the mentalis muscle or at the neck for subtle movement of the cervical muscles. You may be able to confirm the diagnosis of hemifacial spasm by asking the patient if the spasm occurs while sleeping. Hemifacial spasm is the only diagnosis where spasms continue in the patient's sleep.

A tic can involve one side of the face as well. Patients with a unilateral periocular tic show orbital orbicularis

---

Box 9-1

Diagnosis of the Overactive Face

Divide the face into *four quadrants*

First ask yourself if *one* or *both eyes* are involved
- If one eye is involved, ask yourself if the whole side of the face is involved
  - If the eye alone is involved, the problem is probably myokymia
  - If one eye and the whole side of the face are involved, the diagnosis is probably hemifacial spasm
- If you have identified spasm in both eyes, the patient has either a form of blepharospasm or a facial tic
  - Rule out a cause of reflex spasm
  - If the patient with bilateral eyelid spasm is younger than 50 years of age, the spasm is probably a tic
  - If the patient is 50–60 years or older, the spasm is probably essential blepharospasm
- If the *upper and lower face* are involved, the patient has Meige syndrome
- Facial tics can be unilateral or bilateral
  - The movements involve a group of muscles under voluntary control. In most cases, you can trick the patient into stopping the tic for a minute or so to confirm the diagnosis.

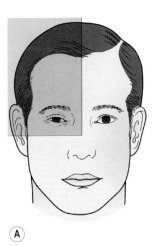 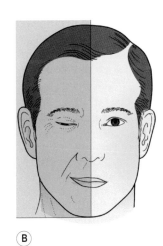 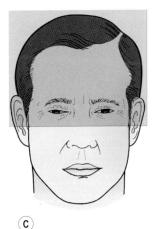 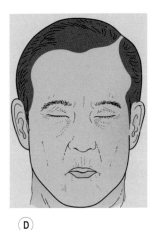

(A)　　　　(B)　　　　(C)　　　　(D)

Figure 9-7 The diagnosis of facial spasm. Divide the face into quadrants to determine the diagnosis. (**A**) Orbicularis myokymia: one quadrant of face; spasm limited to a few muscle fibers on the upper or lower lid. (**B**) Hemifacial spasm: two quadrants, entire side of face; intermittent spasm of one side of the face, including all branches of the facial nerve. Look for subtle involvement of the chin, neck, and brow. (**C**) Essential blepharospasm: two quadrants, upper half of face; bilateral involuntary closure or spasm of eyelids including orbital orbicularis and corrugator superciliaris. (**D**) Meige syndrome: four quadrants, entire face and often neck; "essential blepharospasm" and lower facial involvement, pursing of lips is common.

activity because it is difficult to lightly blink one eye voluntarily. In most patients, it is easy to identify a tic because the movements seem somewhat bizarre and for some reason you get the idea that the patient is actually doing it. Sometimes I will pass by the examination room a few times to see if the movements are occurring in my absence. Frequently, when I enter the room, the facial movements of the tic will start.

If you have identified spasms in both eyes, the patient has either a form of blepharospasm or a facial tic. If the patient with bilateral eyelid spasms is younger than 50 years old, the diagnosis is probably a tic. In all patients, you should rule out the possibility of a reflex blepharospasm from some cause of ocular irritation. The reflex spasm is usually obvious in a young patient but may be more difficult to identify in an older patient who may have an element of dryness in the eye. Ask if the patient has any sensation of a foreign body or burning in the eye. If there is a question of surface irritation causing the spasm, a drop of topical anesthetic should relieve the spasm. If you remain uncertain about the possibility of a reflex component, try lubricants or punctal plugs.

Essential blepharospasm occurs as a degenerative disorder seen mainly in patients older than 60 years. It may occur in the 50s, however. Initially, essential blepharospasm can start out as increased blinking. Over time, the spasms become more forceful. Typically, the symptoms decrease when the patient is busy with an activity such as work or a hobby. Symptoms seem to be worst when the patient is at rest or while the patient is driving or reading. Frequently patients will note that they pry their eyelids open to be able to drive. Sometimes patients will tell you that their eyes feel much more comfortable if they are just closed. On examination, you will see an increased rate of blinking in the early stages of the disease. Usually the orbital orbicularis muscle will be involved. In later stages, the corrugator muscle will pull the eyebrows toward the midline and spasms will be sustained. Often lower facial involvement will be noted with mild abnormal movements of the face, frequently lip pursing. If present, this lower facial movement will help to confirm the diagnosis of essential blepharospasm. As we said earlier, patients with lower facial involvement and blepharospasm are said to have *Meige syndrome*.

Treatment of the overactive face

Botulinum toxin

The treatment of facial spasm was revolutionized by the introduction of botulinum toxin (Botox®, Allergan Pharmaceuticals, http://www.botoxmedical.com). The toxin serotype A is produced by *Clostridium botulinum* and is a potent muscle-paralyzing agent. Subcutaneous injection of botulinum toxin into the eyelids and eyebrow provides symptomatic relief of spasm for 3–6 months, depending on the disease process. Botulinum toxin is the primary treatment of hemifacial spasm and essential blepharospasm.

Orbicularis myokymia

Orbicularis myokymia is a self-limited condition. The spasm usually lasts a few days and rarely more than a week. Botulinum toxin can be used, but be careful that you do not miss a more serious diagnosis if the myokymia persists.

Facial tics

Facial tics are treated with reassurance. In most children, the tic is simply a way to get attention from the parents. I encourage the parents to ignore the tic, if possible. If the tic persists for more than a few months, I recommend that the family discuss the situation with the family pediatrician as the tic may be a sign of a more serious problem in the family or at school.

Adults with facial tics are told that the movement problem is not a serious medical problem and that it may be stress related. If they agree with this assessment and express an interest in counseling, arrangements are made. Botulinum toxin injections are not recommended for facial tics.

Hemifacial spasm

If you diagnose hemifacial spasm, you should order a *magnetic resonance imaging (MRI) scan of the brain* to rule out any mass that may be causing compression of the facial nerve. A mass seen on an MRI scan is very rare. I have seen this only once, in a 20-year-old man with hemifacial spasm caused by an epidermoid tumor of the skull base. His spasm resolved upon removal of the mass. In most cases, the scan will be normal or will show a long dilated basilar artery in proximity to the facial nerve where it exits the brainstem, the so-called *dolichoectatic basilar artery*.

In healthy patients aged 50–60 years or younger, microvascular decompression of the facial nerve (the Janetta procedure) should be considered. In this low-risk intracranial operation, a pad is placed between the artery and the nerve. The reported success rate for this procedure varies, but can be as high as 75%.

Botulinum toxin is the treatment of choice for most patients with hemifacial spasm. Five units of botulinum toxin are administered subcutaneously in five sites around the periocular region (Figure 9-8). The choice of sites can be individualized after the initial injection. Most patients with hemifacial spasm have an element of facial weakness, making the effects of the injections last longer than for patients with essential blepharospasm; 4–6 months is common. Remind your patients to use artificial tears frequently throughout the day and lubricating ointment at night for the first few weeks after injection to prevent corneal exposure.

Essential blepharospasm

Essential blepharospasm is a difficult disorder to treat completely. Most of your patients will see improvement with either botulinum toxin injections or surgical myectomy, but very few will be completely asymptomatic after treatment. The disease tends to be progressive and becomes a lifelong condition that will affect your patient for the rest of his or her life. I urge all patients to subscribe to the Benign Essential Blepharospasm Research Foundation newsletter (637 North 7th Street, Suite 102, PO Box 12468, Beaumont, TX 77726-2468, USA, bebrf@blepharospasm.org).

No oral medication has been proven to be effective for treatment of essential blepharospasm. Most patients will see considerable improvement from botulinum toxin injections. Initially 5 units of botulinum toxin are administered subcutaneously in five sites in the periocular area (Figure 9-9). Injections are given subcutaneously above and below the

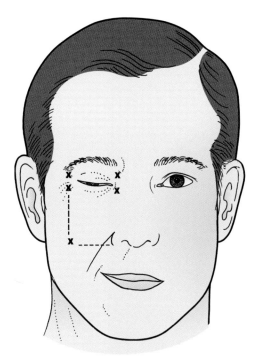

Figure 9-8 Sites of administration of botulinum toxin (Botox®) for hemifacial spasm. Inject 5 units of botulinum toxin underneath the skin at each site (25 units total). Avoid injecting inferior to the lateral ala of the nose to prevent drooping of the lip.

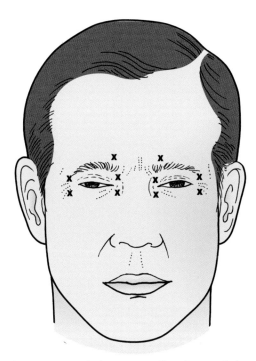

Figure 9-9 Sites of administration of botulinum toxin for essential blepharospasm. Inject 5 units of botulinum toxin underneath the skin at each site (25 units total on each side).

medial and lateral canthal tendons. No injection is made within the orbital bony rims. An additional 5 units is given above the head of the brow in the area of the corrugator and procerus muscles. Patients note the effect of the toxin over the following 48 hours. After the first injection, I check the patient in 1 week. After subsequent injections, I don't see the

patient before the next injection unless there is a problem. The effects of botulinum toxin last approximately 3–4 months. In some cases, you can modify the position of the injection to improve the effect or decrease a particular area of weakness (usually the mouth). I generally do not increase the dose. I will cut the dose in half for a patient who seems particularly sensitive.

Botulinum toxin has been used safely for 20 years. Many patients have temporary dryness related to the paralysis of the orbicularis muscle and resultant decreased blinking. Corneal exposure can be avoided by using topical lubricants for the first 2 or 3 weeks after injection. You will notice some loss of animation to the face after botulinum toxin injection, as you would expect. Patients rarely complain of this. You will also notice that the "crow's feet" and other wrinkles of the skin around the eye diminish as the orbicularis muscle is not pulling on the skin (this is the basis for the use of botulinum toxin injections to eliminate glabellar wrinkles in the patient seeking cosmetic improvement). A small number of patients will get upper eyelid ptosis or double vision secondary to botulinum toxin-induced paresis of the levator muscle or extraocular muscles. Ptosis and diplopia are troublesome side-effects, which may last for 6 weeks, but will resolve completely with time.

Most patients see reduction in the blepharospasm after the initial dose of botulinum toxin. If the injections seem to lose their effectiveness over time, *apraxia of eyelid opening* may be developing. As you know, during eyelid closure, the orbicularis muscle contracts and the levator muscle relaxes. Although we think of essential blepharospasm as a condition related to spasm of the orbicularis muscle, there is an element of uncontrolled levator muscle relaxation involved as well. Remember that many of your patients with essential blepharospasm may tell you that they feel better with their eyes closed. This is because it is a struggle for them to overcome the inhibition of the levator muscle seen with essential blepharospasm. Early in the disease process, the orbicularis spasm predominates and botulinum toxin reduces the spasm. If apraxia develops, the patient may perceive that the injections are no longer working. If this is the case when you ask the patient to close the eyes, you can see that the orbicularis muscle is still weak and spasm is not the main cause of the inability to open the eyes. Recently some relief of apraxia of eyelid opening has been obtained using frontalis sling surgery.

Surgical myectomy was popularized in the early 1980s before the use of botulinum toxin. In this procedure, the orbital orbicularis, the corrugator, and procerus muscles, and portions of the preseptal and pretarsal orbicularis muscles are resected from the upper eyelid. In addition, anatomic problems related to the constant spasm, such as dermatochalasis, eyelid ptosis, and brow ptosis, can be corrected at the same time. Surgical myectomy has been refined over recent years and remains an option for patients who don't get a satisfactory effect from botulinum toxin injections. Myectomy does not eliminate apraxia of lid opening, however. Approximately half of all patients undergoing myectomy continue to require botulinum toxin injections postoperatively, often at a reduced dose or frequency. Although the role for surgical myectomy is small, selected patients with essential blepharospasm will benefit from this procedure.

At this point you should:

- Understand the mechanism and presentation of orbicularis myokymia, facial tics, hemifacial spasm, and essential blepharospasm.
- Imagine a patient in your office with some facial spasm. While you listen to and watch the patient, use this information to make the diagnosis. Remind yourself of the "facial quadrant" scheme.
- Botulinum toxin (Botox®) injections are the mainstay of treatment for hemifacial spasm and essential blepharospasm. You should know how to treat these disorders. What are the main side effects of botulinum toxin?

Weakness of the facial muscles

Medical conditions associated with facial weakness

If you study the facial movements of your patients, you will soon see abnormalities of decreased facial movement. The most common medical condition that you will see is the "mask-like" facies of the patient suffering from *Parkinson disease*. Many of these patients will be seeing you for unrelated problems. Some will be seeing you for "watery" eyes or corneal exposure symptoms related to a decreased rate and force of blinking.

The other patients you may see with decreased facial expression are those with *myopathic ptosis*. As you recall, these patients include those with oculopharyngeal dystrophy, chronic progressive external ophthalmoplegia (CPEO), and myotonic dystrophy. Often the patient is unaware that the facial movements are decreased. Generally, these patients have no problems with decreased facial movement, but may develop corneal exposure after ptosis surgery.

Facial nerve palsy: history

The most common cause of decreased facial movement that you will see is facial nerve palsy. The most common form of facial weakness is *Bell's palsy*. Other causes include *local trauma* and *facial tumor* or *acoustic neuroma resection*. You should pay particular attention to the corneal sensation if the facial palsy is the result of an acoustic neuroma resection. Because the fifth, seventh, and eighth nerves leave the brainstem in close proximity, resection may compromise fifth nerve function, making corneal exposure more difficult to manage.

The treatment that you offer depends, in part, on how permanent the palsy is likely to be. Talk with your otolaryngology colleague who is taking care of the patient with you and find out the *likelihood of recovery*. Perhaps a tumor resection required cutting the facial nerve, meaning there is no chance of recovery. Surgical repair offering a long-term solution will be needed. Alternatively, the nerve may have been contused, and full recovery is anticipated. Lubrication alone may be appropriate.

Facial nerve palsy: physical examination

The deficit in function ranges from mild paresis to complete paralysis (Figure 9-10). After accidental or surgical trauma,

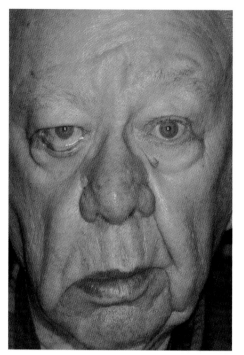

Figure 9-10 Complete right facial nerve paralysis. Note loss of melolabial fold, ectropion, and brow ptosis.

the weakness may be confined to one or more branches. The loss of function to the frontalis muscle is particularly common after operations involving the temporal scalp because the innervation to the frontalis muscle is provided by a single nerve, the frontal nerve.

The eye findings associated with facial nerve palsy include:

- Corneal exposure
- Incomplete blink
- Lagophthalmos
- Lower eyelid ectropion
- Brow ptosis

The degree of functional abnormality depends on the amount of paralysis and the patient's age. It makes sense that more paralysis means more functional disability. Younger patients with more tissue support have lesser degrees of brow ptosis and ectropion (Figure 9-11, A). The amount of corneal exposure also depends on the quality of the patient's tear film and Bell's phenomenon. If a good *Bell's phenomenon* is present, patients may have little or no corneal exposure despite incomplete closure (Figure 9-11, B).

Watch the patient blink during your history. Pay attention to:

- Blink rate
- Completeness of the blink

Most patients with a facial nerve palsy will have a normal blink rate, but the quality, or completeness, of closure will be reduced. You can see during the slit lamp examination that the fluorescein staining occurs inferior to where the lid excursion ends. *Lagophthalmos*, especially if the cornea is visible between the eyelids, suggests the need for lubricating ointment at night.

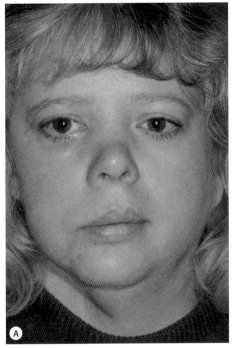
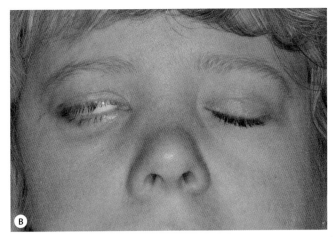

Figure 9-11 A young patient with right facial nerve palsy after parotid tumor and neck dissection. (**A**) Despite a moderate weakness of the facial nerve, there is little functional disability. Note slight retraction of the upper and lower eyelids resulting from mild orbicularis weakness. There is no horizontal lid laxity, so no ectropion is present. Minimal brow ptosis is present. (**B**) A strong Bell's phenomenon and topical lubricants prevent corneal exposure.

There are two special problems related to facial nerve palsy. We have already mentioned both of them (acoustic nerve resection and aberrant regeneration of the facial nerve). *Resection of a large acoustic neuroma may result in both fifth and seventh nerve weakness.* This is a bad combination. Without normal corneal sensation, the blinking is reduced further because the patient "feels" no need to blink. The patient has no perception of dryness, and severe corneal exposure can go without symptoms. Treat the patient with neurotrophic keratitis and facial nerve palsy aggressively. Use extra lubricants. Do protective lid operations early. Follow the patient regularly. Ask the patient to call you as soon as possible if the eye becomes infected.

After injury to the facial nerve, aberrant regeneration may occur. Ask each patient you see who has recovered from a facial nerve palsy to purse the lips closed while you watch for movements in the orbicularis muscle (see Figure 9-1). You are likely to see this present in one of three ways. First, you may see this as an incidental finding. Second, you may be seeing a patient who complains of a drooping eyelid. If there is any hint of a facial asymmetry, check for aberrant regeneration. The increased tone of the orbicularis muscle will narrow the fissure, closing both the upper and lower eyelids a small amount. This finding is frequently misdiagnosed as an acquired ptosis. Likewise, I have yet to see a patient who recognized that the lid closure was related to any other facial movement. Lastly, you may be seeing a patient without obvious facial nerve palsy who is complaining of visual loss from a brow ptosis. Lift up the brow and make sure that there is not an element of tonic closure to the eyelids, contributing to the visual loss with the brow ptosis.

Treatment of facial nerve palsy

The treatment of facial nerve palsy depends on the degree of anatomic dysfunction and the patient's needs. Corneal exposure, ectropion, and brow ptosis commonly need to be addressed.

Corneal exposure: medical treatment

Corneal exposure should be managed initially with frequent doses of artificial tears or ointments. New "gel" formulations provide longer lasting protection without affecting the vision as much as thicker ointments. Emphasize to your patients that drops should be used before the eye becomes irritated. Most commonly, patients wait until the eye is sore to put drops in. Drops used once or twice a day do little to protect the cornea. Significant corneal exposure requires drops at least once every 2 hours. Indoors, moving air, from fans or heating vents, should be avoided. Outdoors, eyeglasses that protect the eye from the wind (moisture chamber glasses) should be worn to protect the eye from wind. Cellophane wrap placed on a lubricated eye helps to prevent corneal exposure at night. Taping the eye closed should be avoided. If the eye opens at night, the tape can rub against the eye. If corneal exposure cannot be managed medically or the facial paralysis is likely to be long term, a surgical solution is needed.

Corneal exposure: surgical treatment

Corneal exposure can be treated surgically by using static or dynamic procedures. *Static procedures narrow the palpebral aperture a fixed amount.* The aperture can be narrowed horizontally using a tarsorrhaphy or vertically by raising the lower eyelid. *Dynamic procedures improve lid closure.* The most commonly used dynamic procedure is implantation of gold weights in the upper eyelid. In recent years, there has been a shift away from permanent tarsorrhaphy to gold weight implantation. Static and dynamic procedures are often used in combination.

Static procedures include:

- Tarsorrhaphy
  - Temporary: suture, botulinum toxin (Botox®)
  - Permanent lateral tarsorrhaphy
  - Permanent medial tarsorrhaphy
- Elevation of lower eyelid
  - Retractor disinsertion without graft
  - Retractor disinsertion with graft

Dynamic procedures include upper eyelid gold weight implantation or palpebral springs. Although springs can give movement to a weak eyelid, they are prone to extrusion and are rarely used.

Tarsorrhaphy

Temporary suture tarsorrhaphy

If you anticipate improvement over a few weeks, a temporary tarsorrhaphy is appropriate. The simplest temporary tarsorrhaphy uses a suture to close a portion of the eyelids. Usually the lateral one third of the lids is closed (Box 9-2).

A *temporary suture tarsorrhaphy* includes:

1. Instill topical anesthetic and inject local anesthetic into the eyelids
2. Cut two 5 mm pieces of *a narrow red rubber catheter* to use as bolster material
3. Pass one arm of a 5-0 nylon suture
   A. Through the bolster material,
   B. Then into the lower lid skin 5 mm below the lid margin, emerging through the meibomian glands,
   C. Into the opposite lid margin,
   D. Out the skin 5 mm below the upper lid margin, and
   E. Through the second bolster.
4. Repeat this procedure with the other arm of the suture
5. Tie a slip knot over the bolster (Figure 9-12)

The temporary suture tarsorrhaphy can be placed anywhere along the lid margins. The suture tarsorrhaphy can be opened

to inspect the cornea by untying the slip knot. The nylon suture can be left in place for 2 weeks. When corneal healing has occurred, the suture can be removed and the lids will open naturally. If you need to close the eye completely for a few weeks, but want to inspect the cornea at intervals, the *"drawstring" tarsorrhaphy technique*, devised by my colleague, Tom Oetting, is a clever way to do it. You will use the same technique described above but, rather than tie the suture, you will use an additional piece of bolster with more narrow suture placement to keep the lids opposed. You can easily slide the bolsters apart to view the cornea. If you need to close the lids again, just slide the bolsters closed (see Figure 9-13).

A more permanent suture tarsorrhaphy can be made by creating an *intermarginal adhesion*. Before passing sutures through the lid margin, use a scalpel to remove the surface epithelium of the opposing lid margins (Figure 9-14). Use the same suturing technique as described above. You will want to add an additional one or two double-armed sutures to create a tight closure. The sutures are removed after 10 days. In the majority of patients, the tarsorrhaphy remains intact. The lids can be opened later if function returns. Little lid deformity is created.

Botulinum toxin temporary tarsorrhaphy

Botulinum toxin can be used to close the eyelids. A 25-gauge needle is passed through the central aspect of the upper lid immediately inferior to the superior orbital rim. The needle is passed against the orbital roof for 1–2 cm. *Five to 10 units of botulinum toxin* are injected. After 48 hours, the upper lid rests closed and remains so for a period of several weeks to several months. The results of botulinum toxin tarsorrhaphy are somewhat unpredictable, however. Repeat injection may be necessary.

Permanent lateral tarsorrhaphy

A more *permanent lateral tarsorrhaphy* can be made by splitting the anterior and posterior lamellae of the lid margin,

---

Box 9-2

Temporary Suture Tarsorrhaphy

- Administer topical and local anesthesia
- Cut four 5 mm pieces of a small red rubber catheter to use as bolsters
- Pass one arm of a 5-0 nylon suture
  - Through the bolster material
  - Then into the lower lid skin 5 mm below the lid margin, emerging out the lid margin through the meibomian glands
  - Into the opposite lid margin
  - Out the skin 5 mm above the upper lid margin and
  - Through the second bolster
- Repeat this procedure with the other arm of the suture
- Tie a slip knot over the bolster on the upper eyelid

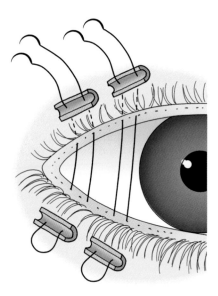

Figure 9-12 Temporary suture tarsorrhaphy. Double-armed 5-0 nylon sutures are passed through the meibomian gland orifices and tied with a temporary tie over rubber bolsters.

de-epithelializing the eyelid margin, and sewing the layers together (Box 9-3).

The steps of the permanent lateral tarsorrhaphy are:

1. Administer topical and local anesthetics
2. Split the lateral one third of the upper and lower lid margins
   A. Use a no. 15 blade to incise the lid margins along the gray line for the lateral one third of the upper and lower eyelids. Keep the plane of the incision parallel to the posterior surface of the tarsus (Figure 9-15, A and B).
   B. Use Westcott scissors to separate the anterior and posterior lamellae 4 mm proximal to the lid margins.
   C. Some bleeding may occur. Use bipolar cautery, if necessary.
3. De-epithelialize the margins of the posterior lamella

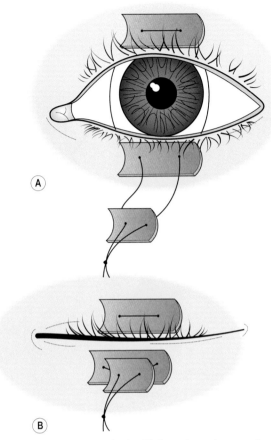

Figure 9-13 Drawstring tarsorrhaphy. (**A**) Open drawstring tarsorrhaphy. (**B**) Closed drawstring tarsorrhaphy. (Based on The Drawstring Temporary Tarsorrhaphy Technique, Kitchens J, Kinder J, Oetting T, *Arch Ophthalmol* 120:187–190, 2002.)

Box 9-3

Permanent Lateral Tarsorrhaphy

- Administer topical and local anesthesia
- Separate the anterior and posterior lamellae of the eyelid
  - Use a no. 15 blade to incise the lid margins along the gray line for the lateral one third of the upper and lower eyelids
  - Use Westcott scissors to separate the anterior and posterior lamella 4 mm proximal to the lid margins. Some bleeding may occur
- De-epithelialize the margins of the posterior lamellae
- Sew the posterior lamellae together
  - Use three 5-0 Vicryl sutures to sew the upper and lower posterior lamellae together
- Sew the anterior lamellae together
  - Use absorbable sutures, placing the eyelashes in an everted position

---

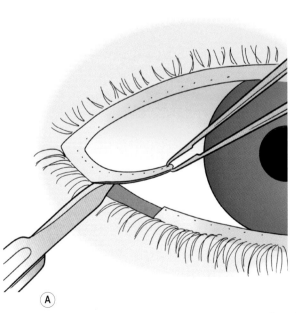

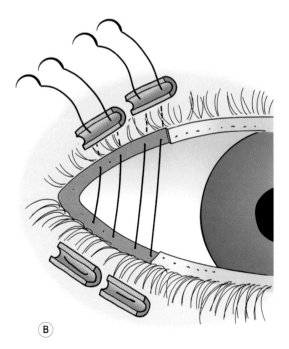

Figure 9-14 Intermarginal adhesion tarsorrhaphy. (**A**) Remove the epithelium from the lid margin. (**B**) Suture rubber bolsters in place to close the eye.

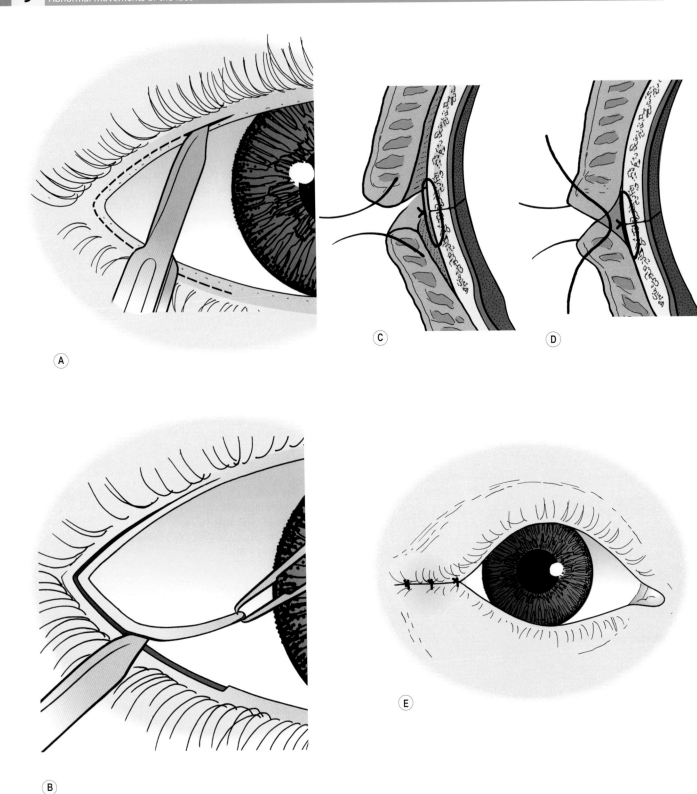

Figure 9-15 Permanent lateral tarsorrhaphy. (**A** and **B**) Incise the lid margin at the gray line using a scalpel blade. Use Westcott scissors to split the anterior and posterior lamellae at the gray line. Remove the epithelium from the margin of the posterior lamella for approximately the lateral one third of the lid. (**C**) Suture the posterior lamellae together using a 5-0 Vicryl suture on a spatula needle. (**D**) Suture the anterior lamellae together using a 7-0 Vicryl suture, everting the eyelashes. (**E**) Completed permanent lateral tarsorrhaphy.

4. Sew the upper and lower posterior lamellae together
   A. Use three interrupted 5-0 Vicryl sutures (Figure 9-15, C).
5. Sew the upper and lower anterior lamellae together
   A. Use interrupted absorbable sutures (Figure 9-15, D).
   B. Evert the eyelashes with the closure (Figure 9-15, E).

This is a very effective way to make a permanent tarsorrhaphy. No bolsters are used, and no suture removal is required. At a later date, the lids can be opened, but some lid margin deformity may follow, so use this procedure only if you are sure that you want a strong long-term tarsorrhaphy.

Medial tarsorrhaphy

One of the most useful but little-known tarsorrhaphies is the *medial tarsorrhaphy*. In this operation, the canalicular portions of the eyelids are sewn together. The medial tarsorrhaphy technique is modified from the usual tarsorrhaphy because the lid margin cannot be split in the area of the canaliculus (Box 9-4).

The steps of the medial tarsorrhaphy are:

1. Prepare the patient
   A. Administer topical anesthetic.
   B. Mark a V-*shaped incision* just peripheral to the canaliculi to the upper and lower lid (Figure 9-16, A).
   C. Inject local anesthetic.
2. Make small myocutaneous flaps at the canthus
   A. Place a *Bowman probe* into the canaliculus.
   B. Use a no. 15 blade, Westcott scissors, or a Colorado needle to cut through the skin and muscle adjacent to the canaliculus. Repeat this on the opposite lid, taking care not to cut the canaliculus itself. Connect the arms to form a V (Figure 9-16, B).
   C. *Dissect a small skin and muscle flap* away from the canaliculi. Be careful not to damage the canaliculi.

Box 9-4

Medial Tarsorrhaphy

- Prepare the patient
  - Administer topical anesthetic
  - Mark a V-shaped incision just peripheral to the canaliculi to the upper and lower lid
  - Administer local anesthetic
- Make small medial canthal skin and muscle flaps
  - Place a Bowman probe into the canaliculus
  - Use a no. 15 blade, Colorado needle, or Westcott scissors to cut through the skin and muscle adjacent to the canaliculus
  - Repeat this on the opposite lid, taking care not to cut the canaliculus itself
  - Dissect a small skin and muscle flap away from the canaliculi
- Suture the medial portion of the eyelids together
  - Suture the upper and lower edges of the muscle together using three interrupted 5-0 Vicryl sutures. You will notice that the canaliculi are inverted
  - Suture the skin edges together anterior to the lid margin

---

3. Suture the medial portion of the lids together
   A. Use three interrupted 5-0 Vicryl sutures in the muscle to close the tarsorrhaphy (Figure 9-16, C and D).
   B. You will notice that the canaliculi are inverted.
   C. Use a 5-0 fast absorbing gut or 7-0 Vicryl suture to close the skin (Figure 9-16, E).

The medial tarsorrhaphy gives a horizontal and vertical narrowing of the palpebral fissure without interfering with the vision or dramatically changing the appearance of the eyelids. Medial tarsorrhaphy can be used with other procedures such as lateral tarsorrhaphy, gold weight implantation, or elevation of the lower eyelid.

Lower eyelid elevation

The lower eyelid can be elevated from its normal position at the limbus. This improves corneal exposure by raising the height of the tear lake and decreasing the distance that the upper lid has to travel to meet the tear film. The lower lid retractors can be extirpated (or recessed) through a transconjunctival (or transcutaneous approach) under local anesthesia. One or 2 mm of elevation of the lid margin is possible with surgical extirpation of the lower eyelid retractors alone. Spacer grafts can push the lower eyelid up further. Hard palate mucosal grafts are a reliable spacer for pushing the lower eyelid 2–3 mm higher. As an alternative to hard palate, commercially available products, such as AlloDerm or Enduragen™, can be used instead. Enduragen™ sheets are made from porcine dermal collagen (1 cm × 4 cm × 1 mm thick, http://www.porexsurgical.com). AlloDerm sheets are made from acellular human dermis (1 cm × 4 cm × 0.79–1.79 mm thick, http://www.lifecell.com). In cases where you need to raise the lower eyelid more than 3 mm, I prefer ear cartilage grafts. The techniques for harvesting hard palate or ear cartilage are discussed next. Placing the graft is similar for all the materials and is outlined briefly in the following paragraphs.

Hard palate can be harvested under local or general anesthesia. The tissue is not difficult to harvest, but usually I have an oral surgery colleague do the harvesting. The dental lab will also make a "splint" that snaps into place that will protect the roof of the mouth while the wound heals, which makes the patient much more comfortable. A single graft is taken from either side of the roof of the mouth lateral to the midline well anterior to the soft palate (Figure 9-17). The ideal graft size is 10–12 mm by 25–30 mm. The trick of harvesting this graft is to remove all the mucosa and submucosa, but leave periosteum and fat in place. If you harvest the graft yourself, be careful not to extend to the soft palate, especially laterally. The greater palatine artery emerges from a foramen of the same name. You will be faced with some brisk bleeding. Similarly, you should avoid the incisive foramen in the midline anteriorly. One graft can be harvested from each side. After harvesting, place some antibiotic ointment on the wound and snap the dental plate into position and the mouth portion is done. We have the patient use Peridex mouthwash (chlorhexidine gluconate) three times per day and pain medicine as needed. Trim any remaining fat off the graft before placing it in the eyelid.

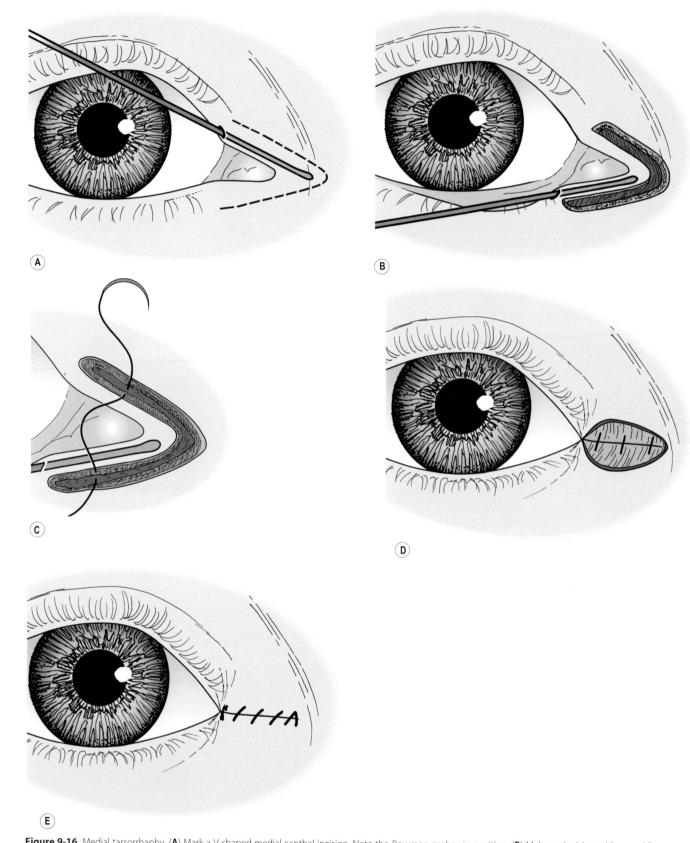

(A)

(B)

(C)

(D)

(E)

Figure 9-16 Medial tarsorrhaphy. (**A**) Mark a V-shaped medial canthal incision. Note the Bowman probes in position. (**B**) Make an incision with a no. 15 blade or a Colorado needle. Form a skin and muscle flap with Westcott scissors. Note the probe in the canaliculus to help prevent inadvertent laceration of the canaliculus. (**C** and **D**) Close the muscle layer with interrupted 5-0 Vicryl sutures. (**E**) Suture the upper and lower edges of the skin using a running 7-0 Vicryl suture or 5-0 fast absorbing gut.

Under local or general anesthesia, you will remove (or recess) the lower eyelid retractors through a transconjunctival incision with lateral canthotomy and cantholysis. This is a standard approach for lower eyelid surgery, one that you should learn because it is used for many procedures. Place a 4-0 silk traction suture in the lower eyelid margin. Inject local under the conjunctiva to balloon it up a bit. Make a canthotomy using a microdissection needle. Next, release the eyelid from the rim by cutting the crus of the lateral canthal tendon. We did the same technique for the lateral tarsal strip procedure. Remember, strum the crus before cutting it. Now evert the eyelid over a Jaeger eyelid speculum and make an incision along the lower edge of tarsus from the punctum to your lateral incision. Make thin passes, cutting through the conjunctiva and the lower eyelid retractors. You will know that you are through the retractors when you see the underlying orbicularis muscle. Next, you will dissect the conjunctiva off the retractors. Use either the microdissection needle or Westcott scissors extending the plane into the fornix. Don't worry if you make a small button hole. Now use your nondominant hand to "pull"

the retractors off the orbicularis muscle, dissecting in this plane to Lockwood's ligament. Remember the fat and the septum will be anterior to your plane of dissection. At this point, you can either cut out the retractors or just let them recess into the fornix. You are ready to place the graft of your choice.

Shape the graft in a long ellipse with a sharp taper at the ends. Trim the length by laying the graft into the wound and cut to size. You need to overcorrect the height significantly, usually about 10 mm high. Some surgeons have a formula. I usually put in as much height as I can fit, but you will learn what works for you. Using 7-0 Vicryl, place interrupted sutures at the lateral and medial edges of the wound to hold the graft in place, then place a few interrupted sutures connecting the lower edge of the graft to the edge of the lower eyelid retractors. The only remaining suturing to be done is sewing the graft to the inferior edge of tarsus. It is very important that you line up the graft exactly with the tarsus and sew carefully so that there are no rough edges or sutures exposed that may abrade the cornea. Use a running 6-0 fast absorbing gut suture for this part or carefully bury any 7-0 Vicryl sutures that you use (Figure 9-18). Reattach the lateral canthus as you would with a lateral tarsal strip using a double-armed 4-0 Mersilene suture. If the eyelid seems too short to reach the bony rim, just attach it to any soft tissue that will hold it in place. Remember a tight lid may slide inferiorly off the eye. Put the lower eyelid on traction and patch for a few days. The technique is the same for any of the commercially prepared materials or the hard palate.

When you sew an ear cartilage graft in place, you must cover it with the conjunctiva. The retractor recession and cartilage graft placement can also be done from the anterior transcutaneous approach, which makes it easy to keep a conjunctival cover intact. Ear cartilage also tends to thicken the eyelid. It also retains its shape so any twist or curl in the cartilage may show up as a slight elevation on the surface of the overlying eyelid skin. Consequently, I rarely use this for any correction of eyelid retraction following a cosmetic procedure unless absolutely necessary. There is virtually no shrinkage of the cartilage, so size the graft so that where you

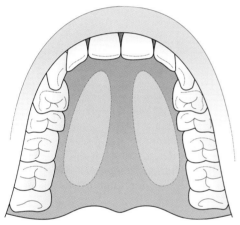

Figure 9-17 Site of hard palate graft harvest.

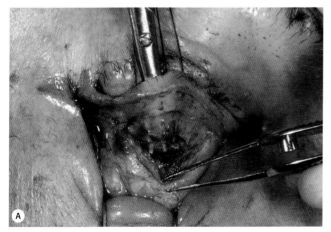

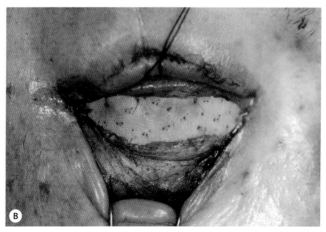

Figure 9-18 Lower eyelid recession with spacer graft. (**A**) Lower eyelid retractors are removed or recessed. (**B**) Graft material is sewn in place.

see the eyelid margin at the end of the case is where you want it to be forever. For the right patient and given the inherent limitations, ear cartilage is a powerful lower eyelid elevator.

The elevation of the lower eyelid does not interfere with the patient's vision or alter the patient's appearance. Occasionally, lower eyelid elevation can interfere with reading in downgaze. Lower eyelid elevation is often combined with gold weight implantation.

Gold weight implantation

A *gold weight* can be implanted into the upper lid to improve eyelid closure. Preoperatively, test weights are applied to the eyelid with benzoin solution to select the correct size weight. I put in the most weight possible creating about 1 mm of eyelid ptosis. You will find that most patients do well with a 1.2 gm weight (Box 9-5).

The steps of gold weight implantation into the upper eyelid are:

1. Prepare the patient
   A. Use a topical anesthetic.
   B. Mark an upper eyelid skin crease 1–2 mm higher than normal.
   C. Inject a local anesthetic.
2. Dissect a pretarsal pocket
   A. Place a 4-0 silk suture in the upper lid margin for traction.
   B. Make a skin crease incision with either a no. 15 blade or a Colorado needle (Figure 9-19, A).
   C. Dissect the skin and muscle off the tarsus inferiorly, stopping 2–3 mm above the eyelashes. You will *create a pretarsal pocket* (Figure 9-19, B).
3. Sew the weights into position
   A. Sew the weight onto the tarsus with 5-0 Dacron or polyester sutures.

   B. Make sure that there is *no tension on the skin* overlying the weight.
   C. The upper edge of the gold weight usually sits at the top edge of the tarsal plate, or slightly above (Figure 9-19, C).
4. Close the wound
   A. Close the orbicularis muscle with interrupted 7-0 Vicryl sutures (Figure 9-19, D). This layer may not be necessary, but you do not want the weight to become exposed.
   B. Close the skin with a running 5-0 fast absorbing gut suture (Figure 9-19, E).

You will find the use of gold weights to be relatively easy and effective. The gold weight procedure eliminates or reduces the need for use of daily lubricants. The lid closure effect of gold weights is gravity dependent, so ointment at bedtime is necessary. The implants do not change the patient's appearance, but sometimes the outline of the weight is visible on the pretarsal skin. Extrusion can occur, but is uncommon. Gold weights can be used with other procedures such as a medial tarsorrhaphy or lower eyelid elevation. The combination of weight implantation and lower eyelid elevation has almost eliminated the use of permanent large lateral tarsorrhaphies (Figure 9-20). In an occasional patient for whom a large weight does not provide enough closure, I will recess the levator aponeurosis to create a slight ptosis before placing the weight. As far as I know, this technique has not been published. Gold weights are available from MedDev Corporation (http://www.meddev-corp.com, 800 543 2789) (Figure 9-21).

MedDev makes two different profile weights—the Contour™ and the ThinProfile™ eyelid implants. I prefer the thinner implant for most patients because the outline of the implant is less visible. Platinum eyelid implants are made for the rare patient who is allergic to gold. Externally applied weights, *Blinkeze™* external lid weights, are useful for patients who have a temporary need or for some reason prefer no surgery.

Box 9-5

Gold Weight Implantation

Preparation

- Instill topical anesthetic
- Mark an upper eyelid skin crease 1–2 mm higher than normal
- Inject local anesthetic
- Prepare and drape the patient

Dissect the pretarsal pocket

- Use a 4-0 silk upper lid traction suture
- Make a skin crease incision with either a no. 15 blade or a Colorado needle
- Separate the pretarsal orbicularis muscle off the tarsus down to 2 mm above the lid margin to create a "pretarsal pocket"

Sewing the weights into position

- Usually one weight is sewn onto the tarsus with Dacron or Polyester sutures (most commonly 1.2 gm weight)
- Make sure there is no stress on the skin overlying the weight

Closure

- Close the orbicularis muscle with interrupted 7-0 Vicryl sutures
- Close the skin with a running 5-0 fast absorbing gut suture

---

Treatment of ectropion

Lower lid paralytic ectropion is common in patients with facial nerve palsy. The ectropion can be repaired using the standard *lateral tarsal strip procedure*. The medial spindle operation will add additional inversion of the punctum, if needed.

In many cases, the tearing associated with facial nerve palsy will decrease after the lateral tarsal strip procedure. Reflex causes of tearing, including the inflamed or keratinized conjunctiva of the lower lid, will be eliminated. The lacrimal pump action will be improved as well. Some patients will remain symptomatic in the cold or wind.

Additional procedures to correct the anatomic and functional abnormalities are often performed at the same time. A common combination is the lateral tarsal strip procedure, gold weight implantation, correction of brow ptosis, and facial sling. Elevation of the lower eyelid using a retractor extirpation operation with a graft can be performed with or without a medial tarsorrhaphy (see Figures 9-18 and 9-20). The periocular and cheek drooping can be corrected by

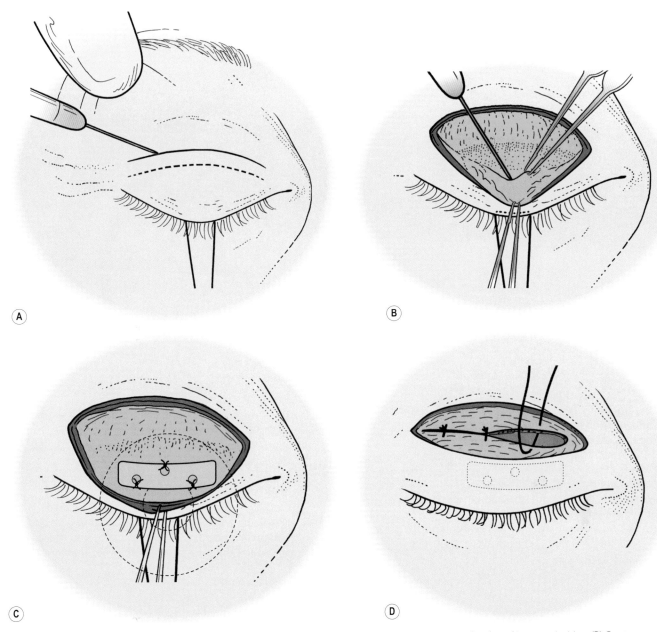

Figure 9-19 Gold weight implantation. (**A**) Mark an upper lid skin crease slightly high. Pass a traction suture and make a skin crease incision. (**B**) Create a "pretarsal pocket" exposing the anterior surface of the tarsus. (**C**) Suture the weight to the tarsal plate with 5-0 Dacron (usually a 1.2 gm weight). (**D**) Close the orbicularis muscle with interrupted 7-0 Vicryl sutures. (**E**) Close the skin with a running 5-0 fast absorbing gut suture. (**F**) Lateral view of weight in place in pretarsal pocket. Note layered closure of skin crease.

lifting the midface (malar fat pads and adjacent tissues). The midface lift is performed through either a transconjunctival or a subciliary lower eyelid incision. Permanent sutures attach the elevated soft tissue to the orbital rims and temporalis fascia. To correct the lower facial droop, a sling procedure is necessary.

Brow ptosis repair

Brow ptosis is common with facial nerve palsy. The eyebrow loses its support with the loss of the frontalis muscle activity. Frequently the eyebrow droops over the superior orbital rim,

obstructing the vision. There are several types of browplasties available (Figure 9-22):

- Direct
- Transblepharoplasty
- Midforehead
- Pretrichial
- Coronal
- Endoscopic

As is the case with most problems that have many surgical options for treatment, there is not a single perfect operation.

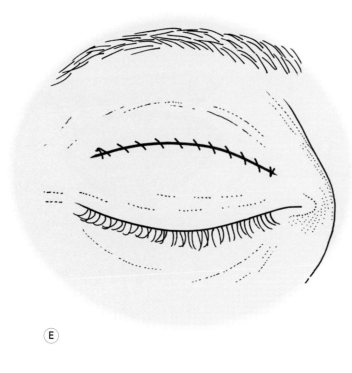

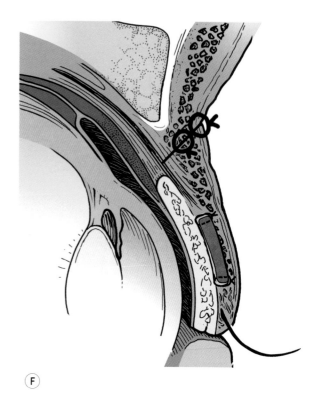

Figure 9-19 Continued.

Procedures in the hair are more involved, but the scar is hidden. The lower the incision on the forehead, the stronger the lift, but more scarring is present.

The most commonly performed browplasty for facial nerve palsy is the *direct browplasty*. The direct browplasty is a simple and straightforward technique to raise the brow above the visual axis. An ellipse of skin and muscle is removed directly above the eyebrow. The wound is closed with attachment of the subcutaneous tissues to the periosteum (Box 9-6).

The steps of the direct browplasty are:

1. Prepare the patient
   A. Mark the area of proposed tissue excision above the eyebrow.
      (1) The *lower incision line* is drawn 1 mm above the eyebrow hairs. This line starts at the head of the brow and extends beyond the tail of the brow in an upward direction for about 1 cm.
      (2) The *vertical height* of the tissue resection is determined with the patient in the sitting position with the brow manually elevated to its normal position.
      (3) A ruler is placed at the brow and the brow is allowed to relax. The millimeters of brow drop are multiplied by 1.5 to determine the vertical height of tissue to be excised. The excision ranges from 10 to 15 mm in most elderly patients. This allows for a slight overcorrection of the brow.
      (4) The *upper incision line* is marked accordingly (Figure 9-23, A–C).
   B. Administer topical and local anesthetics.
2. Excise skin and muscle
   A. *Use a no. 15 blade or Colorado needle to incise through the skin and subcutaneous tissue down to the underlying frontalis and orbicularis muscles.* I don't attempt to

bevel the wound parallel to the brow hairs, as suggested by some surgeons (Figure 9-23, D).
   B. Apply cautery as needed, but *try to avoid damaging the hair follicles.*
   C. *Medially, remove only skin and subcutaneous tissue to avoid damage to the supraorbital nerve.*
   D. *Centrally and laterally, excise the muscle down to the periosteum* with Stevens scissors (Figure 9-23, E). In patients without facial nerve palsy, avoid muscle resection lateral to the brow to avoid damage to the frontal nerve.
3. Close the wound
   A. *Suture the muscle layer to the underlying periosteum with interrupted 4-0 PDS or Prolene sutures to maintain the position of the elevated brow, if the brow ptosis is paralytic* (Figure 9-23, F).
   B. Close the *subcutaneous layer* with interrupted *4-0 PDS sutures.*
   C. Close the *skin* with a *running 5-0 Prolene suture.* The blue color of the Prolene suture contrasts with the brow hairs, facilitating suturing and eventual suture removal.

Although the direct browplasty is a good procedure for facial nerve paralysis, there are some problems with it. Inevitably, some numbness is present even though the skin excision avoids the supraorbital neurovascular bundle. The skin incision tends to "feminize" the eyebrow. The elliptical excision creates a typical female arched brow. The upper brow hairs are lost at the incision line, creating a sharp manicured look for the eyebrow. In most patients, the brow incision is visible for a long period of time.

No browplasty will restore function to the paralyzed brow. Some facial asymmetry will remain postoperatively.

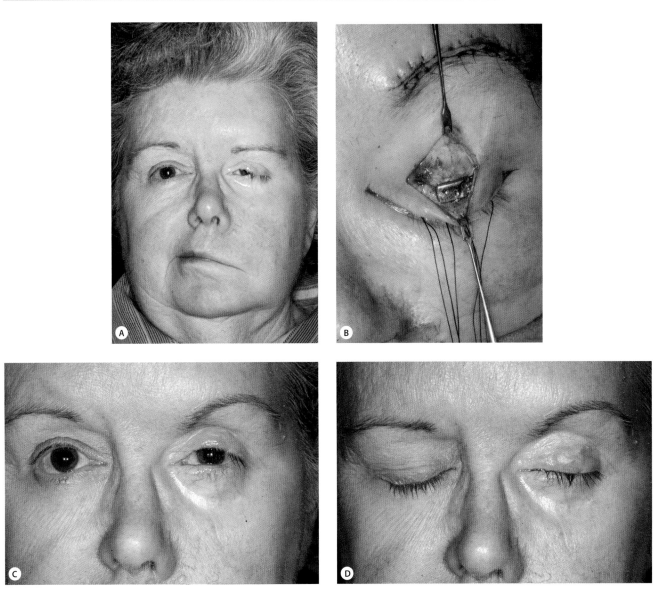

Figure 9-20 Rehabilitation of facial nerve palsy. (**A**) Left facial nerve palsy. A large lateral tarsorrhaphy is in place to protect the cornea. (**B**) Tarsorrhaphy taken down followed by upper lid gold weight implantation, direct browplasty, and lower lid elevation with ear cartilage. (**C**) Postoperatively, corneal exposure, peripheral field, and appearance are improved. (**D**) Good closure after rehabilitation.

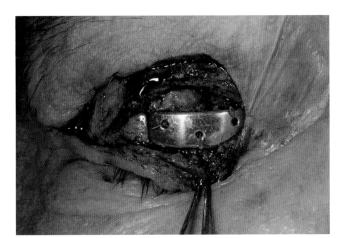

Figure 9-21 Gold weight—1.2 gm gold weight placed in right upper eyelid for severe corneal exposure due to facial nerve palsy. This patient is undergoing levator aponeurosis recession at same time. Note edge of the aponeurosis superior to the weight.

You and your patient should be pleased if the visual axis is cleared and the brow height is symmetric or slightly high with the face at rest.

The *midforehead lift* lifts the brow using an incision placed in a horizontal forehead furrow. The midforehead lift has the advantage of lifting the entire lower forehead and removing some of the glabellar folds that commonly occur. Several variations of the midforehead lift have been described. Some variations are essentially the same technique as a direct brow lift, but placed more superiorly. My preferred variation of the midforehead lift involves creating the plane of dissection within the subcutaneous tissue anterior to the frontalis muscle and extending inferiorly to the brow. The brows are lifted using a "hang back" suture from the periosteum joined to the subcutaneous tissue of the eyebrow. The anterior dissection in the subcutaneous tissue minimizes hypesthesia of the forehead. The incision across the forehead may be broken at the midline to improve camouflage. The midforehead lift avoids the feminizing look of the direct browplasty and can

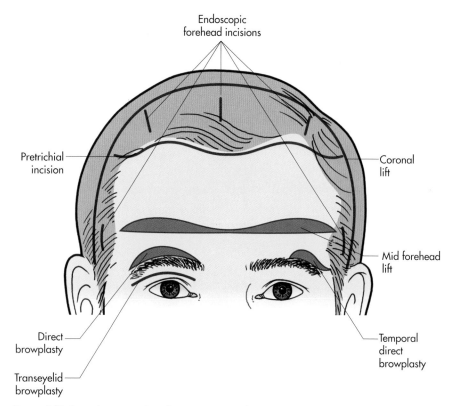

Endoscopic forehead incisions

Pretrichial incision

Coronal lift

Mid forehead lift

Direct browplasty

Temporal direct browplasty

Transeyelid browplasty

Figure 9-22 Browplasty operations. From superior to inferior: coronal, pretrichial, endoscopic, midforehead lift, direct, temporal direct, and transblepharoplasty.

Box 9-6

The Direct Browplasty

- Prepare the patient
  - Mark the area of proposed tissue excision above the eyebrow
  - Instill topical and local anesthetics
- Excise skin and muscle
  - Use a no. 15 blade or Colorado needle to incise through the skin and subcutaneous tissue down to the underlying frontalis and orbicularis muscles
  - Apply cautery cautiously
  - Medially, remove only skin and subcutaneous tissue to avoid damage to the supraorbital nerve
  - Centrally and laterally, excise the muscle down to the periosteum using Stevens scissors. *In patients without palsy, avoid lateral muscle resection and fixation to periosteum*
- Close the wound
  - Suture the muscle layer to the underlying periosteum with 4-0 Vicryl sutures (Ethicon J464 P-3 needle) in paralytic cases only
  - Close the subcutaneous layer with interrupted 4-0 PDS sutures (Ethicon Z496G 19mm PS-2 reverse cutting 3/8 curve, clear)
  - Close the skin with a running 5-0 Prolene suture (Ethicon 8698 P-3 needle)

lift the loose glabellar skin. The midforehead lift is more complicated and tends to give a less efficient lift than a direct forehead lift. You will find that the primary use for a midforehead lift is for men with deep forehead furrows. Most patients with facial nerve weakness do not have deep furrows to hide the skin incision.

The *transblepharoplasty browpexy* described in association with dermatochalasis repair is not powerful enough for lifting the ptotic eyebrow associated with seventh nerve palsy. Brow and scalp tissue are "pushed" upward rather than "pulled" upward and excised as in other browplasty procedures. With the transblepharoplasty browpexy, it is difficult to address the medial aspect of the brow. The position of the supraorbital neurovascular bundle precludes dissection of the head of the eyebrow without creating numbness of the forehead.

The *coronal forehead lift* elevates the eyebrow and forehead through an incision placed either at the hairline or posteriorly in the hair, extending from ear to ear. The coronal lift offers the advantage of eliminating forehead wrinkles and restoring the smooth contours of the glabella and medial canthus by lifting the entire forehead. The scalp incision is made full thickness to the periosteum. Numbness occurs from the incision line posteriorly to the crown of the head. The coronal forehead lift has been largely replaced by the use of endoscopic forehead lift procedures. The *pretrichial forehead lift* is similar to the coronal lift, with the exception that the incision is made at the hairline. This incision is useful for patients who do not want the hairline raised after a brow lift.

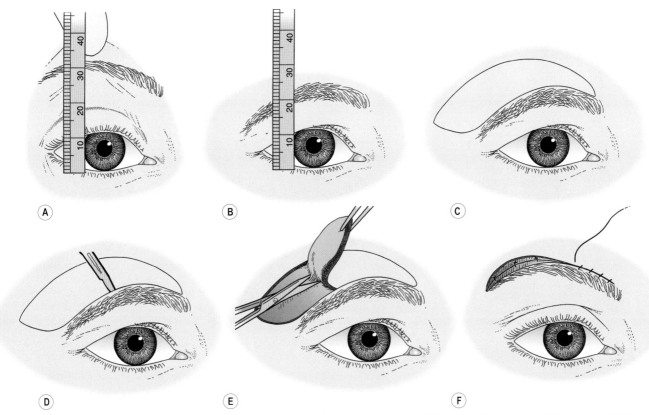

Figure 9-23 Direct browplasty. (**A**) Elevate the brow to the desired position with some overcorrection. (**B**) Place a marker at the top of the brow and let the brow drop. (**C**) Mark an ellipse of tissue to be removed (the normal range of excision is 10–15 mm). (**D**) Make a skin incision through the subcutaneous tissue to the frontalis and orbicularis muscles. (**E**) Excise the skin and muscle to the periosteum. Do not excise muscle over the head of the brow to avoid anesthesia of the forehead. In patients without facial nerve palsy, avoid muscle resection lateral to the brow to avoid damage to the frontal nerve. (**F**) Layered closure. In patients with paralytic ptosis, suture the muscle to the periosteum. In other patients, close the subcutaneous layer with interrupted sutures and the skin with a running suture. Note the position of the brow is overcorrected more for patients with paralytic brow ptosis.

The *endoscopic forehead lift* elevates the eyebrow and forehead through vertical incisions made above the hairline. This procedure has its primary use in patients undergoing cosmetic surgery. The vertical orientation of the incisions minimizes numbness of the scalp. All scars are hidden in the hair. Although the endoscopic forehead lift is effective for treatment of facial nerve palsy, this procedure requires familiarity with the endoscope and moderately advanced soft tissue surgical techniques.

Facial sling

For patients with long-standing lower facial ptosis, a fascial sling can improve facial asymmetry, decrease drooling, and open the nostril. Many suspension materials have been used: autogenous, banked, and synthetic materials. My largest experience is with banked fascia lata. Using this technique, three strips of fascia are attached at three or more places in the lower face, threaded through the subcutaneous plane, and then anchored to firm tissues on the facial skeleton superiorly. Typically, the fascia is sutured to the deep tissues at the modiolus (corner of the mouth), the melolabial fold, and at the lateral ala. The strips are anchored to the deep temporalis fascia, the lateral rim orbital periosteum, and the

inferior orbital rim periosteum respectively (see Figures 9-24 and 9-25).

Treatment of aberrant regeneration of the facial nerve

The synkinetic movements of the face resulting from aberrant regeneration of the facial nerve may be merely an interesting or unusual clinical finding or may require treatment. The most common indication for treatment is narrowing of the fissure that is bothersome for vision. If the synkinesis is mild or if there is also true ptosis of the eyelid, levator aponeurosis advancement may lift the lid enough to reduce symptoms. This operation will not eliminate the synkinetic movements, however.

If the closure of the eye is severe or if there are bothersome facial spasms with any facial movement, botulinum toxin injections will "disconnect" the synkinetic movements and quiet the face. I use the same dose and location of injection as for hemifacial spasm. This patient is at high risk for developing corneal exposure because you will be weakening an already weakened orbicularis muscle. Follow the patient closely and encourage the use of lubricants every few hours for the first few weeks after injection.

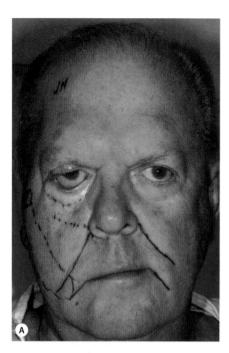

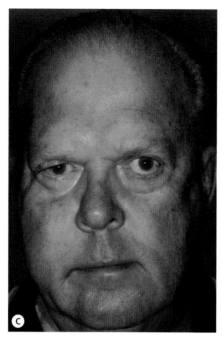

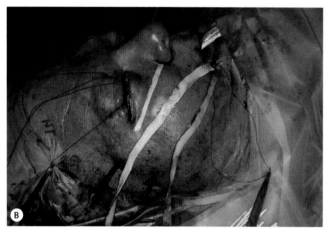

Figure 9-24 Facial nerve paralysis—facial sling. (**A**) Facial nerve paralysis with corneal exposure due to lower eyelid ectropion and incomplete blink despite gold weight implantation. "Hemiproptosis" and cheek descent complicated ectropion (see Figure 3-2 also). Dotted lines show planned suspension. (**B**) Fascial strips shown in position before implantation. (**C**) After facial sling, midface lift, right lower retractor recession, ear cartilage graft, and lateral tarsal strip. Exposure relieved.

Checkpoint

- You will have no problem recognizing facial nerve palsy. What are the main eye problems associated with facial nerve palsy?
- Review in your mind the treatment for corneal exposure (medical, static, and dynamic surgical treatments).
- Don't forget about the medial tarsorrhaphy and raising the lower lid if gold weight implantation is not enough. Remember to check corneal sensation.

- What are the most common treatments for paralytic brow ptosis? What is the treatment for paralytic ectropion? You should be able to do these operations. As you gain more experience, you may choose to add lower facial slings and endoscopic brow lifts to your treatments for facial palsy.
- How can you recognize aberrant regeneration of the facial nerve?

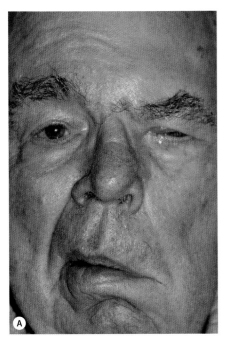 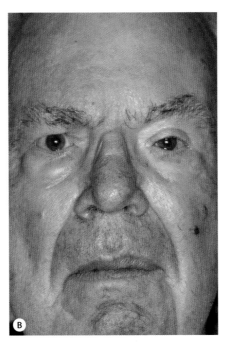

Figure 9-25 Facial nerve palsy. (**A**) Severe facial droop, ectropion, corneal exposure, brow ptosis, and difficult nasal breathing. (**B**) Asymmetry improved with lower and midfacial sling (using fascia lata) and unilateral endoscopic browplasty. Gold weight placed in upper eyelid. Lateral tarsal strip and lower eyelid recession with ear cartilage spacer in left lower eyelid. Nasal breathing markedly improved (from Nerad JA, Carter KD, Alford MA, *Rapid diagnosis in ophthalmology—oculoplastic and reconstructive surgery*, Philadelphia: Elsevier, 2008, p. 86, figure 4.22abc, Facial nerve palsy).

Major points

All muscles of the face are innervated by the facial nerve. The branches of the facial nerve are:

- Cervical
- Mandibular
- Buccal
- Orbital
- Frontal

Disorders of overactive facial muscles include:

- Orbicularis myokymia
- Facial tics
- Hemifacial spasm
- Essential blepharospasm

Orbicularis myokymia is an involuntary twitch of a portion of the orbicularis muscle. The cause is often fatigue or stress related. The problem is self-limited.

Hemifacial spasm is an involuntary spasm of one side of the face. It is usually caused by vascular compression of the facial nerve near its exit from the brainstem. Treatment is usually botulinum toxin (Botox®) injections. Intracranial microvascular decompression of the facial nerve should be considered for healthy patients under age 60 years.

Essential blepharospasm is an involuntary spasm of the eyes caused by a progressive central nervous system abnormality. Lower facial involvement, known as Meige syndrome, may occur. Most patients show considerable improvement after botulinum toxin injections.

The diagnosis of these disorders can be made based on the:

- Age of the patient
- Character of the spasm
- Location of the spasm

It is helpful to divide the face into quadrants:

- One eye only: orbicularis myokymia
- One side of the face: hemifacial spasm
- Two eyes: essential blepharospasm
- Eyes and lower face: Meige syndrome

Apraxia of lid opening, the inability to open the eye, is the most common cause of apparent failure of botulinum toxin injection.

The most common cause of weak facial muscles is facial nerve palsy. Other causes include the myopathic ptoses and Parkinson's disease.

Eye problems caused by facial nerve palsy include:

- Corneal exposure
- Incomplete blink
- Lagophthalmos
- Lower eyelid ectropion
- Brow ptosis

Aberrant regeneration of the facial nerve causes synkinetic facial movements. Palpebral fissure narrowing caused by tonic contraction of the orbicularis muscle may be mistaken for an acquired ptosis.

Major points Continued

Treatment of corneal exposure caused by facial nerve palsy includes:
- Ocular lubricants
- Static surgical procedures to narrow the palpebral fissure, including medial and lateral tarsorrhaphy and elevation of the lower eyelid
- Dynamic procedures to improve eyelid closure including gold weight implantation

Pay special attention to facial nerve palsy associated with decreased corneal sensation. Your patient will not know when the eye is in trouble. Neurotrophic keratitis will delay healing.

Lower eyelid ectropion is most commonly treated with the lateral tarsal strip procedure.

Brow ptosis is most commonly repaired with a direct browplasty. Other procedures are options.

The effects of aberrant regeneration of the facial nerve can be reduced with botulinum toxin injections or ptosis repair.

Suggested reading

1. Adams GG, Kirkness CM, Lee JP: Botulinum toxin A induced protective ptosis. *Eye* 1(pt 5):603–608, 1987.

2. Albert DM, Lucarelli MJ: Blepharospasm and hemifacial spasm. In *Clinical atlas of procedures in ophthalmic surgery*, pp. 397–399, Chicago: AMAP, 2004.

3. American Academy of Ophthalmology: *Basic and clinical science course: orbit, eyelids, and lacrimal system*, sect. 7, pp. 226–228, San Francisco: The American Academy of Ophthalmology, 2006/2007.

4. Anderson RL, Gordy DD: The tarsal strip procedure. *Arch Ophthalmol* 97(11):2192–2196, 1979.

5. Anderson RL, Patel BC, Holds JB, Jordan DR: Blepharospasm: past, present and future. *Ophthalmol Plast Reconstr Surg* 14(5):305–317, 1998.

6. Collin JRO, ed.: *A manual of systemic eyelid surgery*, 3rd edn, pp, 38, 139–148, Edinburgh: Churchill Livingstone, 1989.

7. Cook TA, Brownrigg PJ, Wang TD, Quatela VC: The versatile midforehead browlift. *Arch Otolaryngol Head Neck Surg* 115:163–168, 1989.

8. Dutton JJ: Botulinum-A toxin in the treatment of craniocervical muscle spasms: short- and long-term, local and systemic effects. *Surv Ophthalmol* 41(1):51–65, 1996.

9. Ellenbogen R: Transcoronal eyebrow lift with concomitant upper blepharoplasty. *Plast Reconstr Surg* 71(4):490–499, 1983.

10. Faucett DC, Essential blepharospasm. In Yanoff and , eds, *Ophthalmology*, pp. 695–697, Mosby, 2004.

11. Jordan DR, Patrinely JR, Anderson RL, Thiese SM: Essential blepharospasm and related dystonias. *Surv Ophthalmol* 34(2):123–132, 1989.

12. Kitchens J, Kinder J, Oetting T: The drawstring temporary tarsorrhaphy technique. *Arch Ophthalmol* 120:187–190, 2002.

13. McCord CD, Doxanas MT: Browplasty and browpexy: an adjunct to blepharoplasty. *Plast Reconstr Surg* 86(2):248–254, 1990.

14. Nerad J: Abnormal movements of the face. In *The requisites—Oculoplastic surgery*, pp. 193–214, St Louis: Mosby, 2001.

15. Nerad JA, Carter KD, Alford MA: Essential blepharospasm. In *Rapid diagnosis in ophthalmology—oculoplastic and reconstructive surgery*, pp. 120–123, Philadelphia: Mosby Elsevier, 2008.

16. Nerad JA, Carter KD, Alford MA: Hemifacial spasm. In *Rapid diagnosis in ophthalmology—oculoplastic and reconstructive surgery*, pp. 124–125, Philadelphia: Mosby Elsevier, 2008.

17. Nerad JA, Carter KD, Alford MA: Facial nerve palsy/ Aberrant regeneration of the facial nerve. In *Rapid diagnosis in ophthalmology—oculoplastic and reconstructive surgery*, pp. 126–129, Philadelphia: Mosby Elsevier, 2008.

18. Putterman AM: Botulinum toxin injections in the treatment of seventh nerve misdirection. *Am J Ophthalmol* 110(2):205–206, 1990.

19. Sadiq SA, Downes RN: A clinical algorithm for the management of facial nerve palsy from an oculoplastic perspective. *Eye* 12(pt 2):219–223, 1998.

20. Townsend DJ: Eyelid reanimation for the treatment of paralytic lagophthalmos: historical perspectives and current applications of the gold weight implant. *Ophthalmol Plast Reconstr Surg* 8(3):196–201, 1992.

21. Ward JB, Shore JW, McKeown CA: Essential blepharospasm. In McCord CD, Tanenbaum M, Nunery WR, eds, *Oculoplastic surgery*, 3rd edn, ch. 12, pp. 319–340, New York: Raven Press, 1995.

22. Wearne M, Sandy C, Rose G, Pitts J, Collin J: Autogenous hard palate mucosa: the ideal lower eyelid spacer? *Br J Ophthalmol* 85(10):1183–1187, 2001.

23. Wesley RE, Jackson CG, Glasscock ME III: Management of facial palsy. In McCord CD, Tanenbaum M, Nunery WR, eds, *Oculoplastic surgery*, 3rd edn, ch. 10, pp. 263–283, New York: Raven Press, 1995.

24. Wuebbolt GE, Drummond G: Temporary tarsorrhaphy induced with type A botulinum toxin. *Can J Ophthalmol* 26(7):383–385, 1991.

CHAPTER 10

Diagnosis and Management of the Patient with Tearing

Introduction

When you see a patient with tearing, the goal is to determine the cause of the tearing problem and the appropriate treatment. A pathologic condition may occur anywhere along the path of tear production to drainage. If you know the specific questions to ask during the history taking, you will get a good idea of the cause of the tearing and the severity of the problem. I think of a "watery" eye as a different problem than a "tearing" eye. The watery eye can be caused by a number of problems that are usually not specifically related to obstruction of the lacrimal drainage system. The tearing eye is almost always the result of canalicular or nasolacrimal duct obstruction. The *patient's age* is a good clue to the probable cause of the problem. A tearing eye in a 60-year-old patient almost always has a different cause than a tearing eye in a child.

After you have a good idea from the history of what the problem is, the physical examination will confirm your suspicion or point you to another diagnosis. If eyelid or eyelash problems are not seen during the examination, the cause is lacrimal drainage obstruction. This will be confirmed by the *lacrimal system vital signs: the dye disappearance test, palpation of the canaliculi, and irrigation of the nasolacrimal duct*. When you know the site of obstruction, the treatment choice is clear.

There are many conditions that can cause the patient to seek your help for a problem with tearing. The examination can be long if you do not know what you are looking for. If you master the concepts in this chapter, you will be able to easily diagnose the majority of lacrimal drainage problems. The treatments are successful in most patients.

Anatomy and function

Production, distribution, and drainage of tears

Let's review briefly the function and anatomy of the lacrimal system. Think of tear *production, distribution,* and *drainage* as the three processes required for normal lubrication of the eye.

Three layers of tears are produced to form the tear film. The majority of the tear film is produced by the lacrimal gland. Additional aqueous tears are produced by the glands of Wolfring and Krause. The middle aqueous layer adheres to the eye with the help of an inner mucous layer from the conjunctival goblet cells. Evaporation of the aqueous layer is reduced by a layer of oil superficial to the aqueous film produced by the oil glands of the eyelid. As you already know, these glands are primarily the meibomian glands of the tarsus and the Zeis glands associated with the eyelashes at the eyelid margin. All the glands producing the tear film must be healthy to keep a healthy thick layer of tears on the eye. Any problem in one layer may upset the system. An example is the eye irritation caused by blepharitis. In theory, the aqueous and mucous layers are okay, but the oil layer is not.

The lacrimal pump and reflex tearing

How are the distribution and drainage of tears related? Normal eyelid function is required for both. Normal blinking spreads the tears across the eye. The same normal blinking "pumps" the tears into the sac and down the nasolacrimal duct, the so-called "lacrimal pump." Any abnormality in the *frequency* or *quality* of the blinking will affect the distribution of tears. You have seen examples of both reduced frequency and quality of blinking. Patients with Parkinsonism blink only occasionally, causing symptoms of eye irritation and watery eyes. Patients with facial nerve palsy have a poor-quality blink. By this, I mean that the *blink is not complete*— the inferior cornea does not get wet. Ocular irritation resulting from conjunctival and corneal exposure is the result. The irritation may cause reflex tearing resulting in a watery eye. With facial nerve palsy, the *strength of the blink* is also decreased, reducing the force of the lacrimal pump. If the lid is ectropic, or the pump is very poor, a tearing eye may occur. Two causes of the watery eye are:

- Reflex tearing
- Poor lacrimal pump

Reread the last two paragraphs. The concepts of poor-quality tear production, inadequate distribution of tears, and reduced lacrimal pump function are difficult to understand when you are learning to estimate their contribution to a patient's problem. Anatomic blockage of the lacrimal system is easier to diagnose and easier to fix.

Anatomic sites of obstruction

Normal tear drainage depends on a functioning lacrimal pump and an intact lacrimal drainage system (Figure 10-1). As you recall from Chapter 2, the tears enter the upper and lower puncta and travel in a short vertical portion of the puncta for 1 or 2 mm before entering the horizontal portion of the canaliculi. The canaliculi enter the lacrimal sac at an angle, which forms a sort of valve (called the *common internal punctum*). The lacrimal sac sits in the lacrimal sac fossa bounded by the anterior lacrimal crest (maxillary bone) and the posterior lacrimal crest (lacrimal bone). The sac narrows inferiorly, forming the nasolacrimal duct (membranous nasolacrimal duct). The duct passes inferiorly through a bony canal (osseous nasolacrimal duct) to open beneath the inferior turbinate into the inferior meatus of the nose. The valve of Hasner at this opening prevents retrograde flow of tears or air up into the duct from the nose. An abnormality anywhere along this path can delay or block the drainage of the tears, usually causing a tearing eye. Anatomic obstruction can occur in the canaliculi or the nasolacrimal duct.

Our job is to figure out where the abnormality exists.

History

The "watery" eye versus the "tearing" eye: the significance of true epiphora

The definition of true epiphora—"tears on the cheek"

As you have seen earlier, I try to divide the patient's complaint into the watery eye or the tearing eye. The *watery eye* does not spill tears onto the cheek. The *tearing eye* has true *epiphora*, meaning that tears overflow onto the cheek. Make sure that you understand this difference. When your patient tells you the eye waters, *ask* "Do the tears flow down your cheek or do they stay in your eye?" You will be surprised how many patients tell you that they have tearing, but no tears overflow.

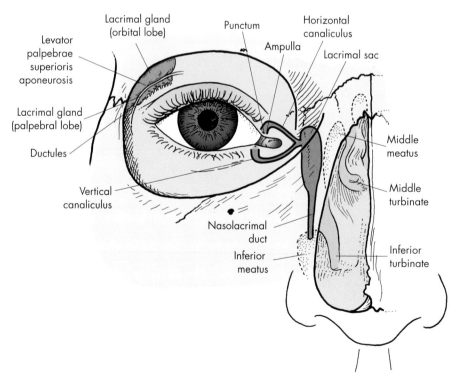

Figure 10-1 The anatomy of the lacrimal system.

What do the answers to these questions mean? The watery eye can be caused by a number of problems. Most of these problems are related to poor tear film, causing ocular irritation (or reflex tearing). There may be a subtle problem with one of the layers of the tears or the distribution of the tears, as we said above. These conditions improve with medical management such as lid hygiene and use of artificial tears and lubricating ointments. Watery eyes caused by an abnormal lid position or a poorly functioning pump are usually easy to diagnose on physical exam. *The tearing eye (true epiphora) is usually caused by poor drainage of tears though the lacrimal system.* There are exceptions to this but, in the absence of other obvious problems causing reflex tearing (an inflamed eye or trichiasis, etc.) or a lacrimal pump problem (ectropion or a facial nerve palsy), *epiphora means obstruction and an operation will be required to eliminate the tearing.* I'll repeat this concept because it is important: in the absence of a cause of reflex tearing or obvious lacrimal pump problem, epiphora means obstruction of the lacrimal drainage system.

The presence of epiphora depends on how complete the obstruction is and how many tears are being made. If the tears flow down your patient's cheek, ask "Do the tears flow down your cheek inside when you are resting or mainly when you are outside in cold and wind?" Everyone's system makes more tears in the wind or cold (a tear drainage stress test of sorts). If tearing is present only in the wind and cold, the obstruction is more likely "partial" or not complete. Remember that *young patients' systems make more tears than those of older patients*, so tear overflow will be seen more readily in younger patients than in older patients with the same anatomic problem. In fact, the lacrimal gland of many older adults makes so few tears that epiphora will not be present despite a complete blockage of lacrimal drainage. With nasolacrimal duct obstruction, these patients may exhibit signs of chronic dacryocystitis (mucopurulent drainage) or acute dacryocystitis (painful swelling of the medial canthus), but have no tearing. On the other hand, a young patient may have bothersome epiphora with only slight eversion of one punctum. An older patient with the same punctal eversion will not notice any epiphora.

Checkpoint

- Remind yourself of one or two problems that can affect tearing:
  — Production
  — Distribution
  — Drainage
- Make a sketch of the normal anatomy of the lacrimal drainage system
- What is the clinical difference between a watery eye and a tearing eye (epiphora)?
- What diagnosis does epiphora imply?
- Remember the questions:
  — "Do the tears flow down your cheek or do they stay in your eye?"
  — "Do the tears flow down your cheek inside when you are resting or mainly when you are outside in cold and wind?"

Findings suggesting lacrimal system obstruction

Things are getting a bit complicated, so let's go back to the general rules. Epiphora (tears on the cheek) implies a blockage in the drainage system. Watery eyes suggest a tear film or subtle blinking problem.

We have already discussed the significance of epiphora. There are always exceptions but, in most patients, nasolacrimal duct (NLD) obstruction will initially occur as a unilateral problem. A history of dacryocystitis means that a NLD obstruction is present. Onset after conjunctivitis suggests that the puncta or the canaliculi have become obstructed as a result of a viral infection (one of the few bilateral onsets). Onset after facial fracture or nasal surgery implies damage to the nasolacrimal duct (Box 10-1).

Watery eyes: findings suggesting other causes of tearing

As we discussed in the earlier sections, a patient may complain of watery eyes. No true epiphora is present. The exact meaning of this complaint can vary from patient to patient. Watery eyes may mean ocular irritation, mucoid discharge, a large tear lake, or just the feeling that the patient needs to blot the eyes. Sometimes even patients with low tear production will complain of watery eyes.

Because the main cause of watery eyes is poor tear film resulting in ocular irritation, the symptoms are usually bilateral. In some situations, the watery eyes may be explained by lacrimal pump problems including lid laxity or mild ectropion. These conditions are also usually bilateral in an older patient. Watery eyes may be caused by an incomplete blink related to facial nerve palsy. This is an exception to the general rule that epiphora occurring unilaterally is usually due to a NLD obstruction. However, the diagnosis of a palsy is usually clear.

When a patient complains of watery eyes without true epiphora, ask if the symptoms are bilateral and if any ocular irritation is present. Look for findings during the examination that confirm a poor tear film or inadequate lacrimal pump (Box 10-2).

Causes of tearing by age

If a patient has true epiphora, you can predict the type of blockage based on the patient's age (Figure 10-2). You will

---

Box 10-1

Findings Suggesting Obstruction of the Lacrimal System

- Epiphora
- Unilateral symptoms
- History of dacryocystitis
- Onset after:
  - Conjunctivitis
  - Facial fracture
  - Nasal surgery
    — History of nasal surgery

Box 10-2

Watery Eyes versus Tearing Eyes

Watery eyes

- No tears on cheek
- A nonspecific complaint
- Related to poor tear quality or poor tear distribution
- Treated with lid hygiene or use of artificial tears or ointment

Tearing eyes

- Epiphora or tears overflowing onto cheek
- Suggests obstruction of the lacrimal drainage: blocked nasolacrimal duct or canaliculus
- Usually treated with an operation to restore drainage

find that the following list is a great place to start for diagnosing the cause of lacrimal obstruction:

- Children
  - Congenital nasolacrimal duct obstruction
- Young adults
  - Trauma—canalicular laceration or facial trauma
  - Canalicular disease—usually postherpetic viral cause
- Middle-aged adult
  - Dacryolith—usually episodes of recurrent epiphora
- Older adults
  - Primary nasolacrimal duct obstruction

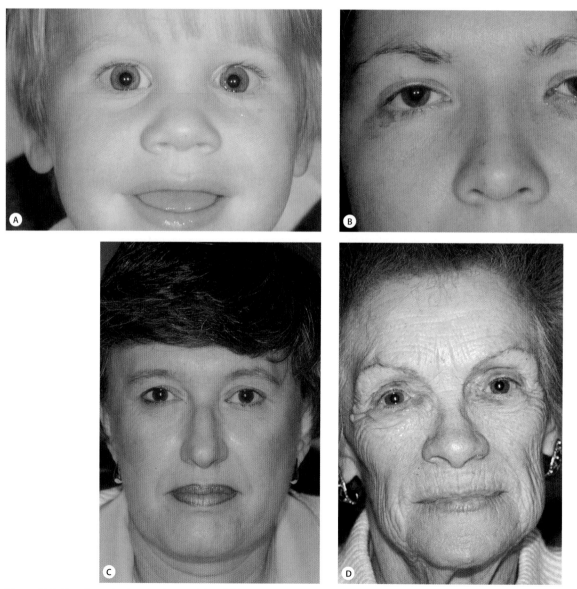

Figure 10-2 The diagnosis of tearing by age. (**A**) A child with congenital nasolacrimal duct obstruction. (**B**) A young adult with canalicular obstruction caused by viral conjunctivitis (the other cause in this age group is trauma). (**C**) A middle-aged woman with recurrent tearing resulting from a dacryolith. (**D**) An older adult with tearing caused by primary acquired nasolacrimal duct obstruction.

Children

A *child* who is seen with a tearing eye, often associated with mattering, has a *congenital nasolacrimal duct obstruction* until proven otherwise. This obstruction presents in the first month or two of life. Sometimes the mattering is present throughout the day. In other children, the mattering may be present only when they first awaken. The cause of the obstruction is a congenital membrane occurring at the valve of Hasner. In greater than 90% of children, this membrane will rupture spontaneously within the first year of life.

Young adults—canalicular disease or trauma

When a *young adult* is seen with epiphora, the cause is usually related to canalicular obstruction or trauma. *Canalicular obstruction* can occur after viral conjunctivitis. Often this obstruction is in all four canaliculi, causing complete scarring of each canaliculus. In other patients, traumatic lacerations of the eyelid may be associated with *canalicular lacerations*. In these patients, the obstruction is usually focal and in one canaliculus. *Facial fractures* may cause damage to the nasolacrimal duct. As you might expect, trauma is more common in young men than in young women.

Middle-aged adults—dacryolith

A *middle-aged adult*, usually a woman, will describe to you recurrent symptoms of true epiphora. In some cases, the epiphora will be associated with slight pain and tenderness in the medial canthus suggesting mild dacryocystitis. In most patients, the epiphora will resolve spontaneously. Interestingly, some patients may sneeze a small cast of stones out the nose. Passing of the *dacryolith* usually results in resolution of the symptoms. In many patients, these symptoms will be recurrent and may require surgical treatment (Figure 10-3).

Older adults—nasolacrimal duct obstruction

An *older adult*, again usually a woman, will be seen with epiphora resulting from *primary acquired nasolacrimal duct obstruction*. The cause of this scarring in the distal portion of the nasolacrimal duct is not known. Symptoms include epiphora, chronic mucopurulent discharge (chronic dacryocystitis), and acute cellulitis of the lacrimal sac (acute dacryocystitis) (Figure 10-4).

Although these diagnoses by age are generalizations, you will find that they are correct for most patients. The physical examination will prove or disprove your tentative diagnosis.

Checkpoint

- What findings in the history suggest lacrimal duct obstruction?
- What are the two common causes of the watery eye?
- Review the causes of epiphora based on age (very important—don't skip this).

Upper and lower lacrimal drainage systems

Tear drainage can be blocked at any point from the punctum to the valve of Hasner. The lacrimal drainage system can be divided into upper and lower systems. The *upper system* starts at the punctum and includes the canaliculi and the common internal punctum. The *lower system* consists of the lacrimal sac and nasolacrimal duct. Upper system obstruction, at the punctum or in the canaliculus, causes tearing only. Normally, mucoid secretions drain down the duct. Lower system

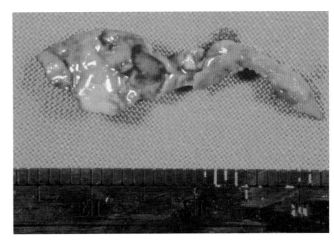

Figure 10-3 An unusually large dacryolith removed from the nasolacrimal sac and duct of a middle-aged woman (Figure 10-1), showing a cast of the entire lacrimal excretory system.

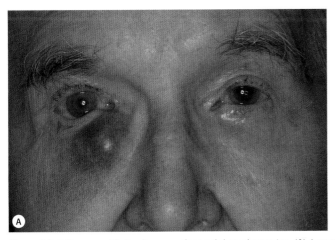
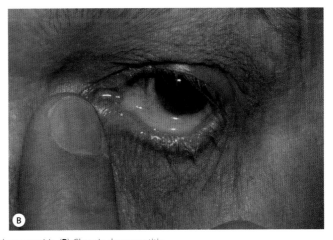

Figure 10-4 Dacryocystitis implies a nasolacrimal duct obstruction. (**A**) Acute dacryocystitis. (**B**) Chronic dacryocystitis.

obstruction, usually in the nasolacrimal duct, causes retention of mucus or pus in the lacrimal sac. Nasolacrimal duct obstruction may present as tearing and/or mucopurulent discharge. Partial obstruction of the nasolacrimal duct commonly occurs. Patients with partial obstruction often have tearing in the cold and wind as discussed earlier. Mucus produced in the sac is drained sufficiently to prevent signs and symptoms of dacryocystitis.

Physical examination

It is almost a cliché, but it is true that the examination starts when the patient walks into the room. You may notice an obvious cause of epiphora such as ectropion, entropion, discharge, ocular inflammation, dacryocystitis, or facial nerve palsy. The patient may have a large tear lake or frank epiphora. The patient may have a tissue in hand. If so, watch to see if the patient wipes the eyes when epiphora is present or merely wipes the eyes as a habit.

The patient with tearing needs a complete eye examination with an emphasis on the eyelid, eyelash, and lacrimal system (Box 10-3).

Eyelid problems

Ectropion and entropion

A number of eyelid problems may cause tearing. Ectropion resulting from any cause may prevent tears from reaching the lower punctum and canaliculus. Minor amounts of ectropion may go unnoticed, but may cause punctal eversion. More severe cicatricial or paralytic ectropion may prevent the lacrimal pump from functioning properly. Entropion is a cause of reflex tearing. If an older patient describes intermittent inward turning of the eyelid that is not seen on the examination, ask him or her to squeeze the eyes tightly. Forceful spasm of the orbicularis muscle may elicit entropion. Patients with cicatricial entropion will have eyelashes or keratinized skin against the ocular surface. Posterior lamellar scarring may be associated with damage to the conjunctiva, causing a poor tear film.

Lacrimal pump problems

Lacrimal pump problems are associated with *lid deformity*, *incomplete blink*, and *involutional laxity of the eyelids*. Scar tissue may cause the lids to be stiff and unable to blink completely and spontaneously. Facial nerve palsy is associated with an incomplete and weak blink that prevents normal lacrimal pump function. In the absence of a strong Bell's phenomenon, corneal exposure may also be present, creating an element of reflex tearing as well.

Probably the most common lacrimal pump problem is related to the laxity of the eyelids associated with aging. These involutional changes do not allow tight apposition of the eyelid against the eye. Lid laxity can be diagnosed by the *lid distraction test* and the *snap test*. The normal lower eyelid cannot be pulled more than 6 mm off the eyeball. If more than 6 mm of distraction is present, the lid is said to be lax. The snap test is performed by pulling the lids downward off the eyeball. A lid with normal tone and no laxity should snap into position spontaneously. Greater amounts of laxity are associated with increasing numbers of blinks required to return the lid to normal position. I usually record the results of the snap test like this: lid returns to position with two blinks (see Chapter 3).

Punctal problems

Eversion of the lower punctum may be subtle and associated with tearing, especially in a young patient (Figure 10-5). *Stenosis* of the punctum often follows eyelid eversion because of the drying of the mucosa. Spontaneous stenosis or closure of the punctum is associated with echothiophate iodide (Phospholine iodide) drops, but may be associated with most antiglaucoma medications. *Congenital punctal atresia* is uncommon but may be present in children, often seen as a family trait. In rare patients, the canalicular system may be normal, but the puncta may be covered with a thin *membrane*. A discharge from a dilated punctum—the "pouting punctum"—should alert you to a diagnosis of *canaliculitis*, an uncommon, but frequently overlooked cause of a mattering eye.

Eyelash problems

Any condition that results in *eyelashes rubbing against the eye* may cause corneal or conjunctival irritation, resulting in reflex tearing. *Marginal entropion* is a common cause of trichiasis (see Chapter 5). Secondary lid margin changes resulting from posterior lamellar shortening may be caused by *chronic blepharitis*. In these patients, reflex tearing is the result of both abnormal lashes and a poor tear film.

Box 10-3

Causes of Tearing by Age

Children
- Congenital nasolacrimal duct obstruction

Young adults
- Trauma—canalicular laceration or facial trauma
- Canalicular disease—usually postherpetic viral cause

Middle-aged adults
- Dacryolith—usually recurrent symptoms

Older adults
- Primary acquired nasolacrimal duct obstruction

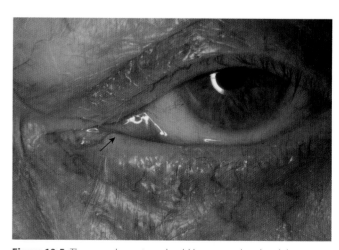

Figure 10-5 The normal punctum should be apposed to the globe. Punctal eversion (*arrow*) may be subtle and a cause of epiphora, especially in a young patient.

Checkpoint

- At this point in the examination, you have eliminated eyelid or eyelash problems as a cause of tearing. What are some eyelid and eyelash problems that can cause tearing?
- You have established that the patient has true epiphora and have made a tentative diagnosis based upon the patient's age.
- The lacrimal examination will confirm your tentative diagnosis.

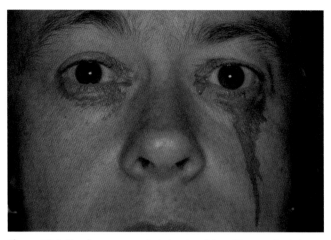

Figure 10-6 Dye disappearance test showing delay of fluorescein drainage and overflow of dye unilaterally.

The lacrimal examination

Rule out dacryocystitis first

Although the lacrimal system examination may seem daunting at first, it is really quite easy and quick when you get familiar with it. *One short cut is to look for signs of dacryocystitis if you suspect a nasolacrimal duct obstruction. The diagnosis of nasolacrimal duct obstruction is made if*:

- Signs of acute dacryocystitis are present
- You can express pus from the lacrimal sac
- A mucocele is present

Any one of these three findings diagnoses nasolacrimal duct obstruction. No further testing is necessary. The signs of acute dacryocystitis include swelling, erythema, and tenderness in the medial canthus. Any purulent or mucoid discharge that can be manually expressed from the sac is diagnostic for NLD obstruction. A mucocele is diagnosed when a palpable cystic mass is present in the medial canthus. A mucocele results when obstruction at both the nasolacrimal duct below and the common internal punctum above causes the lacrimal sac to fill with mucus.

Slit lamp examination

After you have checked the obvious signs of nasolacrimal duct obstruction, move the slit lamp into position and *evaluate the tear lake*. If lacrimal obstruction is present, the tear lake will be enlarged. Obstruction of the nasolacrimal duct will often cause a large tear lake with mucoid debris seen in it. This results from reflux of mucopurulent material in the sac into the tear lake. A block at the puncta or canaliculi results in a large tear lake without any debris present. Remember to evaluate the lacrimal lake before placing any drops in the eye. Next take a look at the cornea to rule out any obvious corneal pathologic changes. Watch the patient blink spontaneously and see how much of the cornea is covered with a blink. Look at the lid margins for signs of blepharitis or marginal entropion. Evaluate the position of the punctum. The normal punctum is not easily visible without slight manual eversion of the eyelid.

Lacrimal system vital signs

Next check the lacrimal system vital signs (Box 10-4):

- Dye disappearance test
- Palpation of the canaliculus
- Lacrimal irrigation

The *dye disappearance test* (Figure 10-6) is one of the most important lacrimal tests that you will do. After instilling a drop of topical anesthetic, place a well-formed drop of 2% fluorescein into each conjunctival fornix. After 5 minutes, check to see how much dye is retained in the eye. The yellow dye will spontaneously clear from a normal eye. The dye disappearance test is very good for confirming lacrimal obstruction. A normal result is recorded as spontaneous symmetric dye disappearance. An abnormal result is recorded as dye retained in the right or left eye. This test is most valuable when symptoms of epiphora are asymmetric. This is a very good test to use in both children and adults. In most patients, the results of the tests are obvious. However, in some older adults, the conjunctiva will stain with fluorescein in both eyes. Nevertheless, you may be able to evaluate the size of the tear film as an indicator of spontaneous tear drainage.

Next, demonstrate the patency of the upper and lower canaliculi using a lacrimal probe. This diagnostic test should not be confused with therapeutic nasolacrimal duct probing. To emphasize this distinction, we call this diagnostic procedure *canalicular palpation* (Figure 10-7, A). A 0 Bowman probe is carefully placed in the canaliculus (Figure 10-8). The lid should be pulled temporally and the probe directed toward the sac. If you meet resistance or the lid moves with the probe, you are probably pushing against the wall of the canaliculus and may cause a false passageway. The probe should pass easily to the lacrimal sac, where a *hard stop* should be present. This hard stop represents normal passage of the probe into the sac against the lacrimal bone. A *soft stop* is said to be present if a soft tissue obstruction at the lacrimal sac is encountered (Figure 10-9).

Careful passage of a 0 or 00 Bowman probe should not cause pain. A mild to moderate amount of tenderness may be encountered as the probe passes through the common internal punctum. *Under no circumstances, should you probe the nasolacrimal duct as a diagnostic procedure.*

Lacrimal irrigation (Figure 10-7, B) will tell you if the NLD is normal, partially obstructed, or closed. Using a lacrimal irrigation cannula in the lower canaliculus (not the sac), you should be able to irrigate saline or water easily into the nose without any reflux around the cannula or out the upper canaliculus (normal NLD). If you can't irrigate at all, make

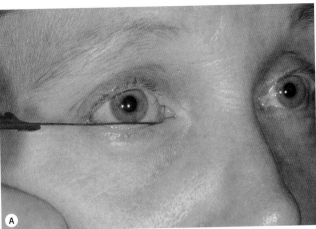
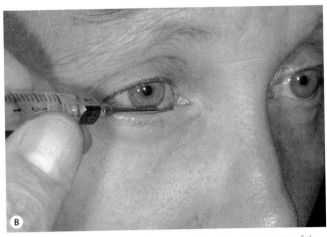

Figure 10-7 Lacrimal examination. (**A**) Canalicular "palpation" using a 0 or 00 Bowman probe (Storz E4200–E4205 for a complete set) to test patency of the canaliculus. (**B**) Lacrimal irrigation, using a lacrimal cannula (Storz E4406 or E4404) to test patency of the nasolacrimal duct. No reflux through the opposite canaliculus should be present.

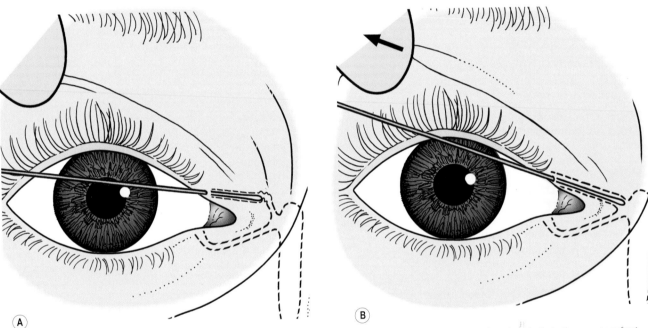

Figure 10-8 Introducing an instrument into the canaliculus. (**A**) Stabilize the lid with a finger. The probe should be placed vertically in the punctum for 1–2 mm. The lid should be pulled temporally and the probe directed toward the canthal angle. If the eyelid moves with palpation of the canaliculus, you are either hitting an obstruction or pushing against the wall of the canaliculus, risking a false passageway. (**B**) Stop. Pull the lid temporally again and redirect the probe.

sure the cannula is properly placed and is not against the wall of the canaliculus. Any reflux is abnormal, suggesting resistance to flow down the duct. If the patient doesn't taste the fluid in the throat, occlude the upper punctum with a cotton-tipped applicator (an assistant can help with this) and irrigate again. If you can irrigate into the nose with pressure on the syringe, the patient has a partially obstructed or narrow duct (*functional obstruction*). If you can't irrigate with pressure on the syringe, the duct is closed (*anatomic obstruction*). After you are comfortable with the irrigation process, try this: when your patient has a functional obstruction, try to irrigate with progressively more pressure until you get a bit of reflux. This will give you an idea of how much fluid the NLD can drain—another form of tear drainage stress test.

You may notice that the historically recommended Jones' test for epiphora (that you may have read about elsewhere) is not recommended. It is time consuming and inaccurate.

Nasal examination

The last portion of the lacrimal examination includes a nasal examination. Three options for illumination and exposure are available. A hand-held illuminated speculum is a handy office tool (Welch Allyn no. 26030 illuminator and speculum or no. 26035 speculum only). Alternatively, a nonilluminated speculum may be used for exposure and a headlight can be worn to provide illumination. If you do many lacrimal operations, you may want to purchase a fiberoptic nasal endoscope, which will permit you to do the best intra-

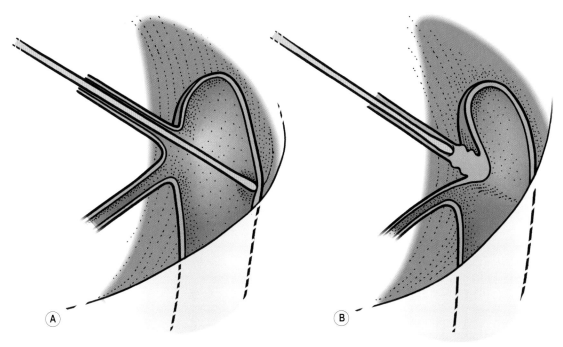

Figure 10-9 (**A**) A "hard stop" with canalicular palpation indicating a normal canaliculus. (**B**) A "soft stop," indicating obstruction of the canaliculus.

Box 10-4

Lacrimal System Vital Signs
- Dye disappearance test
- Palpation of canaliculi
- Irrigation of lacrimal system

---

nasal examination. Regardless of the technique, intranasal tumors or mucosal abnormalities should be ruled out (Box 10-5).

On rare occasions, the examination does not fit with the history. The patient gives a history typical of primary acquired NLD obstruction (PANDO), but you cannot demonstrate an obstruction. In these patients, dacryoscintigraphy can be helpful. In this nuclear medicine procedure, a labeled tear-drop is placed in the conjunctival cul de sac. Its passage into the nose is imaged over time. This test is similar in concept to the dye disappearance test. It gives an estimate of the physiologic drainage of tears. If any delay is noted, a dacryo-cystorhinostomy (DCR) is recommended. The only other imaging test that I use is a computed tomography (CT) scan when a lacrimal sac tumor is suspected.

Checkpoint

- What are the lid distraction and lid snap tests?
- What are three signs of NLD obstruction seen on the external examination that will short cut your lacrimal system examination?
- What are the lacrimal system vital signs? (don't skip this one)
- What is the difference between a "hard stop" and a "soft stop"?

At this point, you have determined the cause of the tearing and are ready to make a plan to correct the problem.

Box 10-5

Lacrimal Examination
- Confirm diagnosis suggested by history of epiphora
- Confirm diagnosis suggested by age
- Rule out lid or lash problems
- Diagnosis of nasolacrimal duct obstruction is made if:
  - Acute dacryocystitis is present
  - Mucopurulent material can be expressed from the sac
  - A mucocele is present
- Perform a slit lamp examination
  - Large tear lake
  - Debris in tear lake
  - Punctal position and patency
  - Cornea and lid margins
- Evaluate lacrimal system vital signs
  - Dye disappearance test
  - Palpation of canaliculi
  - Lacrimal irrigation
- Do not probe the nasolacrimal duct
- Perform a nasal examination

Treatment

Treat eyelid and eyelash problems first

Ectropion, entropion, and lacrimal pump problems

In all cases, eyelid and eyelash problems should be treated before lacrimal surgery. Standard treatments for ectropion and entro-pion should be used. Conditions affecting the lacrimal pump should be treated. Lid deformities such as cicatricial entro-pion should be treated with skin grafts. Incomplete blinking can be treated with topical lubricants and gold weight place-ment in the upper lid. Laxity of the lower lid can be repaired

---

Box 10-6

Treatment of Lacrimal Pump Problems

Lid deformity—treat deformity

Incomplete blink of upper lid

- Lubricants
- Gold weight

Laxity of lower lid

- Lateral tarsal strip

Facial nerve palsy

- Lubricants
- Lateral tarsal strip operation plus additional procedures

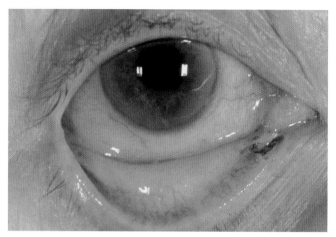

Figure 10-10 The three-snip punctoplasty. A triangle is removed from the posterior wall of the canaliculus. Snip 1 is in the vertical portion of the canaliculus. Snip 2 is along the horizontal portion of the canaliculus edging slightly posteriorly. Snip 3 is the diagonal cut connecting snips 1 and 2.

using standard horizontal lid tightening procedures. Additional procedures are available for facial nerve palsy and are covered in a later chapter. In most patients, the lacrimal pump can be improved, but it is often difficult to eliminate all symptoms of tearing (Box 10-6).

After appropriate treatment of the eyelid abnormalities, the lacrimal symptoms should be re-evaluated. Before we move on to treatment of NLD obstruction, we will discuss treatment of punctal problems. Instruments and sutures of special interest in lacrimal surgery are listed in Boxes 10-16 and 10-17.

Punctal stenosis

Stenosis of the punctum can be treated with dilation; however, the effect of punctal dilation is usually temporary. Substitution of an alternative antiglaucoma medication for an offending drug is appropriate if possible. Although punctoplasty procedures are described, I find that I seldom use them. *Two-snip and three-snip punctoplasties* are possible. The two-snip punctoplasty consists of a V-shaped excision of the posterior portion of the punctum and vertical part of the canaliculus. A three-snip punctoplasty is somewhat more useful. In this operation, a small triangle of the posterior wall of the vertical and horizontal portion of the canaliculus is excised.

The steps of the *three-snip punctoplasty* are:

1. Vertical cut of punctum: "snip 1"
   A. Place a Westcott scissors in the vertical portion of the canaliculus and cut inferiorly.
2. Horizontal cut of the canaliculus: "snip 2"
   A. Turn the scissors 90 degrees and slide one tip in the horizontal portion of the canaliculus.
   B. The scissors will be parallel to the lid margin.
   C. Make a 2 mm cut slightly posterior to the lid margin. It is important to place this horizontal cut posteriorly; otherwise you will disturb the normal appearance of the lid margin.
3. Diagonal cut of the canaliculus: "snip 3"
   A. Grasp the cut corner and make a diagonal cut, removing a posterior triangle of canaliculus.
   B. The excised area should not be visible when looking at the lid margin.
   C. The mucosa of the inside of the canaliculus should be visible from the posterior aspect of the eyelid (Figure 10-10).

In some patients, you will find that the stenosis of the punctum is associated with stenosis of the canaliculus as well. For these patients, intubation of the entire nasolacrimal system with silicone stents is appropriate. Make sure that stents will not be required before you perform a punctoplasty procedure. Once the integrity of the punctum is disturbed, stents can erode the remaining canaliculus (Box 10-7).

Punctal eversion

Eversion of the punctum is most commonly caused by laxity in the lower eyelid. The lid distraction or snap test will demonstrate if laxity is present. Before proceeding with any lid tightening procedure, be sure that there is no anterior lamellar shortening pulling the puncta outward. *If cicatricial causes are present, a full-thickness skin graft* is usually required. If laxity alone is present, evaluate the potential effectiveness of the lateral tarsal strip procedure during the slit lamp examination. While viewing the punctum, place your index finger at the lateral canthus and simulate tightening the eyelid. If the punctum returns to normal position, a horizontal lid tightening procedure will be effective. If the punctum remains somewhat everted, consider adding a medial spindle operation. If no horizontal lid laxity is present, use the *medial spindle operation* alone. This is a rare situation, however.

The *medial spindle procedure* is simple to perform and quite effective. It is a combination of a posterior lamellar shortening procedure and a mechanical inversion of the lid margin with an absorbable suture (see Chapter 3).

The *medial spindle operation* includes:

- Patient preparation
- Excision of a diamond of conjunctiva
- Closure of the conjunctiva to invert the punctum
- A lateral tarsal strip operation (usually)

The steps of the *medial spindle operation* are:

1. Prepare the patient
   A. Instill topical anesthetic drops.
   B. Inject local anesthetic into the inferior fornix of the medial conjunctiva.

C. Inject local anesthetic under the skin at the orbital rim inferior to the punctum.

2. Excise a diamond of conjunctiva
   A. Place a no. 1 Bowman probe into the canaliculus and evert the lid margin.
   B. *Excise a "diamond" of conjunctiva* (and theoretically lower eyelid retractors) inferior to the punctum and the tarsal plate (3–4 mm by 3–4 mm) (Figure 10-11, A).
      (1) Make the diamond-shaped excision by grasping the conjunctiva with a Paufique forceps and using Westcott scissors to excise a V of conjunctiva inferiorly. Cut a similar V of conjunctiva superiorly so the two incisions form into a diamond. The excised area of conjunctiva will be closed vertically, shortening the posterior lamella and turning the punctum inward.
      (2) Take care not to cut the vertical portion of the canaliculus when performing the excision.

3. Close the conjunctiva to invert the punctum
   A. Use a double-armed *5-0 chromic suture* (Ethicon 792G G-3 needle) to close the diamond, incorporating a pass through the lower lid retractors in the center of the diamond excision (Figure 10-11, B). (You will not always be able to recognize retractors.)
   B. Next pass the two arms of the suture back-handed through the apex of the diamond adjacent to the punctum. This part of the operation theoretically advances the lower lid retractors to the top of the diamond.
   C. The remainder of the closure involves collapsing the diamond and passing the sutures out through the eyelid. Pass each suture arm through the inferior apex of the diamond and continue the full-thickness pass through the lid, exiting at the junction of the eyelid and cheek skin. The suture pass can be visualized as a *spiral* if viewed laterally (see Figure 10-11, C). The conjunctival suture passes close the posterior lamellar, resulting in a posterior lamellar shortening. The full-thickness pass of the suture through the eyelid, emerging inferiorly, causes a mechanical inversion of the punctum. A significant mechanical inversion of the punctum will occur when the sutures are pulled tightly on the skin side of the eyelid.

4. Do a lateral tarsal strip operation (usually)
   A. Cut the needles of the spindle suture off and clamp the suture ends out of the way. If a lateral tarsal strip operation is also being done (as is usually the case), it should be performed at this point.
   B. The medial spindle suture should be tied after the strip is sewn into position. The amount of inversion can be titrated by tying the suture with more or less tension. At the conclusion of the medial spindle procedure, a slight overcorrection (inversion) is desired.

The chromic suture will fall out on its own in approximately 7–10 days. The overcorrection will reduce spontaneously, leaving the punctum in its normal position. Remember that the medial spindle operation must be performed before

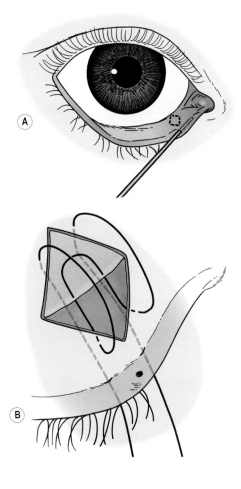

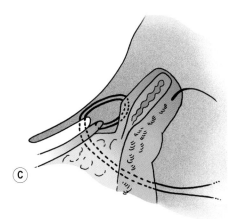

Figure 10-11 The medial spindle operation. (**A**) Place a no. 1 Bowman probe in the canaliculus and evert the medial aspect of the lower eyelid. Excise a diamond of conjunctiva and lower lid retractors inferior to the punctum. (**B**) Close the diamond using a double-armed 5-0 chromic suture through the retractors, through the superior apex of conjunctiva, and through the lower edge of the conjunctiva, continuing full thickness through the eyelid and emerging superior to the inferior orbital rim. (**C**) Lateral view showing closure of the diamond using the "spiral" suture to create slight inversion of the punctum.

the eyelid is tightened with a lateral tarsal strip operation. Once the lateral tarsal strip sutures are tied, the medial eyelid cannot be everted to perform the medial spindle operation (Box 10-8).

Canaliculitis

Patients with canaliculitis most commonly complain of a persistent discharge or red eye. In some cases, this is confused with "tearing," but true epiphora is not usually present. Usually, you will see canaliculitis in an older patient. Often the patient has been treated with antibiotic drops for some time before the correct diagnosis is made. On your external examination, you will see a swelling and erythema of the canalicular portion of the eyelid (Figure 10-12). In some cases, this finding is subtle. Usually it is an easy diagnosis, if you remember to think of canaliculitis in the differential diagnosis of a watery or discharging eye (no one comes in saying the inside corner of my eyelid is "red and swollen").

Canaliculitis arises from an aerobic infection, most commonly *Actinomyces israeli*. The organism burrows into the canalicular wall creating an ideal microclimate for survival buried out of the range of any topical drops. To treat, you will need to curette the canaliculus. Usually you can do this through the dilated punctum. In some cases, you will need to open the punctum using a one-, two-, or three-snip punctoplasty. Be meticulous about cleaning the entire lining of the canaliculus, which will likely be quite dilated. Keep curetting until you do not retrieve any more "stones." Irrigate the canaliculus with saline or penicillin G (100,000 units/cc). Topical antibiotic drops are reasonable postoperatively, but the primary treatment appears to be surgical removal of the infection. Occasionally, reoperations are required.

Box 10-7

Three-Snip Punctoplasty

Vertical cut (snip 1)

- Use Westcott scissors to open the posterior portion of the punctum and ampulla of the canaliculus

Horizontal cut (snip 2)

- Rotate the scissors and cut 2–3 mm along the horizontal portion of the canaliculus
- Stay posterior so the cut is not visible anteriorly

Diagonal cut (snip 3)

- Excise a triangle of tissue off the posterior portion of the canaliculus
- The mucosa of the canaliculus should be visible

Box 10-8

The Medial Spindle Operation

Patient preparation

- Instill topical anesthetic
- Inject local anesthetic into the conjunctiva and skin on the medial one third of the lid

Conjunctival diamond excision

- Evert the lid margin with a Bowman probe
- Excise a diamond of conjunctiva and lower lid retractors

Closure of diamond

- Pass a double-armed 5-0 chromic suture through
  - lower lid retractors,
  - then apex near punctum,
  - then apex inferiorly,
  - and out full-thickness through the lid
- Do a lateral tarsal strip operation for most patients
- Tie sutures to invert the punctum slightly

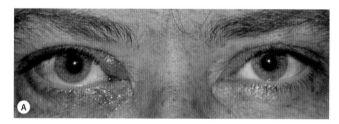

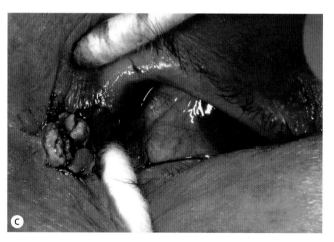

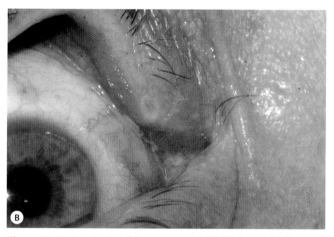

Figure 10-12 Canaliculitis of the upper eyelid. (**A**) Discharge of right eye. Erythema and swelling of right upper canaliculus. (**B**) "Pouting punctum"—punctum is dilated. Pressure on canaliculus expresses pus. (**C**) "Sulfur granules"—stones curetted from patulous canaliculus typical of *Actinomyces*, after 3-snip punctoplasty (different patient than in parts A and B).

Treatment of congenital nasolacrimal duct obstruction

Congenital nasolacrimal duct obstruction is caused by the persistence of a membrane at the valve of Hasner. In greater than 90% of patients, this membrane will spontaneously rupture within the first year of life. Treatments include:

- Massage and antibiotic drops
- NLD probing
- NLD probing with lacrimal system intubation
- Dacryocystorhinostomy

Massage and antibiotic drops

Massage of the lacrimal sac is recommended as a conservative treatment while waiting for spontaneous rupture of the obstruction to occur. Massage throughout the day will empty the contents of the sac and reduce the amount of discharge. An antibiotic drop used two or three times a day will help. In some cases, massage may build up enough pressure in the sac so that the membrane is broken. Although we recommend massage commonly, you will find that *most parents do not perform lacrimal sac massage correctly or often enough to make much difference.* Most parents massage the side of the nose rather than posteriorly in the area of the lacrimal sac. Feel your own lacrimal sac fossa. You must push your index finger posterior to the anterior lacrimal crest to empty the sac. It is helpful to show the parents of your patients how to massage the sac effectively. How often massage should be done varies from child to child. The idea is to massage as often as necessary to empty the sac. In some children, this may be as often as every 2 hours.

If you have children, you can imagine the burden of trying to keep up with massage several times a day. It is not long before the child will cry in anticipation of the massage when he or she sees a finger coming toward the face. Consequently, if discharge is a significant problem and massage is ineffective, I recommend probing earlier rather than later (don't wait until 1 year of age). This is not the "textbook" recommendation, but is a practical solution for many families.

Nasolacrimal duct probing

If spontaneous resolution of the tearing and mattering does not occur by 1 year of age, *nasolacrimal duct probing* should be performed. In most cases, this procedure is performed under general anesthesia in an outpatient setting.

Nasolacrimal duct probing includes:

- Patient preparation
- Infracture of the inferior turbinate
- Dilation of the punctum
- "Hard stop" pass into the sac
- Passage of the probe into the nasolacrimal duct
- Confirmation that the probe is in the nose

The steps for nasolacrimal duct probing are:

1. Prepare the patient
   A. Spray a vasoconstricting agent in the nose. Like all other lacrimal operations, it is important to prepare the nose with a vasoconstricting agent so you will minimize bleeding and maximize visualization in the nose. In the preoperative holding area, spray the involved side of the nose with a nasal decongestant spray such as oxymetazoline hydrochloride 0.05% (Afrin) twice, ten minutes apart.
   B. Pack the nose. After induction of general anesthesia, pack the inferior turbinate with either a small piece of cotton or a small *neurosurgical cottonoid* dampened with oxymetazoline hydrochloride. You may need to cut the cottonoid so that it is narrow enough to slide under the inferior turbinate easily. You should use a *fiberoptic headlight and a pediatric nasal speculum* to visualize the inside of the nose. *Bayonet forceps* are useful to place the pack in the nose. You will get the best decongestion and intraoperative view if you pack medially and laterally to the inferior turbinate. Remember, lateral to the inferior turbinate means that the pack is under the inferior turbinate (Figure 10-13, A). When you perform a DCR, you will be packing the area around and under the *middle* turbinate. No local anesthetic is necessary. Clear any discharge from the patient's eyelids, but no formal prep is necessary. Remove the nasal packing.

2. Infracture the inferior turbinate
   A. Look inside the nose again to see how much space there is in the inferior meatus. I place a Freer elevator under the turbinate and rotate it. If there is resistance to this rotation, I perform an *inferior turbinate infracture*. This is easy to do.
   B. With the elevator under the turbinate held in your dominant hand and the nasal bridge in your nondominant hand, push the turbinate toward the nasal septum. You will feel the turbinate "give" a bit or sometimes crack. I am not aware of any study that has definitely proven that turbinate infracture is a helpful procedure, but it is a common practice (Figure 10-13, B).

3. Dilate the punctum
   A. Next proceed with careful punctal dilation. *You must avoid creating a false passageway.*
   B. Sit at the head of the bed and stabilize the lower eyelid with your index finger and thumb of your nondominant hand. Place the punctal dilator into the *vertical portion* of the lower punctum.
   C. Carefully rotate the punctal dilator to a position parallel with the lid margin. Give slight lateral traction on the eyelid. Gently pass the probe toward the medial canthus into the *horizontal portion* of the canaliculus. If you meet any resistance to the probe, you should stop to avoid creating a false passageway. It is not necessary to push the probe very far into the canaliculus.
   D. I perform probings through the lower punctum only. Dilation and passage of the probe into the canaliculus are easier in the lower eyelid than in the upper eyelid.

4. Make a *hard stop* pass through the canaliculus
   A. The nasolacrimal duct probing is best done with a larger probe such as a *no. 1 Bowman probe*. Place the probe into the *vertical portion* of the canaliculus while stabilizing the lid with the same lateral traction you used for dilation of the punctum (Figure 10-13, C).

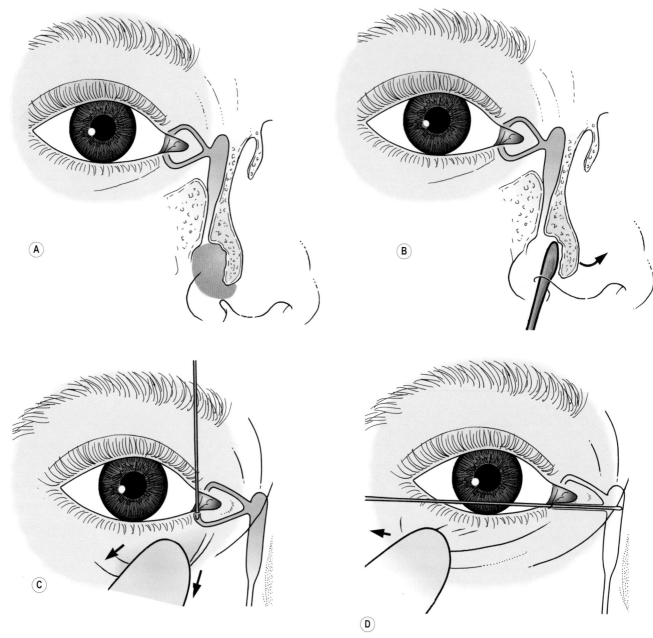

Figure 10-13 Nasolacrimal duct probing. (**A**) Pack under the inferior turbinate using a trimmed neurosurgical cottonoid. (**B**) Infracture of the inferior turbinate, if the meatus is tight. Push the Freer elevator against the turbinate until you feel it give or crack. (**C**) Vertical entrance of no. 1 Bowman probe into the punctum. (**D**) With lateral traction on the lower lid, rotate the probe 90 degrees and pass it along the horizontal portion of the canaliculus to a "hard stop." (**E**) Rotate the probe 90 degrees in the coronal plane and pass the probe into the nose, aiming slightly posterior and lateral (at the lateral ala of the nose). Feel for a slight "pop" (not always palpable). (**F**) Curving the probe to fit over the brow facilitates passage. (**G**) You must confirm that the probe has passed into the nose with either direct visualization or irrigation of fluorescein-tinged saline. In this case, the probe is visualized under the inferior turbinate on the left side using an endoscope.

B. Turn the probe 90 degrees and pass it along the *horizontal portion* of the canaliculus (Figure 10-13, D). Give lateral traction on the eyelid.

C. If you see the *lid move* as you pass the probe, you are running into a soft tissue obstruction, a *soft stop*. You should not advance the probe any further. Reorient the probe and try again. In an unobstructed canaliculus, the probe should pass easily into the sac and hit the medial wall of the lacrimal sac fossa resulting in a *hard stop* (see Figure 10-9). Make sure that you understand the concepts of soft and hard stops discussed here and earlier in this chapter.

5. Pass the probe into the nasolacrimal duct
   A. You will not be able to see inside the sac so *you need to visualize in your mind what is happening*. The goal is to pass the probe atraumatically down the duct into the inferior meatus. The orientation of the duct lies in the coronal plane of the face, perhaps somewhat more posterior and slightly lateral. Think about where you placed the pack under the inferior meatus. That is where you are aiming. In your mind, visualize the tip of the probe in the sac.
   B. Without moving the tip of the probe off the medial wall of the sac, rotate the probe into the coronal

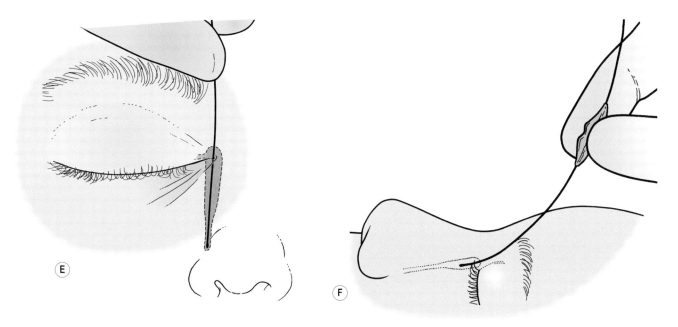

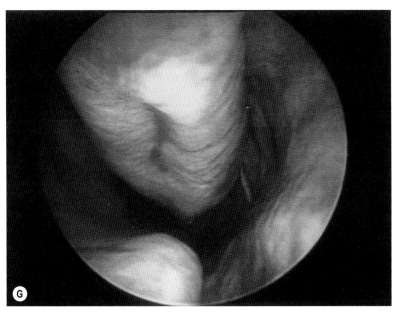

Figure 10-13 Continued.

plane (Figure 10-13, E). Imagine that you are sliding the probe down into the neck of a funnel as the probe passes from the sac into the duct. Continue to pass the probe down the duct. The nasolacrimal duct is shorter than you think, usually less than 15 mm (sometime you might find it helpful to place the probe on the outside of the patient and actually see how short the duct is).

C. It won't be long before you feel a *small "pop"* as you penetrate the membrane of the duct. If you cannot advance the probe, you are probably hitting the floor of the nose. You will not always feel a definitive "pop."

D. Sometimes it is difficult to get the proper orientation of the probe if the brow is prominent. I find it

helpful to hold the probe against the medial canthus and bend the probe in a *curved fashion* so that it can pass easily into the nose (Figure 10-13, F).

6. Confirm that the probe is in the nose
   A. You must confirm that the probe has passed into the inferior turbinate. This can be done either by *direct visualization* or by *irrigation of fluorescein-tinged solution* into the nose.
      (1) *Direct visualization.* Over the years, as I have gotten more proficient in looking in the nose, I often choose the direct visualization route. Again, using a headlight and nasal speculum, it is usually possible to look under the inferior turbinate and see the metal probe in position. Most times, you can see the probe in the nose

by direct view, especially if you use a Freer elevator to push the turbinate away and place a suction tip in the inferior meatus.

(2) This is a good time to recheck the position of the inferior turbinate. If the inferior meatus is too narrow, it is reasonable to perform an infracture of the turbinate as described above.

(3) If you are interested in using a *nasal endoscope*, this is an easy way to see the probe in the nose (Figure 10-13, G).

(4) *Fluorescein irrigation.* An alternative to direct visualization is irrigation using fluorescein-tinged fluid. An irrigation syringe is passed through the lower punctum into the canaliculus. With a suction tip in the inferior turbinate, irrigate fluorescein-stained saline down the nasolacrimal duct (put some fluorescein strips in saline to make the irrigation fluid yellow). The yellow fluid will easily be seen in the tubing of the suction. Remember children usually don't have a cuffed endotracheal tube so don't irrigate more than you have to and suction out as much of the irrigation fluid as you can.

7. Apply antibiotic ointment
   A. At the conclusion of the procedure, put some topical antibiotic ointment into the conjunctival cul de sac. Tell the parents to use the ointment three or four times a day for 1 week.
   B. Explain to the parents that a bloody tear or small amount of blood from the nose is not unexpected.
   C. I usually see the patients 1 month postoperatively. The majority of patients will be symptom free (Box 10-9).

Nasolacrimal duct intubation with stents

For 90% of patients undergoing nasolacrimal duct probing, the outcome is successful. If tearing or mattering continues, intubation of the nasolacrimal duct using silicone stents is the next step. The technique of passing stents through the nasolacrimal system is similar to that of passing a Bowman probe down the tear duct. One stent is placed in each canaliculus, and the stents are retrieved and brought out through the nose. They are tied in a knot, forming a loop through the nasolacrimal system. There are several types of stents available. The most commonly used stents are *Crawford silicone stents* (set 28-0185, JEDMED Instrument Co., http://wwwjedmed.com).

The *nasolacrimal duct intubation procedure* includes:

- Patient preparation
- Dilation of the punctum
- Passage of the stents into the canaliculus and NLD
- Retrieval of the stents
- Tying the stents

The steps of the nasolacrimal duct intubation procedure are:

1. Prepare the patient
   A. Use general anesthesia in an outpatient setting.
   B. The preparation of the nose is the same as that for nasolacrimal probing. During the preparation, you

---

Box 10-9

Nasolacrimal Duct Probing Procedure

Patient preparation
- Oxymetazoline hydrochloride 0.05% (Afrin) spray in the preoperative area
- General anesthesia
- Nasal packing in inferior turbinate
- Clean off any mattering on lids

Punctal dilation and canalicular "palpation"
- Perform punctal dilation (stabilize lid with lateral traction to avoid a false pass)
- Remove nasal packing
- Infracture inferior turbinate if meatus is tight
- Place 1-0 Bowman probe into punctum vertically
- Rotate and advance in the horizontal canaliculus (stabilize lid with lateral traction to avoid a false pass)
- Feel a "hard stop" at the lacrimal sac fossa

Nasolacrimal duct intubation
- Rotate the probe 90 degrees; make a curve in the probe
- Pass the probe down the duct about 15 mm (not very far)
- Confirm the presence of the probe under the turbinate:
  - Direct visualization
  - Endoscopic view
  - Suction fluorescein-tinged saline irrigation fluid
- Apply topical antibiotic ointment

Follow-up

---

should determine whether the inferior turbinate needs to be infractured.

2. Dilate the punctum
   A. Slightly more aggressive punctal dilation is necessary to allow the entrance of the olive tip of the Crawford stent. You must be careful not to create a false passage with the dilator.

3. Pass the stents into the canaliculus and NLD
   A. I often pass a no. 1 Bowman probe through the duct before positioning the stents. This gives me information about the anatomy of the system more easily than with the metal probes on the stents, which are thinner and less malleable. They are somewhat more difficult to pass than the no. 1 Bowman probe.
   B. Repeat the probing technique with one arm of the stent.

4. Retrieve the stents
   A. Once the stent is in the nose, the olive tip on the end of the stent can be retrieved with either a
      (1) Crawford hook (JEDMED Instrument Co. no. 28-0186, http://www.jedmed.com).
      (2) Anderson Hwang grooved director (JEDMED Instrument Co. no. 28-0189, http://www.jedmed.com).
      (3) A small hemostat.
   B. My preference is to use the grooved director (Figure 10-14, A and B). This is a very atraumatic way to retrieve the stents. A slotted hood on the end of a grooved director is used to hook the olive tip of the Crawford stent.

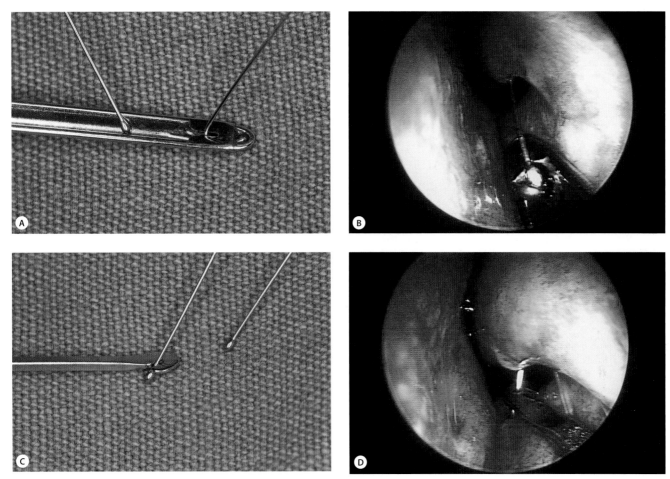

Figure 10-14 Stent retrieval techniques. (**A**) Tse–Anderson grooved director (similar to the newer Hwang-Anderson grooved director). The olive tip of the Crawford stent slides in the groove to catch in the hood of the director. (**B**) Endophoto of the Crawford stent, in the inferior turbinate, engaged in the Tse–Anderson grooved director. (**C**) Crawford hook with the tip of Crawford stents. (**D**) Endophoto of a Crawford stent, in the inferior turbinate, engaged in a Crawford hook.

C. The Crawford hook (Figure 10-14, C and D) is a simpler, but more traumatic, way to retrieve the stent.

D. Some surgeons prefer the use of a hemostat.

E. If you are able to use an endoscope easily, visualization of the stent makes retrieval much easier.

5. Consider these tips for retrieval of the stent

A. Unless you are using an endoscope or can see the stent directly, *retrieval of the stent is all by touch.*

B. You must first make sure that you are actually in the inferior turbinate. When an instrument is placed in the inferior turbinate, it extends out the nose perpendicular to the plane of the operating table. The inferior meatus is very narrow so that the instrument will hold securely in place.

C. Once the *grooved director* is in position, you must locate the metal olive tip of the stent.

　(1) In most cases, the tip is against the lateral wall of the nose inferior to where the duct opens.

　(2) Push the grooved director against the lateral wall of the nose and slide it anteriorly and posteriorly a few millimeters to see if you can feel the stent.

　(3) If you can feel the stent or see the stent move in the punctum above, push the grooved director

against the lateral wall of the nose and retract the stent from above a few millimeters.

　(4) Confirm that the grooved director is against the lateral wall of the nose and advance the stent inferiorly again.

　(5) Pull the grooved director anteriorly, and the tip should catch in the slot.

　(6) Once the olive tip is engaged, offer some general resistance on the stent at the punctum above to "set" the olive tip in the grooved director. Advance the grooved director out of the nose, and the stent will follow. Be careful to pull the stent out slowly.

D. The *Crawford hook* can be used in a similar fashion.

　(1) Make sure that you know where the open side of the hook is facing. A flat area on the handle of the hook is opposite to the open end of the hook. Place your index finger on this marked area on the handle.

　(2) Place the Crawford hook in the nose as you would the grooved director. Turn the closed side of the hook against the lateral wall of the nose and see if you can palpate the probe. If you can palpate the stent, advance the hook a few millimeters and rotate the open end of the hook

against the lateral wall of the nose. Pull the hook anteriorly, and you should be able to hook the olive tip of the stent.

   (3) If the hook doesn't come out of the nose easily, it may have attached itself to the nasal mucosa so try to carefully loosen the hook rather than pull harder.

  E. Both the grooved director and the Crawford hook techniques take some practice. *If you can't find the stent, make sure that it is not placed too far down the duct into the nose. Perhaps the biggest mistake is that the stent has been advanced too far into the nose and has turned posteriorly, parallel to the floor of the nose toward the nasopharynx.* If you don't find either of these stent retrieval techniques easy, you may want to try the Ritling intubation system, which may make retrieval easier

6. Tie the stents

  A. After the upper and lower canalicular stents have been passed out the nose, spread the eyelids open to properly position the stent in the canthus.

  B. With a small needle holder, reach into the nostril and grasp both stents anterior to the tip of the inferior turbinate. Withdraw the stents from the nose and tie a 1-1-1 square knot on the needle holder. Release the needle holder and let the knot retract into the nose (Figure 10-15).

  C. Cut the ends of the stent so that they hang out from under the turbinate, but not outside the nose.

  D. Remember not to tie the stents under traction or the knot will retract up in the duct. A new stent set is available that has a suture within the lumen of the tubing (Crawford intubation set with suture, JEDMED Instrument Co. no. 28-0184, http://www.jedmed.com). You can strip the tubing off the suture and tie the suture rather than the stent. This facilitates stent removal because you can pull the

stent out more easily from above as there is no knot in the tubing itself (Box 10-10).

  E. Some surgeons prefer to suture the stents to the lateral wall of the nose or to secure a sleeve or piece of silicone around the knot to prevent prolapse. I have found this generally unnecessary. If you do choose to secure any material to the stent to prevent prolapse, be aware that excessive tension on the stents will cause punctal erosion and eventual unroofing of the canaliculi.

7. Use antibiotic ointment three times per day for 1 week

8. Follow-up

  A. Leave stents in place for 6 months.

  B. A small amount of tearing will often remain with the stents in place, especially when the child has a cold. No discharge should be seen, however.

  C. Remind the parents that tears do not flow through the stents and that any residual tearing usually resolves when the stents are removed.

Stents can be removed in two ways. You can cut the tubing in the canthus and withdraw the stent through the nostril. This takes some practice if the patient is awake. Alternatively, the stent can be prolapsed out from above by pulling the stent out one of the canaliculi. The loop can easily be cut, but you must pull the knot out the canaliculus, which will hurt for a second or so. There is a small risk that the stent can break and leave some of the tubing in the sac. This is unlikely, especially if you tie a small knot when initially placing the stent. If one end does break, you can pull the other end of the stent out. Try to master one of these office techniques. It seems unnecessary to use general anesthesia to remove a stent as some surgeons do. The newer stent set described above is an option if you have trouble removing the stent with a knot in it.

Prolapse of the stents (outside the lids) (Figure 10-16) occurs in a small number of patients. In these patients, the stents cannot be repositioned because the knot is up in the duct. Patients are horrified when this happens, so warn them of this small risk. If prolapse occurs, ask that the loop be taped to the cheek. The stents must be removed from above as described. Usually the intubation will be successful even if the stents come out early.

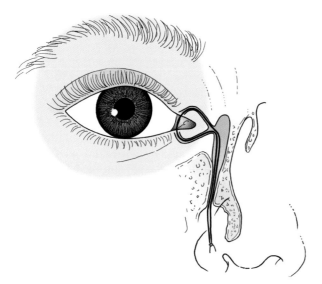

Figure 10-15 Bicanalicular nasolacrimal duct intubation with silicone stents. A 1-1-1 knot is tied in the nose.

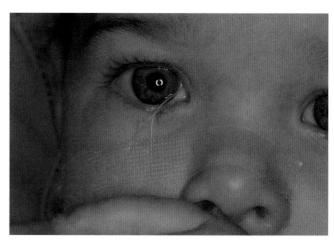

Figure 10-16 Prolapsed stent. Ask mom to tape it to the baby's nose.

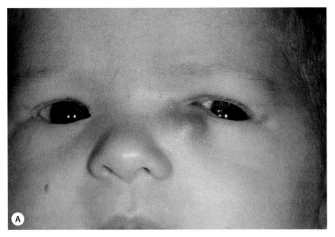

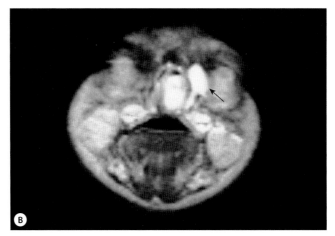

Figure 10-17 Congenital dacryocystocele. (**A**) Congenital dacryocystocele—clinical appearance. (**B**) Magnetic resonance image showing a dacryocystocele. Notice the large sac (*arrow*) and the nasolacrimal duct filled with fluid.

Unusual congenital lacrimal system problems

Dacryocystocele

A dacryocystocele forms when both the nasolacrimal duct and the common internal punctum are closed in utero. The mucus produced within the sac expands the sac and duct. At birth, a newborn has a mass in the medial canthus (Figure 10-17). This mass is the same as that seen in an adult with a mucocele of the lacrimal sac. Often the congenital dacryocystocele will become infected within the first few days of life if not treated.

This is an uncommon condition. However, it is important that you recognize it because pediatricians are unfamiliar with dacryocystocele and may identify it as an encephalocele when they refer the patient to you. A dacryocystocele is more inferior than most encephaloceles and is not associated with other abnormalities such as telecanthus. If there is any question, you may obtain a CT scan, although this is usually not necessary. An interesting presentation of dacryocystocele is respiratory distress. The dilated nasolacrimal duct may extend into the nose, resulting in a nasal mass. Because newborns are obligatory nasal breathers, the mass may cause some difficulty in moving air through the nasal passages.

A dacryocystocele is usually treated with simple probing in the office. Some surgeons prefer to put the child under general anesthesia and do probing. At the same time, any redundant soft tissue underneath the inferior turbinate can be removed. I have found that simple probing while holding the child down is successful for most dacryocystoceles. I use general anesthesia, stent placement, and nasal tissue excision only for the rare child in whom simple probing fails.

Punctal atresia

Other rare, more subtle, congenital abnormalities will cause tearing. You may never see one of these, but the fact that these abnormalities exist should remind you to look at the puncta of children before you schedule a routine probing. A *congenital punctal membrane* can be opened with a sharp punctal dilator. This is a rare problem, however. More commonly (but still rare), *one or more puncta are absent*, a condition known as *punctal atresia* (Figure 10-18). This condition is usually associated with incomplete development of the

Box 10-10

Nasolacrimal Duct Intubation

Patient preparation

- Oxymetazoline hydrochloride 0.05% (Afrin) spray in the preoperative area
- General anesthesia: can be done with a mask
- Nasal packing in inferior turbinate: wear a headlight
- Clean off any mattering from lids

Infracture of turbinate

- Remove nasal packing
- Infracture inferior turbinate if meatus is tight

Punctal dilation

- Use wide punctal dilation (stabilize lid with lateral traction to avoid a false pass)

Introduction of the stents

- Initial probing with no. 1 Bowman probe is optional
- Place olive tip of Crawford silicone stent into vertical portion of the canaliculus
- Rotate and advance in the horizontal canaliculus (stabilize the lid with lateral traction to avoid a false pass)
- Feel a "hard stop" at the lacrimal sac fossa
- Rotate the probe 90 degrees; make a curve in the probe
- Pass the stent down the duct about 15 mm

Retrieval of stents

- Options include:
  - Grooved director
  - Crawford hook
  - Hemostat
  - Endoscope
- Repeat procedure with other end of stent placed in upper canaliculus
- Tie loosely and cut stent in nose, leave in place 6 months

entire canaliculus in the affected eyelid. Punctal atresia is a dominant trait, so you will often see the condition in the parent with the child. If only one punctum is affected on each side, no treatment will usually be necessary. If both puncta are absent, a DCR with Jones tube placement can be performed at age 5.

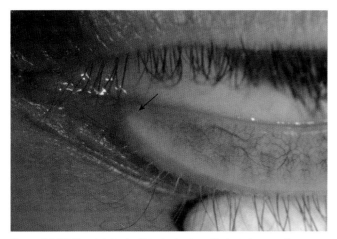

Figure 10-18 Punctal atresia. Note lacrimal papilla, but absence of punctum (*arrow*).

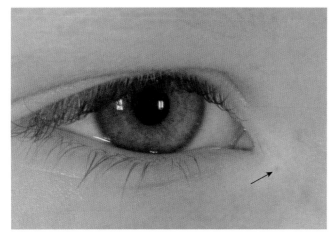

Figure 10-19 Congenital fistula of the lacrimal sac (*arrow*).

Lacrimal sac fistula

Another unusual condition presenting with tearing in a child is the *lacrimal sac fistula* (Figure 10-19). Apparent epiphora results from a small inconspicuous opening, or dimple, inferior to the medial canthus. A congenital lacrimal sac fistula is treated with excision of the fistula and intubation of the lacrimal system.

Treatment of tearing in adults

Overview

In children, tearing is almost always associated with NLD obstruction. As we have already seen, in adults, the diagnosis is not as simple. Bilateral conditions associated with ocular discomfort and no true epiphora are managed with topical lubricants. Other causes of reflex tearing such as entropion or trichiasis must be addressed. Pump problems resulting from seventh nerve palsy or lid scarring should be addressed before lacrimal drainage procedures are performed in most patients. Lower eyelid tightening using a lateral tarsal strip type procedure and gold weight placement in the upper eyelid is a common remedy for pump problems caused by seventh nerve palsy. In most patients, there is postoperative improvement, but often incomplete resolution.

Lacrimal drainage problems may arise at the puncta, canaliculi, or nasolacrimal duct. Punctal eversion is treated with a lateral tarsal strip operation alone or in combination with a medial spindle operation as described previously. Punctal stenosis is treated by discontinuing treatment with any offending eye drop, if known. Punctoplasty or silicone stent intubation of the lacrimal system usually gives a long-term cure. It is common for the lower lid punctum to be stenotic with long-standing ectropion. The punctum usually returns to normal after appropriate repositioning of the eyelid.

Canalicular obstruction can be repaired if the obstructed area is localized. In most patients with obstruction following a viral infection, canalicular reconstruction is not possible, and Jones tube placement (discussed later in this chapter) is necessary.

Acute and chronic dacryocystitis

As we said earlier, any sign of dacryocystitis during the physical examination is an automatic diagnosis of nasolacrimal duct obstruction. Patients with *chronic dacryocystitis* presenting with mucopurulent discharge but with no signs of cellulitis should be treated with topical antibiotics and DCR. Patients with *acute dacryocystitis* should be treated with oral or parenteral antibiotics. You may want to do a culture and sensitivity test to target your antibiotic therapy. In most cases, treatment with a cephalosporin is adequate.

If a *lacrimal sac abscess* is present, incision and drainage of the lacrimal sac through an external incision will speed recovery. This is usually done with the patient under local anesthesia, but will probably be painful. A small stab incision using a no. 11 blade is made in the area of the abscess (Figure 10-20). A small length of gauze is placed in the wound to promote drainage over the following few days. Most patients are admitted for the administration of intravenous antibiotics.

Acute dacryocystitis in children is rare, but does occur (Figure 10-21). If an abscess if present, you should drain the abscess, culture, and give intravenous antibiotics. If only cellulitis is present, give oral or intravenous antibiotics, depending on the severity. Your patient should complete a 10 day course of oral antibiotics. Following resolution of the infection, my habit has been to treat with tear drainage surgery. Most cases are treated with probing and stents. I cannot say that probing alone would not work, although the presence of infection seems to suggest a significant block. Occasionally, DCR is necessary. Most pediatric DCRs can be performed endoscopically after you get experience. An external DCR incision site looks large on a young child.

Treatment of suspected dacryolith (middle-aged woman)

NLD obstruction caused by a *dacryolith* or lacrimal stone is one of the more interesting, but poorly understood, causes of NLD obstruction. As we said earlier, this condition usually occurs in middle-aged women. Often, the tearing resolves spontaneously, and there is no recurrence of symptoms. Patients may be seen with signs of mild acute dacryocystitis. Oral antibiotic therapy is usually sufficient. I try to treat these patients without a DCR unless the problem is recurrent. If more than two episodes occur within a year, a DCR is a

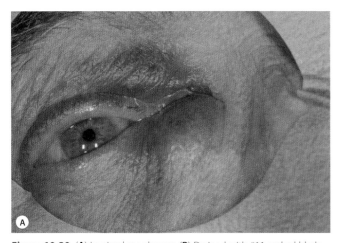
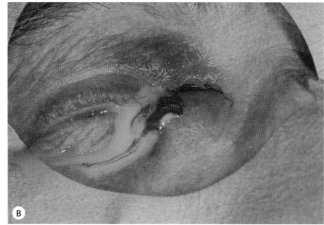

Figure 10-20 (**A**) Lacrimal sac abscess. (**B**) Drained with #11 scalpel blade.

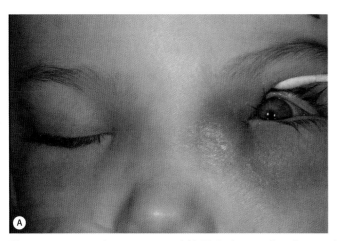
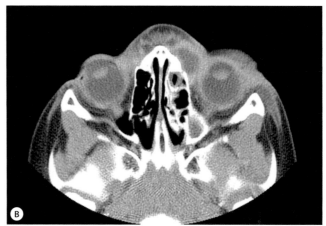

Figure 10-21 Acute dacryocystitis in a child. (**A**) Erythema and swelling over lacrimal sac abscess. Acute dacryocystitis in a child is an unusual presentation for congenital nasolacrimal duct obstruction and an unusual cause of orbital cellulitis in childhood (almost always caused by sinus disease). (**B**) Axial CT—lacrimal sac abscess with diffuse inflammation of orbit. Drained surgically, initially. Later treated with probing and nasolacrimal duct intubation.

reasonable therapeutic option. Sometimes very large stones or casts of the lacrimal system are removed (see Figure 10-3, Box 10-11).

The dacryocystorhinostomy

Introduction

The dacryocystorhinostomy, or DCR, is a difficult procedure for most ophthalmologists to learn. The surgery requires techniques that are unfamiliar to most ophthalmologists. Today, the majority of patients with NLD obstruction are treated with an *external DCR*. You may be familiar with this procedure. The obstructed NLD is bypassed by forming an anastomosis of the lacrimal sac and nasal mucosa through a nasal ostium created by an external skin incision. The *endoscopic DCR* is an alternative to the external approach. In this procedure, the ostium and anastomosis are made from

the inside of the nose, using an endoscope. The endonasal technique is more direct, and in some ways simpler, but demands a more complete understanding of intranasal anatomy. Initially, the endoscope adds a new level of complexity to the procedure, but eventually using it becomes routine. Both external and endonasal DCR procedures are much easier if you can learn to prepare the nose preoperatively to prevent intraoperative bleeding.

Preoperative nasal preparation for DCR

In this section, we will discuss decongestion of the nose and anesthetic injection for DCR.

1. **Gather equipment and medications** (A list of instruments to use is provided in Box 10-16)
   A. You will need some special equipment before you perform a DCR. Have at hand an *atomizer, fiberoptic headlight, bayonet forceps, nasal speculum,* and *neurosurgical cottonoids.*

Dacryocystitis

Acute dacryocystitis

- You have already diagnosed nasolacrimal duct obstruction
  - Don't probe!
  - Don't irrigate!
- Treatment
  - Dicloxacillin as an outpatient (or admit for intravenous antibiotics)
  - Drain and culture, if abscess forms
  - Dacryocystorhinostomy when inflammation resolves

Chronic dacryocystitis

- You have already diagnosed nasolacrimal duct obstruction
  - Don't probe!
  - Don't irrigate!
- Treatment
  - Topical antibiotics
  - Dacryocystorhinostomy

B. You will also need *0.05% oxymetazoline hydrochloride (Afrin) spray and 2% lidocaine (Xylocaine) with 1:100,000 epinephrine mixed with 0.5% bupivacaine (Marcaine)*.

2. Perform preoperative decongestion of the nose
   A. *The first step to successful lacrimal surgery is excellent nasal decongestion.* Without thorough nasal decongestion, visualization in the nose and hemostasis will be difficult and surgery will be long and "painful" for you.
   B. *Begin decongestant therapy with oxymetazoline hydrochloride nasal spray in the preoperative area 15 minutes ahead of surgery.* In the operating room, spray the nose once again.

3. Use general or local anesthesia
   A. I suggest that you perform your first few DCRs with patients under general anesthesia. When you are confident of your ability to control bleeding easily and do the surgery quickly, local anesthesia is preferred.
   B. If you are using local anesthesia, you must provide both nasal decongestion and anesthesia. Spray the nose with the lidocaine containing epinephrine using the atomizer.

4. Mark the skin incision
   A. If you are using the external approach, mark a skin incision on the nose halfway between the nasal bridge and medial canthus as the nose spray takes effect.
   B. Start at the level of the medial canthus and draw the incision inferiolaterally toward the lateral alae of the nose for 12 mm (Figure 10-22, A). You should palpate the anterior lacrimal crest and, in some patients, move the incision somewhat closer to the crest.

5. Inject local anesthetic
   A. In any patient undergoing DCR, with either the external or the internal approach, you should *inject 2% lidocaine with epinephrine* into:

(1) The tissue around the incision site (Figure 10-22, B).
(2) The sac.
(3) The skin around the canaliculi.
(4) The mucosa of the lateral nasal wall adjacent to the anterior tip of the middle turbinate.
(5) The mucosa of the middle turbinate.

6. Pack the nose
   A. After injection of local anesthetic, *pack the nose with cottonoids dampened with oxymetazoline hydrochloride.* One-half inch by 3 inch neurosurgical cottonoids are good for this. The packing should be placed in the middle meatus against the lateral wall of the nose (Figure 10-22, C).
   B. Cocaine 5% is an excellent topical anesthetic and vasoconstrictor. However, it should be used with caution, especially in elderly patients or in any patient undergoing general anesthesia, because many of the inhalation agents sensitize the heart to arrhythmia, making a combination of cocaine and any injection containing epinephrine dangerous.

7. Position the patient
   A. Before starting the surgery, place the patient in the *reverse Trendelenburg position* (with the head up 10–15 degrees).
   B. Check the height of your operating stool.

8. Prep and drape the patient
   A. If your patient is under general anesthesia, include the eye to be operated on and ipsilateral nostril in the surgical field.
   B. If the patient is under local anesthesia, it is best to include the whole face in the field.

9. Scrub while the decongestants are working
   A. Remember to put a headlight on if you are using an external approach. On your way out to scrub, discuss with the nursing staff the orientation of the operating table and video unit (for endoscopic approaches), if you haven't done so already (Box 10-12).

The external DCR

Before performing an external DCR, you should follow the steps outlined above for nasal preparation. After you have injected anesthetic and packed the nose of the patient, scrub while the nursing staff prepare and drape the patient. When you return to the operating room, sit by the side of the head to be operated on (see Box 10-13).

The procedure can be broken down into these steps:

- Expose the sac
- Create the osteotomy
- Form the flaps, suture the posterior flaps, intubate the system, and close the anterior flaps
- Close the incision

1. Expose the sac
   A. You will find that *exposure of the sac* is important because visualization of the tissues in the ostium is difficult for the novice surgeon.

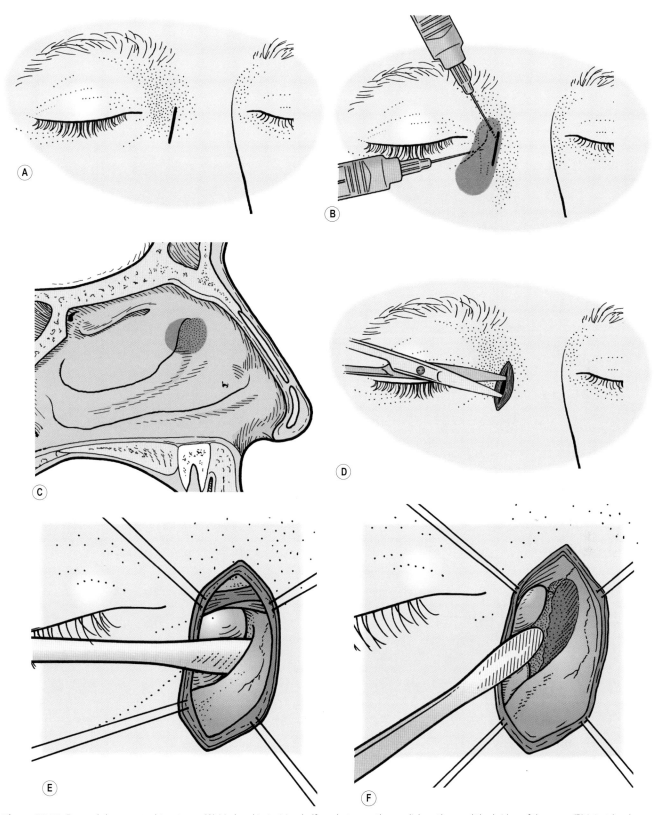

Figure 10-22 External dacryocystorhinostomy. (**A**) Mark a skin incision halfway between the medial canthus and the bridge of the nose. (**B**) Inject local anesthetic with epinephrine into the subcutaneous tissues at the incision site and into the sac (approached from the lateral side posterior to the anterior lacrimal crest). (**C**) Position of the packing for DCR in the middle meatus. Lateral view. (**D**) Spread the orbicularis muscle with a Stevens scissors to expose the periosteum. (**E**) Expose the anterior lacrimal crest. Note the surgical landmark, the innominate suture. Elevate the sac from the fossa with a Freer elevator. (**F**) Start the ostium. Note the suture line between the thick maxilla and the thin lacrimal bones shown. Use a Freer elevator to break through the thin lacrimal bone.

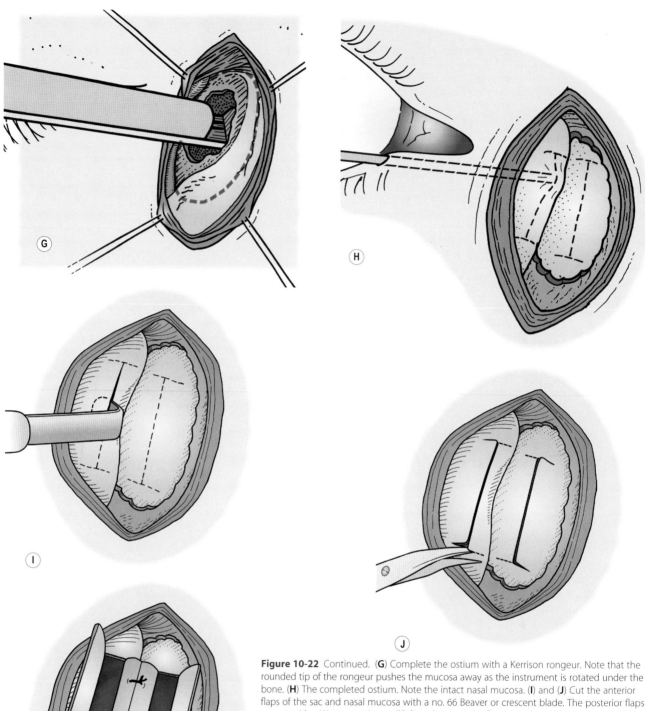

Figure 10-22 Continued. (**G**) Complete the ostium with a Kerrison rongeur. Note that the rounded tip of the rongeur pushes the mucosa away as the instrument is rotated under the bone. (**H**) The completed ostium. Note the intact nasal mucosa. (**I**) and (**J**) Cut the anterior flaps of the sac and nasal mucosa with a no. 66 Beaver or crescent blade. The posterior flaps are cut with a Westcott scissors. (**K**) Sew the posterior flaps together with one or two 4-0 chromic sutures. (**L**) and (**M**) Pass the stents into the nose. Tie a piece of 4-0 silk suture from the traction sutures around the stents in the ostium to prevent prolapse. Close the anterior flaps with the same 4-0 chromic suture. (**N**) Close the orbicularis muscle with two or three 5-0 Vicryl sutures. Close the skin with an absorbable suture.

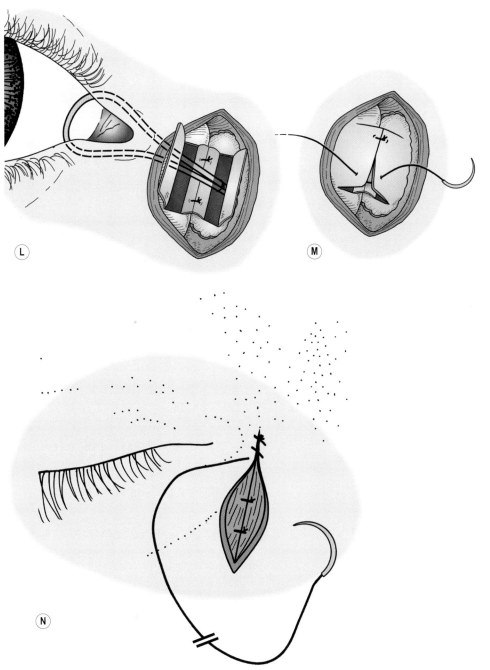

Figure 10-22 Continued.

B. Make the skin incision *using a no. 15 blade or Colorado needle*. Try to cut through the thick nasal skin, but not into the underlying muscle.

C. Using a Stevens scissors in your dominant hand, *spread the orbicularis muscle* parallel to the muscle fibers. Continue spreading deeply until you see the white periosteum (Figure 10-22, D).

D. Pass two 4-0 silk *traction sutures* on each side of the wound for exposure.

   (1) Pass the sutures into the orbicularis muscle, but not through the skin.

(2) Broad bites of the orbicularis muscle will help with hemostasis.

(3) If the angular artery or vein is visualized, be careful not to pass the needle through it.

(4) Have the scrub nurse load the needles forehanded for the edge of the wound closest to the eye, and back-handed for the edge of the wound away from the eye.

(5) Clamp the sutures to the drapes using hemostats.

Box 10-12

Preoperative Nasal Preparation for Dacryocystorhinostomy

Equipment and medicines

- Atomizer
  - Oxymetazoline hydrochloride 0.05% (Afrin) nasal spray
  - Lidocaine (2% Xylocaine) spray with 1:100,000 epinephrine
- Fiberoptic headlight
- Bayonet forceps
- Nasal speculum
- Neurosurgical cottonoid (0.5 inch by 3 inch) or cotton ball

Patient preparation

- Decongestants
  - Spray the nose with decongestant (oxymetazoline hydrochloride nasal spray) in the preoperative area
  - Spray oxymetazoline hydrochloride again on arrival in the operating room
  - If using local anesthesia, spray the nose with lidocaine using an atomizer
- Mark incision on nose
- Local anesthesia (in all patients): inject lidocaine with epinephrine into:
  - Tissue around incision site and canaliculi
  - Lacrimal sac
  - Lateral nasal wall mucosa adjacent to the anterior tip of the middle turbinate
  - Mucosa of the middle turbinate
- Pack the nose with cottonoids dampened with oxymetazoline hydrochloride
  - In middle meatus (under middle turbinate)—one cottonoid
  - Around tip of turbinate—one cottonoid
- In a young healthy patient, you may substitute cocaine 5% spray for the oxymetazoline hydrochloride spray
- Elevate head of the bed 15–20 degrees
- Prep and drape the patient, leaving the whole face in the field if under local anesthesia

E. Elevate the periosteum.
  (1) Take a *Freer elevator* in your dominant hand and a small *Baron suction tube* (5FR, Storz N0610) in your nondominant hand. Use the suction tube to retract the sides of the wound open and use the Freer elevator to clean any remaining muscle off the periosteum.
  (2) Incise the periosteum parallel to the incision with the sharp edge of the elevator. Reflect the periosteum toward the anterior lacrimal crest using the Freer elevator.
  (3) You will probably encounter some bleeding from the *innominate suture* 2 or 3 mm anterior to the anterior lacrimal crest. You may want to use bone wax applied with a cotton-tipped applicator to stop this bleeding (Figure 10-22, E)
  (4) Carefully elevate the periosteum from the edge of the anterior lacrimal crest and lift the entire contents of the lacrimal sac fossa off the bone.

2. Create the osteotomy
  A. Once you have elevated the lacrimal sac from the underlying bone, use the suction tube in your nondominant hand to *retract the sac tissue* so you can see the floor of the lacrimal sac fossa clearly.
  B. Identify the suture line between the thinner lacrimal bone and thicker maxilla (Figure 10-22, F). This occurs slightly more than halfway back in the lacrimal sac fossa.
  C. Use your Freer elevator to gently break open the suture line. Be careful not to disturb the underlying nasal mucosa.
  D. Next use a Hardy sella punch (90 degree) to start the ostium.
    (1) Place the punch in the hole. Use the blunt end of the punch to push the nasal mucosa away from the bone. Then close the blades to cut the bone. Retract the punch to clean the bone from the punch jaws.
    (2) Move anteriorly to enlarge the ostium. Put the sella punch in the ostium as though you are placing a key in a lock. Remember, the end of the punch is designed to push the soft tissues off the back of the bone. Once against the mucosa, *rotate* the punch (*like turning the key*) under intact bone to enlarge the ostium.
  E. Enlarge the osteotomy with Kerrison rongeurs.
    (1) As the size of the ostium is enlarged, use consecutively larger Kerrison rongeurs (Storz N1951, N1952, and N1953) to complete the bone removal (Figure 10-22, G). The Kerrison rongeurs are much stronger than the sella punch and will allow quick removal of the thicker maxillary bone anteriorly.
    (2) The ostium is completed when the entire lacrimal sac mucosa is adjacent to nasal mucosa (Figure 10-22, H). The ostium size is approximately 15 mm by 15 mm, but varies from patient to patient. The important point is to remove enough bone to easily connect the mucosal flaps.
  F. Remove *a small spine of bone* often present at the neck of the sac. This bone is best removed with a rongeur that looks like a pair of pliers, known as a Belz lacrimal sac rongeur (Bausch and Lomb Surgical, Storz, no. E4590).

3. Form the flaps, suture the posterior flaps, intubate the system, and close the flaps
  A. Use a no. 1 Bowman probe passed through the canaliculus into the sac. Look inside the ostium to see the probe tent up the sac.
  B. *Cut the anterior sac flap.*
    (1) Use a *no. 66 Beaver blade or crescent blade* to make an incision along the long axis of the sac (toward the duct).
    (2) Turn the blade 90 degrees to cut the anterior lacrimal sac flap at both ends of the sac incision.
  C. Cut the opposite anterior nasal mucosa flap.
    (1) Incise the nasal mucosa using the same no. 66 blade, cutting parallel to the initial sac incision.

(2) Again, turn the blade 90 degrees to cut the nasal mucosa at each end of the incision, completing the anterior nasal mucosal flap (you haven't put the blade down yet) (Figure 10-22, I).

D. Cut the posterior flaps.

(1) Exchange the blade for a Westcott scissors to cut the *posterior sac flap* and *posterior nasal flap.*

(2) Use the scissors to cut perpendicular to the initial long axis cuts to form the posterior sac and nasal flaps (Figure 10-22, J).

(3) At this point, you will have made four flaps of mucosa. You will notice that the posterior flaps are apposed. You will soon pass sutures through these flaps to connect them.

(4) The nasal packing should be visible and can be removed through the nose.

E. Suture the posterior flaps.

(1) You will now be connecting the lacrimal sac mucosa to the nasal mucosa. This is a difficult concept in the beginning, but in essence *you are making a tunnel of mucosa from the sac into the nose.* The posterior flaps form the back wall of this tunnel.

(2) Use a 4-0 chromic gut suture on a short half-circle needle (the Ethicon 798G G-2 micropoint cutting needle is essential) to suture these flaps together (Figure 10-22, K).

(3) Usually two sutures are best. When you look in the wound, you will now see the back wall of what will be a mucosal tunnel between the sac and the nose.

F. Pass the Crawford stents through the canaliculi into the ostium and pull them out the nose.

(1) Either an open grooved director or a hemostat will help you to retrieve the stents out of the nose (Figure 10-22, L).

(2) At this point, I cut off a 3 inch piece of one of the 4-0 silk traction sutures and tie it around the stent in the ostium. *This will prevent postoperative stent prolapse.* To do this, reach through the incision with an empty needle holder and grasp the two arms of the silicone stent inferior to the ostium. Pull the stents out from the wound and tie the silk suture around them, cutting the ends of the suture short. Let the stent retract back into the wound. The silk suture will shorten the loop of the stent, preventing prolapse.

G. Tie the ends of the stent together in the nose.

(1) After you have tied the silk suture, reach through the nostril and grasp the stents with the empty needle holder where you would like the knot to be.

(2) Retract the stents out of the nostril. Pull the wire probes off the stent and tie the stents together at the needle holder.

(3) Remove the needle holder and allow the stent to retract in the nose. Cut the ends of the stent.

H. Close the anterior flaps.

(1) *Use the same P-2 needle.* Sometimes it is easier to use a back-handed pass of the needle. Pass the suture through the sac flap first and then use the needle to hook the anterior nasal mucosal flap from underneath.

(2) Use two sutures to close the anterior flaps (Figure 10-22, M).

4. Close the incision

A. The remainder of the closure is simple. Remove the 4-0 silk traction sutures. Sometimes there will be some additional bleeding at this point that requires cautery.

B. Use two or three interrupted *5-0 PDS sutures Ethicon Z844G* to close the muscle layer.

C. Try using an *absorbable skin suture for the skin layer.* A running stitch is fine as suturing in this area leaves little scarring (Figure 10-22, N).

5. Provide postoperative care

A. Put topical *antibiotic ointment* in the conjunctival cul de sac and on the wound.

B. I like to give a 1 week course of *cephalexin* (*Keflex*) to reduce the already low wound infection rate to zero postoperatively. I see the patient 1 week postoperatively.

C. Remove the stent in 6 months. It is easy to cut the stent in the canthus and pull the stent out of the nostril.

D. Prolapse of the stent rarely occurs if you tie a suture around the stents as described above.

Nasolacrimal duct intubation for functional obstruction

Silicone stent intubation of the nasolacrimal duct is an alternative to DCR for functional obstruction of the nasolacrimal duct in adults. Remember the definition of a functional block: anatomically the duct is open on irrigation, but the tears do not seem to pass into the nose spontaneously under normal conditions. Presumably intubation of the system dilates a somewhat stenotic duct. The reported success rate for adult nasolacrimal duct intubation is about 75%. This procedure should not be used for a true anatomic block where no irrigation can pass into the nose. The technique has been studied very little, and I use it only when I am uncertain about the exact cause of the tearing, but feel that some narrowing of the duct may be a contributing factor. As with any DCR, I leave the stents in place for approximately 6 months. I have colleagues who remove the tubes at any time from 3 to 12 months, so you will want to use your own judgment on this (Box 10-13).

The endonasal DCR

The indications for endonasal DCR are the same as those for an external DCR. As with other DCR operations, I suggest that you perform your first endonasal procedures with patients under general anesthesia until you become comfortable with the anatomic structures and hemostasis. When doing the endonasal approach, pay special attention to the preparation of the nose because any bleeding makes this procedure much more difficult. Put the patient in the reverse Trendelenburg position, elevating the head of the bed 10–15 degrees. Use the same nasal spray and liberal injection of local anesthetic with epinephrine followed by nasal packing as for the exter-

Box 10-13

External Dacryocystorhinostomy

Preparation

- Local anesthesia is preferred
- Elevate head of the bed 15–20 degrees
- Use nasal spray, injection, and packing
- Mark the skin incision and inject local anesthetic at the incision and sac
- Prepare and drape the patient
- Sit at the side of the head to be operated on

Exposure of sac

- Incise the skin
- Spread with Stevens scissors
- Use 4-0 silk traction sutures in the orbicularis muscle for exposure
- Use a Freer elevator (dominant hand) and suction (nondominant hand) to incise and reflect the periosteum off the anterior lacrimal crest
- Use bone wax for bleeding in the innominate suture
- Elevate the sac from the lacrimal sac fossa

Osteotomy

- Use the suction tube in the nondominant hand
- Use the Freer elevator or hemostat in the dominant hand to open bone in the suture line
- Use a 90 degree Hardy sella punch to start the ostium
- Do "keyhole" enlargement of the ostium
- Complete the ostium with a Kerrison rongeur
- Remove any spine of bone inferiorly with a Belz rongeur

Flap formation and intubation

- Insert a 1-0 Bowman probe in the canaliculus to the sac
- Tent the sac and incise with a no. 66 Beaver blade on long axis of sac
- Turn the blade 90 degrees to cut the anterior sac flap
- Incise the nasal mucosa parallel to the initial sac incision
- Turn the blade 90 degrees to cut the anterior nasal flap
- Use Westcott scissors to cut the posterior sac and nasal flaps
- Remove nasal packing

Closure of the flaps and wound

- Suture posterior flaps with 4-0 chromic using a short half-circle needle (Ethicon 798 G-2 needle)
- Pass stents into the ostium and out the nose
- Tie suture around the stent inferior to the ostium to prevent prolapse
- Suture the anterior flaps
- Tie and cut stent in the nose
- Cut the traction sutures and close the orbicularis muscle with 5-0 PDS sutures
- Suture the skin with running 5-0 fast absorbing gut

Oral and topical antibiotic

nal DCR. Have the nurses prep and drape the patient while you scrub. If the patient is under local anesthesia, remember to leave eyes, nose, and mouth in the surgical field.

You should sit on the patient's right side, placing the video monitor off the patient's left shoulder. Your position is the same for both left and right eyes if you are right-handed. If you are left-handed, you should operate from the patient's left side (Figure 10-23).

Before you start the procedure, *connect and check all the equipment*. This includes the endoscope light and video unit, the light pipe (which you will insert into the canaliculus), the suction tubing, and the bipolar cautery tool. You will also need an antifogging agent to apply to the tip of the endoscope.

You need to become familiar with how the endoscope works. It is best to hold the endoscope in your nondominant hand. Cradle it from below (Figure 10-24, A). Aim the endoscope at a familiar object so that you can orient the camera to make the picture on the video monitor upright. Some endoscopes have a focusing ring, which will require some adjustment when the scope is in the nose.

Remove the nasal packing. Next inspect the nasal cavity with the endoscope light on near maximum intensity. Use your nondominant hand to insert the endoscope into the nose so that the scope rests against the anterior edge of the nostril (Figure 10-24, B). Look at the patient and aim the scope toward the medial canthus. Now look at the monitor for the familiar landmarks inside the nose, including the inferior and middle turbinate (Figure 10-24, C). Keep the endoscope resting against the anterior part of the nostril. This will steady the scope and allow you to place other instruments into the nose posteriorly to the scope.

Now have the circulating nurse turn the endoscope light on standby. With the light pipe illumination off, have your assistant pass the light pipe into the superior canaliculus until a hard stop is reached (Figure 10-25, A). Aim the endoscope in the nose (illumination is off) to see the light pipe shining through the sac wall and floor of the fossa. Move the light pipe in all directions to get an estimate of the position of the entire sac. With the endoscope light back on, use a Freer elevator to infracture the middle turbinate, if necessary, to get a good view of the lateral wall of the nose. Be gentle when moving the middle turbinate, because it is connected at the cribriform plate. Theoretically, vigorous fracture could cause a cerebrospinal fluid leak. At this point, you should know where the sac is and have a good view of the nasal mucosa directly lateral to it. This is important as the next step is to incise and remove this nasal mucosa.

There are fewer steps for the endonasal DCR than for the external DCR. The endonasal approach is easier than the external approach once you master using the endoscope (see Box 10-14). The endonasal DCR includes:

- Removing the nasal mucosa
- Forming the osteotomy
- Placing the stents

The steps of the endonasal DCR are:

1. Remove the nasal mucosa
   A. *Locate the position of the sac* by visualizing the glow of the light pipe with the endoscope light off (Figure 10-25, B and C).
   B. Use a *crescent blade* (Alcon 6600 crescent blade or Beaver angled 55 degree 373807) from a cataract instrument set to perform an elliptical incision of the nasal mucosa that roughly outlines the sac (Figure 10-25, D and E). If a crescent blade is not available, a no. 66 Beaver blade (376600) will work well.

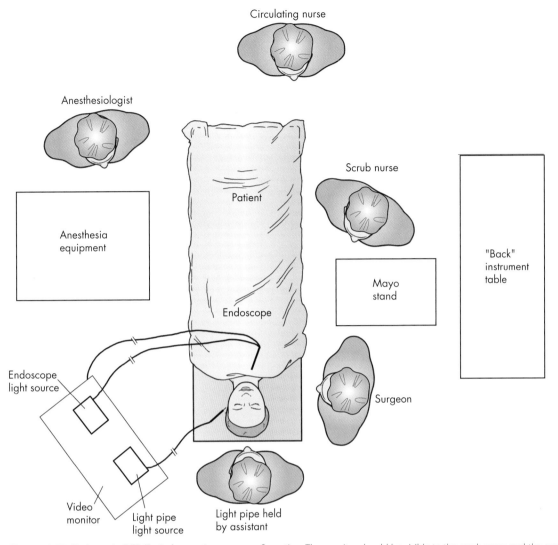

Figure 10-23 Endoscopic DCR. Typical operating room configuration. The monitor should be visible to the scrub nurse and the surgeon. Right-handed surgeons stand at the right side of the patient for left- and right-sided operations.

(1) Usually, this incision is made with the endoscope light on, but you may want to experiment with the light off so you can learn where the position of the sac is.

(2) As you learn to do this operation with the endoscope, you may find that you are losing track of the blade as you pass it into the nose. Try this: before you put any instrument into the nose, pull the endoscope back to get a broad view of the nasal cavity. You will quickly be able to see the other instrument as it enters the nose and can then advance the scope and the blade (or any other instrument) together with the scope, "watching" the instrument advance forward.

C. Next *use a Freer periosteal elevator to elevate this mucosa off the nasal wall. A pediatric upturned ethmoid forceps (N2984 or N0965 Hartman–Herzfeld ear forceps) can be used to tear the mucosa away once it is elevated* (Figure 10-25, F).

2. Form the osteotomy

A. Use the *Freer elevator to penetrate the thin bone of the fossa,* being careful not to damage the underlying sac. Sometimes you can see the *suture line between the thin lacrimal bone and the maxillary bone.* If not, feel for the thin bone.

B. As you would with an external DCR, *use a right-angle Hardy sella punch to remove the anterior portion of the fossa* (Figure 10-25, G and H).

C. Switch to a small Kerrison rongeur when room allows.

(1) Remove the bone anteriorly until the sac is exposed.

(2) You can move the light pipe around in the sac to point to any bone that requires removal.

D. In contrast to the external DCR, *no formal flaps are made.* The remainder of the procedure involves opening the medial wall of the sac into the nose and placing stents.

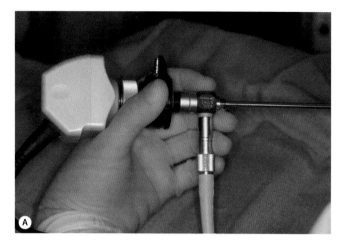

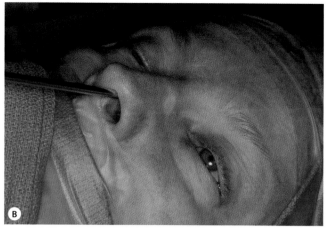

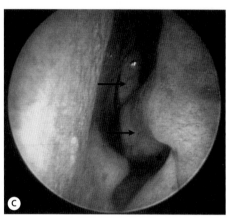

Figure 10-24 (**A**) Hold the endoscope in your nondominant hand. (**B**) It is helpful to steady the endoscope against the nostril. (**C**) Normal intranasal anatomy (left side of nose). Superior arrow is middle turbinate. Inferior arrow is inferior turbinate. Asterisks show middle meatus and inferior meatus. Projecting spur from septum toward inferior meatus is also seen.

(1) *Tent up the sac using the light pipe or probe.* Using the crescent blade again, cut a posterior incision along the vertical axis of the sac (Figure 10-25, I). The light pipe should present itself through this incision.

(2) If you can make a similar incision anteriorly, the flap can be removed. It is often easier to take the small forceps (pediatric upbiting ear forceps) and tear the sac flap away, because it is difficult to make the second cut. This will open the interior of the sac to the nose (Figure 10-25, G).

3. Place the stents
   A. Use Crawford stents passed into the nose as with an external DCR (Figure 10-25, K and L).
   B. Under endoscopic view, use an open-ended grooved director or hemostat to retrieve the stents (Figure 10-25, M).
   C. It is not possible to tie a suture around the stents as you do in an external DCR.
      (1) Instead, you can slip a no. 270 silicone sleeve (Labtician Ophthalmics, S 3019, http://www.labtician.com), cut to a 3 mm length, onto the stents and slide it up near the ostium. This will effectively shorten the loop of the stents and prevent prolapse.
      (2) After the sleeve is positioned, cut and tie the stents as you would for an external procedure.

4. Provide postoperative care and follow-up
   A. Place topical antibiotic ointment into the conjunctiva. No oral antibiotics are required.
   B. The stents are removed at 6 months. You must remove the stents through the nostril, as you cannot pull the sleeve out through the canaliculus above (Box 10-14).

Treatment of canalicular obstruction

Canalicular reconstruction

Canalicular obstruction can be repaired if the obstructed area is localized. A small obstruction can be excised and the canaliculus repaired over stents, as is done for canalicular lacerations (see Chapter 13). Localized obstruction may occur after trauma, but it is rare after viral infection or chemotherapy use. For these latter patients, canalicular reconstruction is usually not possible and Jones tube placement is necessary.

DCR with jones tube placement

If the canalicular system is occluded and there is no hope of reconstruction, a Jones tube is required. This is a Pyrex tube that carries the tears from the conjunctival cul de sac through a DCR ostium into the nose, bypassing the obstructed canaliculi. The Jones tube can be placed in conjunction with a

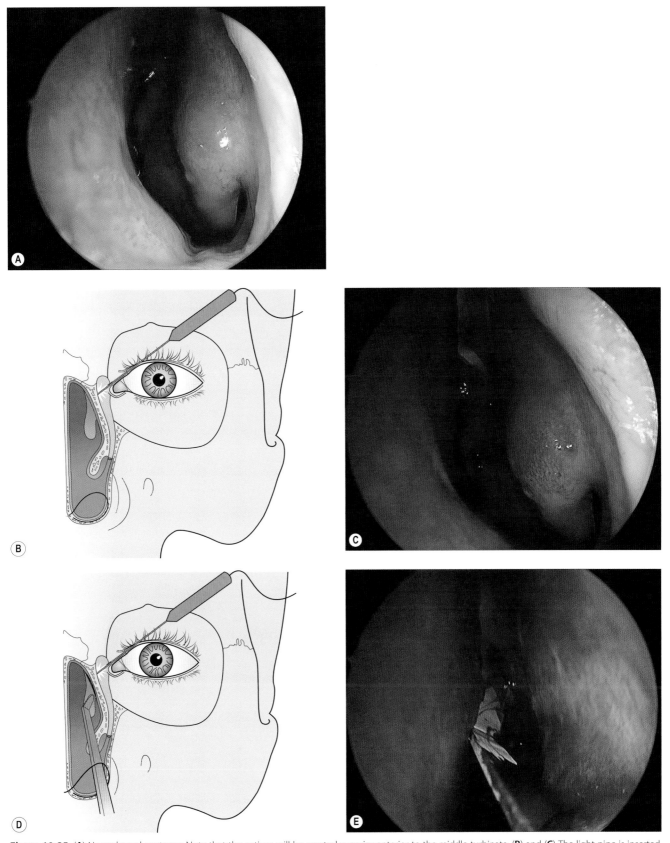

Figure 10-25 (**A**) Normal nasal anatomy. Note that the ostium will be created superior anterior to the middle turbinate. (**B**) and (**C**) The light pipe is inserted into the canaliculus and the glow of the light is visible from within the nose. (**D**) and (**E**) A crescent blade or 6600 Beaver blade is used to incise the nasal mucosa. (**F**) A Freer elevator (not shown) is used to elevate the mucosa and a pediatric ethmoid forceps is used to tear the nasal mucosa free from the underlying bone. (**G**) and (**H**) Either a drill or rongeur is used to remove the bone and expose the underlying lacrimal sac. (**I**) The light pipe can be pushed forward to tent up the sac mucosa. (**J**) A 5910 Beaver blade and pediatric ethmoid forceps are used to cut and tear away the sac mucosa (not shown). The light pipe is visible protruding from the sac opening. (**K**) (**L**) and (**M**) The stents are passed into the nose from above and retrieved. A 2–3 mm piece of Watzke sleeve is cut and slid over the stent below the ostium and the stent is tied (not shown).

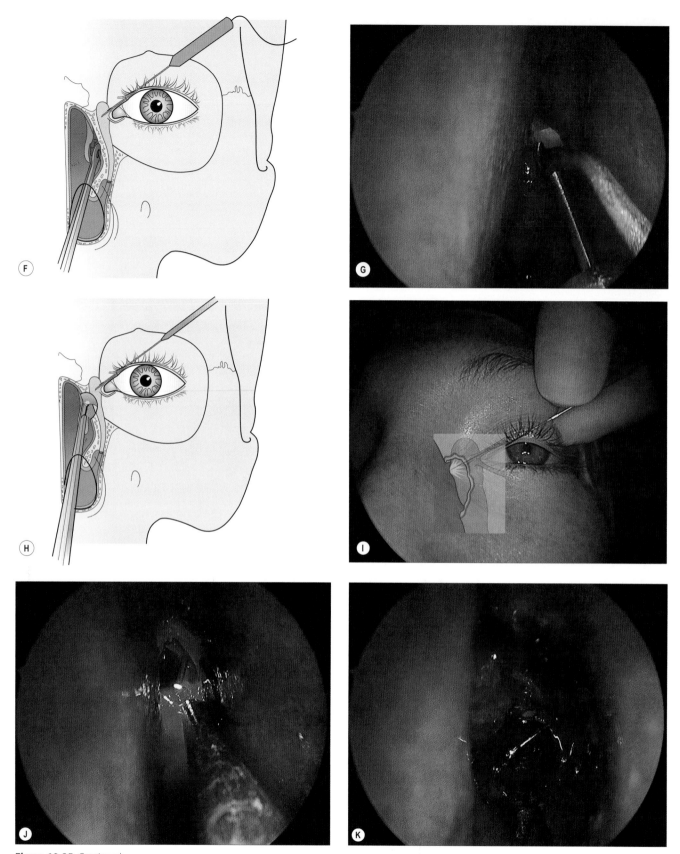

Figure 10-25 Continued.

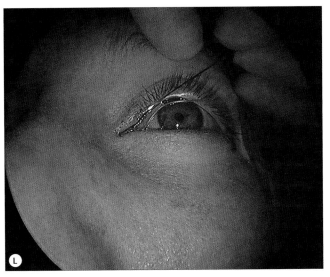

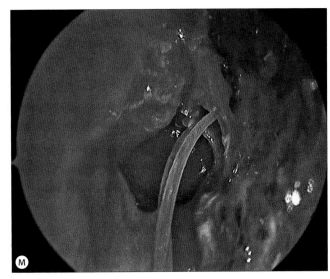

Figure 10-25 Continued.

Box 10-14

Endonasal Dacryocystorhinostomy Procedure

Preparation

- Administer local or general anesthesia
- Elevate head of the bed 10–15 degrees
- Use nasal spray, injection, and packing
- Prepare and drape the patient
- Sit at the patient's right side; place the monitor off the patient's left shoulder

Connect and check equipment

- Endoscope light and video unit
- Light pipe
- Suction tube
- Cautery tool
- Antifogging agent

Inspect the nasal cavity

- Insert the light pipe into the upper canaliculus and turn on
- Inspect the interior of the nose with the endoscope light on
- Turn the endoscope light on standby to view light pipe illumination of the sac
- Infracture the middle turbinate if necessary

Osteotomy

- Turn the endoscope light on
- Make an elliptical mucosal incision with a crescent blade or a no. 66 Beaver blade

- Use a Freer elevator to lift the mucosa
- Penetrate bone of the fossa at the suture line and remove the thin lacrimal bone posteriorly
- Use a Hardy sella punch to remove the anterior portion of the fossa
- Move the light pipe in all directions to outline the sac

Flaps

- There are no formal flaps!
- Tent up the sac with the light pipe
- Use a crescent or no. 66 Beaver blade to incise the sac posteriorly down to the duct
- Use pediatric upbiting ear forceps to tear off the mucosa anteriorly

Stents

- Pass stents into the nose
- Retrieve stents with an open grooved director or hemostat using endoscopic view
- Pass a no. 270 silicone sleeve onto stents near the ostium
- Tie and cut stents in the nose

Topical antibiotic ointment, no oral antibiotic

---

standard external or endonasal DCR. In some situations, the Jones tube is added after a DCR. In my experience, the Jones tube is never quite as good as the natural tear drainage system but, for most patients, it is far better than having epiphora.

The critical factor in the success of a Jones tube is proper positioning during insertion. There is not much space between the lateral wall of the nose and the septum in most patients. Examine the nose preoperatively. If there is not enough room for the tube to protrude into the nose without pushing against the septum, a septoplasty should be considered. In

some patients, removal of the anterior portion of the turbinate will be required to make space for the intranasal end of the tube. It is not very often that you will see a Jones tube on a CT scan, so I have included this image for you to get an idea of the tube position (Figure 10-26).

Notice the position of the normal lacrimal sac on the right side and the DCR ostium on the left side. The Jones tube is extending from the medial canthus through the ostium. A portion of the middle turbinate has been removed to make more room for the tube, but the lumen is still touching the nasal septal mucosa, not an ideal position.

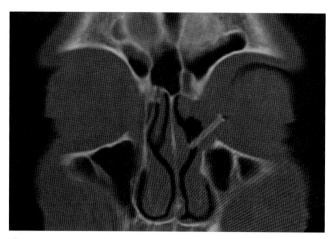

Figure 10-26 CT scan showing a Jones tube in position. Note that a middle turbinectomy has been performed.

Jones tube placement includes:

- DCR
- Determining the tube position and length
- Placing the tube
- Suturing the tube in position

The steps in Jones tube placement are:

1. Perform a DCR
   A. An ostium is required to pass the Jones tube into the nose. Either an external or an endonasal DCR can be used.
   B. The Jones tube is usually placed at the time of the DCR, but can be positioned later if a DCR has been performed in the past (Boxes 10-15 to 10-17).
2. Determine the tube position and length
   A. Both the conjunctival and the nasal ends of the tube should be positioned accurately.
      (1) The tube should *enter the conjunctiva between the plica and the caruncle* slightly inferior to the lower lid margin.
      (2) The tube should be *angled slightly inferiorly* into the nose, *emerging through the ostium anterior to the tip of the middle turbinate.*
   B. *The position, angle and length of the Jones tube can be determined by placing a 20-gauge needle attached to a 5 ml syringe through the conjunctiva into the nose.* The intranasal position of the needle should be checked to see if the tube opening is obstructed. If so, the needle should be redirected until the appropriate position, free of obstruction, is obtained. If the middle turbinate prevents the tube from projecting into the nose, *the anterior part of the middle turbinate can be excised using a rongeur.* Inject the turbinate with local anesthetic with epinephrine before excision. Disturbance of the air flow in the nose can result, so do this only when necessary. Postoperative bleeding can be a problem in some patients, so excise a conservative amount.
   C. After the ideal position has been determined with the needle, determine the appropriate length of the tube. To enlarge the soft tissue opening, slide a 375210 Beaver blade into the nose adjacent to the

needle (sharp side away from eye). Place a hemostat on the needle at the medial canthus and withdraw the needle. *The distance from the needle tip to the hemostat will be a good guide for choosing the proper length of Jones tube* (Figure 10-27, A). Usually a 4 mm flange, 17 mm length tube is appropriate.
   D. Slide a Quickert lacrimal intubation probe (Storz E4220 1) along the side of the blade and remove the Beaver blade. You will slide the Jones tube over the Quickert probe into the nose.

3. Place the tube
   A. Select the tube size and length that matches the length of the measured 20-gauge needle—average seems to be 17 mm straight Jones tube for adults. I use only the 4 mm flange and rarely use an angled tube.
   B. You will need a suture to secure the conjunctival end of the tube, so wind a double-armed 6-0 Vicryl suture (Ethicon J-570) around the tube near the flange on the end of the tube. Tie this suture onto itself, leaving the needles on the suture.
   C. Push the Jones tube over the Quickert probe into the nose. Sometimes the conjunctiva can impede the passage of the Jones tube as there is a flange on the end of the glass tube. The gold dilator in the Jones tube set will help to stretch the opening if necessary.
   D. Push the Jones tube into position against the conjunctiva and caruncle. Check the position of the tube in the nose.
   E. The Jones tube should ideally protrude into the nose 3 mm or more with a slight inferior tilt. The nasal end of the tube should not be obstructed by the

Box 10-16

Instruments of Special Interest for Lacrimal Surgery
Evaluation, probing, and intubation of the lacrimal system

- Bowman lacrimal probe (Storz E4200–E4205 for complete set, JEDMED Instrument no. 58-0220)
- Lacrimal irrigation cannula (Storz E4404)
- Welch Allyn battery-powered illuminated nasal speculum
  - Illuminator and speculum (Welch Allyn 26030)
  - Speculum only (Welch Allyn 26035)
- Nasal speculum (Storz N2105 (adult), N2108 (infant))
- Oxymetazoline hydrochloride 0.05% nasal spray (Afrin)
- Pontocaine or lidocaine (Xylocaine) to use in atomizer as a nasal spray
- Fiberoptic headlight
- Nasal mucosa bayonet forceps (Storz P0525)
- Neurosurgical cottonoids or unrolled cotton balls
- Ziegler double-ended lacrimal dilator (curved) (Storz E4336, JEDMED Instrument no. 58-0280)
- Crawford silicone stents (JEDMED Set 28-0185)
- Quickert grooved director (Storz E 4220 15)
- Anderson Hwang slotted grooved director (JEDMED 28-0189)
- Crawford hook (JEDMED 28-0186)

Repair of canalicular laceration
- For pigtail probe repair
  - Pigtail probe (Storz E4251 C)
  - Precut polyethylene tubing (Storz E4251 B)
  - 6-0 nylon suture (Ethicon 1698 P-3 needle)
- For bicanalicular repair
  - Standard intubation instruments (see above)
- For monocanalicular repair
  - Collarette Monoko, FCI Ophthalmics, S1-1710u
  - Mini Monoko, FCI Ophthalmics, S1-1500u

Dacryocystorhinostomy (DCR)/Jones tube
- Standard preparation drugs and equipment (see above)
- Colorado microdissector needle or no. 15 blade
- Knapp lacrimal sac retractor (Storz E4538)
- Freer elevator (Storz N2348)
- Baron suction tube (5 French, Storz N0610)
- Hardy sella punch, upbiting, 2 mm, Walter Lorenz Surgical no. 80-1340 and no. 80-1341 (90 degree)
- Kerrison rongeurs (Storz N1951, N1952, and N1953)
- Belz lacrimal sac rongeur (Storz E4590)
- No. 66 Beaver blade to cut anterior flaps
- Westcott tenotomy scissors, curved right, blunt tips, to cut posterior flaps (Storz E3320 R)
- Endoscope and monitor
- Vitrectomy light pipe
- Crescent blade for cutting nasal and sac mucosa in endonasal DCR (Alcon 6600 crescent blade or Beaver Angled 55 degree 373807)
- Struempel ear forceps: small forceps useful for tearing flaps off in endonasal DCR (Storz N0962)
- Standard intubation equipment (see above)
- No. 270 silicone sleeve to prevent stent prolapse (Labtician Ophthalmics, S 3019)
- Jones tube placement
  - Jones tube set (Weiss Scientific Glass Blowing, http://www.guntherweiss.com)
  - Quickert lacrimal probe
  - Beaver blade 375210
  - 20-gauge needle

Box 10-17

Sutures for lacrimal surgery
- 4-0 chromic: medial spindle operation (Ethicon 793G G-3 needle, double-armed)
- 4-0 Mersilene S-2: short half-circle needle (S-2), braided polyester, for lateral tarsal strip operation (Ethicon 1779G, double-armed)
- 4-0 silk: skin and muscle traction suture (Ethicon 789 G-3 reverse cutting needle)
- 4-0 chromic: for sewing flaps during external DCR (Ethicon 798G G-2 micropoint half-circle needle)
- 5-0 PDS: for closure of orbicularis muscle wound (Ethicon Z844G)
- 5-0 fast absorbing gut: used as skin suture (Ethicon 1915G PC-1 needle)
- 6-0 Vicryl: to secure Jones tube in place (Ethicon J-570G S-14 needle)
- 6-0 nylon (Ethicon 1698G P-3 needle) for pigtail probe procedure

septum or turbinate. If you are not satisfied with the placement of the tube, change it. *It is nearly impossible to change the position of a Jones tube after healing has occurred, so this is the best chance to get a good functioning tube.*

F. On rare occasions, a good fit cannot be obtained without removing the tip of the middle turbinate. You can do this with injection of local anesthetic with epinephrine and a rongeur. Bleeding can be a problem, however.

4. Suture the tube in position
   A. After the proper position and length of the tube are confirmed, pass the Vicryl sutures through the surrounding conjunctival tissue to pull the tissue snugly around the tube. Tie the suture to secure the tube in position (Figure 10-27, D).
   B. If too much conjunctival tissue pulls around the neck of the tube, you may want to trim some conjunctiva or some of the caruncle before tying the suture.

5. Provide postoperative care and follow-up
   A. Instil a *topical antibiotic.* Use an *oral antibiotic* if a DCR has been performed simultaneously.
   B. There is little maintenance required for the typical Jones tube. The tube should remain in position for the remainder of the patient's life. Occasionally, the tube will become clogged. If the tube gets obstructed, it is easy to exchange a Jones tube using the plastic guide provided in the Jones tube set.
   C. Other operations are rarely needed.

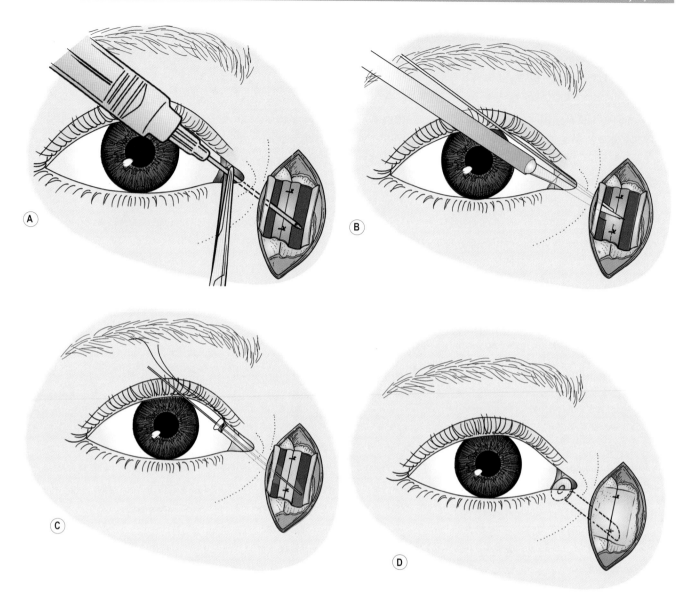

Figure 10-27 Jones tube placement. In the example, an external DCR is used. The same technique can be used with an endoscopic approach. (**A**) After the posterior flaps of the DCR are sewn closed, place a 20-gauge needle between the plica and the caruncle and push it into the ostium. After verifying the correct position, slide a 375210 Beaver blade alongside the needle (sharp edge away from the eye). Clamp and remove the needle. (**B**) Slide a Quickert probe alongside the blade and remove the blade. (**C**) Push the Jones tube over the Quickert probe into position. (**D**) Jones tube in position. The anterior flaps are sewn and the wound is closed. A double-armed 6-0 Vicryl suture is wrapped around the neck of the tube and sewn to the plica.

Major points

Is true epiphora present?

- Listen to the patient to differentiate "watery" eyes from "tearing" eyes
  - Watery eyes result from a variety of problems not usually related to nasolacrimal duct obstruction
  - True tearing means tear overflow onto the cheek—epiphora
  - Epiphora suggests lacrimal duct obstruction
- The patient's history will tell you if nasolacrimal duct obstruction is present:
  - Epiphora, rather than a watery eye
  - Unilateral symptoms

- History of dacryocystitis
- Onset after conjunctivitis, facial fracture, or nasal surgery
- Sometimes patients will confuse the blur of a "dry" eye with a watery eye

You can often guess the diagnosis by age

- Children
  - Congenital nasolacrimal duct obstruction
- Young adults
  - Canalicular disease—usually postherpetic
  - Trauma—canalicular laceration or facial fracture
- Middle-aged adults
  - Dacryolith

Major points Continued

- Older adults
  - Nasolacrimal duct obstruction

Do a physical examination to confirm the diagnosis you suspect from history and age

- Look for problems with the lids, lashes, and puncta first
- Short cut your lacrimal examination by asking yourself, "Is dacryocystitis present?"
  - Signs of acute dacryocystitis are present
  - You can express pus from the sac
  - Mucocele is present
  - If dacryocystitis is present, there is no need for more testing
- Do a dye disappearance test first with 2% fluorescein. This test is very helpful to confirm your suspicion of decreased drainage
- "Palpate" the canalicular system with a 0 or 1-0 Bowman probe to show that the drainage problem is not in the canaliculi
- Irrigate the lacrimal system to demonstrate obstruction or resistance to flow
- Do not probe the nasolacrimal duct
- For most patients, the information you obtain from your history and their age will be confirmed during the physical examination

Treatment of congenital nasolacrimal duct obstruction

- Obstruction of the valve of Hasner is the cause
- Use massage and topical antibiotic
  - Make sure parents are really massaging the sac, not the nose
  - Don't be afraid to probe early if mattering is a big problem
- Most spontaneously resolve by the end of the first year of life
- If no resolution, do a nasolacrimal duct probe and infracture the turbinate
- If probing fails, repeat the nasolacrimal duct probe and intubate with a stent
- Children rarely need a dacryocystorhinostomy

Treatment of adult nasolacrimal duct obstruction

- Dacryocystorhinostomy is the procedure of choice
  - The endonasal approach reduces morbidity, but is slightly less effective
  - The external approach is still the gold standard
- Nasolacrimal duct intubation with stents alone is an option for functional obstruction. Never do a nasolacrimal duct probe without stents in adults
- If a canaliculus is obstructed, attempt repair with stents
- If unable to reconstruct a canaliculus, a Jones tube will be required

Suggested reading

1. Albert DM, Lucarelli MJ: Lacrimal surgery. In *Clinical atlas of procedures in ophthalmic surgery*, pp. 320–339, Chicago: AMAP, 2004.

2. American Academy of Ophthalmology: *Basic and clinical science course: orbit, eyelids, and lacrimal system*, sect. 7, pp. 251–284, San Francisco: American Academy of Ophthalmology, 2006/2007.

3. Anderson RL, Gordy DD: The tarsal strip procedure. *Arch Ophthalmol* 97(11): 2192–2196, 1979.

4. Carter KD, Nerad JA: Primary acquired nasolacrimal duct obstruction. In Bosniak S, ed., *Principles and practice of ophthalmic plastic and reconstructive surgery*, vol. 2, ch. 77, pp. 784–796, Philadelphia: WB Saunders, 1996.

5. Codere F, Gonnering R, Wobig JL, Dailey RA: Surgery of the tear sac. In Wobig JL Dailey RA, eds, *Oculofacial plastic surgery: face, lacrimal system, and orbit*, pp. 167–189, New York: Thieme, 2004.

6. Collin JRO: Lacrimal surgery. In *A manual of systematic eyelid surgery*, 3rd edn, pp. 165–176, Philadelphia: Butterworth Heinemann Elsevier, 2006.

7. Dutton JJ, ed.: *Atlas of ophthalmic surgery*, vol. II, pp. 220–248, St Louis: Mosby, 1992.

8. Dutton JJ: *Atlas of clinical and surgical orbital anatomy*, pp. 139–148, Philadelphia: WB Saunders, 1994.

9. Levine MR: Dacryocystorhinostomy. In Levine MR, ed.: *Manual of oculoplastic surgery*, 3rd edn, pp. 51–59, Boston: Butterworth-Heinemann, 2003.

10. Linberg JV, McCormick SA: Primary acquired nasolacrimal duct obstruction: a clinicopathologic report and biopsy technique. *Ophthalmology* 3:1055–1063, 1986.

11. McCord CD, Tanenbaum M, Nunery WR, eds: *Oculoplastic surgery*, 3rd edn, pp. 341–378, New York: Raven Press, 1995.

12. Nerad JA, Carter KD, Alford MA: Disorders of the orbit: infections, inflammations, neoplasms, vascular abnormalities. In *Rapid diagnosis in ophthalmology— oculoplastic and reconstructive surgery*, pp. 160–239, Philadelphia: Mosby Elsevier, 2008.

13. Nerad JA: Eyelid causes of tearing. In Bosniak S, ed, *Principles and practice of ophthalmic plastic and reconstructive surgery*, vol. 2, pp. 762–776, Philadelphia: WB Saunders, 1996.

14. Nerad JA: Eyelid malpositions. In Linberg JV, ed., *Contemporary issues in ophthalmology: lacrimal surgery*, ch. 4, pp. 61–89, New York: Churchill Livingstone, 1988.

15. Nowinski TS, Anderson RL: The medial spindle procedure for involutional medial ectropion. *Arch Ophthalmol* 103(11):1750–1753, 1985.

16. Zide BM, Jelks GW: *Surgical anatomy of the orbit*, pp. 33–39, New York: Raven Press, 1985.

CHAPTER 11

Diagnosis of Malignant and Benign Lid Lesions Made Easy*

Chapter contents

Introduction

Periocular skin lesions are commonly seen in practice. It will be easy to get lost in this chapter, so read this introduction carefully. It will give you an overview of the information in the whole chapter. The main goal of the evaluation of a lid lesion is to rule out malignancy. The most common skin malignancy is basal cell carcinoma. Because basal cell carcinoma causes more than 90% of skin cancers, it is essential for you to confidently diagnose basal cell carcinoma. The easy way to diagnose basal cell carcinoma is to learn the characteristics of epithelial cell malignancy:

- Ulceration
- Lack of tenderness
- Induration

- Irregular borders and asymmetric shape
- Telangiectasia
- Pearly borders
- Loss of lid margin architecture

We will talk about these features in detail, so don't memorize them now. If any of these features of malignancy are present, a biopsy should be performed to rule out malignancy. If none of these characteristics of malignancy is present, it is highly unlikely that the lesion is malignant. Once you have excluded malignancy, the important part of the evaluation is over. Spend time understanding these characteristics of malignancy rather than trying to learn the names of all the benign lesions that may occur. Get a picture in your mind of what these lesions look like. "Don't lose sight of the forest while trying to learn all the trees." Eventually, you will be able to name the majority of benign lesions as well.

The skin has two layers, the epidermis and the dermis. Basal cell and squamous cell carcinomas arise from the epidermis. The dermis contains the skin appendages or adnexa ("added on"). The adnexae include hair follicles, oil

*The content of this chapter has been presented in course format at the annual meeting of the American Academy of Ophthalmology for the past several years.

(sebaceous) glands, and sweat glands. The most common adnexal malignancy is sebaceous cell carcinoma. This malignancy does not have a characteristic appearance. Sometimes a yellow pigmentation of sebaceous cell carcinoma may be noted. A chronic unilateral blepharoconjunctivitis or an eyelid margin lesion extending from the posterior lamella onto the skin should suggest a possible diagnosis of sebaceous cell carcinoma.

Pigment cells are found at the base of the epidermis. Pigment cell malignancy, or melanoma, is unusual in the periocular area, but may occur. We will describe the characteristics of pigmented lesions that should make you suspect melanoma.

After you are familiar with the characteristics of epithelial cell malignancies—basal cell and squamous cell carcinomas—you are not likely to miss a cutaneous malignancy. Although any adnexal malignancy (almost always sebaceous cell carcinoma) is rare, you should keep the diagnosis in mind. All the other lesions are benign. Eventually, you will recognize the names of all the benign epithelial, adnexal, and melanocytic skin lesions (the "Aunt Minnies").

Let's talk about Aunt Minnies. How do you recognize your aunts and uncles at a family reunion? How do you tell your Aunt Minnie from your Aunt Blanche from your Aunt Muriel? They all look different and you have seen them many times before. We take this daily form of pattern recognition for granted. It is no different for lid lesions. After you see a lesion and learn its name, you will eventually be able to recognize it again. We will discuss this concept again later in this chapter.

The last section of the chapter deals with biopsy techniques, including both incisional biopsy (removing a portion of the tumor) and excisional biopsy (removing the entire tumor). Three important techniques are the shave biopsy, the punch biopsy, and cyst marsupialization. These techniques will be discussed in detail.

Skin anatomy

Layers of the skin

The eyelid skin is the thinnest skin in the body. This skin contains two layers:

- Epidermis
- Dermis

The epidermis is the continually dividing superficial layer of the skin that covers the body. The dermis is the deep layer of the skin. Other than in the eyelid, there is a layer of subcutaneous fat deep to the dermis (Figure 11-1). The eyelid skin is tightly bound to the underlying orbicularis muscle.

Cells destined to become the surface of the skin start as undifferentiated basal cells along the junction of the epidermis and dermis. As these epidermal cells differentiate and move toward the skin surface, they lose their nuclei, flatten, and become keratinized. The most common skin malignancy, basal cell carcinoma, arises from these undifferentiated cells in the basal layer. Because these cells are not producing keratin, basal cell carcinomas do not have excessive keratin production, or hyperkeratosis, as part of their clinical picture. In contrast, squamous cell carcinoma arises from more superficial epidermal skin cells, known as squamous cells, which produce keratin. Consequently, squamous cell carcinoma is associated with hyperkeratosis.

Appendages of the skin

The dermis contains the skin appendages or adnexa (Figure 11-1). The adnexa are the specialized tissues added on to the skin including:

- Sebaceous glands
- Sweat glands
- Hair

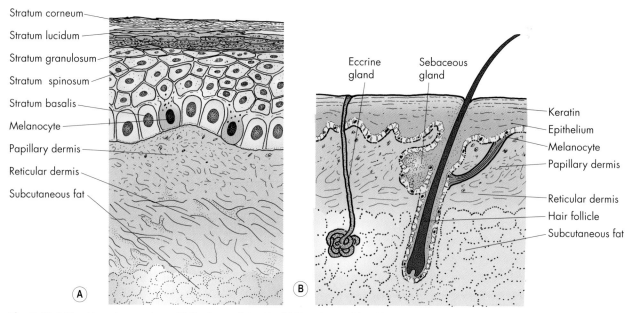

Figure 11-1 The skin and appendages. (**A**) The layers of the skin. (**B**) The adnexa of the skin.

Each adnexal tissue contains specialized cells that may create both solid or cystic cell proliferations. Common tumors arising from the adnexa include chalazia and various cysts. Chalazia arise from the specialized sebaceous glands of the tarsal plate, the meibomian glands. The most common cyst in the periocular area, the apocrine hidrocystoma, arises from the apocrine sweat glands along the lid margin. We will talk about this later. For now, just remember that there can be solid and cystic tumors of each adnexal tissue.

The dermis also contains a number of other tissues including vascular, fibrous, and neural elements. Each of these tissues may give rise to tumors that are rarely seen in the eyelids. You are not likely to see many of these lesions so they will not be covered in this text (Box 11-1).

Malignant tumors of the epidermis

Characteristics of malignancy

This is the most important section of this chapter. Remember that the main goal of evaluating a lid lesion is to rule out malignancy. The most common skin malignancy is basal cell carcinoma, which arises from the epidermis. Basal cell carcinoma represents more than 90% of lid malignancies. If you can recognize basal cell carcinoma, you will be able to recognize the majority of skin cancers affecting the eyelids. Review the characteristics of skin malignancy listed in Box 11-2. Remember these characteristics and you will have little difficulty in diagnosing cutaneous malignancies.

Ulceration

Ulceration is commonly seen in malignant tumors of the epidermis. Malignant cells grow rapidly, tending to outgrow their blood supply, causing areas of central ulceration. Despite areas of ulceration, often associated with bleeding, malignant lesions do not tend to be painful, nor are they tender to touch. Think of this in terms of the bowel tumors that you saw in medical school. Despite the tumor being very large and irregular, often with areas of necrosis, the patient had no pain from the tumor itself. Pain only

developed when the tumor caused another problem such as a bowel obstruction or perforation.

Induration

All malignancies, including skin cancers, tend to be firm or indurated, so palpate each skin lesion (remember the firm bowel tumor). Benign lesions such as cysts and other epithelial lesions feel soft, similar to the surrounding skin.

Irregularity

Malignant tumors are composed of cell populations that grow at different rates. These varying growth patterns create lesions with irregular margins and asymmetric shapes. The margins of malignant lesions tend to be scalloped. Benign lesions tend to have smooth borders. Irregular borders make the shape of the lesion asymmetric so that it is not easy to imagine folding the lesion in half on itself.

Pearly borders and telangiectasia

Pearly borders and telangiectasias are pathognomonic for basal cell carcinoma. Heaped up edges often surround an area of central ulceration. With the slit beam focused on the edge of these lesions, there appears to be a translucency to the lesion itself allegedly from the proliferating cells in the basal layer of the epidermis. Telangiectasias refer to the dilated and irregular vessels accompanying the pearly margins of the basal cell carcinoma. Review the photographs of typical basal cell carcinomas and make sure in your mind that you recognize all the features of epithelial cell malignancy (Figure 11-2).

All the characteristics of malignancy are not always seen in each tumor. When one or more characteristics of malignancy exist, consider a biopsy.

Loss of eyelid margin architecture

A skin malignancy may destroy the normal architecture of the lid margin. Often the tumor outgrows its blood supply, leading to ulceration and subsequent destruction of surrounding tissue. This characteristic destruction of tissues does not occur with benign lesions. Suspect malignancy when an area of lash loss or lid margin destruction is present.

Remember, the goal is to diagnose malignancy. When your diagnostic skills become more sophisticated, you may

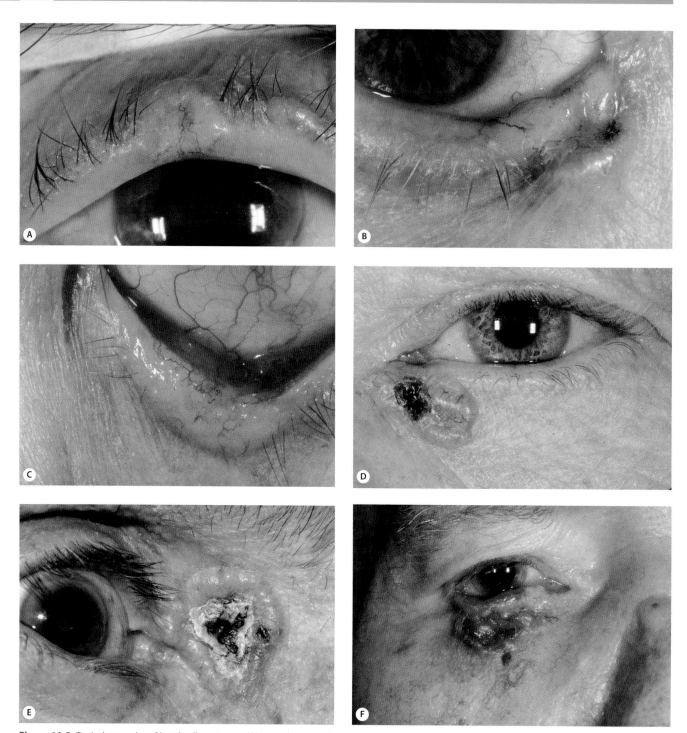

Figure 11-2 Typical examples of basal cell carcinoma. (**A**) Note the classic features—pearly margins and telangiectasias—in this small nodular basal cell carcinoma on the upper eyelid margin. (**B**) Pearly margins and an irregular shape are prominent in this basal cell carcinoma. Note the central ulceration and loss of the lid margin architecture. (**C**) This basal cell carcinoma is pearly white and has typical telangiectasias. Note the indurated thickening of the lid margin. The eyelashes are gone, and the lid margin is altered. The tumor margins are not distinct in this example. (**D**) A more nodular basal cell carcinoma with distinct pearly margins, telangiectasias, and central ulceration. (**E**) Nodular basal cell carcinoma with crusting over central ulceration. (**F**) The most obvious feature of this basal cell carcinoma is ulceration. (**G** and **H**) Morpheaform or nodular type. This type of basal cell carcinoma has less apparent clinical margins. The telangiectasias in (**G**) and thickening of the skin strongly suggest a basal cell carcinoma and should prompt a biopsy. The sclerosing changes in (**H**) pulling the eyelids away from the eye suggest a biopsy. The defect after excision of these diffuse lesions may be large.

be able to tell the type of skin cancer based on the location and how the lesion affects the lid margin. Study the skin carefully during the slit lamp examination. Use the slit lamp as the equivalent of the gynecologist's colposcope used to diagnose potential malignancies of the cervix. Remember

that squamous cell carcinoma tends to be the most superficial of skin cancers initially, and often only scaling is seen in its early phases. Basal cell carcinoma begins a little deeper with rolled edges at the periphery "pulling" normal skin into the lesion. You will not see keratinization on the

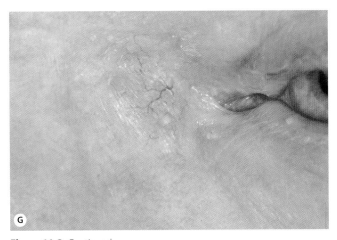

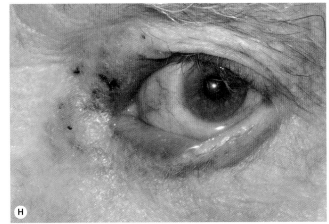

Figure 11-2 Continued.

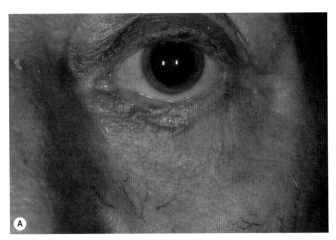

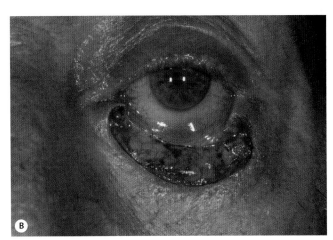

Figure 11-3 (**A**) Basal cell carcinoma with diffuse margins. Note light irises and weathered skin on cheek. (**B**) Large defect after excision.

examination. Because basal cell and squamous cell carcinomas are epithelial lesions, they affect the anterior lamella initially. Sebaceous cell carcinoma affects the posterior lamella first in most patients. Look at the area of distortion or destruction of the lid margin for these clues to the type of malignancy. Don't lose sight of the goal: learning to differentiate malignant from benign lesions first.

Basal cell carcinoma

Basal cell carcinoma, like squamous cell carcinoma, is related to ultraviolet or actinic damage. Consequently, basal cell carcinoma is most common in fair-skinned patients whose skin tends to burn rather than tan in the sun. The lower lid and medial canthus are the most commonly affected locations, probably related to getting more sun exposure than the upper lid. The hallmarks of basal cell carcinoma are pearly borders with telangiectasia. Central ulceration is common. The lesions are not painful and not tender to touch. The border and contour of the lesion are generally irregular. Destruction of normal lid architecture occurs when the lesion involves the lid margin. Lashes are often lost. Hyperkeratosis is not a common finding associated with basal cell carcinoma, because these tumors arise from cells in the basal layer of the epidermis.

Basal cell carcinoma and squamous cell carcinoma may be recognized by the company that they keep. Other signs of actinic damage to the skin, especially in a patient with light skin and blue eyes, should heighten your suspicion of a skin malignancy. Look for signs of sun damage on your patient's face to help you diagnose basal cell carcinoma (Figure 11-3).

A rare genetic disorder, basal cell nevus syndrome, predisposes patients to multiple basal cell carcinomas. This autosomal dominant syndrome, also known as Gorlin's syndrome, is also associated with palmar pits, jaw cysts, and skeletal abnormalities.

Squamous cell carcinoma

Squamous cell carcinoma may resemble basal cell carcinoma clinically. Although differentiating between these two lesions may not always be clinically possible, there should be little doubt about the presence of an epithelial malignancy based on the characteristics outlined above. Squamous cell carcinoma is much less common than basal cell carcinoma, representing less than 5% of lid tumors. If you have to guess the diagnosis, you should guess basal cell carcinoma because it is so much more common.

Squamous cell carcinoma can appear as a nodule or an indurated plaque with some hyperkeratosis. Often the scaly

303

skin will fall off—strongly suggesting a squamous cell cancer or its precursor, actinic keratosis (discussed later in this chapter). Ulceration is sometimes present. Generally, the pearly margins and telangiectasia of basal cell carcinoma are not seen.

Squamous cell carcinoma is usually more aggressive than basal cell carcinoma. The margins of squamous cell carcinoma may be diffuse, resulting in a large area of subclinical tumor involvement (Figure 11-4). Neurotrophic spread (along nerves) occurs in squamous cell carcinoma but is uncommon in basal cell carcinoma. Squamous cell carcinoma in the periocular area with the presence of cranial nerve palsy suggests neurotrophic spread into the cavernous sinus.

Like basal cell carcinoma, squamous cell carcinoma arises in sun-damaged skin. The features of cutaneous actinic damage, such as deep wrinkles, skin thinning, generalized telangiectasia, and mottled pigmentation, may be seen (see Figure 11-19). Scaling keratotic lesions, actinic keratoses, the precursors of squamous cell carcinoma, are often present.

Keratoacanthoma

Keratoacanthoma is considered to be a low-grade squamous cell carcinoma. This tumor has a characteristic appearance different than that of most squamous cell carcinomas. A large lesion with a central crater filled with a keratin plug is typical. The lesion often appears in a few weeks and may spontaneously resolve. This lesion is discussed under the section, "Sun-Damaged Skin and Related Conditions." You will see an illustration of this later.

Malignant tumors of the dermis are very rare and are not considered here. The dermis contains the adnexa of the periocular skin. Sebaceous cell carcinoma is the most common adnexal malignancy and is discussed next.

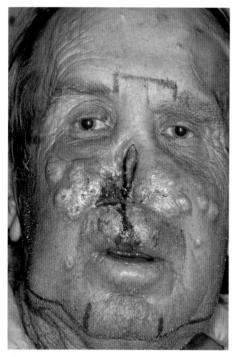

Figure 11-4 Recurrent squamous cell carcinoma. Note the large size, diffuse margins, and hyperkeratinization. This lesion was considered unresectable because of the size and degree of neurotrophic spread. The patient underwent a course of radiation therapy.

Malignant tumors of the adnexa: sebaceous cell carcinoma

Sebaceous glands in the periocular area

Basal cell, squamous cell, and sebaceous cell carcinomas comprise greater than 95% of the malignancies of the eyelids. Sebaceous cell carcinoma is rare, representing between 1% and 5% of eyelid cancers. Sebaceous cell carcinoma arises within the sebaceous glands of the skin and therefore is referred to as an adnexal malignancy. As a reminder, the sebaceous glands in the periocular area are the following:

- Meibomian glands located within the tarsal plates
- Glands of Zeis associated with the eyelash follicles
- Sebaceous glands of the periocular skin
- Sebaceous glands in the caruncle
- Sebaceous glands associated with eyebrow follicles

The presence of specialized sebaceous glands in the periocular area such as the meibomian glands and glands of Zeis makes the occurrence of sebaceous cell carcinoma in the periocular area more common than anywhere else in the body.

Clinical characteristics

Sebaceous cell carcinoma has no characteristic appearance; consequently, it is known as a "masquerader." You won't see many sebaceous cell cancers, but be suspicious if you see a unilateral blepharoconjunctivitis or a chronic or recurrent chalazion. In my experience, the classic recurrent chalazion is the more unusual presentation. An inflamed or swollen lid with conjunctivitis is more common. This blepharoconjunctivitis may present as a chronic condition (Figure 11-5). In some patients, many medical or surgical treatments will have been tried without relief, and the diagnosis of sebaceous cell carcinoma will not have been considered. Biopsy should be performed for chronic unilateral blepharoconjunctivitis or recurrent chalazia. In some cases, the conjunctival spread will predominate, so don't forget to evert the eyelid. In other patients, sebaceous cell carcinoma may present as a more subtle thickening of the lid and lid margin (Figure 11-6). You should consider the diagnosis if you see

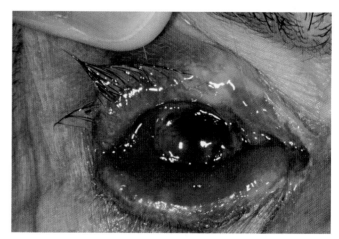

Figure 11-5 Sebaceous cell carcinoma presenting as an advanced unilateral chronic blepharoconjunctivitis.

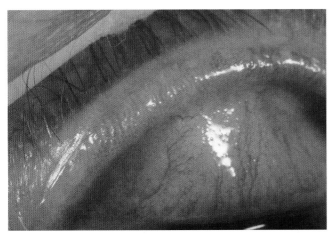

Figure 11-6 Sebaceous cell carcinoma. Note the subtle thickening of the lid margin. These lesions often have a yellowish hue. This is seen in thin lines along the eyelid margin, giving a "tigroid" appearance to the thickened tissue.

a lid margin lesion that appears to arise from or extend over the margin onto the tarsal conjunctiva. The presence of any yellowish material within a malignant-appearing lesion should suggest the diagnosis of sebaceous cell carcinoma.

Biopsy technique

Full-thickness lid biopsy has been recommended for the diagnosis of sebaceous cell carcinoma. When there is diffuse thickening of the lid with no obvious mass, it is a good idea to do a full-thickness lid biopsy. A full-thickness specimen gives the pathologist an opportunity to see the architecture of both affected and normal lid tissues, including the conjunctival epithelium. If a large mass is present, a generous incisional biopsy of the mass itself is usually diagnostic and a full-thickness biopsy is not necessary. Small biopsies of conjunctiva alone may be difficult to interpret. Oil red-O stain on fresh tissue has also been recommended for the diagnosis of sebaceous cell carcinoma. Although oil red-O does stain the sebaceous material within the tumor, the histologic and cytologic features of the tumor (including the typical foamy cytoplasm seen in the dysplastic sebaceous cells) are diagnostic in most cases without special staining.

Remember that sebaceous cell carcinomas are rare tumors. If you suspect a sebaceous cell carcinoma, be sure to let the pathologist know. General and dermatologic pathologists see few, if any, of them. When there is any question about the diagnosis of a sebaceous cell carcinoma, consultation with an ophthalmic pathologist is appropriate. He or she is likely to have the most experience and should be able to provide the most accurate diagnosis.

Unusual growth characteristics

Sebaceous cell carcinoma has two unusual growth characteristics that make removal difficult. The first is pagetoid spread. Intraepithelial sebaceous cell carcinoma may spread superficially over large areas of the conjunctiva. Secondly, sebaceous cell carcinoma appears to arise from multifocal noncontiguous tumor origins. These characteristics make excision of sebaceous cell carcinoma more complicated than that of the more common cutaneous malignancies. Basal cell

and squamous cell carcinomas arise from a single origin and tend to spread radially. Clinical margins can be approximated and then confirmed with frozen sections. With sebaceous cell carcinoma, the true pathologic margins are often not clinically visible because of the pagetoid spread. Noncontiguous tumor origins make intraoperative margin confirmation of tumor removal unreliable, because the surgical margin may be free of tumor, but another focus of tumor may be just beyond the first margin.

Tumor excision

For these reasons, excision of sebaceous cell carcinoma is somewhat specialized. Preoperatively, map biopsies of the conjunctiva are done to determine the probable peripheral extent of any pagetoid spread. From the results of these permanent section biopsies, a surgical excision is planned.

At the time of excision, generous margins are taken to include the involved areas of the tarsus, lid margin, skin, and conjunctiva. There is some controversy about the usefulness of frozen sections in sebaceous cell carcinoma as pagetoid spread may be difficult to identify using this technique because of poor resolution and tissue artifacts of freezing. For this reason, I use a permanent section, evaluated overnight, to determine if margins are clear of tumor. This is somewhat tedious, but gives the best accuracy in terms of tumor removal. The defect is then reconstructed using the usual techniques of repair. Because sebaceous cell carcinoma often involves the upper lid, reconstruction is often complicated.

Sebaceous cell carcinoma is an uncommon tumor. It is difficult to diagnose because of its many manifestations. It is difficult to excise because of pagetoid spread and noncontiguous tumor origins. Unlike with basal cell carcinoma and squamous cell carcinoma, there is a possibility of regional lymph node metastasis (Figure 11-7). In most patients, no regional disease is present at the time of diagnosis. Fortunately, local resection is usually curative. If all four lids are involved or orbital fat is invaded, orbital exenteration is required. Death caused by sebaceous cell carcinoma is possible, but rare.

Benign lesions arising in the sebaceous glands include chalazia, sebaceous hyperplasia, and sebaceous adenoma. These lesions will be discussed later in the chapter.

Checkpoint

- At this point in this chapter, you should be able to diagnose the majority of malignant lid lesions you will encounter in practice
- The diagnosis of most cutaneous malignancies is based upon recognition of the clinical characteristics of malignancy that will help you identify basal cell carcinoma and squamous cell carcinoma
- Important! What are the clinical characteristics of skin malignancy?
- What growth characteristics make sebaceous cell carcinoma difficult to resect?
- Chronic unilateral conjunctivitis or a "chalazion" resistant to treatment should alert you to the possible diagnosis of sebaceous cell carcinoma

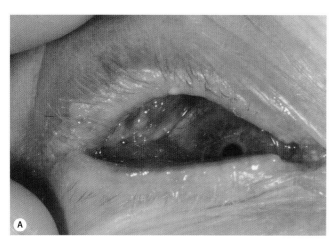

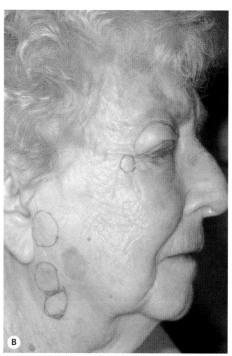

Figure 11-7 An unusually aggressive sebaceous cell carcinoma. (**A**) A large mass of tumor is seen in the superior fornix originating from the upper lid tarsus. (**B**) Regional and "in transit" lymphatic metastases were present. Despite orbital exenteration, neck dissection, and radiation therapy, the patient died a few months after diagnosis.

Box 11-3
Pigmented Skin Lesions—Concepts to Remember
• Most pigmented lesions are not melanomas
• Any skin lesion may be pigmented
• Not all pigmented lesions are nevi
• Not all nevi are pigmented

Pigmented lesions: ruling out melanoma

General concepts

Although eyelid melanomas are rare, we are all concerned about the possibility of a pigmented lesion being a melanoma. This section will help you to differentiate benign from malignant pigmented lesions of the skin. Let's start with these basic concepts (Box 11-3).

- The majority of pigmented lesions will not be melanoma
- Any type of skin lesion may be pigmented depending on the patient's skin coloring
- Not all pigmented lesions are nevi (Figure 11-8, A)
- In fact, not all nevi are pigmented (we will cover this later) (Figure 11-8, B)

Characteristics of benign pigment cell tumors

Benign lesions grow in a controlled manner with the cell population under normal biologic controls. Features of benign pigmented lesions include:

- Uniform color
- Regular smooth borders
- Symmetric shape

Small variations in color from light brown to brown are normal. In general, benign lesions appear to have smooth edges and symmetric shape (Figure 11-9).

Characteristics of malignant pigment cell tumors: melanoma

Because many of the pigmented lesions seen on the face are not of pigment cell origin, the characteristics of epidermal malignancy emphasized earlier should be applied to any pigmented lesion. These serve as a starting point for diagnosing malignancy.

Several clinical features that should make you suspect that a pigmented lesion is a melanoma are listed in Box 11-4.

The recent onset of a pigmented lesion or a change in the color, shape, or size of any existing lesion suggests an uncontrolled pattern of growth. This may signal the start of melanoma. Pigmented lesions that have irregular margins also suggest uncontrolled growth. An asymmetric shape, such that the lesion cannot be folded on itself, suggests a diagnosis of melanoma (Figure 11-10, A). Many melanomas will have several colors within the lesion, ranging from a light white or tan to very dark black (Figure 11-10, B). In between are shades of red and blue, hence the term red, white, and blue sign as an indication of melanoma. Large pigmented lesions (>6 mm in diameter or the size of a traditional wooden pencil eraser) may be associated with melanoma. Strongly consider a biopsy for any pigmented tumor larger than 1 cm in diameter.

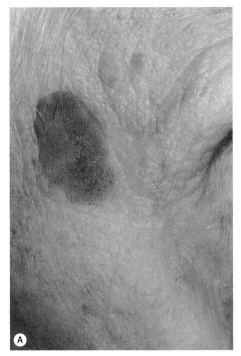

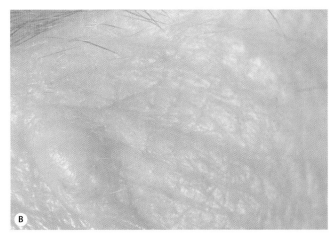

Figure 11-8 Pigmentation of skin lesions. (**A**) A pigmented nonpigment cell tumor—a seborrheic keratosis. (**B**) A nonpigmented pigment cell tumor—a compound nevus.

Figure 11-9 A benign nevus. Note the uniform color, smooth border, and symmetric shape.

Benign tumors of the eyelid

"Aunt minnies": pattern recognition of benign skin lesions

The majority of tumors in the periocular area are benign. Given the large number of tissues within the skin, you can imagine that there are a huge number of possible benign cell proliferations. Here is where you need to step back and get the big picture again. There are many benign proliferations arising from the epithelial tissues. Add to those the lesions arising from the tissues of the adnexal structures: the hair

---

Box 11-4
Characteristics of Pigment Cell Malignancy: Melanoma
• Recent onset of pigmented lesion
• Change in existing pigmented lesion
• Irregular margins
• Asymmetric shape
• Color change or presence of multiple colors
• Large size greater than 6 mm in diameter

follicles and associated erector pili muscles, the various sebaceous glands in the periocular tissue including the meibomian glands and Zeis glands, and the apocrine and eccrine sweat glands. Finally, add all the other tissues within the dermis: fibrous, vascular, and neural tissues. Each of these tissues can give rise to a benign periocular tumor. Fortunately, a relatively small number of tumors occur commonly. With time, you will be able to recognize them by their characteristic appearance.

You have already been introduced to the term Aunt Minnie. A medical school professor of mine called pulmonary lesions that were diagnosed by sight or pattern recognition on chest X-ray Aunt Minnies. Take a look at the Aunt Minnie in Figure 11-11. This Aunt Minnie is a rare skin tumor known as a cylindroma; several collectively form a "turban tumor." Once you have seen a patient with cylindromas, you will always recognize these lesions. You may not remember that these benign tumors are thought to arise from sweat glands and that the multiple form of cylindroma occurs as a familial disease, but you will recognize that the tumor is benign (none of the characteristics of malignancy that we discussed are present). You, undoubtedly, will

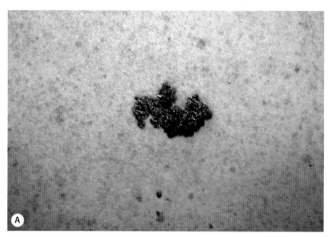

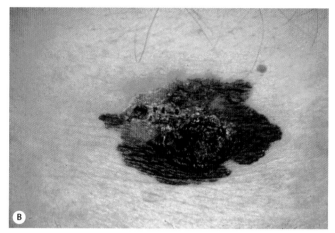

Figure 11-10 Cutaneous melanoma. (**A**) Note the irregular margins and asymmetric shape. (**B**) Note the variation in color (courtesy of Duane Whitaker, MD).

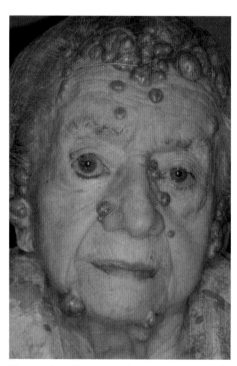

Figure 11-11 "Aunt Minnie" pattern recognition of cylindroma, a type of sweat gland tumor, also known as a "turban tumor." (from Krachmer JH, Mannis MJ, Holland EJ, eds: *Cornea and external disease: clinical diagnosis and management*, St Louis: Mosby, 1997).

remember the diagnosis of cylindroma and the name "turban tumor" once you have seen it.

The majority of benign lid lesions are like this. After you have seen one and learned to recognize it, you will be able to recognize others that look just like it. That is not to say that an understanding of the cell origin or the histopathology of the lesion is not important. But the most important point to understand is that the lesion is benign. Remember the big picture. This lesion has none of the clinical characteristics of malignancy that we have discussed. When you evaluate a patient with a lid lesion, first focus on whether the lesion is benign or malignant. After you have seen the common lesions several times, you will learn the names.

Checkpoint

- When evaluating a lid lesion, determine if the clinical features suggest malignancy. If so, plan a biopsy. If none of the characteristics of malignancy is present, the lesion is probably benign
- What are the characteristics of malignant epidermal skin lesions?
- What are the characteristics of the malignant pigment cell tumor—melanoma?
- For many lesions, you will have "sight or pattern recognition" and will know its "Aunt Minnie" name. For other lesions, you will have to be content with just knowing that it is not malignant

We will discuss the "Aunt Minnies" of benign lid lesions that arise from the epithelium, from the adnexa, and from pigment cells. Other more unusual lesions arising from vascular, fibrous, and neural elements will not be discussed.

Benign epidermal tumors

Acrochordon

Acrochordon or fibroepithelioma is the name given to the common pedunculated, flesh-colored skin lesions that may arise anywhere on the skin of the face. These "skin tags" occur commonly on the neck, axilla, groin, and eyelids (Figure 11-12). On the lid, they are usually small 2–3 mm flesh-colored pedunculated lesions. They may be removed by simply snipping them off at the base with a small ring scissors or Westcott scissors. If the lesion is very pedunculated, no local anesthetic is required to remove it.

The term squamous papilloma is a clinical term used to describe any pedunculated papillomatous lesion occurring on the skin. This is a descriptive clinical term and does not have a diagnostic meaning. A variety of lesions including acrochordon, nevi, seborrheic keratosis, and actinic keratosis are sometimes described as squamous papillomas (Figure 11-13). If a biopsy is required, it is important to sample the base of the lesion.

Seborrheic keratosis

Seborrheic keratoses are extremely common, asymptomatic, benign proliferations of normal epithelial cells. Probably you have seen these, but may not have known the name. These lesions appear as greasy, or shiny, lesions with a "stuck-on" appearance. They look like a small ball of a child's modeling clay was pressed against the skin and stuck in place. On the thinner skin of the eyelid, these lesions appear wrinkled. On the thicker areas of the skin including the cheek and forehead, the lesions have the more typical greasy, "stuck-on" appearance.

Seborrheic keratoses occur as individual or multiple lesions. The color varies from flesh color to tan, depending on the amount of pigment in the patient's skin. Larger and flatter lesions show keratin pits, which are pores filled with keratin (Figure 11-14).

Seborrheic keratoses are quite superficial, although they appear thick in many cases. They can be removed by a shave-type superficial biopsy, leaving the deep layers of the skin intact.

Cutaneous horn

The term cutaneous horn is a descriptive, not a diagnostic, term. The "horn-like" curved, hard projection from the skin is a collection of keratin that may arise from any number of benign or malignant skin lesions. It is important to perform a biopsy at the base of the horn to determine the definitive diagnosis (Figure 11-15).

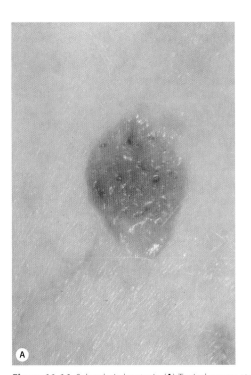

Figure 11-12 Acrochordon, "skin tag" (from Krachmer JH, Mannis MJ, Holland EJ, eds: *Cornea and external disease: clinical diagnosis and management*, St Louis: Mosby, 1997).

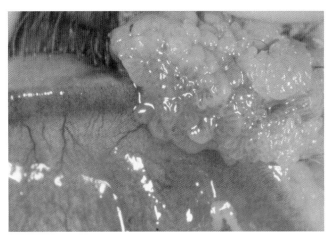

Figure 11-13 Squamous papilloma: a clinical, not histopathologic, diagnosis.

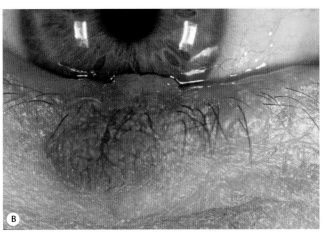

Figure 11-14 Seborrheic keratosis. (**A**) Typical greasy, stuck-on appearance of this lesion occurring on the cheek. (**B**) More crenated and sometimes pedunculated lesion occurring on the thin eyelid skin (see **Figure 11-35**).

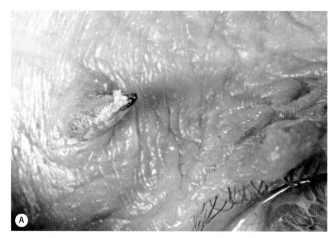
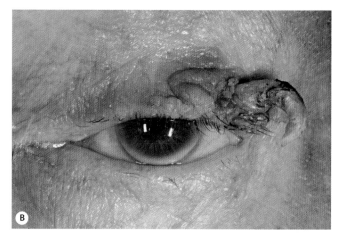

Figure 11-15 Cutaneous horn. Remember to perform a biopsy at the base of the lesion. (**A**) Typical small lesion that frequently flakes off. (**B**) Large lesion, ignored for several months. Diagnosis of tissue taken at base of the lesion was squamous cell carcinoma.

Sun-damaged skin and related conditions

Actinic damage

The thin skin of the eyelid is susceptible to ultraviolet damage. This ultraviolet damage is largely responsible for the aging changes of the face. Consider the effects of sun damage on your own skin by comparing your face to the unexposed areas of your body. Sun is largely responsible for any difference in the appearance of your skin because the age and genetic composition in each part of your body is identical.

You will see that sun-damaged skin occurs most commonly in fair-skinned patients with blonde or red hair and blue eyes. The sun-damaged skin appears thin with deep wrinkles and furrows (Figure 11-16, A). Changes in pigmentation include diffuse mottling or brownish patches known as solar lentigo. The vessels of the dermis are visible due to loss of surrounding collagen in elastic tissue (Figure 11-16, B). Sometimes an impressive difference in the amount of sun damage between the lower face and forehead can be seen in patients who work outdoors and who protect their forehead with a cap (Figure 11-16, C). Scaling and inflamed lips associated with sun-damaged skin are known as actinic cheilitis.

The most important clinical point about actinic skin damage is that patients with clinical signs of sun-damaged skin are at risk for development of basal cell and squamous cell carcinomas. Learn to recognize sun-damaged skin. It is unusual for a patient to develop skin cancers without surrounding evidence of sun damage.

Actinic keratosis

Actinic keratosis is a premalignant skin lesion, the precursor to squamous cell carcinoma. These lesions appear in the context of sun-damaged skin on the face, hands, bald scalp, and ears. Patients identify these lesions as gritty areas to touch that come and go over time. This roughness is a result of excessive keratin production (the same hyperkeratosis we talked about with squamous cell carcinoma), which tends to flake off only to return later. Clinically, the lesions appear as flesh-colored, yellowish, or brownish plaques, depending on the degree of hyperkeratosis. Sometimes the lesions are associated with some erythema of the skin. The lesions are

usually multiple. The upper lid is rarely a site of actinic keratosis because of shading of the skin by the prominence of the superior brow.

The presence of actinic keratosis indicates sun-damaged skin and the possibility of the development of other skin cancers such as basal cell and squamous cell carcinomas (Figure 11-17). If left untreated, actinic keratosis may turn into squamous cell carcinoma.

Patients with actinic keratoses should be under the care of a dermatologist, who can treat these lesions and monitor them for the formation of squamous cell carcinoma. The usual treatment of actinic keratosis is cryotherapy. Excision or topical 5-fluorouracil (5-FU) is also used in selected patients.

Keratoacanthoma

Keratoacanthoma is an uncommon dome-shaped epithelial tumor. Clinically, the lesion starts as a small flesh-colored papule, usually on the lower lid. You will diagnose this tumor by its rapid growth over a few weeks. You will see a dome-shaped nodule with a characteristic central keratin-filled crater (Figure 11-18, A). The clinical history and examination are usually typical. Keratoacanthomas commonly occur in middle-aged to elderly men with considerable sun-damaged skin.

The incidence of keratoacanthomas and squamous cell carcinomas is increased in immunosuppressed patients (Figure 11-18, B). This fact should reinforce the point that "abnormal" cells are forming continually, but that normal "immunosurveillance" destroys these cells before they develop. When you see a patient who is chronically immunosuppressed, be on the lookout for squamous cell carcinomas and other tumors. A genetic loss of immunosurveillance occurs with basal cell nevus syndrome (discussed above). In this autosomal dominant syndrome, a mutation in a tumor suppressor gene, the *PATCHED* gene (PTC on chromosome 9q22), has been identified. Similarly, a loss of DNA repair enzymes is responsible for the high incidence of tumors in xeroderma pigmentosa.

Keratoacanthomas are said to resolve spontaneously within 6 months. Although keratoacanthoma has long been regarded as a benign self-limited lesion, many pathologists now regard the tumor as a form of low-grade squamous cell

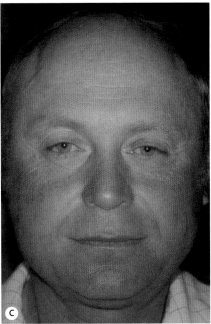

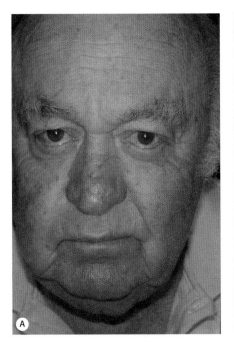

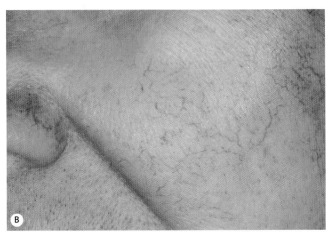

Figure 11-16 Sun-damaged skin. (**A**) Note the deep wrinkles, irregular surface of the skin, and dry lip (actinic cheilitis). (**B**) Actinic damage to the skin causes collagen loss, which allows dermal vessels to be visible. (**C**) Sun damage to the lower face. The patient wears a cap with a bill, which protects the forehead skin.

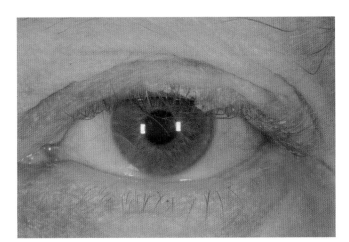

Figure 11-17 Actinic keratosis. Note the scaly appearance to the lesion, which feels gritty to the touch. This lesion is uncommon on the eyelids, but common on the sun-exposed areas of the face, hands, and ears.

carcinoma (Figure 11-18, B). You may want to put keratoacanthoma on your list of malignant epidermal tumors. In practice, given the rapid growth and large size that these lesions may attain, keratoacanthomas are generally removed surgically with margins free of tumor. Success has been reported with the use of topical or intralesional 5-FU or cryotherapy as well, but I have no personal experience with either of these treatments.

Benign adnexal lesions

The skin adnexae commonly give rise to benign skin lesions of the periocular area. These lesions, often cystic, are rarely confused with skin malignancies and have a typical appearance that is usually easily recognized ("Aunt Minnies"). Benign lesions of a single type of gland often have cystic and solid counterparts, such as the solid syringoma and the cystic hidrocystoma of the eccrine sweat glands. Sebaceous and sweat glands commonly produce benign lesions on the lids.

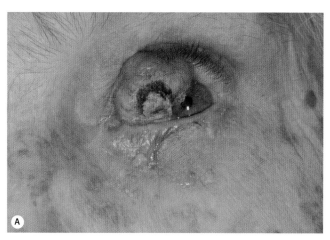

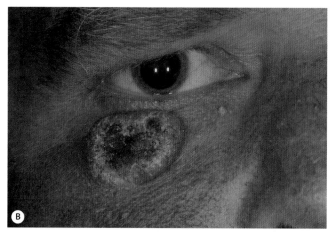

Figure 11-18 Keratoacanthoma. (**A**) Note the central crater filled with keratin. (**B**) Typical appearance of a keratoacanthoma in an organ transplant patient taking cyclosporine and prednisone. This lesion was removed and histologically determined to be a low-grade squamous cell carcinoma.

A chalazion or the common "stye" is a good example of the benign adnexal lesion encountered commonly in everyday practice. Lesions related to hair follicle origin are rare.

Benign adnexal tumors of sebaceous gland origin

Hordeolum and chalazion

As discussed earlier, the eyelids are a unique site of specialized sebaceous glands. These glands include the meibomian glands of the tarsal plate, the Zeis glands associated with the eyelashes, and the sebaceous glands associated with the eyebrow hairs, caruncle hairs, and vellus hairs of the skin.

There is a considerable amount of confusion regarding the nomenclature of these lesions related to the sebaceous glands of the eyelid. Don't get too concerned with what you call these lesions. You probably already have names for them. Two factors help me to categorize these common lesions:

- Which glands are involved?
  — Glands of Zeis
  — Meibomian glands
- What is the chronicity of the lesion?
  — Acute: hordeolum
  — Chronic: chalazion

The first factor addresses which glands are involved. In the eyelid itself, this means either the glands of Zeis associated with the eyelashes along the lid margin or the meibomian glands of the tarsal plate. The second factor is related to the chronicity of the lesion. If the pathologic process such as inflammation, infection, or obstruction causes an acute condition in either the meibomian gland or gland of Zeis, I like to use the term hordeolum. This term suggests a staphylococcal infection, but the role of infection in this process is not clearly identified. An acute condition related to the meibomian glands is called an internal hordeolum. An acute event related to the glands of Zeis is called an external hordeolum. The external hordeolum is what most patients call a stye. With treatment using antibiotics, warm wet lid compresses, and lid scrubs, the majority of these lesions will resolve.

If the acute event becomes chronic, I am inclined to use the term chalazion, suggesting chronic retention of material

> **Box 11-5**
>
> **Hordeolum and Chalazion**
> **Glands of Zeis**
> - Acute: external hordeolum (most common "stye")
> - Chronic: "marginal" chalazion
>
> **Meibomian glands**
> - Acute: internal hordeolum
> - Chronic: chalazion

within the sebaceous gland. The chronic cystic retention of material within the meibomian gland is called simply a chalazion or a deep chalazion (Figure 11-19).

These lesions contrast with the chronic process that occurs along the lid margin involving the Zeis glands, which I am inclined to call a marginal chalazion. There is no widespread agreement about this terminology. The important concept is to understand which glands are involved and the degree of acute versus chronic inflammation present (Box 11-5).

If a chalazion develops, incision and drainage will result in a prompt cure. Alternatively, injections of a small amount of a steroid such as betamethasone 6 mg/ml (Celestone) may result in resolution.

My preference for treating the firm, painless, chronic nodule of a deep chalazion is incision and drainage. This is a simple technique commonly performed by general ophthalmologists. The majority of deep chalazia will "point" on the back of the tarsal plate and should be opened posteriorly. If the chalazion points toward the skin, I will open the lesion on the skin side. For most anterior lesions, any incision and drainage performed from the posterior approach tears through the skin no matter how careful you are.

The procedure for drainage of a deep chalazion is outlined below:

1. Anesthesia
   A. Instill topical anesthetic.
   B. Inject 2% lidocaine (Xylocaine) with 1:100,000 epinephrine subconjunctivally proximal to the tarsal plate. A similar injection is given under the pretarsal skin.

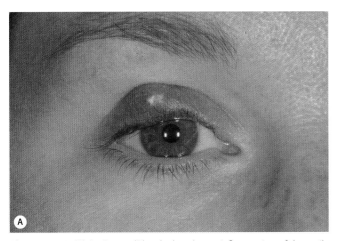
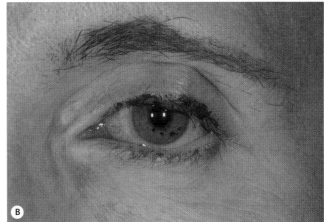

Figure 11-19 (**A**) An "internal" hordeolum (acute inflammation of the meibomian gland) is treated with warm, wet compresses. (**B**) A chalazion (chronic inflammation of the meibomian gland) needs incision and drainage.

2. Incision
  A. Position a chalazion clamp and evert the eyelid. Tighten the clamp to provide stabilization of the lid and hemostasis (Figure 11-20, A).
  B. Use a no. 11 blade to make a cross-shaped incision into the lesion on the tarsal plate (Figure 11-20, B).
3. Curettage
  A. Use a chalazion curette of appropriate size to scrape out the contents of the cyst (Figure 11-20, C).
  B. Excise the corners of the cross-shaped incision with Westcott scissors (Figure 11-20, D).
  C. Apply thermal cautery to the wound edges for hemostasis (Figure 11-20, E).
  D. Instill a small amount of antibiotic ointment.
  E. If there is no bleeding, the eye need not be patched. If there is a persistent amount of oozing, tape a patch into position for 6–12 hours.

Marginal chalazia are approached in a similar fashion with a single incision placed across the lesion. Take care not to cut all the way through the lid margin. Scrape the contents of the cyst with a small chalazion curette. Cautery is usually not necessary. A patch is optional. Generally, patients are treated with antibiotic ointment for a few days postoperatively.

Epidermal inclusion cyst

Epidermal inclusion cysts appear as round elevated cysts usually measuring 3–8 mm (Figure 11-21). These cysts arise in association with a hair follicle. The term sebaceous cyst has been used to describe these lesions. This term is incorrect because the cysts contain keratin rather than sebaceous material (therefore, the term epidermal inclusion cyst).

Frequently, a pore on the top of the cyst will be present. These cysts are best treated by marsupialization of the cyst and removal of the cyst contents (see Figure 11-37).

Milia

Milia are small 1–3 mm superficial white cysts occurring on the eyelids and periocular area. Milia are tiny epidermal inclusion cysts. These cysts arise in association with the root of the vellus hairs of the skin. There should be no confusion between milia and any malignant lesion of the eyelid. The treatment of milia includes opening the surface of the lesion with a small hypodermic needle and expressing the cyst contents (marsupialization) (Figure 11-22).

Sebaceous hyperplasia

Sebaceous hyperplasia is a common lesion arising from the solid proliferation of sebaceous glandular elements. This solid-appearing shiny yellow papule commonly occurs on the forehead, cheeks, and nose where sebaceous glands are prominent. Sebaceous hyperplasia is unusual on the thin skin of the eyelid. This lesion is slow growing and, in most patients, has been present for many years. Its raised, irregular margins with central umbilication may resemble a basal cell carcinoma, but the presence of the lesion without change for many years suggests a nonmalignant proliferation (Figure 11-23). Some have described the appearance of a sebaceous hyperplasia lesion as a "flower petal."

Sebaceous adenoma

Another solid proliferation of sebaceous glands is called sebaceous adenoma. These yellow superficial epidermal nodules are rare. They may be confused with seborrheic keratoses or basal cell carcinoma. Their importance for our purpose is their association with Torre's syndrome, where patients with multiple sebaceous adenomas may have adenocarcinoma of the colon.

Benign adnexal tumors of sweat gland origin

Types of sweat glands

You learned this in medical school, but have probably forgotten it. Two types of sweat glands exist in the body. Eccrine sweat glands are thermal regulatory glands distributed throughout the entire surface of the skin. The primary role of eccrine sweat glands is thermoregulation. The evaporation of sweat from the surface of the skin cools the body. Emotional stimuli may cause secretion of the eccrine glands, especially those glands concentrated on the palms of the hands ("sweaty palms") or the soles of the feet. Like eccrine glands elsewhere in the body, eccrine sweat glands on the eyelid have a true duct with the secretory portion of the gland lying deep in the dermis (see Figure 11-1).

Apocrine sweat glands are specialized scent glands. They are concentrated in the axilla, groin, and anogenital area.

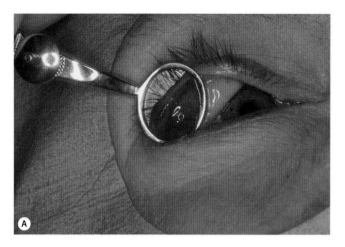

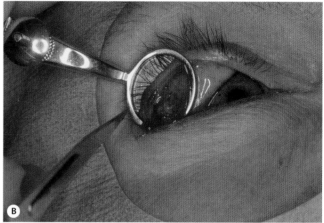

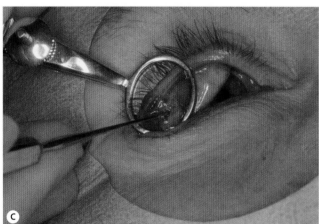

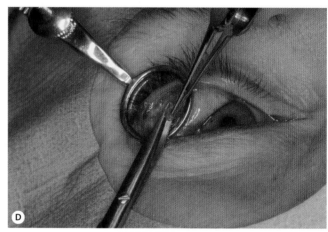

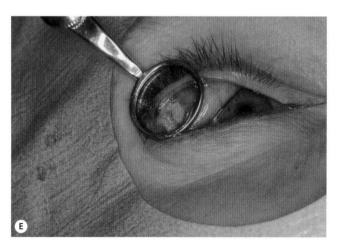

Figure 11-20 Incision and drainage of a chalazion (see Figure 11-19, B). (**A**) A chalazion clamp is in place. Note the chalazion "pointing" posteriorly. (**B**) A cross-shaped incision is made with a no. 11 blade. (**C**) The internal contents of the cyst are removed with a curette. (**D**) The "corners" of the incision are excised to promote drainage and eliminate any tissue mass. (**E**) The wound is cauterized lightly and left open to drain.

Modified apocrine sweat glands include the mammary gland of the breast, the ceruminous glands of the external auditory canal, and the apocrine glands of the eyelid associated with the eyelashes known as the glands of Moll. Like the eccrine glands, the secretory portion of the gland is located deep in the dermis. Unlike eccrine sweat glands, apocrine glands secrete by cellular decapitation so that the apocrine sweat has some cellular debris in it. This debris is sometimes seen layered out as sediment in apocrine gland cysts along the eyelid margin.

Both cystic and solid forms of sweat gland lesions can exist on the eyelid. The most common sweat gland lesions are cystic, so-called sudoriferous cysts (a generic term for a cyst arising from a sweat gland). Many varieties of rare sweat gland tumors can exist in the eyelid, including sweat gland carcinomas. Only the lesions commonly seen in practice will be discussed (Box 11-6). These include the eccrine sweat gland lesions (syringomas and eccrine hidrocystoma) and one apocrine lesion (apocrine hidrocystoma).

Syringoma

Syringomas are cellular proliferations of eccrine sweat gland epithelium. These small, multiple papules occur bilaterally. They are common on the lower lids, especially in women.

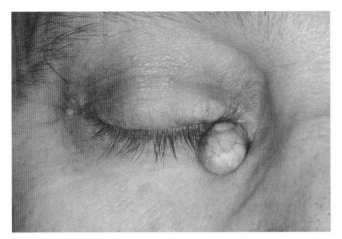

Figure 11-21 Epidermal inclusion cyst.

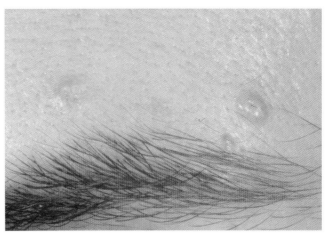

Figure 11-23 Sebaceous hyperplasia. Two lesions are present in the thick skin above the brow in this patient. The lesion on the left is sebaceous hyperplasia. The lesion on the right is a nevus.

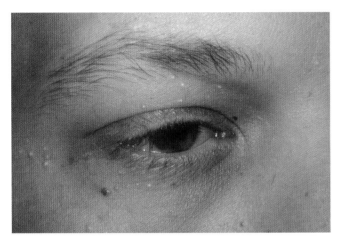

Figure 11-22 Milia.

<hr/>

Box 11-6

Benign Sweat Gland Tumors

Eccrine sweat glands

- Thermoregulatory function
- Generally distributed across the eyelid skin
- Tumors
  - Solid—syringoma
  - Cystic—eccrine hidrocystoma

Apocrine sweat glands

- Scent glands
- Glands of Moll on lid margin
- Tumors
  - Solid—apocrine adenoma (rare)
  - Cystic—apocrine hidrocystoma (common)

<hr/>

The lesions tend to be flesh-colored or slightly yellow (Figure 11-24, A). Their appearance is noted at puberty. The features of syringomas are entirely benign and should not be confused with any eyelid malignancy. The multiple lesions presenting are due to the general distribution of eccrine sweat glands over the entire surface of the skin. These multiple small lesions arise deep within the dermis of the skin. Their appearance can be improved by individual excision of the more prominent lesions. Some success has been obtained with laser resurfacing of these lesions.

Eccrine hidrocystoma

The eccrine hidrocystoma is the cystic equivalent of syringoma. Multiple small cysts filled with clear fluid usually present on the lower lid (Figure 11-24, B). Initiating stimuli include heat, humidity, and perspiration. The individual cysts can be opened, but tend to recur when aggravating factors are encountered. These cysts are uncommon.

Apocrine hidrocystoma

Of the sweat gland tumors, the apocrine hidrocystoma is by far the most common. You should become familiar with this lesion. Remember the apocrine sweat glands of the eyelid are the glands of Moll. These glands are present along the lid margin in association with the eyelashes. The majority of

apocrine hidrocystomas occur as single lesions along the lid margin (Figure 11-25). The lesions may be small, measuring 1–2 mm in diameter but, in some cases, may grow to be 1 cm or larger in size. The cyst is filled with translucent material. Commonly, debris from the apocrine cellular decapitation will be present, layered in the bottom of the cyst. Deeper lesions may have a bluish color.

Apocrine hidrocystomas can be removed by complete excision. An easier form of treatment is marsupialization of the cyst. Removal of cysts will be discussed in the section, "Biopsy Techniques."

Benign pigment cell lesions

Melanocytic nevus

To recognize and understand nevi, melanoma, and other pigmented lesions, let's start with this statement. Pigmented lesions and pigment cell lesions are not necessarily the same thing. The color of a lid lesion is determined by an individual patient's skin color rather than by the presence of pigment cells in the lesion.

We will explore this further, because some understanding is important for you to be comfortable with diagnosing

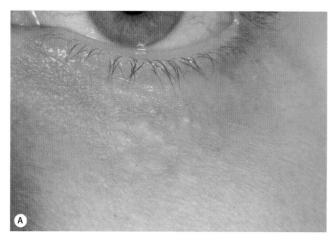

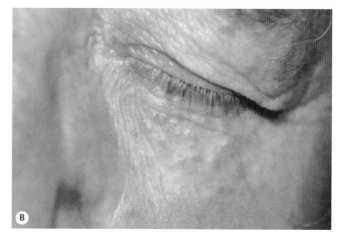

Figure 11-24 Eccrine sweat gland lesions. (**A**) Syringomas of the lower eyelids: cellular proliferation of an eccrine sweat gland. (**B**) Eccrine hidrocystoma of the lower eyelids (rare on the eyelids): cystic enlargement of the eccrine sweat glands.

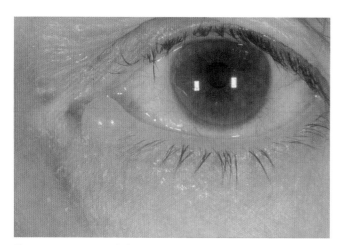

Figure 11-25 Apocrine hidrocystoma occurring along the medial lid margin.

Checkpoint

- Don't confuse pigment cell lesions (those derived from melanocytes such as nevi and melanoma) with pigmented lesions
- Any type of skin lesion may contain melanin and be pigmented
- We will soon see that the converse is also true: not all melanocytic lesions are pigmented

pigmented lesions of the skin. Melanocytes, the pigment-producing cells, are found in the basal layer of the epidermis. Melanin is the pigment produced in small intracellular structures within the melanocyte called melanosomes. Packets of melanin within melanosomes are phagocytized by keratinocytes in the skin. It is the number of melanosomes and the amount of melanin in the melanosome that has been incorporated into the keratinocytes that actually determine the color of the skin. The number of melanocytes within the skin does not determine the color of the skin. In fact, black and white people have the same density of melanocytes within the skin (approximately 1 melanocyte per 10 basal layer cells) (Figure 11-26). However, when compared with white people, black people have larger and greater numbers of melanosomes packed with more melanin within the individual keratinocyte.

Think of skin pigmentation in this simple way. Melanocytes are the melanin factories. Melanin is produced and packaged within containers, the melanosomes. The melanosomes are shipped out to the customers, individual skin cells (keratinocytes), which consume the melanin. The amount of melanin in the skin cell determines the skin color. The same concepts apply to pigmentation of skin lesions.

The familiar mole is a collection of melanocytes forming nests within the skin. The lesions are more precisely known as melanocytic nevi (nevocellular nevi, benign acquired nevi). A melanocytic nevus has a life cycle. Nevi are not normally present at birth. Young children develop small oval or round light to dark brown macules. Development of nevi is accelerated during puberty. This young flat nevus, "a teen-aged nevus," is known as a junctional nevus (Figure 11-27, A). With time, the nevus retains its color and becomes more raised, evolving into a dome shape. This middle-aged nevus is known as a compound nevus (Figure 11-27, B).

With time, the nevus becomes more raised, sometimes even developing a sessile or verrucous component. As the nevus ages, it tends to lose its color, often returning to light brown or flesh color. This "elderly" nevus is referred to as an intradermal nevus (Figure 11-27, C). Loss of skin pigmentation is normal in older patients. Although as ophthalmologists, we generally are not aware of the loss of skin pigment in our older patients, we certainly recognize the development of graying hair that is a part of the general loss of pigment with age.

Nevi of all "ages" are quite common. The concept of the evolving nevus or the life cycle of a nevus is important when evaluating patients. You will notice that the majority of young children you see have few or no nevi. As the children get older and enter puberty, flat brown nevi will appear. In adulthood, these lesions tend to become more raised and retain their color. In older patients, the majority of nevi will lose their color completely. The raised pale "older" or intra-dermal nevus is often not recognized to be a nevus because of the loss of pigmentation. Look carefully at your patients and you will soon recognize the examples throughout the

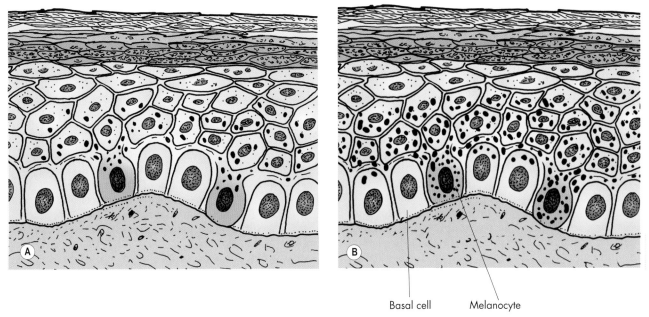

Basal cell   Melanocyte

Figure 11-26 Pattern of pigmentation of the skin: (**A**) White skin. (**B**) African American skin. Each contains the same number of melanocytes. Darker skin is the result of more melanin within each keratinocyte (drawings prepared with assistance from Chris Arpey, MD, Duane Whitaker, MD, and Lynette Watkins, MD).

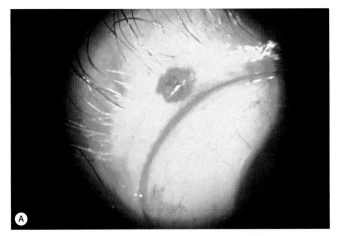

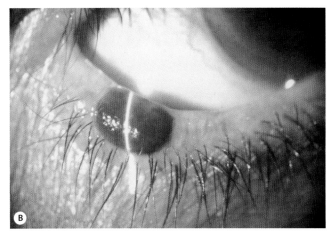

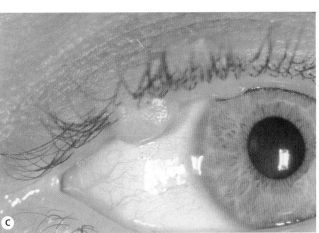

Figure 11-27 The life cycle of a nevus. (**A**) A "teenaged" nevus—the junctional nevus. (**B**) A "middle-aged" nevus—the compound nevus. (**C**) An "elderly" nevus—the intradermal nevus (from Krachmer JH, Mannis MJ, Holland EJ, eds: *Cornea and external disease: clinical diagnosis and management*, St Louis: Mosby, 1997).

whole nevus life cycle. When you are familiar with the clinical appearance of these lesions and the life cycle concept, the histologic terminology will become easy too (Box 11-7).

As nevi "age," they migrate into the deeper layers of the skin. Junctional nevi are found at the junction of the epidermis and the dermis. Compound nevi extend from the epidermis into the dermis, and intradermal nevi lie completely within the dermis (Figure 11-28).

The majority of nevi require no treatment. Should a nevus show a dramatic change in color or shape, a biopsy should be performed (see "Punch Biopsy" later in this chapter). This might be a good time to go back and review the features of a pigmented lesion that would make you suspect melanoma.

Occasionally, a patient will want a nevus excised for other reasons. Complete removal of a nevus with any pigmentation theoretically would require excision to at least the level of the dermis and epidermis. Excision of these lesions is possible with a deeper excision. In practice, many nevi that are objectionable to patients are elevated nonpigmented nevi. These intradermal "older" nevi can be shaved off. This shave biopsy (see "Shave Biopsy" later) will leave nevus cells remaining, but the lack of pigment makes them unapparent.

Congenital nevus

The presence of a nevus at birth is abnormal. Congenital nevi may range in size from a few millimeters to a very large area covering an entire anatomic region such as the thorax. The color is generally fairly uniform, sometimes very dark. Numerous coarse hairs may be present (Figure 11-29).

Congenital nevi carry a small risk of development of malignancy. The risk is related to the size of the nevus, with larger nevi having a greater risk of malignant degeneration. The lifetime risk of malignancy ranges between 5% and 10%. Removal of all congenital nevi should be considered. In practice, some small periocular congenital nevi are not removed.

An unusual form of congenital nevus is the so-called kissing nevi. This form of congenital nevus develops on the

Box 11-7		
Types of Nevi		
Presentation age	**Clinical characteristics**	**Type of nevus**
Birth	No nevi present	—
Birth	Nevus present	Congenital nevus
Teenaged child	Brown flat nevus	Junctional nevus
Teenaged child	Darker dome-shaped nevi	Compound nevus
Older adult	Elevated nonpigmented nevi	Intradermal nevus

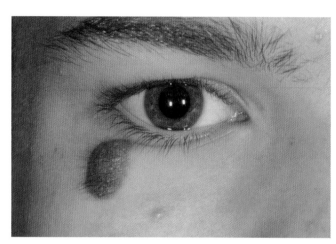

Figure 11-29 Congenital nevus. Note the coarse hairs.

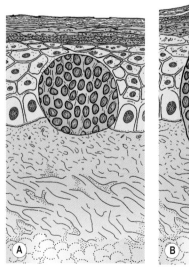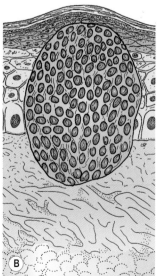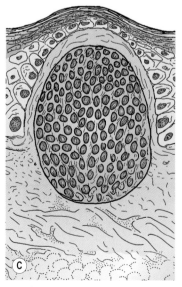

Figure 11-28 Descent of the nevi into the dermis with age. (**A**) Junctional nevus: found at the junction of the epidermis and dermis. (**B**) Compound nevus: seen extending from the epidermis into the dermis. (**C**) Intradermal nevus: found within the dermis (drawings prepared with assistance from Chris Arpey, MD, Duane Whitaker, MD, and Lynette Watkins, MD).

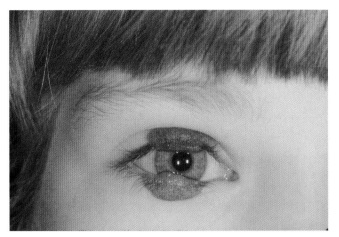

Figure 11-30 "Kissing nevi"—a form of congenital nevus.

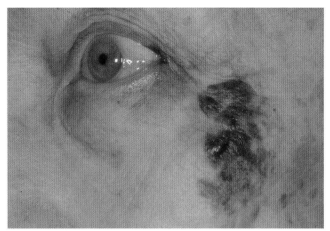

Figure 11-31 Lentigo maligna and lentigo maligna melanoma. Malignant transformation of lentigo maligna to lentigo maligna melanoma. Note that the dark raised areas have turned into a malignancy.

eyelids while they are fused in utero. The lesion is seen as nevi opposite one another on the upper and lower eyelids. In general, these lesions are small and are kept under observation, rather than excised (Figure 11-30). Malignant degeneration is theoretically possible, but rare.

Lentigines

Lentigines are acquired light brown to brown macules. These lesions are caused by an increase in the number of melanocytes in the affected area of the skin.

Lentigo simplex is a small, well-circumscribed brown macule. In contrast to freckles, lentigo simplex lesions do not darken with sun exposure. There is no clinical significance to these lesions other than identifying their benign nature. In extremely rare situations, multiple lentigo lesions around the eyes and mouth are associated with Peutz–Jeghers syndrome. This autosomal dominant condition is associated with intestinal polyps, which may become malignant.

Lentigo senilis is a benign, expanding macule associated with aging. These "age spots" or "liver spots" are light to dark brown and develop on the sun-exposed areas of the face and forearms of whites. These lesions generally do not occur until after the fifth decade of life and continue to enlarge in size up to several centimeters. Many patients have these asymptomatic spots. Lentigo senilis lesions do not have the highly irregular borders or extreme color changes associated with malignant degeneration.

Lentigo maligna (Hutchinson's melanocytic freckle or idiopathic acquired melanosis) is a premalignant acquired pigmentation of the skin, usually on the forehead or cheek (Figure 11-31). These lesions tend to have more irregular borders and more uneven pigmentation. They start in the fourth and fifth decade. In most patients, small lesions are indistinguishable from other more benign lentigines. They are observed until a change in size, color, or contour suggests biopsy. If left untreated over a variable period of time, often decades, malignant nodules may form in up to 50% of these lesions (known as lentigo maligna melanoma). When these lesions are recognized as possible lentigo maligna, biopsies should be performed and the lesions should be removed if possible. Often the histologic extent of the lentigo maligna extends well beyond the clinically apparent lesion, which makes excision somewhat difficult and the resultant defect unpredictable.

Other benign pigmented lesions

Freckles or ephelides are the familiar, well-circumscribed red–brown macules occurring on the face, shoulders, chest, and back. The onset of freckles is usually in childhood. A diagnostic feature is that exposure to sunlight darkens the freckles. You probably know of some children or adults who have very obvious freckles in the summer. Freckles result from hyperpigmentation along the basal cell layer. There is no change in the number of melanocytes present.

Remember, freckles are not growths of pigment cells (melanocytes). Freckles represent extra pigment (melanin) in areas of normal/skin cells (keratinocytes). There should be no confusion of freckles and any potential pigmented malignancy. Removal is not a practical undertaking as there are usually such a large number present. Cosmetics may cover the freckles. Use of sunscreen prevents the darkening of freckles associated with sun exposure.

Biopsy techniques

Incisional biopsy

A biopsy is called incisional if only a portion of the lesion is removed. In contrast, a biopsy is called excisional if the entire lesion is removed (Figure 11-32). Incisional biopsies are usually performed to sample a lesion for diagnosis. A typical example is a suspected basal cell carcinoma. Local anesthetic with epinephrine is injected into the lesion or tissue around the lesion. A representative portion of the lesion is removed with a scalpel blade or scissors. The tissue should be handled carefully. It is a good idea to hold the tissue in one area, rather than grasping the sample in many areas causing crush artifact. The best place to sample the tumor is at the periphery of the lesion. It is always a good idea to include some normal tissue with the edge of the lesion, as interpretation is often easier. The center of the lesion should not be sampled, especially if there is central ulceration. Histopathologic interpretation may yield only necrotic tissue. If the quality of the biopsy is not considered, adequate additional tissue should be removed. Remember, the success of the biopsy is not at the end of the procedure, but when the tissue comes back with an accurate diagnosis.

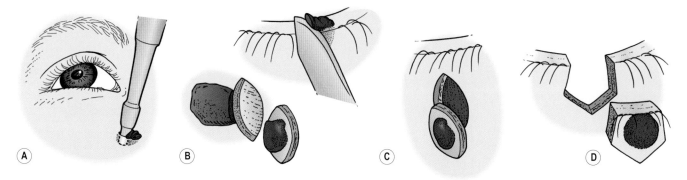

Figure 11-32 Biopsy types. (**A**) Punch biopsy. (**B**) Lid margin shave biopsy (incisional). (**C**) Incisional biopsy. (**D**) Full-thickness eyelid excisional biopsy.

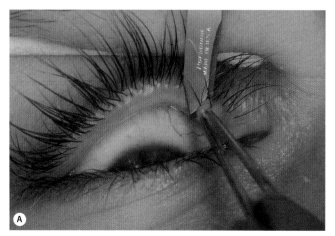

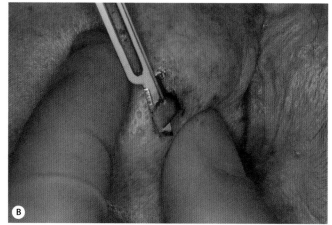

Figure 11-33 Shave biopsy techniques. (**A**) Lid margin dermal nevus. Stabilize the lid and "saw" lightly, taking care not to leave a notch. (**B**) Cheek or forehead lesions. Pinch the thick skin between your fingers and "saw" lightly. Avoid the temptation to lift the lesion with forceps as you can make a depressed scar.

Shave biopsy

Another use for incisional biopsy is to remove a portion of a benign lesion, as in a so-called shave biopsy. A nevus on the lid margin of an older patient (probably an intradermal nevus—an older, more elevated nevus without much pigment) may be disfiguring or irritating to the eye. Although the lesion extends deep into the dermis, it is easy to "shave" the lesion off flush with the lid margin (Figure 11-33, A). All of the lesion is not removed, so the biopsy is an incisional biopsy. The visible part of the lesion is gone, however. There are situations in which a shave biopsy is actually an excisional biopsy. We will discuss this later in the text.

Punch biopsy

Another useful incisional biopsy technique is the punch biopsy. This technique is most useful for diagnosis of a pigmented lesion, likely to be a melanoma. A disposable skin dermatome (like a corneal trephine) is used to "core" out a sample of the lesion (Figure 11-34). The diagnosis and the depth of the lesion can be determined with this simple technique. Remember that the thickness of a melanoma is a prognostic indicator for survival.

Excisional biopsy

An excisional biopsy is performed when you want to remove the entire lesion. We alluded to a situation above where a

lesion could be completely excised with a shave biopsy. What type of lesion could undergo a shave biopsy that would result in complete excision of the lesion or at what locations within the layers of the skin? The lesion would have to be a superficial lesion for a shave to remove the entire tumor. A good example is a seborrheic keratosis. Although these lesions sometimes look thick like they may involve the deep layers of the skin, they are superficial epithelial lesions that can be removed with a shave type of excisional biopsy (Figure 11-35).

In these patients, inject the surrounding skin with local anesthetic with epinephrine. Use a no. 15 scalpel blade to shave the lesion off. It is helpful to stabilize the skin around the lesion by stretching it tight or by pinching the lesion and the surrounding tissue (see Figure 11-33, B). I find it helpful to use a light touch on the blade and lots of sawing back and forth across the lesion. You must be careful not to shave the lesion below the level of the skin surface. Knowing what a lesion is and its depth will help to plan the best procedure to remove the lesion. This same "pinching and sawing" shave technique is applicable in the example above where we suggested a shave incisional biopsy for a nevus.

Another common situation involving an excisional biopsy is to remove a cutaneous malignancy, such as a basal cell carcinoma. In the case of a well-demarcated nodular type of basal cell carcinoma, draw a ring 3–5 mm away from the clinical margin of the tumor (Figure 11-36). Excise the tumor and the surrounding normal appearing tissue. Assess the edge of the sample for the presence of tumor cells, usually with a frozen section technique. When the surgical margins are free of malignancy, the excisional biopsy is complete. The resultant defect will usually require reconstruction for closure. In many instances, the ophthalmologist will do the excisional biopsy and the hospital pathologist will do the frozen section interpretation intraoperatively. This is a well-accepted technique, but requires a significant amount of "down time" while the frozen section results are processed and interpreted. Remember that removal of a skin malignancy without histologic confirmation of surgical margins free of tumor is not an acceptable practice.

Mohs' micrographic tumor excision technique

The Mohs' micrographic tumor excision technique or Mohs' surgery is a form of specialized excisional biopsy for skin

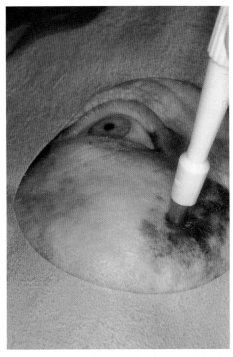

Figure 11-34 Punch biopsy of melanoma of the skin (from Warren RC, Nerad J, Carter KD: Punch biopsy techniques. *Ophth Arch Ophthal* 108(6):778–779, 1995).

malignancies. This technique is usually performed by a dermatologist who is trained in this specialty. After removal of a debulking layer, narrow margins of surrounding tissue including the sides and the base of the tumor bed are removed for frozen section analysis. A careful map of the tumor excision site is made. The interpretation of the frozen section specimen is performed by the excising surgeon. If any tumor remains, the surgeon goes back to the exact site and removes more tissue. The process is repeated with small areas of excision until all tumor tissue has been excised. The use of Mohs' excision produces the highest cure rate with the smallest amount of normal tissue removed.

An additional advantage of working with a Mohs' surgeon is that the excising and the reconstructing surgeons are different people. The job of the surgeon performing the Mohs' excision is to remove the tumor. If a reconstructive surgeon, such as you, is available to do the repair, the Mohs' surgeon has no hesitation in performing one more excision that might make the defect more difficult to reconstruct. You and I might subconsciously hesitate if we are performing both excision and reconstructive surgery.

Mohs' surgery is especially useful around the eyelids, where small amounts of tissue excision may involve important anatomic structures and affect normal function of the lids. This technique is also valuable for removing squamous cell carcinomas or recurrent or morpheaform basal cell carcinomas in which clinical margins may not accurately predict the histologic extent of the tumor. The Mohs' excision technique is not as useful for sebaceous cell carcinomas because frozen section analysis of conjunctiva may not accurately confirm the pagetoid spread commonly seen. Similarly, Mohs' surgery is not ideally suited for melanoma because of problems with interpretation of pigmented lesions using frozen section testing.

Cyst excision and marsupialization

Cysts, especially apocrine hidrocystomas, are very common on the lid. You remember that apocrine hidrocystomas are those cysts, sometimes with a bluish tinge, that arise from the apocrine sweat glands associated with the lashes, the glands of Moll. There are two options for cyst removal: excision or marsupialization (Figure 11-37). Excision requires removal of the cyst with its epithelium intact. Closure of the skin follows. Excision is difficult to perform

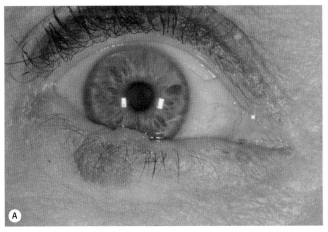
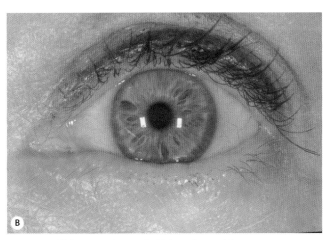

Figure 11-35 Shave biopsy—excision of seborrheic keratosis. (**A**) Preoperative appearance. (**B**) Postoperative result, 10 days after excision.

because the cyst wall often breaks with attempted dissection. If parts of the cyst wall are left behind and the skin is closed, a recurrence of the cyst is possible. An easier technique is to marsupialize the cyst. The top is cut off the cyst and the contents drain spontaneously. No attempt is made to close.

The lining of the cyst returns to normal epithelium within 1 or 2 weeks. This same technique is applicable for all types of cysts, including epidermal inclusion cysts and eccrine hidrocystomas. Marsupialization of cysts is a safe and effective way to remove both small and large cysts.

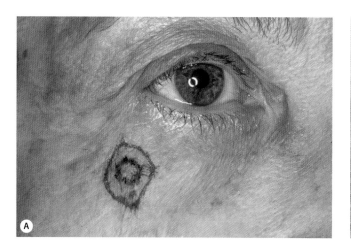

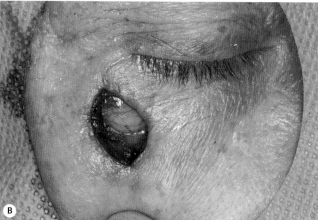

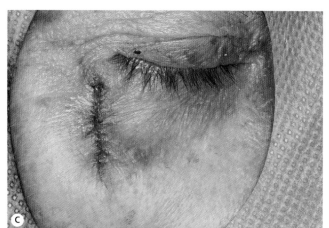

Figure 11-36 Excisional biopsy of a small nodular basal cell carcinoma. (**A**) Mark the clinical margins of the nodule. Draw a ring 3–4 mm peripheral to the lesion. (**B**) The tissue is excised and sent for analysis of the margins. (**C**) Close the wound, leaving a vertical scar to minimize tension on the lower eyelid.

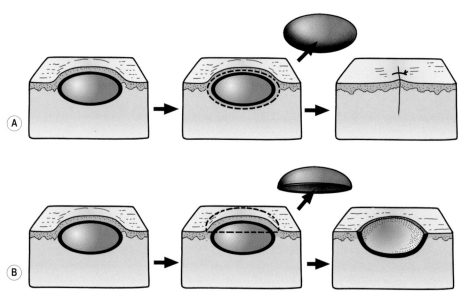

Figure 11-37 Options for surgical treatment of cysts. (**A**) Cyst excision removing all epithelium. (**B**) Cyst marsupialization leaving epithelium at the base of the lesion.

Major points

Remember the basic skin anatomy:

- Layers: epidermis and dermis
- Adnexae: hair, oil glands, and sweat glands
- Pigment cells

Most skin cancers are from the epidermis: basal cell and squamous cell carcinoma.

Most adnexal lesions are benign. The only adnexal malignancy to worry about is sebaceous cell carcinoma. It is rare.

The presentation of a sebaceous cell carcinoma can be:

- Eyelid mass involving the eyelid margin and extending to the posterior lamella
- Thickened eyelid (often with yellow color)
- Chronic unilateral blepharoconjunctivitis
- A recurrent chalazion is the "textbook" presentation, but it occurs rarely in my experience

Remember not to lose sight of "the forest for the trees." There are so many lesions, it is easy to lose track of what you are trying to do for your patient. The main goal in diagnosing lid lesions is to rule out malignancy. The most common malignancy is basal cell carcinoma. Malignant lesions typically grow in an "uncontrolled manner." The characteristics of malignancy include:

- Ulceration
- Induration
- Irregularity
- Lack of tenderness
- Loss of lid margin architecture
- Telangiectasia
- Pearly borders

When a malignancy is suspected, an incisional biopsy should be performed.

Melanoma of the eyelids is rare. Do an incisional biopsy of a pigmented lesion using these guidelines:

- Recent onset of a pigmented mass
- Change in color, shape, or size
- Irregular margins
- Asymmetric shape
- Multiple shades or colors: "red, white, and blue sign"
- Large lesions: >6 mm

When you have ruled out malignancy by the clinical examination or biopsy, you have done the most important job for your patient. The diagnosis of the common benign lesions is usually by sight or pattern recognition (Aunt Minnies). After you have seen them and get to know them, you will always recognize them.

Benign epidermal skin lesions include:

- Acrochordon: skin tag
- Seborrheic keratosis
- Cutaneous horn

Learn to recognize sun-damaged skin. If sun damage is present, your patient is at risk for basal cell and squamous cell carcinomas. Actinic damage causes stiff, translucent skin, with deep furrows and visible dermal vessels. Pigmentary irregularities (dyschromias) are common.

In sun-damaged skin, you may recognize the scaly plaque of actinic keratosis as a premalignant form of squamous cell carcinoma.

You already know the most common of the benign adnexal lesions:

- "Styes" and chalazia (from sebaceous glands)
- Epidermal inclusion cyst
- Milia
- Sebaceous hyperplasia: you have seen this yellowish lesion on the forehead, but probably didn't know the name
- Apocrine hidrocystomas: cysts from the sweat glands, glands of Moll

You won't miss a melanoma using the guidelines for biopsy above. Recall that:

- Periocular melanomas are rare
- Pigmented lesions are common
- Any skin lesion may be pigmented
- Not all pigmented skin lesions are nevi

You will be able to easily recognize nevi by the age of the nevus.

- Teenaged nevus: flat and pigmented (junctional nevus)
- Middle-aged nevus: raised, pigmented (compound nevus)
- Elderly nevus: raised, no pigment (intradermal nevus)

A variety of useful biopsy techniques are easily learned. The shave biopsy and punch biopsy are two examples. A portion of the tumor is removed with an incisional biopsy. Complete removal of skin lesions is carried out with an excisional biopsy.

Using the principles outlined in this chapter, you should be able to recognize the majority of malignant lesions that you will see. Gain confidence that you will recognize the malignant lesions. Perform a biopsy if you are unsure. Don't get bogged down in all the details the first time through this chapter. There are too many lesions to learn them all at once. Learn the characteristics of malignant lesions first. Develop an understanding of the layers of the skin and the adnexal anatomy next. Finally, aim to learn all the names of the benign lesions. You will be impressed by how much of this information will be useful to you every day when seeing patients.

Suggested reading

1. American Academy of Ophthalmology: Basic and clinical science course: orbit, eyelids, and lacrimal system, sect. 7, pp. 167–187, San Francisco: American Academy of Ophthalmology, 1998/1999.

2. Conlon MR, Leatherbarrow B, Nerad JA: Benign eyelid tumors. In Bosniak S, ed., *Principles and practice of ophthalmic plastic and reconstructive surgery*, ch. 31, pp. 323–341, Philadelphia: WB Saunders, 1996.

3. Doxanas MT: Malignant epithelial eyelid tumors. In Bosniak S, ed., *Principles and practice of ophthalmic plastic and reconstructive surgery*, ch. 32, pp. 342–351, Philadelphia: WB Saunders, 1996.

4. Doxanas MT, Green WR: Sebaceous gland carcinoma: review of 40 cases. *Arch Ophthalmol* 102:245–249, 1984.

5. Doxanas MT, Iliff WJ, Iliff NT, Green WR: Squamous cell carcinoma of the eyelids. *Ophthalmology* 94:538–544, 1987.

6. Grossniklaus H, McLean IW: Cutaneous melanoma of the eyelid. *Ophthalmology* 98:1867–1873, 1991.

7. Howard GR, Nerad JA, Carter KD, Whitaker DC: Clinical characteristics associated with orbital invasion of cutaneous basal cell and squamous cell tumors of the eyelid. *Am J Ophthalmol* 113:123–133, 1992.

8. McCord CD, ed.: Management of eyelid neoplastic disease. In *Eyelid surgery: principles and techniques*, ch. 25, pp. 312–329, Philadelphia: Lippincott-Raven, 1995.

9. Mohs FE: Chemosurgery for skin cancer. *Arch Dermatol* 112:211–215, 1976.

10. Nerad JA, Whitaker DC: Periocular basal cell carcinoma in adults 35 years of age and younger. *Am J Ophthalmol* 106:723–729, 1988.

11. Sacks EH, Lisman RD: Diagnosis and management of sebaceous gland carcinoma. In Bosniak S, ed., *Principles and practice of ophthalmic plastic and reconstructive surgery*, ch. 13, pp. 190–195, Philadelphia: WB Saunders, 1996.

12. Stefanyszyn MA, Silbert DI: Malignant eyelid and orbital tumors. In Bosniak S, ed., *Principles and practice of ophthalmic plastic and reconstructive surgery*, ch. 29, pp. 300–306, Philadelphia: WB Saunders, 1996.

13. Tanenbaum M, Grove AS, McCord CD: Eyelid tumors: diagnosis and management. In McCord CD, Tanenbaum M, Nunery WR, eds, *Oculoplastic surgery*, 3rd edn, ch. 6, pp. 145–174, New York: Raven Press, 1995.

CHAPTER 12

Eyelid Reconstruction

Chapter contents

Introduction

If your incisional biopsy of a cutaneous tumor shows malignancy, the next step is excision with documentation of tumor-free surgical margins. Reconstruction follows tumor excision. Unusual malignant eyelid tumors may be controlled with cryotherapy or radiation treatments.

Reconstruction is based upon the surgical principles that you are already familiar with. These principles are covered in the section "Repair of Soft Tissue Trauma," in Chapter 13. The goal of the reconstruction is to restore the normal anatomy and function. You will be impressed by how quickly you can learn successful eyelid reconstruction techniques.

We will begin this chapter with a review of the eyelid and periocular anatomy that is especially important for understanding the concepts involved with lid reconstruction. Use these fundamentals of eyelid anatomy to describe the postoperative excision defect and to plan the reconstruction.

Your choice of reconstructive technique depends on what portions of the eyelid are missing. Smaller anterior lamellar defects can be closed primarily or with some undermining. Larger defects will require a myocutaneous advancement flap or free skin graft. Skin grafts are usually full-thickness grafts to avoid shrinkage. Very large defects away from the lid margin occasionally require repair with a split-thickness graft. The preferred technique for repair of larger anterior lamellar defects is to use a myocutaneous advancement flap. These advancement flaps have several advantages over free skin grafts. We will describe the basic techniques for skin grafting and forming myocutaneous advancement flaps in this chapter.

Full-thickness eyelid defects of up to 25% of the eyelid margin can be repaired by pulling the eyelid margins together and suturing them using a primary eyelid margin repair technique. This is the same technique that you will use to repair many traumatic lacerations of the eyelid margin. Small lid margin defects involving the lateral canthus are repaired using a simple lateral canthoplasty technique such as the lateral tarsal strip operation. Medial canthal defects are more difficult to repair because of the presence of the lacrimal drainage system.

If you find that pulling the edges of the eyelid wounds together creates a great deal of tension, you will need to perform canthotomy and cantholysis to allow the lateral portion of the lid to slide over. Larger full-thickness lid defects require special techniques for closure. Using the

Tenzel flap or Hughes procedure, you will be able to repair lid margin defects of between 50% and 100% of the lower eyelid. If you are interested in having an active practice in skin cancer removal and eyelid reconstruction, you should learn all of the techniques that we have discussed thus far. With some experience, you will learn to modify these procedures and use them in combination. More advanced procedures such as the Mustarde cheek rotation and median forehead flap are used to cover large anterior lamellar defects.

Small upper eyelid defects can be closed using the same principles as those for lower eyelid reconstruction. When more than 50% of the upper lid is missing, the Cutler Beard procedure is necessary. This operation borrows tissue from the lower lid to recreate the upper lid. This procedure is complicated, and you won't want to use it until you can confidently perform the basic procedures.

In this chapter, I will describe the operations that an interested and well-trained ophthalmologist should use in repairing eyelid defects with enough detail that you can perform them. I will describe the more advanced procedures with less detail, but enough that you can learn the concepts.

Fundamentals of eyelid anatomy

Eyelid margin

The eyelid margin is an anatomic structure that we take for granted until we have to repair it. To repair a lid margin defect, you must know the eyelid margin architecture. We have discussed this in detail, but refer to Figure 12-1 to refresh your memory. Recall that the eyelid margin is a flat

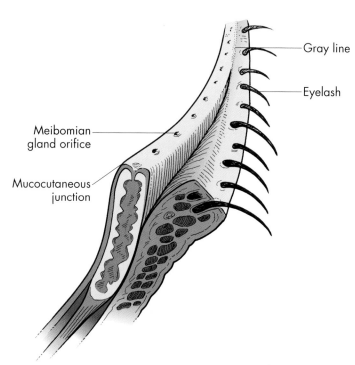

Figure 12-1 The eyelid margin architecture. Landmarks are the mucocutaneous junction, the meibomian gland orifices, the gray line, and the eyelashes. Note that the lid margin can be split into anterior and posterior lamellae, a concept helpful for lid reconstruction.

platform with nearly right angles at the anterior and posterior edges of the eyelid. From posterior to anterior, the anatomic structures that you should know are:

- The mucocutaneous junction
- The meibomian gland orifices
- The gray line
- The eyelash follicles

Precise alignment of the lid margin structures is necessary to repair eyelid margin defects. Tension-bearing sutures should be placed in the tarsal plate. Precise alignment of the lid margin using everting vertical mattress sutures is required to prevent a postoperative lid notch.

Anterior and posterior lamellae

You will recall that the anterior lamella of the eyelid consists of the skin and muscle. The posterior lamella of the eyelid consists of the conjunctiva and tarsal plate. Start to think of eyelid defects in terms of these anatomic building blocks.

In many patients, you can repair posterior lamellar defects by pulling the tarsal plate together as described above. For larger defects, you will need a graft to replace the tarsal plate. The best replacement for missing tarsus is other tarsal tissue either as a free tarsal graft from the contralateral upper lid or as part of a vascularized tarsoconjunctival flap from the upper lid on the same side (as you will see in the Hughes procedure for reconstruction of large lower lid defects). Other substitutes for the tarsal plate are the hard palate mucosa and, rarely, nasal cartilage.

Anterior lamellar defects are repaired with free skin grafts or myocutaneous advancement flaps. You cannot place an anterior lamellar free graft on a posterior lamellar free graft. There must be a vascular bed covering one surface of a graft. You can use a free tarsal graft for posterior lamella covered with a myocutaneous flap for anterior lamella. You can use the reverse, a free skin graft for anterior lamella over a tarsoconjunctival flap for the posterior lamella. Remember, don't use a free graft on a free graft.

Lateral canthus

The lateral canthus is relatively simple anatomically. The upper and lower crus of the lateral canthal tendon extend from each tarsal plate to form the lateral canthal tendon. The lateral canthal tendon inserts at Whitnall's tubercle on the inner aspect of the lateral orbital rim approximately 10 mm below the frontozygomatic suture (Figure 12-2). Although the lateral portion of the eyelid is attached to the rim mainly by the lateral canthal tendon, contributions from the orbicularis, orbital septum, levator aponeurosis, and lower lid retractors provide additional support for the eyelids.

Think of the lateral canthal tendon as a Y. A cantholysis converts the Y of the lateral canthal tendon into a V. To release the lateral aspect of the lid, you must cut the respective crus of the lateral canthal tendon. Think of this as now cutting one leg of the V off the orbital rim (see Figure 13-15). Often you must make some additional cuts when performing the cantholysis to mobilize the lid. These cuts release the septum, orbicularis, and lower lid retractors, the other contributions to the lateral canthus that we just mentioned. You learned to do this when you performed a lateral tarsal strip procedure.

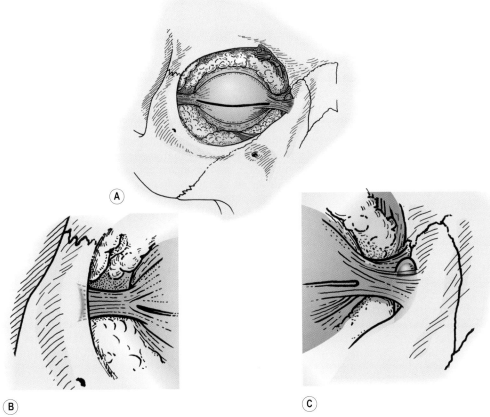

Figure 12-2 (**A**) Canthal tendons. (**B**) The lateral canthal tendon attaches on the inner surface of the lateral rim. (**C**) The medial canthal tendon surrounds the lacrimal sac.

Reconstructing a lateral canthus is simple, anatomically. Remember to reattach the reconstructed tissues on the inside of the lateral orbital rim so that the eyelid margin rests against the curve of the eye. Usually you can reattach the lateral canthus to the periosteum of the bone. If there is no periosteum present, you may have to make small drill holes in the lateral orbital rim to attach the lid.

Medial canthus

The medial canthal tendon is anatomically more complex than the lateral canthal tendon. The anterior and posterior limbs of the medial canthal tendon surround the lacrimal sac (see Figure 12-2). The anterior limb of the medial canthal tendon attaches to the frontal process of the maxilla. The posterior limb of the medial canthal tendon attaches on the posterior lacrimal crest. A tough layer of tissue known as the lacrimal fascia surrounds the sac, fusing with the periosteum of the orbital rim and periorbita of the orbital walls. Disinsertion of the anterior limb of the medial canthal tendon will not change the position of the lower eyelid. An intact posterior limb of the medial canthal tendon will support the canthus and is required to pull the medial aspect of the eyelid posteriorly to follow the curve of the eye.

Attempts to reform the posterior limb of the medial canthal tendon are complicated by the lacrimal sac and canaliculus. If the lacrimal drainage apparatus is intact, it is difficult to provide a posterior point of attachment for a new medial canthus. If the canaliculus has been excised, you can recreate the pull of the posterior limb of the medial canthal tendon using permanent sutures to attach the medial end of any remaining lid to the posterior lacrimal crest.

Description of the postexcision defect

Learn to use these fundamentals of eyelid anatomy to describe the postexcision defect. Consider these examples:

- Full-thickness defect of the central 25% of the lower eyelid
- Full-thickness defect of the lower eyelid involving the lateral 50% of the eyelid, including the lateral canthal tendon
- Anterior lamellar defect over the inferior orbital rim measuring 1 cm by 1.5 cm
- Full-thickness defect of the upper eyelid involving the medial one third of the lid, including the punctum and canaliculus

Each description should bring to mind a picture of the anatomic structures involved and, eventually, the steps you will need to take to reconstruct the eyelid.

Treatment of malignant cutaneous tumors

Biopsy techniques

If you suspect an eyelid malignancy, you already know to perform an incisional biopsy to confirm your diagnosis. The techniques of incisional biopsy were discussed in Chapter 11.

Tumor excision

Frozen section control

The majority of eyelid malignancies are treated by excisional biopsy. All surgical margins should be confirmed histologically to be free of tumor. Frozen section analysis of the margins is usually done before reconstruction. Alternatively, analysis of permanent sections for tumor-free surgical margins may be performed after reconstruction. However, if a margin is found to contain tumor, the reconstruction must be taken down and the excision repeated until tumor-free margins are obtained.

Ideally, your first several excisions for cutaneous malignancies should be performed on well-demarcated small nodular basal cell carcinomas. Outline the area of clinical involvement with the surgical marker. Draw a second ring around the tumor, marking an additional 3 mm of clinically uninvolved skin to be removed. Excise the tumor using the most peripheral marking. Orient the tissue for the pathologist with a suture. If frozen sections show residual tumor, re-excise the area of involvement. When the surgical margins are tumor free, you can reconstruct the eyelid. Often, surgeons will begin reconstruction while the frozen sections are being processed and analyzed. If you need a refresher on the excision technique, refer back to Figure 11-36.

As you gain experience, you may choose to excise larger nodular basal cell carcinomas. As your ability to perform larger, more complicated reconstructions improves, you can excise morpheaform basal cell carcinomas or squamous cell carcinomas (Figure 12-3). Remember that the margins of these more aggressive tumors are indistinct. The postexcision defect can be large in many patients.

Mohs' surgery

If you plan to treat a large number of cutaneous malignancies, you should develop a good working relationship with a surgeon trained in Mohs' excision. Mohs' excision of cutaneous malignancies provides a high cure rate with the minimum amount of excision of normal tissue along with the tumor. The Mohs' surgeon, usually a dermatologist, performs both the excision and the microscopic interpretation of the tissue. The expertise of a Mohs' surgeon can benefit you and your patient. The Mohs' surgeon will return the

patient to you with the malignancy excised, ready for your reconstruction. Mohs' surgery is especially useful for large nodular basal cell carcinomas, morpheaform basal cell carcinomas, squamous cell carcinomas, and any recurrent tumor. The role of Mohs' excision in the treatment of sebaceous cell carcinoma and cutaneous melanoma is controversial because the surgical margins of these tumor excisions are difficult to interpret using frozen section analysis.

Radiotherapy

Radiotherapy has been used extensively in Canada for the treatment of periocular malignancies. The cure rate is said to be high. Skin malignancies are relatively radioresistant so high doses of radiation therapy are required. An obvious advantage is that no reconstruction is required. Disadvantages include no histologic confirmation of complete tumor removal and the side-effects related to radiotherapy. In the United States, the majority of cutaneous malignancies are surgically excised. Radiotherapy is reserved for large recurrent tumors and is often considered palliative in these patients.

Cryotherapy

Cryotherapy, using liquid nitrogen, is used for precancerous actinic keratoses. Small nodular basal cell carcinomas away from the eyelids can also be treated with liquid nitrogen. Long-term follow-up is required to ensure that there is no recurrence.

Checkpoint

At this point, you should know the fundamentals of eyelid anatomy that will guide your reconstruction. As you read the text, try to visualize the defects that are discussed and describe them anatomically.

We have briefly discussed the steps of incisional biopsy and tumor excision with frozen section-controlled margins or Mohs' surgery, and you are ready to learn lid reconstruction techniques.

Anterior lamellar defects

Options for repair

We have used the terms anterior and posterior lamella to describe the layers of the eyelid near the lid margin. In this chapter, we will use the term anterior lamella to also describe skin and muscle defects peripheral to the tarsal plates where no true posterior lamella exists. There are several options for repair of skin and muscle defects in the periocular area:

- Healing by granulation
- Primary closure
- Primary closure with undermining
- Free skin graft
- Myocutaneous advancement flap

We will talk about the advantages and disadvantages of each technique. For many defects, more than one technique may work. You will learn to choose the best technique for the particular defect. Small lesions away from important land-

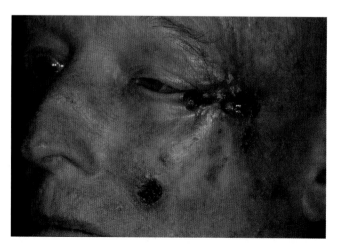

Figure 12-3 Indistinct margins of recurrent squamous cell carcinoma in an elderly man. You can imagine that a postexcision defect will be large.

marks will heal by granulation over time. Although successful in some patients, the healing may take weeks to months. Scar contracture can result in distortion of anatomic landmarks. Primary closure with or without undermining is generally a better option. Myocutaneous advancement flaps are the best choice for larger anterior lamellar defects. Free skin grafts give the least acceptable result, but allow you to cover any size anterior lamellar defect. If you cannot perform a more aesthetically acceptable procedure, you can always use a skin graft, so it is important to learn the technique.

Primary closure

Primary closure can be performed if redundant skin exists adjacent to the defect. Areas of the face that typically have redundant skin include the glabella, the upper lid skin fold, and the temple. There is normally little redundant skin in the lower eyelid or medial canthus. You will also learn to appreciate how the amount of redundant tissue varies from one patient to the next. The patient with wrinkled and sagging skin has plenty of redundancy to help you close small defects. In the patient with sun-damaged, tight skin with no wrinkles despite advancing age, more than primary closure will be required for all but the smallest defects (Figure 12-4).

Primary closure with undermining

Primary closure with undermining is commonly used to close lesions away from the eyelid margin. You must know the level to undermine to mobilize tissue, preserve blood supply, and avoid nerve damage (Box 12-1). Within the orbital rims, any tissue undermining should be done in the preseptal plane. Outside the orbital rims, undermining should be done in the subcutaneous tissue plane. Be especially careful when undermining any tissue in the path of the seventh nerve extending from the tragus of the ear to the tail of the eyebrow. The facial nerve is superficial as it crosses over the zygomatic arch. When closing areas in the forehead or scalp, you should undermine deep to the frontalis muscle in the loose areolar tissue superficial to the periosteum. You will find that extensive undermining is usually necessary to mobilize skin in the scalp or forehead (Figure 12-5).

When closing a wound, always orient the closure to minimize tissue distortion and maximize scar camouflage. Closing a forehead wound parallel to the forehead furrows creates less tissue distortion and a better scar than a vertical closure can provide. Depending on the size of the defect, the eyebrow may be elevated. Remember that tissue is most easily mobilized in a direction 90 degrees from the natural skin creases.

When reconstructing the lower lid, minimize any vertical traction on the eyelid by closing wounds to leave a vertical scar. Although the vertical scar does not blend in with the natural skin creases, this technique will avoid ectropion or lid retraction (Figure 12-6).

Do enough undermining to minimize tension on the skin closure. Use deep anchoring sutures to the underlying periosteum to support the deep tissues and take tension off the subcutaneous and skin closure. Common places to use anchoring sutures are at the periosteum along the inferior and lateral orbital rim. When using anchoring sutures to prevent lower eyelid retraction or ectropion, place the sutures superiorly to overcorrect the lower eyelid or canthal height.

When the tension is off the edges of the wound, use an interrupted deep layer closure with an absorbable suture such as 3-0 PDS in the scalp, 4-0 PDS in the cheek, and 5-0 PDS in the orbicularis muscle. Perform a routine skin closure with slight eversion of the wound edges. Interrupted sutures provide the best wound alignment and eversion. Running sutures can be used when you anticipate that the scar will fall within a natural skin crease.

Free skin grafts

Free skin grafts are harvested from a donor site and transferred to fill an anterior lamellar defect. The vascular supply to the free graft must be provided by the recipient site for the graft to "take" or survive. You will use full-thickness skin grafts routinely in reconstructive eyelid surgery.

Full-thickness skin graft

The term full-thickness skin graft (FTSG) means that an entire thickness of the epidermis and dermis has been removed for transfer. The floor of the donor site is usually subcutaneous fat. The donor site must be closed surgically, which limits the size of the graft available for transfer. All the skin appendages are contained within the donor skin, so

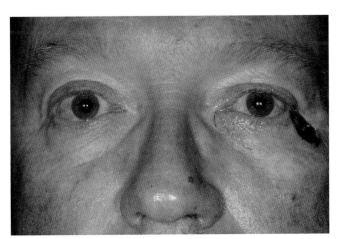

Figure 12-4 Middle-aged man, an outdoor worker, with sun-damaged tight skin. Despite the small size of the defect, extensive undermining was required to pull the stiff, inelastic skin closed.

Box 12-1

Tissue Planes for Reconstruction

When doing any soft tissue surgery think in terms of tissue planes:

- Know the tissue planes well
- What plane do you need to be in?
- What plane are you in?

Common tissue planes to work in are:

- Eyelids: preseptal plane
- Cheek skin: subcutaneous plane
- Forehead: subcutaneous plane, subgaleal plane (posterior to the frontalis muscle)

Avoid danger areas for the facial nerve:

- Over the zygomatic arch
- Greater than 1 cm lateral to the brow

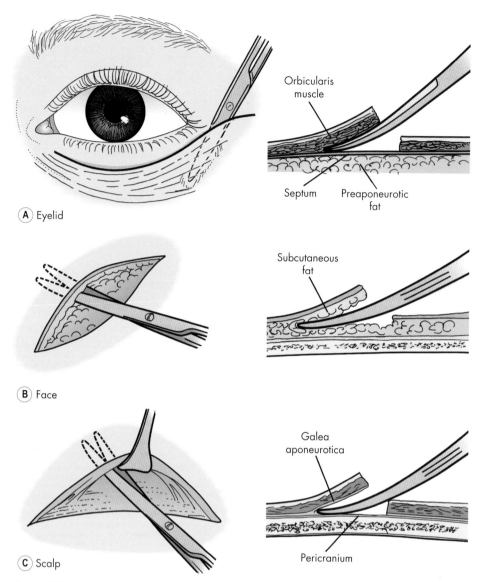

(A) Eyelid

Orbicularis muscle

Septum   Preaponeurotic fat

(B) Face

Subcutaneous fat

(C) Scalp

Galea aponeurotica

Pericranium

Figure 12-5 Dissect in the appropriate tissue plane for developing facial flaps. (**A**) Eyelid—under the orbicularis muscle (preseptal plane). (**B**) Cheek—within the subcutaneous tissue. (**C**) Forehead and scalp—in the loose areolar tissue plane anterior to the periosteum and posterior to the galea or frontalis. For large defects, relaxing incisions may be required in the galea.

you should choose a hairless donor site for obtaining the graft. FTSGs heal with less shrinkage than split-thickness skin grafts, making the full-thickness technique better suited for eyelid reconstruction where shrinkage can cause ectropion, lid retraction, or lagophthalmos.

Donor sites include (Figure 12-7):

- Upper eyelid skin
- Retroauricular skin
- Preauricular skin
- Supraclavicular or upper inner arm skin

When possible, donor skin of the same color, texture, and thickness should be picked for transfer. Upper eyelid skin is the best choice for reconstructing eyelid defects. From a practical point of view, this skin is seldom used for fear of creating upper eyelid skin fold asymmetry or lagophthalmos. When the situation permits, grafts can be taken from both upper eyelids to obtain sufficient skin and maintain symmetry. The results of full-thickness skin grafting with upper eyelid skin are good (refer back to Figure 3-11).

The traditional donor site is retroauricular skin. However, it is difficult to work behind the ear and somewhat uncomfortable for patients postoperatively. Preauricular skin is similar to retroauricular skin in character and is much easier to harvest. Slightly less skin is available, but the 15 mm by 40 mm area from the preauricular site is well suited in size and shape for most eyelid grafting. We discussed the technique of preauricular skin grafting in Chapter 3, so I'll review it only briefly here.

Inject local anesthetic containing epinephrine into the preauricular area. Transfer a template of the defect to the preauricular region. Outline the template on the skin. Incise the skin with a blade or Colorado needle, and create a plane of dissection between the subcutaneous fat and the skin. After removing the skin graft, trim any fat off the graft before suturing it into the defect. Use a running suture to sew the graft into place. Sew a bolster over the graft, and patch the eye for 1 week. Close the preauricular site with subcutaneous interrupted 4-0 PDS sutures and a cutaneous 5-0 Prolene running suture.

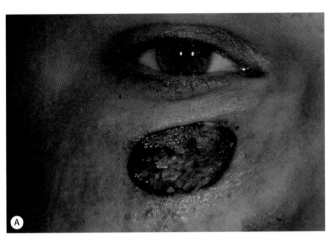

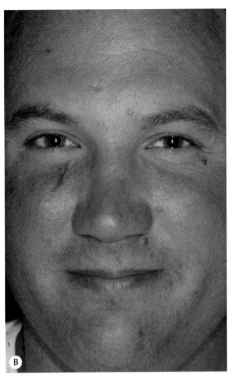

Figure 12-6 Plan the reconstruction to minimize horizontal tension on the lower eyelid to prevent lower lid ectropion or retraction. (**A**) Defect after excision of basal cell carcinoma in a young patient with no redundant tissue. (**B**) Undermining laterally and medially allowed closure without creating vertical tension, avoiding lid retraction or ectropion.

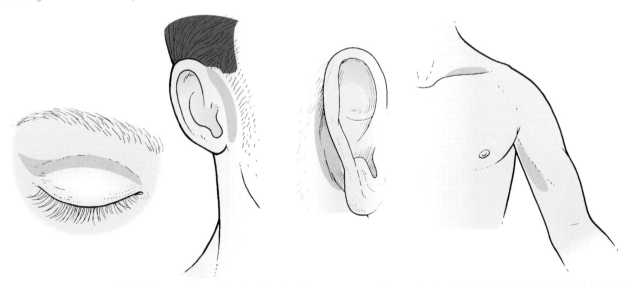

Figure 12-7 Donor sites for full-thickness skin grafting. In order of preference: upper eyelid, preauricular, retroauricular, supraclavicular, and upper arm.

Graft survival is usually high when the FTSG is placed on a healthy bed of tissue. The graft will often look dark at 1 week. Normal color and texture will return several weeks postoperatively. A small amount of shrinkage of the graft is expected (Figure 12-8). FTSGs do not take well on bare bone.

Split-thickness skin graft

You should know about split-thickness skin grafts, although you will seldom use them in eyelid reconstruction. A split-thickness skin graft (STSG) is harvested by leaving the deep layer of the dermis intact. The normal donor site is the thigh. Typically, a power dermatome is set to harvest a layer of skin between 0.012 and 0.020 inch thick from the thigh. The donor site will epithelialize spontaneously over a few weeks. Because the skin appendages are left in the donor site, you can harvest a STSG from hair-bearing skin.

The main advantage of a STSG is that a large area of skin may be harvested because no skin closure is required. Split-thickness skin will usually survive on bare bone, especially if the cortical bone is burred to create some bleeding. The donor skin is thin, and considerable shrinkage is always seen (Figure 12-9). The color, texture, and thickness are often a poor match for eyelid skin. As you might guess from this description, STSGs are used only if the defect is too large for a FTSG and there is no myocutaneous flap that is practical for closure.

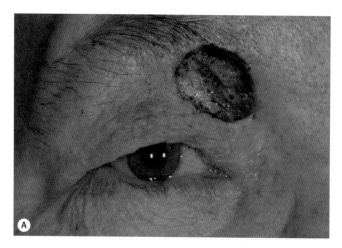

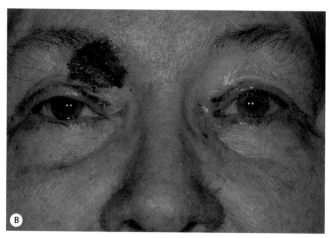

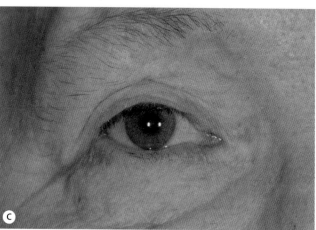

Figure 12-8 Full-thickness skin graft for repair of an anterior lamellar defect of the upper eyelid and brow. (**A**) Defect after excision of a basal cell carcinoma. (**B**) Full-thickness skin graft in place. Dark color is often present and does not suggest poor survival. Note that the full-thickness skin has been harvested from bilateral upper blepharoplasties. (**C**) Result 1 year postoperatively.

Myocutaneous flaps

Advancement of a myocutaneous flap is usually the best choice to repair an anterior lamellar eyelid defect. Use these flaps whenever possible. Myocutaneous flaps in the periocular area are formed of skin and orbicularis muscle that is dissected off the underlying orbital septum and stretched into position over the anterior lamellar defect. Myocutaneous flaps have many advantages over free skin grafts:

- Locally available tissue
- Good match for color and texture
- Near normal innervation
- Carries a blood supply to allow use over bare bone
- High rate of successful healing
- Excellent function

Locally available tissue means that little additional injecting, preparing, and draping are necessary to perform the surgery. Because the tissue is adjacent to the defect, the match for color and texture is good. After healing, near normal sensory and motor innervation returns to the mobilized tissue. Because the myocutaneous flap brings its own blood supply, bare bone or free grafts can be covered. Properly designed myocutaneous advancement flaps on the face rarely become infected or ischemic because the blood supply to the face is so rich. Often it is difficult to see the operative site after complete healing has occurred.

You have already been creating myocutaneous flaps as parts of other procedures. Surgical approaches to the inferior orbital rim for a transcutaneous lower blepharoplasty, fracture repair, and retractor reinsertion are all examples of myocutaneous flaps. You create an upper lid myocutaneous flap each time you perform an upper lid blepharoplasty or ptosis repair. Some specific tips will help you when creating myocutaneous flaps for reconstruction:

- Choose natural skin creases to hide the incision lines
- Know the planes to move into when you advance peripheral to the orbital rims
- Create horizontal tension rather than vertical tension on the lower eyelid
- Develop the flap so that there is little tension on the final closure
- Use anchoring sutures to reduce tension on the skin and to provide vertical support
- Always overcorrect the position of the flap
- Consider tightening the lower eyelid if you are concerned about retraction or you have shortened the anterior lamella

Most skin cancers that you will see occur on the lower eyelids. The most common incision to create a myocutaneous flap is the subciliary incision, which you can extend laterally into a laugh line. As you develop the flap, continue the dissection until there is as little tension on the wound closure as possible. It takes some experience to know how far to undermine. When in doubt, do more dissection to free up the flap. Each patient's tissues will stretch different

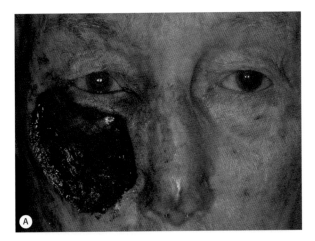

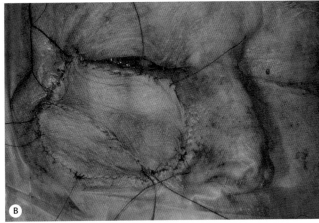

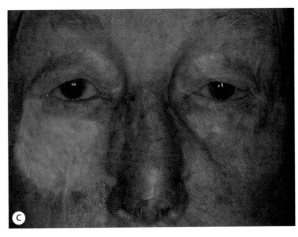

Figure 12-9 Split-thickness skin grafting. (**A**) Preoperative large anterior lamellar defect. (**B**) Split-thickness skin graft in place. (**C**) One year postoperatively, note shrinkage and poor color match of the graft. Note that the lower eyelid was tightened at the time of grafting to help prevent cicatricial lid retraction.

amounts, so there are no exact formulas for determining how far to extend the flap.

If you extend the flap beyond the orbital rims on to the cheek, stay posterior to the orbicularis muscle and enter the subcutaneous plane of the cheek. This is an important concept. Remember, when doing any soft tissue surgery, you must think in terms of tissue planes. Plan the operation based on tissue planes. Ask yourself, "What plane do I need to be in?" During the operation, ask, "What plane am I in?" Be especially careful in danger zones where damage to the facial nerve can occur. Keep your dissection superficial over the path of the facial nerve, from the tragus of the ear to the tail of the brow, especially over the zygomatic arch.

When you close a defect, construct the flap so that any tension on the lower eyelid is horizontal rather than vertical. A simple example is the 2 cm circular anterior lamellar defect in the lower eyelid shown in Figure 12-10. The defect can be closed leaving a vertical scar or a horizontal scar. Although the horizontal scar is more natural, ectropion or lid retraction can be produced. The vertically placed scar puts horizontal traction on the eyelid so the eyelid is not pulled inferiorly or away from the eye.

As you develop the flap, stop and pull the tissue into place to see if you have dissected enough to take the tension off the skin closure. When in doubt, dissect further. After you have freed up enough tissue, place one or more anchoring sutures from the undersurface of the flap to the periosteum at the orbital rims to support the flap position and reduce the tension on the skin closure. Another good place to

anchor is just posterior to the lateral orbital rim in the temporalis fascia. It is always wise to overcorrect the vertical height of the flap at the lateral canthus and along the lower lid margin. As the wound heals, some contracture will occur. Overcorrection by a small, but noticeable amount will prevent lid retraction and lateral canthal dystopia.

You may want to tighten the lower lid when you close the anterior lamella under horizontal tension. Sometimes the posterior lamella will be too "lax" for the tight anterior lamella. In extreme cases, the posterior lamella will bunch up posterior to the tight anterior lamella (the flap). If you think that this will be a problem, do a lateral tarsal strip operation at the time of anterior lamellar closure. I often tighten the lower eyelid with lid reconstruction "low threshold." As you recall, a tight lower eyelid is a stable eyelid. It is less likely to become ectropic or retracted.

As you get experience, you may be able to "bend" the rules a bit. If the defect is small enough, you may be able to close it vertically, leaving a horizontal scar. To do this, you must create redundant tissue in a vertical orientation by undermining the cheek in the subcutaneous plane and lifting the tissue vertically. You will need to use anchoring sutures to prevent the eyelid from being pulled down (Figure 12-11). Place deep 4-0 PDS sutures from the cheek subcutaneous tissues to the lower rim of the periosteum to support the cheek, preventing any traction on the lower eyelid. You may want to put deep sutures from the flap to the lateral canthal periosteum or temporalis fascia. Remember to overcorrect the height of the flap. This technique of undermining and

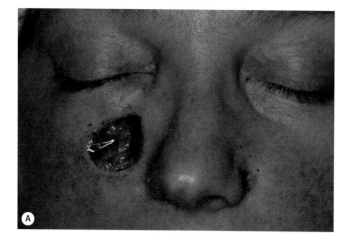

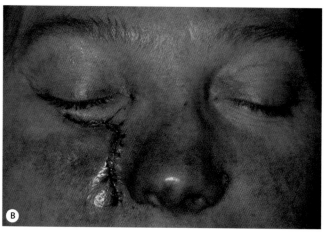

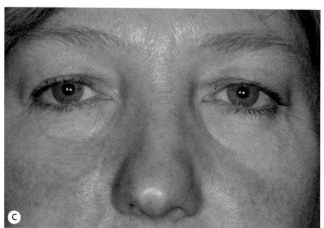

Figure 12-10 Reconstruction to avoid lower eyelid retraction. (**A**) Cheek defect after excision of basal cell carcinoma. (**B**) Flap constructed to avoid vertical tension on lower eyelid. (**C**) Postoperative result 6 months after reconstruction.

anchoring of the soft tissues is a functional midface lift. Although this technique is worthwhile to learn, it is more advanced and will require some technical experience and judgment for you to be able to decide which patients will benefit from it.

Checkpoint

At this point, we have covered the options for anterior lamellar repair. You should always consider primary closure with or without undermining before you try the other options. These options are a free skin graft and a myocutaneous advancement flap.

- What is the difference between full-thickness and split-thickness skin grafts? Which is more suitable for eyelid reconstruction? Which shrinks less? Name three possible donor sites for FTSG.
- Which is the first choice for anterior lamella repair: FTSG or myocutaneous advancement flaps?
- Name three advantages of a myocutaneous advancement flap over an FTSG.
- What is the dissection plane for:
  - Eyelids
  - Cheek
  - Forehead

Repair of full-thickness eyelid defects up to 25%

Primary eyelid margin repair

We will begin our discussion of the repair of full-thickness lid lesions. The primary eyelid margin repair technique is essential for you to learn if you plan to reconstruct any eyelids after tumor excision or trauma. Although many texts, including this one, describe full-thickness eyelid repair techniques by the percentage of eyelid margin removed, you should learn to use all these techniques as a continuum of treatments. In a particular patient, a 33% defect of the lid margin can be closed primarily. In another patient, a 25% defect of the lid margin will require a canthotomy and cantholysis. In the operating room, try to pull the defect together and choose the simplest operation that will close the wound. Follow these guidelines for lower or upper eyelid margin repair:

- Attempt primary closure—if the closure is under too much tension or the lower lid retracts inferiorly under the globe
- Do a canthotomy and cantholysis—if there is still too much tension
- Perform a Tenzel flap procedure, advancing tissue from the temple to form a new lid margin
- If the defect involves most of the lower eyelid, you should start with a Hughes flap procedure

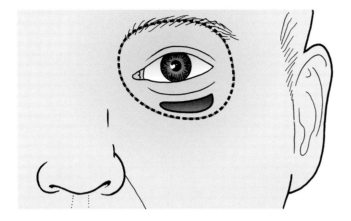

(A)

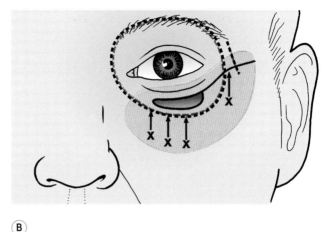

(B)

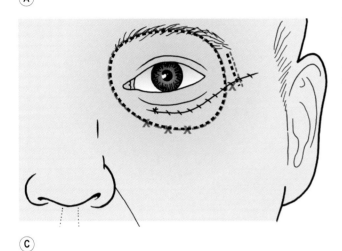

(C)

Figure 12-11 Lower eyelid defect repaired with anchoring sutures. (**A**) Lower eyelid defect. (**B**) Undermine and advance cheek superiorly. Extend the incision laterally into a laugh line at the lateral canthus. (**C**) Use anchoring sutures into the inferior rim periosteum and lateral canthus temporalis fascia to support the tissues and take the vertical tension off the eyelid. In some patients, you may want to support the posterior lamella with a lateral tarsal strip as well.

- If the defect involves most of the eyelid, you should start with a Cutler Beard procedure (an advanced technique)

If you are interested in doing most eyelid reconstructions, you should learn all of these lower eyelid reconstruction techniques. You can use the same primary closure techniques for upper lid reconstruction as well. Don't attempt complete full-thickness lid margin repairs of the upper eyelid until you can do lower lid repairs well. Although the Hughes flap procedure is more complex, it is well within your capability. The Cutler Beard procedure is a more difficult procedure to do correctly. Save this procedure until you have mastered the others.

We will cover the technique of primary repair of the eyelid margin in detail in Chapter 13, but this technique is so important we will introduce it here also. The eyelid margin repair begins with identifying the appropriate anatomic landmarks of the eyelid, especially the landmarks of the lid margin. You may want to review the section on "Fundamentals of Eyelid Anatomy" in this chapter if you don't know this anatomy well. The strength of the closure is in sutures placed in the tarsal plate. Eyelid wound margin eversion is necessary to prevent lid notching.

Eyelid margin repair includes:

- Injecting local anesthetic
- Aligning the lid margin

- Suturing the tarsal plate
- Suturing the lid margin
- Closing the skin

The steps of eyelid margin repair are:

1. Inject local anesthetic
   A. Instill topical anesthetic drops and inject local anesthetic with epinephrine into the wound.
2. Align the lid margin
   A. Use a 7-0 Vicryl vertical mattress suture passed through the meibomian gland orifices to align and evert the lid margin. Keep this suture long for traction on the eyelid (Figure 12-12, A).
3. Suture the tarsal plate
   A. Use two or three interrupted 5-0 Vicryl sutures passed in a lamellar fashion to align the tarsal plate (Figure 12-12, B). The initial lid margin suture will help with the positioning of your tarsal sutures.
4. Suture the lid margin
   A. Go back to the lid margin and place a 7-0 Vicryl vertical mattress suture anterior to the gray line. This suture should align the eyelashes and provide eversion of the lid margin (Figure 12-12, C).

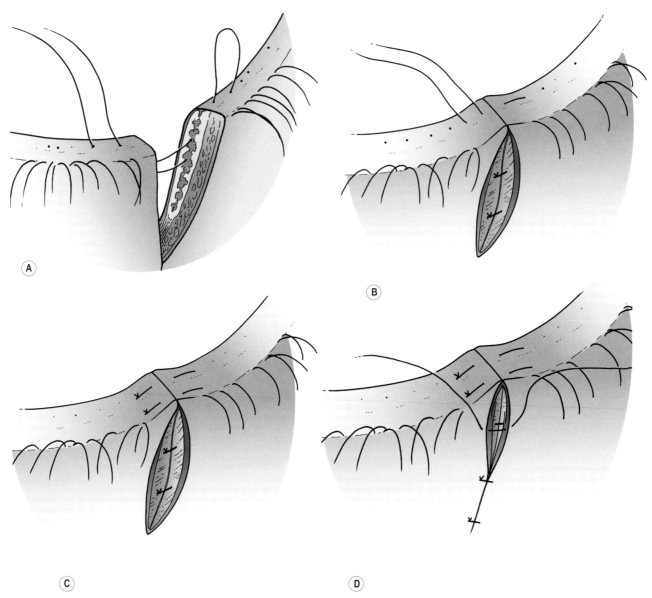

Figure 12-12 Lid margin repair. (**A**) Align the lid margin using a 7-0 Vicryl suture throughout the meibomian gland orifices. (**B**) Suture the tarsal plate with 5-0 Vicryl sutures. (**C**) Complete the lid margin closure, creating eversion of the wound edges with 7-0 Vicryl vertical mattress sutures. (**D**) An additional 7-0 Vicryl suture may be used to align the eyelash follicles. Close the skin with 5-0 or 6-0 fast absorbing sutures.

B. If you are unhappy with the alignment of the lid, replace the suture.

C. An additional suture may be used to help improve the alignment of the eyelashes.

D. I prefer to use 7-0 Vicryl sutures for the eyelid margin. Traditional teaching suggests the use of 6-0 or 8-0 silk sutures, which are left long and require removal later. The 7-0 Vicryl sutures can be cut short and allowed to absorb.

5. Close the skin
   A. The skin can be closed with an interrupted simple or vertical suture using permanent or absorbable sutures (Figure 12-12, D).
   B. If the wound seems under tension, you may want to place 5-0 Vicryl sutures through the orbicularis muscle before closing the skin (Box 12-2).

Lateral canthal defects of less than 25%

Small defects of the lower or upper eyelid involving the lateral canthus can be repaired with the lateral tarsal strip operation. Create a strip from the remaining tarsus and suture it to the periorbita on the inner aspect of the lateral orbital wall. Review the steps of the lateral tarsal strip procedure. Remember that using the P-2 small circle needle is helpful to anchor the strip to the lateral canthus.

If the lid will not stretch to the periosteum of the rim, you can try forming a periosteal strip from the lateral rim to the cut end of the tarsus. Cut a 5 mm high strip of periosteum angled superiorly, starting slightly above where the lateral canthal tendon should be (Figure 12-13). You will need to cover the periosteal strip with a myocutaneous flap to repair the anterior lamella. If the posterior lamella can't be closed using a periosteal strip, you will need to use a free tarsal graft to bridge the gap or a Hughes flap. We will discuss these procedures below.

Sometimes the periosteum on the lateral orbital rim will have to be removed to obtain tumor-free surgical margins. For these patients, there won't be any soft tissue to suture the eyelid to. You will need to drill two holes in the lateral orbital rim to reattach the tarsus. Remember to drill holes that open on the inner aspect of the rim. Overcorrect the canthal height slightly. Use a permanent suture such as 4-0 Prolene to thread through the holes from medial to lateral and tie the suture on the outside of the rim.

Medial canthal defects of less than 25%

Medial canthal defects are more difficult to repair than lateral canthal defects. There are two complicating factors. First, the lacrimal drainage system usually needs to be repaired if there is a medial canthal defect. Second, to anatomically reconstruct the medial canthus, the attachment of the eyelid to the medial orbit needs to be at the posterior lacrimal crest.

Box 12-2

Eyelid Margin Repair

Inject local anesthetic with epinephrine

Align the lid margin
- 7-0 Vicryl suture in the meibomian gland orifices
- Vertical mattress sutures

Suture the tarsus
- 5-0 Vicryl sutures, two to three passed partial thickness

Suture the lid margin
- 7-0 Vicryl sutures in the meibomian glands
- Vertical mattress sutures

Use additional simple interrupted sutures around the lashes as needed

Close the skin
- 5-0 fast absorbing interrupted sutures
- Consider 5-0 Vicryl sutures in the muscle, if under tension

---

In many patients, this is impossible because of the position of the canaliculus, and you may have to settle for a good attachment at the frontal process of the maxilla where the anterior limb is normally positioned.

Many medial defects will damage the lacrimal system. If one canaliculus is cut, try to reconstruct it using either the pigtail probe or Crawford stents. These techniques will be described in detail in Chapter 13. If the punctum has been removed, then the best you can do is to marsupialize the cut end of the canaliculus into the conjunctival fornix. Because most patients with skin cancers are older, you could argue that reconstruction of the canaliculus is not necessary because many patients would not have tearing with one functional canaliculus.

If you choose not to reconstruct the canaliculus, you may be able to get a more anatomic reattachment of the medial canthus by suturing the tarsus to the posterior lacrimal crest (Figure 12-14). Use Westcott scissors to sharply incise the conjunctiva between the plica and the caruncle. Use a Stevens scissors to perform blunt dissection to the medial orbital wall. Use a permanent suture, such as a 4-0 Mersilene suture (Ethicon 1779G, S-2 needle double-armed), to reattach the cut end of the tarsus to the posterior lacrimal crest. This is not easy to do and requires some experience in manipulating the orbital tissues. Nevertheless, it is possible to find the posterior lacrimal crest and anatomically reattach the medial portion of the cut tarsus. Because you are using a permanent suture, you will not have to actually attach the cut end of the tarsus to the posterior lacrimal crest. If the defect is too wide to easily reattach the medial eyelid, you should proceed with a canthotomy and cantholysis to allow the eyelid to move laterally, as described below.

Not infrequently, the entire lacrimal system may be removed during tumor removal. Periosteum and canthal tendons are often removed. In the past, a transnasal wire was used to secure the remaining medial eyelid margin(s) to the bone (Figure 12-15, A). A simpler procedure uses a Y-shaped microplate to attach the remaining eyelid. The plate is attached to the maxillary process of the frontal bone such that the leg of the Y projects across the lacrimal sac fossa.

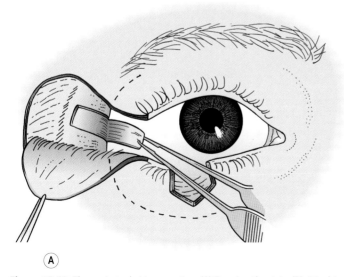

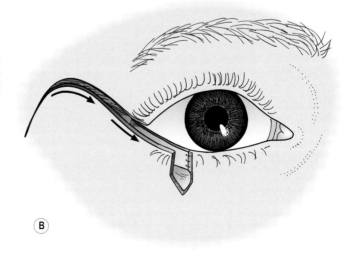

Figure 12-13 The periosteal strip operation. (**A**) Forming the strip. (**B**) Attaching the strip to the remaining tarsal plate. Shown with a Tenzel myocutaneous flap used as an anterior lamellar replacement.

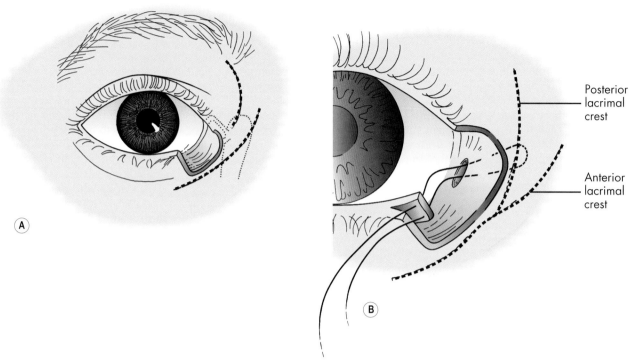

Figure 12-14 Full-thickness medial lid margin defect repair. (**A**) Medial lid margin defect. (**B**) A "medial tarsal strip" is formed and sutured through the plica of the conjunctiva to the posterior limb of the medial canthal tendon.

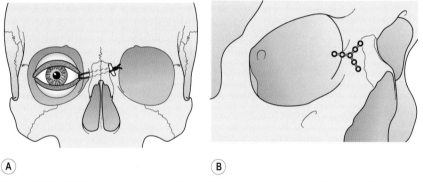

Figure 12-15 (**A**) Transnasal wiring of medial canthus. A stainless steel wire, attached to the anterior limb of the medial canthal tendon, is drawn across the nasal bridge and anchored on the contralateral frontal process of the nasal process of the frontal bone. You will find it helpful to make a bony ostium at the posterior one half of the lacrimal sac fossa to pull the tendon into place. The wire is tied over a cut piece of a 20-gauge needle. (**B**) Miniplate fixation. An easier option is to attach a Y or T micro- or miniplate on intact bone so that the most posterior of the plate holes is near the posterior lacrimal crest about two thirds of the way up. Use a 3-0 or 4-0 Prolene suture to attach the tendon to the plate (see the reconstruction series in Figure 12-27).

Recall that the attachment of the medial canthus is at the posterior lacrimal crest, about two thirds of the way up the fossa. It is always a good idea to overcorrect both the height and the posterior position of the microplate. Use a 4-0 or 5-0 Prolene suture on a free needle to suture the lid tissue to the plate (Figure 12-15, B).

Repair of full-thickness eyelid defects of 25% to 50%

Canthotomy, cantholysis, and eyelid margin closure

The canthotomy and cantholysis are used to release the lateral aspect of the lid to allow the lid margin to be closed under less tension. You will find that these are very useful procedures and, when you know how to use them, you will add this step to many primary lid margin repairs. We will discuss the canthotomy and cantholysis in detail in Chapter 13, but I will introduce them here for you. When you perform a canthotomy and cantholysis, you will be advancing a small amount of skin over the lateral orbital rim medially. The skin will become a portion of the lateral lid margin. Perform the canthotomy in the usual way, but angle the canthotomy incision slightly superiorly. Next, strum the deep tissues and sharply incise the crus of the lateral canthal tendon. Some cautery will be necessary. If additional relaxation is necessary, cut the tissues that are fixing the lid to the rim. You may not recognize these tissues anatomically, but they are portions of the septum and lower lid retractors as they fuse at the lateral canthus (Figure 12-16). If you are unable to perform the eyelid margin closure without tension, you should extend the canthotomy incision to perform the Tenzel flap procedure described below. You will see in the next section why it is important to angle the canthotomy superiorly.

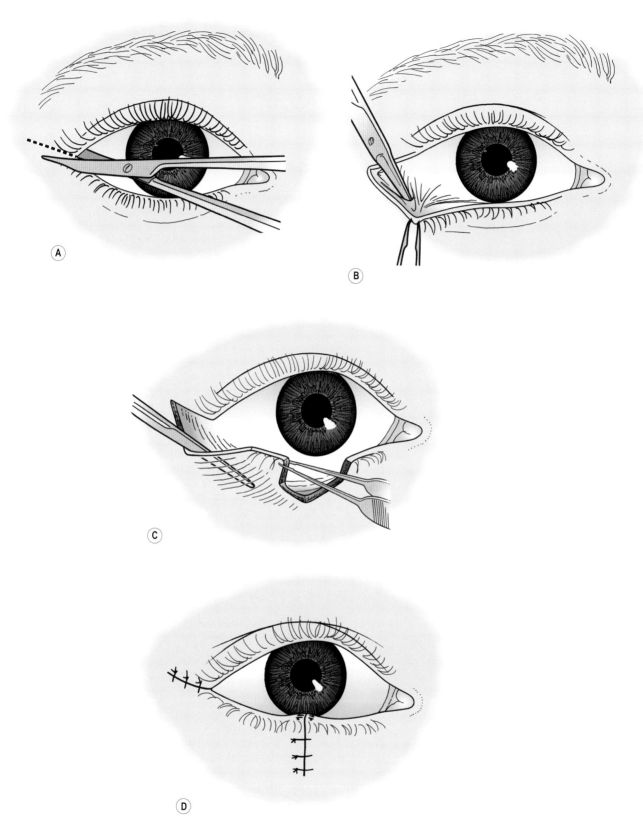

Figure 12-16 Canthotomy and cantholysis for closure of a full-thickness lower eyelid defect. (**A**) Angle the canthotomy superiorly. (**B**) Perform a cantholysis. (**C**) Free the orbital septum and lower lid retractors. (**D**) Perform a primary lid margin repair and close the canthotomy.

Repair of lid defects of 50% to 75%

The Tenzel flap

Early in my career, I did not use the Tenzel flap procedure much for repair of larger full-thickness lower lid defects. If I could not close a primary lid margin defect without a canthotomy and cantholysis, I would perform a Hughes procedure. The Hughes tarsoconjunctival flap operation is a very good procedure, but a second operation is required to complete the reconstruction of the lower lid. The Tenzel flap procedure does not require a second stage. If 50% of the upper or lower lid is missing, a Tenzel flap will work well.

Remember that you should think of closure of the eyelid margin as a series of steps that allow you to mobilize the cut ends of the margin until the wound can be closed without tension. First, try primary closure. If the wound is too tight, do a canthotomy and cantholysis. If the wound is still too tight, move to a Tenzel flap procedure.

The Tenzel flap procedure includes:

- Injecting local anesthetic
- Performing canthotomy and cantholysis
- Forming the flap
- Mobilizing the flap
- Repairing the margin

The steps of the Tenzel flap for reconstruction of the lower eyelid are:

1. Inject local anesthetic
   A. Draw an arched line extending superiorly from the lateral canthus in a curve. Extend the canthotomy incision along the marked incision with a no. 15 blade or Colorado needle (Figure 12-17, A).
   B. Most lid reconstructions can be performed on a cooperative patient with local anesthesia and sedation.
   C. As usual, you will be using local anesthetic with epinephrine added.
2. Perform canthotomy and cantholysis
   A. Perform the canthotomy and cantholysis as described above.
   B. Remember to angle the canthotomy superiorly as the canthotomy incision will continue as the Tenzel flap (Figure 12-17, B).
   C. Perform a lower cantholysis (Figure 12-17, C).
3. Form and mobilize the Tenzel flap
   A. Dissect a myocutaneous flap posterior to the orbicularis muscle (in the preseptal plane). You will see that you will be able to mobilize the skin and muscle medially (Figure 12-17, D).
   B. The originally described Tenzel flap was a small (dime-shaped) flap that did not extend beyond the lateral orbital rim. Using this small flap is possible if you know that a minimal amount of mobilization will be necessary. I prefer to make the longer arched incision to allow as much mobilization as necessary. You will see that the arched incision is the beginning of a larger rotational flap called the Mustarde cheek rotation.

   C. Keep in mind that the frontal nerve passes from the tragus to the tail of the brow. If you have to extend the myocutaneous advancement flap lateral to the lateral orbital rim, you will need to keep your incision superficial to avoid damage to the frontal branch of the facial nerve.
   D. As you create the flap, check to see that the margin can be opposed without tension. After you have achieved satisfactory mobilization of the tissue, place one or two 4-0 PDS sutures to anchor the flap medially on the lateral canthal rim periosteum. Place the anchoring sutures so that the lateral canthus is slightly overcorrected superiorly (Figure 12-17, E). Place the suture on the inner aspect of the rim to pull the lateral canthus posteriorly toward its natural insertion on the inner aspect of the rim.
4. Repair the lid margin
   A. Repair the lid margin in the usual way, supporting the tension of closure on the tarsus using 5-0 Vicryl sutures.
   B. Sew the lid margin with everting mattress sutures using 7-0 Vicryl (Figure 12-17, F).
5. Give postoperative care
   A. Instill topical antibiotics and place a patch over the wound for 24 hours.
   B. You will notice that the lateral portion of the eyelid margin is created by the advancement flap. Some patients will have a small amount of notching where the canthotomy was made (especially if you have not angled the canthotomy incision superiorly). If an irregularity in the lid margin is present, you may want to repair this with one or two 7-0 Vicryl sutures.

Intraoperatively, I am always concerned that the final result will look good. Postoperatively, I am always pleasantly surprised with the final eyelid position and contour. This is a useful operation that you should learn to do for lower and upper eyelid reconstruction (Figure 12-18).

Repair of lower lid defects of 75% or greater

The Hughes procedure

If you know how to do a Hughes procedure, you can fix almost all large lower eyelid defects. The Hughes procedure is used to reconstruct the posterior lamella of a full-thickness lower eyelid defect that is too wide for the use of a Tenzel flap. The procedure provides a flap of tarsus and conjunctiva, from the upper eyelid, which is sewn into the lower eyelid. This tarsoconjunctival flap carries its own blood supply because it remains attached to the upper eyelid for 4 weeks. You must provide an anterior lamella using a myocutaneous advancement flap or full-thickness skin graft. You should learn this procedure because it will give you the flexibility and confidence to take care of larger lower eyelid skin cancers.

The Hughes flap procedure includes:

- Injecting local anesthetic
- Measuring the lower eyelid defect

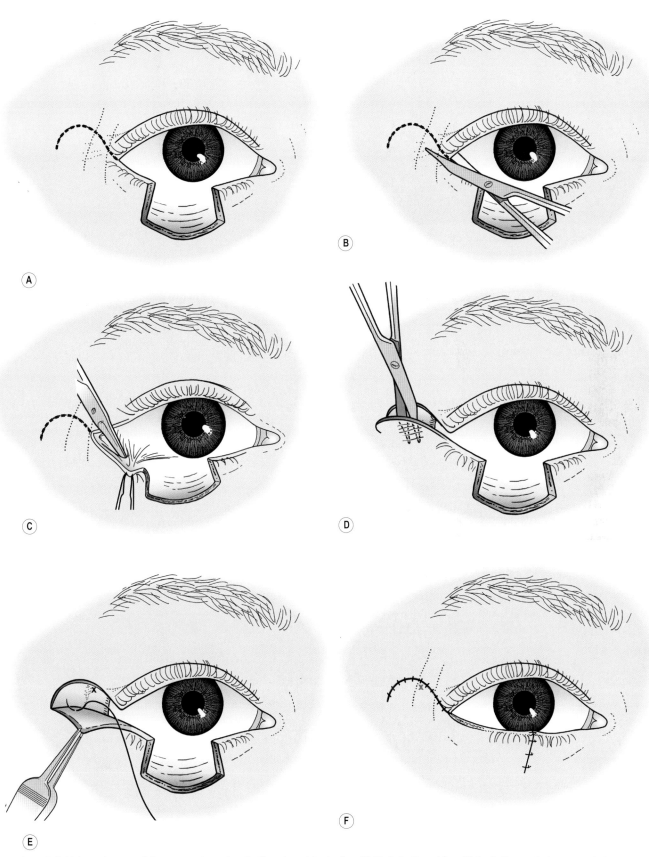

Figure 12-17 Full-thickness lower eyelid reconstruction using the Tenzel semicircular flap. (**A**) Mark the Tenzel flap. (**B**) Angle the canthotomy superiorly. (**C**) Perform a lower cantholysis to release the eyelid. (**D**) Mobilize the flap dissecting in the plane posterior to the orbicularis muscle. (**E**) Anchor the flap at the periosteum of the lateral rim. (**F**) Perform a primary lid margin repair and close the flap.

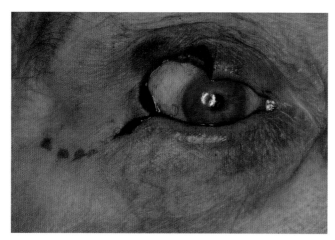

Figure 12-18 Tenzel semicircular flap marked for upper eyelid full-thickness reconstruction.

- Forming the tarsoconjunctival flap
- Suturing the flap into the lower lid defect
- Completing anterior lamellar repair
- Postoperative care

The steps of the Hughes flap procedure are:

1. Inject local anesthetic
   A. The Hughes flap procedure can easily be performed with local anesthesia. As always, use local anesthetic with the addition of epinephrine. Infiltrate the superior and inferior conjunctival cul de sacs.
   B. Infiltrate the skin of the upper lid. Infiltrate the wound edges of the lower lid.
2. Measure the lower eyelid defect.
   A. Examine the edges of the lower eyelid wound. Identify any remaining posterior lamella at the medial and lateral edges of the wound (Figure 12-19, A).
   B. Pull the edges of the wound together with slight to moderate tension. Use a caliper to measure the defect (Figure 12-19, B).
   C. In most patients, you can harvest up to a 20 mm width of tarsus from a normal upper lid. If more length is needed, you can extend the tarsal graft to include conjunctiva on the medial and lateral edges of the graft.
3. Form the tarsoconjunctival flap
   A. Place a 4-0 silk suture in the lid margin and evert the lid over a Jaeger lid speculum (shoehorn).
   B. Use a caliper to place a mark parallel and 3 mm superior to the upper lid margin. You need to leave 3 mm of intact lid margin to prevent upper lid entropion.
   C. Use a Colorado needle or a no. 15 blade for this incision (Figure 12-19, C).
   D. Use Westcott scissors to develop a plane in the pretarsal space superiorly to the top edge of the tarsus (Figure 12-19, D).
   E. You have the option of creating a flap of conjunctiva alone or conjunctiva and Müller's muscle. In most patients, you can dissect a plane between Muller's muscle and conjunctiva, bringing only conjunctiva down with the tarsus.

   F. Dissect high into the fornix. This will help to avoid upper lid retraction postoperatively. If you are finding that your patients have upper lid retraction postoperatively, dissect between Muller's muscle and the conjunctiva more superiorly to avoid advancing the Müller's muscle and the levator aponeurosis when you bring the flap into the defect.
   G. Make vertical cuts into the conjunctiva to complete the formation of the flap (Figure 12-19, D).
4. Suture the flap into the lower lid defect
   A. Identify the inferior margin of conjunctiva and lower lid retractors.
   B. Use 5-0 Vicryl sutures with a spatula needle (Ethicon J571 S-14 needle) to attach the flap to the edges of the remaining posterior lamella of the lower eyelid (Figure 12-19, E).
   C. Make sure that the superior edge of the tarsus is at or slightly above what will be the new lower lid margin.
   D. Suture the inferior aspect of the tarsal graft to the remaining conjunctiva.
5. Complete the anterior lamellar repair
   A. To determine if you will be able to use a myocutaneous advancement flap from the cheek, dissect the edges of the remaining skin and muscle free and pull up toward the upper lid. If there is a moderate amount of redundancy, you will probably be able to use a myocutaneous advancement flap. If not, a full-thickness skin graft will be required.
   B. If there is not adequate skin to drape over the tarsoconjunctival flap (see Figure 12-20), place a full-thickness skin graft harvested from the preauricular area over the tarsoconjunctival flap.
      (1) Place the skin graft slightly superior to the edge of the tarsal graft.
      (2) Use a running suture on the periphery of the graft to secure its position.
      (3) You may want to use mattress sutures from the tarsal graft through the skin graft (Figure 12-19, F).
   C. If there is enough redundant skin and muscle in the remaining lower lid and cheek, you can develop a myocutaneous flap to cover the defect. Use the technique that you are already familiar with to elevate the flap (Figure 12-19, G).
      (1) When you get to the inferior orbital rim, advance into the subcutaneous fat plane and use anchoring sutures to elevate the cheek if necessary (see Figure 12-11).
      (2) Suture the flap into position over the newly reconstructed posterior lamella (Figure 12-19, H).
      (3) Because the tarsoconjunctival flap is supported superiorly, you can advance lower eyelid and cheek tissues with slightly more vertical tension than you would otherwise consider. A Hughes flap will not support a poorly constructed flap with significant vertical tension, however.
6. Give postoperative care
   A. Place topical antibiotic ointment on the wound and tape a patch into position for 1 week.

B. The Hughes flap should be allowed to heal for 3–4 weeks before you undertake the second stage of the operation.

C. During this time, the eyelid will look closed, which should be comfortable for the patient.

The opening of the upper lid, the second stage of the Hughes flap procedure, can be performed under local anesthesia. The injection will be somewhat more painful than normal because there will be some scar tissue in the lid. Inject both the upper lid and the superior edge of the flap. Use Westcott scissors to sharply incise the flap, creating a new lid margin (see Figure 12-19, I). As you would expect, it is better to make this initial cut too high. You can trim more if necessary. I prefer to angle the scissors slightly inferiorly toward

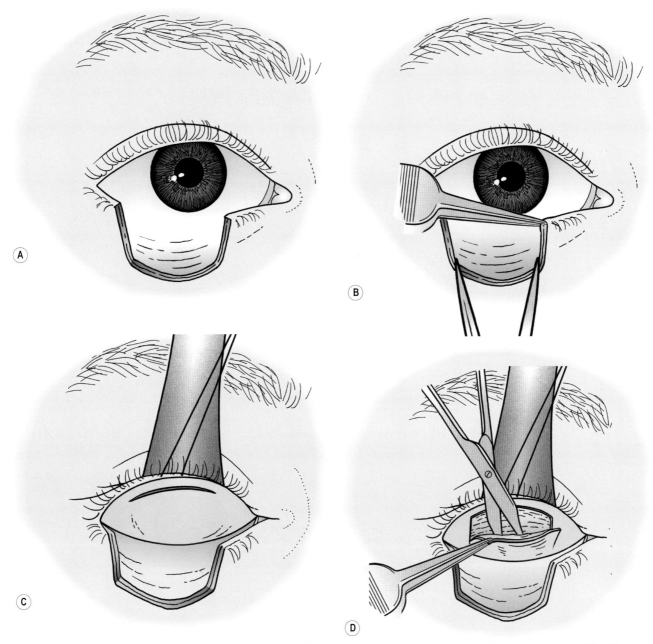

Figure 12-19 The Hughes procedure (tarsoconjunctival advancement flap) for repair of full-thickness lower eyelid defects of greater than 50% of the eyelid. (**A**) A full-thickness lower eyelid defect of greater than 50% of the lower eyelid. (**B**) Bring the wound edges together and measure the lower eyelid defect. (**C**) Place a 4-0 silk traction suture in the upper lid margin. Make a horizontal cut parallel to the lid margin full thickness through the tarsus, preserving 3–4 mm of lid margin. (**D**) Dissect the tarsus off the underlying orbicularis muscle and levator aponeurosis superiorly to the top edge of the tarsus. (**E**) Dissect a tissue plane between Muller's muscle and the conjunctiva up to the superior fornix. Make vertical cuts in the conjunctiva to bring down the tarsal flap. Sew the flap to the edges of the tarsus laterally and medially. Sew the inferior edge of the flap to the lower eyelid conjunctiva or retractors to complete the posterior lamellar repair. (**F**) If there is no redundant anterior lamella in the lower eyelid, use a full-thickness skin graft to cover the flap. (**G**) If there is redundancy in the lower eyelid anterior lamella, dissect a myocutaneous flap inferiorly. (**H**) Advance the flap into position, excising any dog-ears. (**I**) Second-stage procedure: 3–4 weeks later, open the eyelids by excising the flap. Cut slightly above the lower lid margin. (**J**) Use a battery-operated cautery tool for hemostasis and to angle the lid margin with the posterior surface higher than the anterior surface.

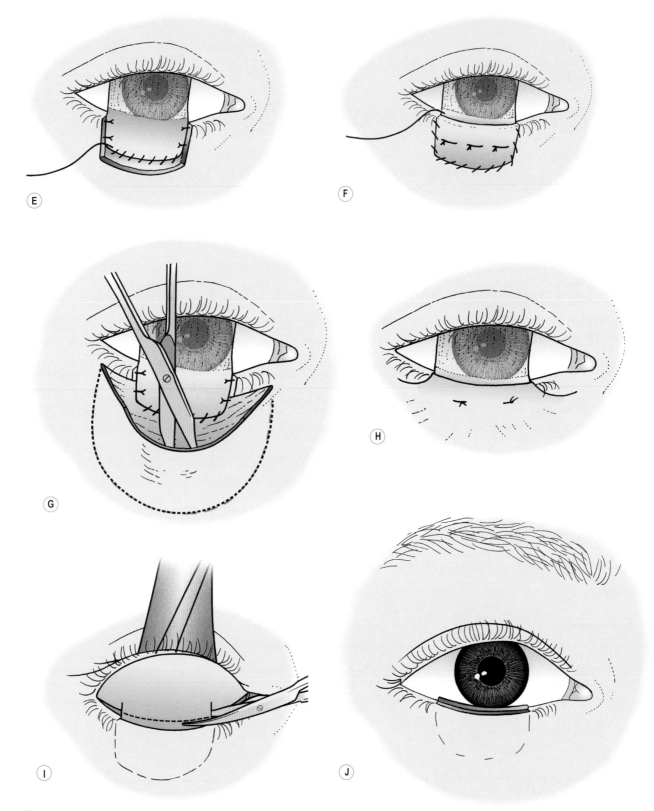

Figure 12-19 Continued.

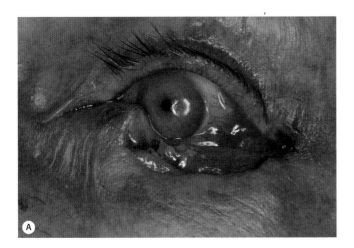

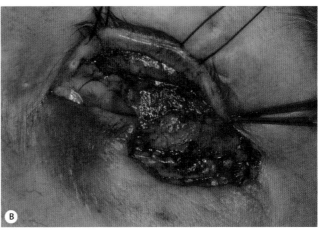

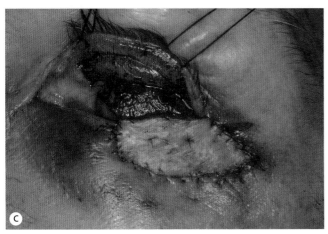

Figure 12-20 The Hughes procedure. (**A**) Full-thickness lower eyelid defect. (**B**) The tarsoconjunctival flap formed and sutured into position for the posterior lamellar reconstruction. (**C**) A preauricular full-thickness skin graft is used to repair the anterior lamella.

the anterior edge of the lid margin. The bevel of the lid margin incision plays a role in where the mucocutaneous junction will form (Figure 12-19, J). In some patients, conjunctiva will heal slightly over the edge of the new lid margin, which can create erythema as a result of drying of the conjunctiva.

After the lower lid is separated, excise the remaining tarsoconjunctival flap at the tarsal plate of the upper lid. Some cautery may be required to stop a small amount of bleeding there. A patch is usually not necessary, unless oozing is present.

You will find the Hughes flap procedure to be very helpful and worth your efforts to learn. Although the Hughes procedure is a two-stage operation and there will be no lashes on the lower eyelid, the results are very good. Most patients will have a functioning lower eyelid that appears normal.

Free tarsal graft

A free tarsal graft can be harvested from the contralateral upper lid to be used as a posterior lamellar replacement for lower eyelid defects. This is an alternative to the Hughes flap or Tenzel-type flaps. The disadvantage of a free tarsal graft is that it does not have a blood supply, so it must be covered with a myocutaneous advancement flap.

The advantage of a free tarsal graft is that it is a one-stage procedure and gives a result very similar to that of the Hughes procedure. The free tarsal graft is harvested similarly to the initial steps of forming the Hughes flap. When the dissection

in the pretarsal space reaches the superior margin of the tarsus, the conjunctiva is cut, freeing the graft. No suturing of the upper lid donor site is required. Usually there are no problems with the donor site. If the upper lid of the donor site is lax, a small "kink" of the upper lid margin can occur as the donor bed contracts during healing. Remember to leave 3 mm of tarsus along the lid margin to prevent upper lid entropion.

You should consider using a free tarsal graft as a posterior lamellar replacement for upper or lower lid defects when you are certain there is adequate anterior lamella to cover the free tarsal graft (Figure 12-21).

Combination procedures

Using the techniques discussed thus far, you will be able to repair most lower and many upper lid defects after removal of cutaneous malignancies. As your surgical experience increases, you will learn to put the various techniques together in combinations that you have not used before. For example, you may encounter a lower lid defect that involves considerably more anterior lamella than posterior lamella. You can apply the technique of primary lid margin repair to the posterior lamella alone, closing the tarsal defect and lid margin. You then have the option of using a myocutaneous advancement flap or a skin graft over the reconstructed posterior lamella. You will find the combination of procedures available to be limited only by sound surgical principles, good technique, and your creativity.

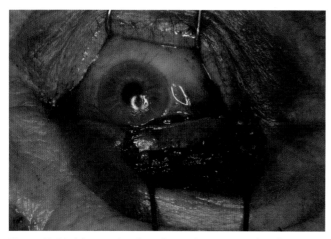

Figure 12-21 A free tarsal graft can be used as a posterior lamellar replacement when there is adequate lamella to cover the graft.

Checkpoint

- You should be able to figure out a technique for reconstructing most lower lid lesions at this point. Review the repair techniques for progressively larger full-thickness defects of the lower lid.
- Primary closure of the lid margin is a part of most full-thickness eyelid repairs. Describe the steps for primary repair of the eyelid margin.
- Why is a medial canthal full-thickness defect more difficult to repair than a lateral canthal defect?
- Picture in your mind the steps of the Tenzel flap procedure. Why is it important to angle the canthotomy incision slightly superiorly?
- For defects involving nearly the entire lower lid, you will usually need to perform a Hughes flap procedure. Remember that this is a two-stage procedure. The posterior lamella is from the upper lid tarsus. The anterior lamella can be replaced with a full-thickness skin graft or a myocutaneous advancement flap. You should learn these techniques if you are going to take care of many skin cancers.
- The free tarsal graft is easier to do, but you will need enough skin to advance over it.

Specialized procedures

The Mustarde cheek rotation

There are some specialized procedures that you should know about, but may not want to perform. The Mustarde cheek rotation is a facial flap that is used to cover large anterior lamellar defects in the lower lid (Figure 12-22, A). An arched incision starting at the lateral canthus is drawn toward the hairline, extending inferiorly anterior to the tragus of the ear. The skin is cut with a Colorado needle or a no. 15 blade. A flap is created in the subcutaneous tissue plane, freeing up a large area of the temple and cheek that will be rotated to fill an anterior lamellar defect (Figure 12-22, B–D). You can use any of the posterior lamellar repair techniques we have discussed thus far in combination with a Mustarde cheek flap.

The Mustarde cheek rotation is no more difficult than many of the procedures we have discussed but, because of the relatively large size of the flap, many less experienced surgeons are reluctant to perform this operation. If you perform this procedure, remember to stay in the subcutaneous cheek plane ("fat up and fat down" when dissecting the flap) and use wide areas of undermining to allow the cheek to be rotated with minimal tension on the flap or skin closure. Use anchoring sutures to overcorrect the height of the flap at the lateral canthus. In some patients, you may use a small back-cut or notch at the inferior extent of the incision to help closure.

The median forehead flap

The median forehead flap is commonly used as an anterior lamellar repair for larger defects of the lower lid and medial canthus, often over bare bone (Figure 12-23, A). The median forehead flap can be combined with other procedures such as the Mustarde cheek rotation for large defects involving the medial and lateral canthus and entire lower lid.

The proposed flap is outlined on the axis of the contralateral supraorbital and supratrochlear neurovascular bundle. The axial blood supply of this flap allows for a long narrow flap to be formed without danger of flap necrosis. A plastic surgical drape can be used as a template. The length of the flap is determined by rotating the template while it is anchored at the contralateral supraorbital notch. In some patients, the median forehead flap will extend to the hairline.

The skin flap is incised with a no. 15 blade or Colorado needle. The plane of dissection is deep, extending to the loose areolar tissue anterior to the periosteum of the frontal bone. The tip of the flap is thinned to the subcutaneous tissue plane. The median forehead flap should not be used to reconstruct the upper lid because a thick and immobile lid will result. The flap is rotated 120–180 degrees into position covering the defect. Deep sutures (4-0 or 5-0 PDS) are used to tack the flap into position. Additional undermining at the base of the flap may be required, but care should be taken not to disrupt the blood supply to the flap. The forehead is closed with aggressive dissection anterior to the periosteum of the frontal bone. A wide area of undermining is necessary to close the forehead wound. Deep 3-0 PDS sutures will be required to close the forehead wound. Subcutaneous and skin sutures are placed (Figure 12-23, B). The closure leaves a large "hump" at the bridge of the nose. This will be removed in a second-stage operation.

The second-stage operation is performed 6 weeks postoperatively. The redundant tissues at the base of the flap are incised and removed. Thinning of the base of the flap can be performed. Additional thinning of the flap can be done after healing is complete and all the swelling is gone.

The median forehead flap is useful to cover a large area of anterior lamella on the bridge of the nose and lower lid. Where the lower lid is missing, the median forehead flap can be lined with mucous membrane of the mouth to reconstruct all layers of the eyelid. By necessity, the median forehead flap leaves a visible vertical scar in the forehead. There is numbness of the forehead caused by disruption of the supraorbital nerve. The median forehead flap should not be

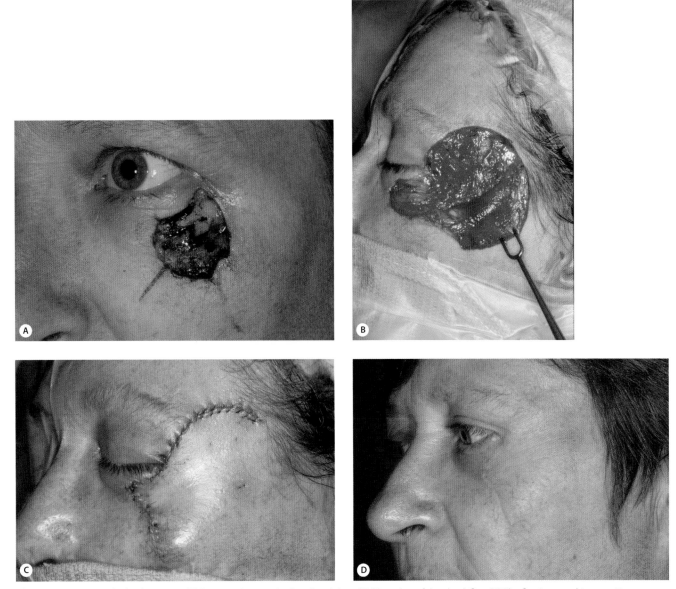

Figure 12-22 Mustarde cheek rotation. (**A**) Preoperative anterior lamellar defect. (**B**) Dissection of the cheek flap. (**C**) The flap is rotated into position. (**D**) Postoperative appearance 3 months after repair.

used to reconstruct the upper lid because a thick and immobile lid will result. The operation requires a planned second-stage revision. Despite these problems, good results can be obtained (Figure 12-23, C).

The glabellar flap

The glabellar flap is useful to reconstruct smaller anterior lamellar defects in the medial canthus. This is not an axial flap, so the length cannot be as long as a median forehead flap. The loose glabellar tissues are incised and undermined (see Figure 2-57). The flap is rotated 90–120 degrees into position. The redundant tissue of the glabella and reduced angle of rotation allow this reconstruction to be completed in a single stage. Good results occur because the thickness, color, and texture match well (Figure 12-24). Thinning of the flap can be performed if necessary.

The Cutler Beard procedure

The Cutler Beard procedure is used to repair large full-thickness defects of the upper lid. The procedure is a two-stage, lid-sharing procedure. A width of full-thickness lower eyelid below the tarsal plate is used to reconstruct the upper eyelid defect. The eyelids are sewn closed for several weeks before the second-stage procedure to open the eyelids is performed. Smaller defects, of up to 50%, of the upper eyelid can be repaired with the Tenzel flap technique, as discussed above.

The width of the upper eyelid defect is measured, and the width is marked on the lower eyelid. A horizontal incision 2 mm below the inferior tarsal plate is made with a blade, and the incision is extended full thickness through the lid with scissors (Figure 12-25, A). The conjunctiva is dissected off the lower lid retractors and sewn to the edge of the upper

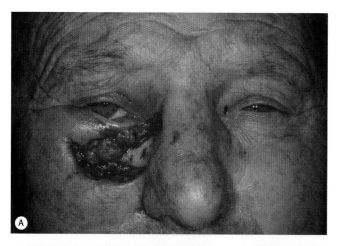

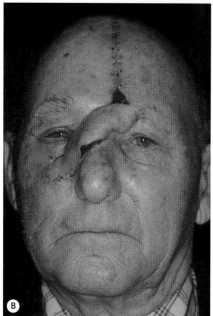

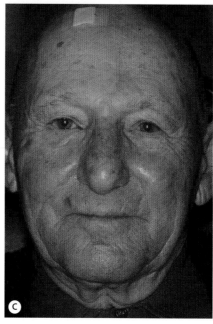

Figure 12-23 Median forehead flap. (**A**) Preoperative medial canthal and lower eyelid defect, exposing bare bone on inferior orbital rim and lateral wall of nose. (**B**) One week after repair, which left a "hump" at the glabella. The flap is based on the axial blood supply of the opposite supraorbital neurovascular bundle. (**C**) The postoperative result after the second-stage procedure 1 year later.

lid conjunctiva and levator aponeurosis (Figure 12-25, B). Although not in the original description, I use a piece of ear cartilage or free tarsal graft to sew on the conjunctiva to add some rigidity to the upper lid. The skin and muscle of the lower eyelid are dissected inferiorly to the rim or into the cheek and brought under the bridge of the lower eyelid and sewn to the skin and muscle of the upper eyelid defect (Figure 12-25, C). The lower lid incision is not closed.

Six to eight weeks later, the lids are separated. The upper eyelid conjunctiva is advanced anteriorly onto the lid margin for 2 mm. The horizontal lower lid incision is sewn to the cut edge of the lower eyelid skin (Figure 12-25, D).

Healing is slow because of lymphedema of the reconstructed tissues. Often one or more additional touch-up procedures are required (Figure 12-25, E). Lower eyelid ectropion is common because the lid has been denervated. Lower eyelid tightening is indicated if the lower eyelid remains lax. Upper eyelid entropion is a problem in many patients. Skin and lanugo hairs of the new eyelid rub on the cornea because

the levator tends to pull the new posterior lamella more than the new anterior lamella. After you see this problem, you will understand why the normal pretarsal tissues adhere to the tarsal plate. Creating a firm attachment of the anterior lamella to the ear cartilage graft helps to prevent this entropion, but the problem remains for many patients.

Large full-thickness defects of the upper eyelid are the most difficult to repair. Many reconstructions will require some slight revision. Save these complex reconstructions until you are confident with the easier ones. If you choose to reconstruct large upper lid defects, you will learn to appreciate the subtleties of the upper eyelid anatomy and function.

I use the Cutler Beard procedure when there are no other options to repair the upper lid defect. Consider other options before using it. Primary closure with or without canthotomy or a Tenzel flap is useful for small defects. If there is upper lid dermatochalasis, try a free tarsal graft for posterior lamellar repair and use the redundant upper lid skin for anterior

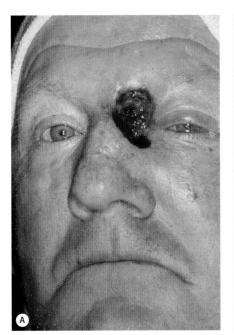
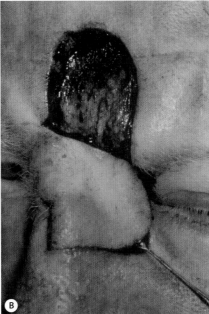
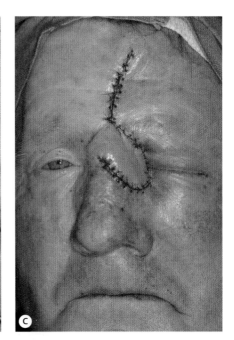
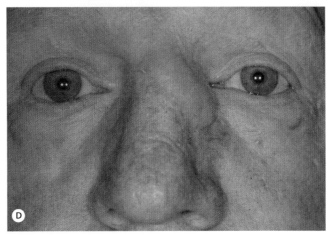

Figure 12-24 The glabellar flap. (**A**) A medial canthal defect. (**B**) The flap is rotated into position. (**C**) The forehead wound is undermined and closed. The flap is sutured into position. (**D**) The postoperative result 3 months after repair before any thinning of the flap.

lamellar repair. If there is not quite enough upper eyelid fold, a clever alternative is using staggered anterior and posterior lamellar grafts. Use a free tarsal graft to fill the posterior lamellar defect. Make a horizontal incision in the upper lid anterior lamella and advance a bipedicle flap of skin and muscle inferiorly to vascularize the free tarsal graft. Place a free skin graft over the defect where you borrowed the tissue for the bipedicle flap (Figure 12-26).

I use this technique rather than a Cutler Beard type procedure whenever possible. It is a one-stage procedure. Revisions are rarely necessary. Lid margin entropion is not a common problem.

Combination procedures

Eyelid reconstruction after tumor excision is always interesting and a great way to learn. In your early stages, you will likely be nervous that you cannot repair a pending defect. As your surgical armamentarium grows, you will be able to combine the simpler reconstructions that you know to fill in

larger defects. The repairs get creative and soon you will find that you are "improvising"—putting steps together that you did not ever do in combination. These cases are some of the most challenging and fun to do in the specialty. Take the large medial lower eyelid defect shown in Figure 12-27 for example. This is a combination of both posterior and anterior lamellar repair. The repair for this case was complex:

- Canthotomy/cantholysis of the upper and lower eyelids
- Medial canthal fixation using a T-shaped microplate screwed to frontal bone
- Mustarde cheek rotation
- Forehead flap
- No canalicular repair—sac was gone
- Full-thickness skin grafts
- Second-stage revision of forehead flap

See if you can follow it. If so, you are on your way to being a great reconstructive surgeon. It doesn't get much more complicated than this.

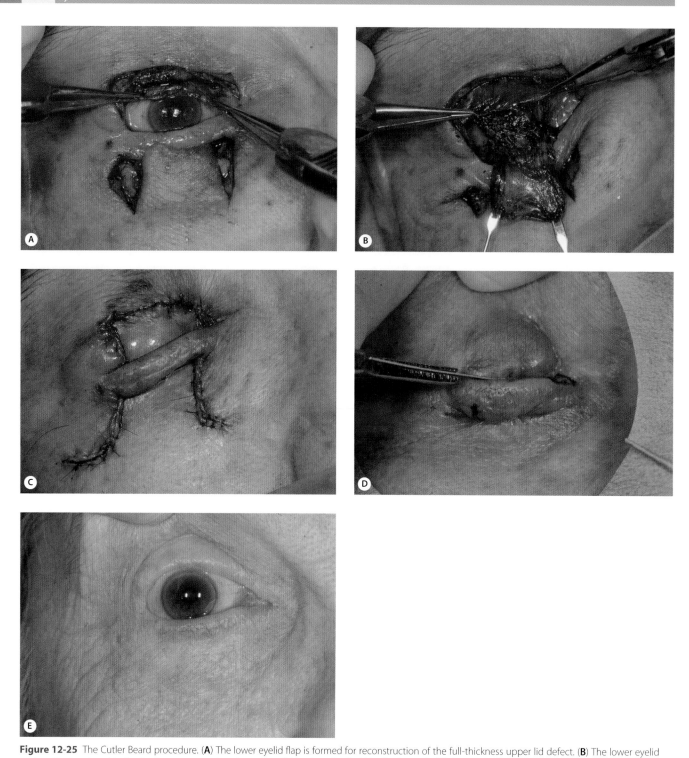

Figure 12-25 The Cutler Beard procedure. (**A**) The lower eyelid flap is formed for reconstruction of the full-thickness upper lid defect. (**B**) The lower eyelid conjunctiva is sutured to the levator aponeurosis and upper eyelid conjunctiva (held in the forceps). (**C**) An ear cartilage graft is sewn into position as a "middle lamella" (not shown). The skin and muscle flap is sewn to the upper eyelid. (**D**) The upper lid is separated with a no. 15 blade 6–8 weeks later. (**E**) The postoperative result 10 months after repair.

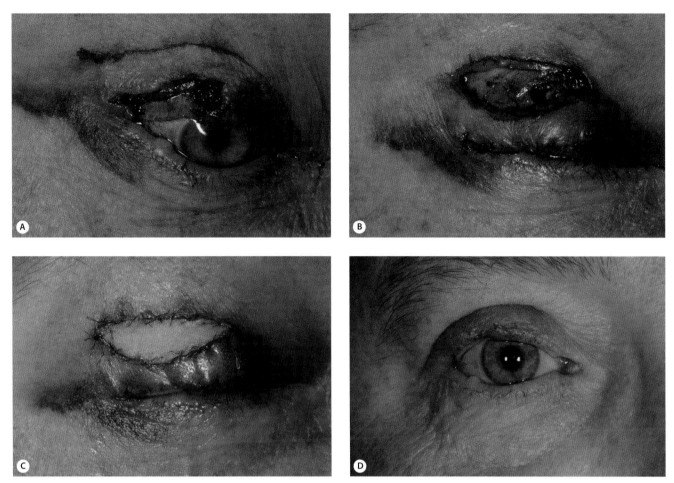

Figure 12-26 Full-thickness upper eyelid reconstruction using staggered anterior and posterior lamellar grafts—an unusual reconstruction, but based on sound surgical principles. (**A**) A free tarsal graft is harvested from the opposite upper tarsus and sewn into position as the posterior lamellar replacement. A bipedicle anterior lamellar flap is marked on the skin fold. (**B**) The bipedicle flap is sutured over the free tarsal graft, creating an anterior lamella defect superior to the flap. (**C**) The defect is repaired with a full-thickness skin graft from the preauricular region. (**D**) Postoperative result 3 weeks after repair.

Checkpoint

By now, you are an expert on lid reconstruction. You have seen all the procedures that you will need. Visualize the defect and the repair:

- Small anterior lamellar defect away from the lid margin
  - Primary closure with no vertical tension on the eyelid
- Larger anterior lamellar defect away from the lid margin
  - Primary closure with undermining, flap, or skin graft
- Full-thickness defect of 25% of the lower or upper eyelid
  - Primary lid margin repair
- Full-thickness defect of 40% of the lower or upper eyelid
  - Primary lid margin repair with canthotomy and cantholysis

- Full-thickness defect of 50% of the lower or upper eyelid
  - Primary lid margin repair with Tenzel flap
- Full-thickness defect of 75% of the lower eyelid
  - Hughes procedure
- Medial canthal and lower lid defect down to bare bone on the nasal bridge
  - Median forehead flap
- Full-thickness defect of the entire upper lid
  - Cutler Beard procedure
  - Free tarsal graft and bipedicle flap

If you did not have any problems deciding what to do for each of the defects above, you are ready to try some lid reconstructions.

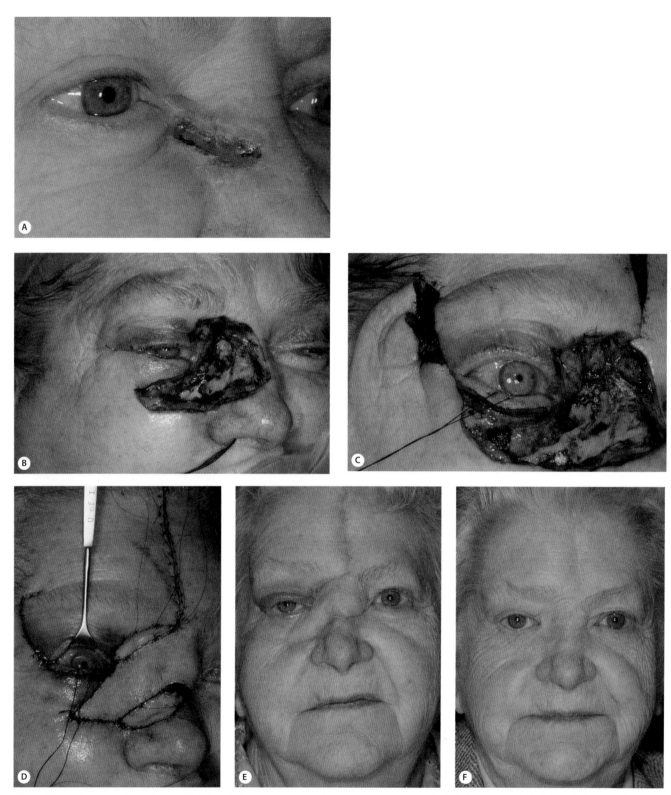

Figure 12-27 Reconstruction series. (**A**) Medial canthal morpheaform basal cell carcinoma. Note the indistinct margins. (**B**) Medial canthal defect. Tissue excised includes skin, muscle, periosteum, medial canthal tendon, lacrimal sac, periorbita, medial one third of the upper and lower eyelids, and cheek tissue over the inferior orbital rim. (**C**) Repair including upper and lower eyelid cantholysis, Mustarde cheek flap, median forehead flap, and T microplate fixation of the medial ends of the upper and lower eyelids to the medial canthus (see **Figure 12-15, B** for a close-up view). (**D**) Eyelid, cheek, and forehead flaps in position. Note additional full thickness skin grafts adjacent to the forehead flap or nose. (**E**) Postoperative view, 1 month after repair. (**F**) Postoperative view, following debulking of the forehead flap, 11 months after initial reconstruction.

Major points

Learn to describe eyelid defects and plan the repair in terms of the fundamentals of eyelid anatomy:

- The eyelid margin
- The anterior and posterior lamellae
- The lateral canthus
- The medial canthus

From posterior to anterior, the anatomic structures that you should know are:

- The mucocutaneous junction
- The meibomian gland orifices
- The gray line
- The eyelash follicles

Confirm the diagnosis of a suspected cutaneous malignancy with an incisional biopsy. Remove the lesion with an excisional biopsy, ensuring pathologically that surgical margins are free of tumor by intraoperative frozen sections or with the help of a Mohs' surgeon.

There are several options for repair of anterior lamellar defects in the periocular area:

- Healing by granulation
- Primary closure
- Primary closure with undermining
- Free skin graft
- Myocutaneous advancement flap

Repair posterior lamellar defects before you repair any anterior lamellar defect.

Granulation is an alternative to surgical repair when the defect is small and away from anatomic landmarks that will be disturbed by scar contraction.

Anterior lamellar defects that cannot be closed primarily are repaired with myocutaneous advancement flaps or free skin grafts. Myocutaneous flaps are preferred over skin grafts.

Skin grafts are used when you cannot bring a flap into position. Full-thickness skin grafts are preferred over split-thickness skin grafts. You cannot place an anterior lamellar free graft on a posterior lamellar free graft.

Donor sites for full-thickness skin grafts include:

- Upper eyelid skin
- Retroauricular skin
- Preauricular skin
- Supraclavicular or upper arm skin

The most practical donor site is the preauricular skin.

Myocutaneous flaps have many advantages over free skin grafts:

- Available local tissue
- Good match for color and texture

- Near normal innervation
- Blood supply allows use over bare bone
- High rate of successful healing
- Excellent function

Know what plane you should be in when developing a flap. Always avoid vertical tension on the lower eyelid. Minimize tension on the skin closure by adequate flap development and the use of anchoring sutures. Always overcorrect the height of the flap at the lid margin and lateral canthus.

Full-thickness defects of the eyelid often involve primary repair of the lid margin. Follow these guidelines for lower or upper eyelid margin repair:

Attempt primary closure. If the closure is under too much tension or the lid retracts inferiorly under the globe:

- Do a canthotomy and cantholysis. If there is still too much tension,
- Perform a Tenzel flap procedure, advancing tissue from the temple to form a new lid margin
- If the defect involves most of the lower eyelid, start with a Hughes flap procedure
- If the defect involves most of the eyelid, start with a Cutler Beard procedure (an advanced technique)

Lateral canthal defects can be repaired with the lateral tarsal strip procedure. If the lid is too tight, use a periosteal strip to attach the remaining lid to the lateral canthus. A free tarsal graft is another alternative for a posterior lamellar graft.

When repairing full-thickness medial canthal defects, repair the canaliculus if necessary. Make an attempt to reattach the medial canthal tendon to the posterior lacrimal crest, if possible.

Advanced reconstructive procedures for anterior lamellar repair include:

- The Mustarde cheek rotation
- The median forehead flap

Full-thickness defects in the upper lid can be repaired using:

- Primary closure
- Primary closure with canthotomy and cantholysis
- The Cutler Beard procedure (for more than half of the upper lid)
- Free tarsal graft and myocutaneous advancement of skin fold
- Staggered anterior and posterior lamellar grafts

Suggested reading

1. American Academy of Ophthalmology: *Basic and clinical science course: orbit, eyelids, and lacrimal system*, sect. 7, pp. 167–191, San Francisco: American Academy of Ophthalmology, 1998/1999.

2. Anderson RL, Gordy DD: The tarsal strip procedure. *Arch Ophthalmol* 97:2192–2196, 1979.

3. Collin JRO: Eyelid reconstruction and tumour management. In *A manual of systematic eyelid surgery*, 3rd edn, pp. 147–164, Butterworth Heinemann Elsevier, 2006.

4. Dailey RA, Habrich D: Medial canthal reconstruction. In Bosniak S, ed., *Principles and practice of ophthalmic plastic and reconstructive surgery*, vol. 2, pp. 387–399, Philadelphia: WB Saunders, 1996.

5. Jackson IT, ed.: *Local flaps in head and neck reconstruction.* St Louis: CV Mosby, 1985.

6. Jordan D: Reconstruction of the upper eyelid. In Bosniak S, ed., *Principles and practice of ophthalmic plastic and reconstructive surgery*, vol. 2, ch. 34, pp. 356–386, Philadelphia: WB Saunders, 1996.

7. McCord CD: System of repair of full-thickness eyelid defects. In McCord CD, Tanenbaum M, Nunery WR, eds, *Oculoplastic surgery*, 3rd edn, ch. 3, pp. 85–97, New York: Raven Press, 1995.

8. McCord CD, Nunery WR, Tanenbaum M: Reconstruction of the lower eyelid and outer canthus. In McCord CD, Tanenbaum M, Nunery WR, eds, *Oculoplastic surgery*, 3rd edn, ch. 5, pp. 119–144, New York: Raven Press, 1995.

9. Nerad J: Diagnosis of malignant and benign lid lesions made easy. In *The requisites—Oculoplastic surgery*, pp. 282–311, St Louis: Mosby, 2001.

10. Patrinely JR, Marines HM, Anderson RL: Skin flaps in periorbital reconstruction. *Surv Ophthalmol* 31(4):249–261, 1987.

11. Rivlin D, Moy RL: Mohs' surgery for periorbital malignancies. In Bosniak S, ed., *Principles and practice of ophthalmic plastic and reconstructive surgery*, vol. 2, pp. 352–355, Philadelphia: WB Saunders, 1996.

12. Weinstein GS, Anderson RL, Tse DT, Kersten RC: The use of a periosteal strip for eyelid reconstruction. *Arch Ophthalmol* 103(3):357–359, 1985.

13. Wesley RE, McCord CD: Reconstruction of the upper eyelid and medial canthus. In McCord CD, Tanenbaum M, Nunery WR, eds, *Oculoplastic surgery*, 3rd edn, ch. 4, pp. 99–117, New York: Raven Press, 1995.

Eyelid and Orbital Trauma

Introduction

The patient's medical condition must be stabilized before you will be able to determine the full extent of any injuries to the eye, orbit, or head. A history that recalls the details of the trauma will help you to determine if a facial fracture or deep orbital penetration is likely to have occurred. Next you will perform a systematic evaluation of the eye and periocular tissues. The presence of any orbital fat in the wound suggests the possibility of deeper injury to the eye, orbit, or brain. These patients need imaging of the orbit and brain.

Trauma is divided into soft tissue injury and bone injury. First, we will discuss the types of soft tissue injuries that you are likely to see. You should learn the techniques for repair of soft tissue injury, including suturing of simple and complex lacerations. With some practice, you can learn the techniques for repair of lid margin and canalicular lacerations.

You will see fractures involving the calvarium, face, and mandible. The facial bones break in predictable patterns associated with specific findings that you will learn to recognize on examination. Common orbital fractures include blowout fractures, zygomaticomaxillary complex fractures, naso-orbital ethmoid fractures, and Le Fort fractures. The symptoms of diplopia and hypesthesia of the infraorbital nerve should make you suspect an orbital floor fracture. On examination, look for decreased eye movements, enophthalmos, or any deformity of the orbital rims or face. After viewing the computed tomography (CT) scan of the facial bones, you will be able to determine the type of fracture and make a plan for repair if necessary.

The surgical approach to the repair of orbital fractures is through a combination of periocular and/or transoral incisions. After anatomic realignment and fixation of the facial skeleton, thin implants are used to reconstruct the orbital floor and medial wall, as needed. In most patients, substantial improvements in the structure and function of the orbit are possible. We will cover the surgical approach for the treatment of a blowout fracture in detail. We won't cover the details of the repair of all facial fractures, but you should learn the principles of repair.

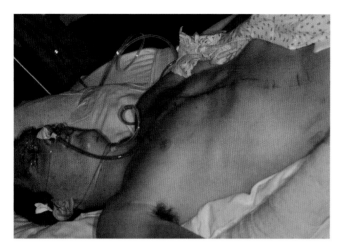

Figure 13-1 Cardiac contusion caused by the seat belt following a motor vehicle accident. His other injuries included a severe eyelid laceration.

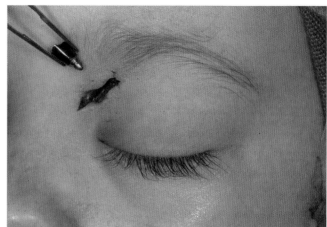

Figure 13-2 Unsuspected foreign body found in a laceration in a child injured at preschool.

Evaluation of the trauma patient

History

Periocular trauma can occur as an isolated injury or as a small part of multisystem trauma. You must make sure that the patient's cardiopulmonary and neurologic status is stable before your evaluation and treatment of any ocular or periocular injury (Figure 13-1). Evaluation of the eye precedes evaluation of the soft tissue and bones. You must prevent further injury to the eye as a result of manipulation of the surrounding tissues.

Try to obtain some history about how the injury occurred. A broad area of superficial involvement may initially look worse than a small puncture wound. The puncture wound may extend deeply, causing injuries to the eye, orbital contents, or brain, a much more serious situation than the superficial abrasion. If it appears possible that there was deep penetration into the orbit, try to determine what instrument caused the injury to give you some information about the depth of penetration and the possibility of the presence of a foreign body that may have broken off. Symptoms of diplopia or hypesthesia of the infraorbital nerve should suggest an orbital fracture. Always be skeptical about the history if alcohol was involved or if the patient is a child. Alcohol use has a way of distorting a patient's perception of the facts. Children may not give an accurate history, fearing they may get in trouble with their parents (Figure 13-2). Your examination will help you decide if the history is plausible and if imaging studies are necessary to rule out injury to deep tissues (Box 13-1).

Take a general medical history to make sure that the patient is able to tolerate local or general anesthesia. You need to know when the patient last ate or drank if you are considering general anesthesia. Inquire about recent tetanus injections.

Photographs

Take photographs of the patient before cleaning the wounds. These photographs should document the severity of the injury for medicolegal documentation. Occasionally, after repair, your patient may be unhappy with your best attempts to

---

Box 13-1

Examination for Periocular Soft Tissue Trauma

Ensure stable neurologic and cardiopulmonary status

Eye examination

Eyelid examination

- Lid margin laceration
- Canalicular injury
- Anterior lamellar injury
  - Presence of preaponeurotic fat in the wound
  - Levator muscle or aponeurosis damage

Periocular examination

- Describe injury and extent
- Check facial nerve function
  - Trunk injury
  - Frontal nerve injury

---

reconstruct the facial injuries. These photographs can remind the patient of the severity of the initial injury. In some cases, photographs may provide some legal defense of your efforts.

Examination of the soft tissues

The eye

We won't go into much detail about examining the eye. Remember that eye injuries commonly occur with facial trauma. As always, measuring the vision is an essential part of the eye examination. You must explain any acuity measurement that is not normal. This can be difficult if the patient is lethargic, intoxicated, or otherwise uncooperative. Remember to check the visual acuity on both sides. In an uncooperative patient, a vision of 20/20 OD and 20/100 OS is much more suggestive of an injury to the visual system than an acuity of 20/100 OU. If you can't explain the decrease in visual acuity as being caused by an injury to the eye itself, consider the possibility of damage to the optic nerve, a traumatic optic neuropathy. We will discuss traumatic optic neuropathy in more detail in the section on facial fractures later in this chapter.

The eyelids

Next inspect the eyelids. Note the location, extent, and severity of injury to the soft tissues. Draw a diagram to describe the soft tissue injury. Develop a routine for examination of the soft tissue. Start with inspection of the continuity of the lid margins. Pay special attention to the lid margins medial to the puncta so you will not miss a canalicular laceration (Figure 13-3). If you suspect a canalicular laceration, pass a 1-0 or smaller Bowman probe through the punctum and inspect the canaliculus. You may be surprised to know that most canalicular lacerations do not occur from direct trauma of the medial lid. Most are the result of an avulsion or tear that occurs when the lid or cheek is pulled laterally. This explains why the patient who has been punched with a fist on the zygoma can be seen with a lower canalicular laceration.

Examine the anterior lamella of the eyelids. The presence of orbital fat in a wound means that the orbital septum has been violated and that there is a possibility of deeper orbital injury. Observe the upper eyelid movement to ensure that the levator muscle has not been damaged.

Next examine the more peripheral periocular areas. If a laceration has occurred near the trunk of the facial nerve, check for normal facial movements. If you suspect that the nerve has been damaged, primary nerve reanastomosis by a surgeon trained in this procedure may be required. If the injury is near the brow, check to make sure that the frontal nerve branch is intact. Clearly document any abnormality.

Soft tissue injuries

Soft tissue injuries are classified as:

- Contusion
- Abrasion
- Avulsion
- Puncture
- Laceration
  — Simple or complex
  — Superficial or deep

Contusions and abrasions do not require surgical repair. Cleaning and use of topical antibiotics and ice are appropriate. Avulsions imply a tearing of the tissue, sometimes separating with loss of tissue. Tearing often occurs with injuries

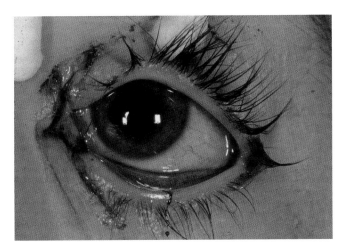

Figure 13-3 Canalicular lacerations of upper and lower eyelids.

on pavement, but loss of tissue is extraordinarily rare. Remember that wounds usually spread open, making them look like tissue may be lost. Punctures are caused by long sharp objects that create small entrance wounds, but may extend deeply. Lacerations are caused by sharp objects. "Clean cuts" or simple lacerations require only single-layer closure and heal with minimal scarring. Complex lacerations have extensive "jagged" edges that extend into deeper layers of tissue. These lacerations may require several hours of layered closure but, with good technique, the results can be spectacular (Figure 13-4). Canalicular and lid margin lacerations require special techniques that you can master with some instruction and practice.

Checkpoint

At this point, you should be able to evaluate the patient with soft tissue facial injuries. You have established that the patient's neurologic and cardiopulmonary status is stable. You have evaluated the eye. The history gives you an idea about what injuries you might expect. You should be able to describe the injuries.

- Recall the steps of a systematic evaluation of the soft tissues. Write down the information in Box 13-2 and memorize it.
- What would make you suspect that a canalicular laceration has occurred? What are the possible mechanisms for this injury?
- What is the significance of fat in an eyelid wound? What layers of the eyelid have been disrupted? What are you concerned about?
- When you evaluate a patient, consider the type and mechanism of soft tissue injury. This information will help you to develop a plan for repair.
- Don't forget to evaluate for deep injuries that may involve the eye or brain.

Repair of soft tissue trauma

Preparation

Small, simple lacerations are usually repaired with local anesthesia in adults and children. New tissue adhesives are available that show promise for repairing small lacerations without anesthesia, which can be especially helpful in

---

Box 13-2

Soft Tissue Injuries

- Contusion
- Abrasion
- Avulsion
- Puncture
- Laceration
  - Simple or complex
  - Superficial or deep
  - Lid margin
  - Canalicular

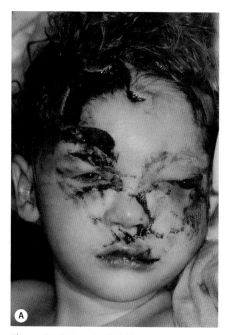
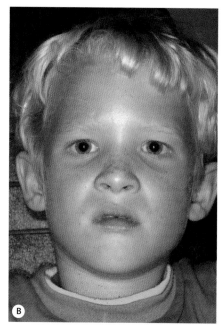

Figure 13-4 Complex facial lacerations caused by a dog bite. (**A**) Initial injury. (**B**) Final result after repair and scar maturation.

children. More complex lacerations should be repaired with general anesthesia. Facial lacerations should be repaired within 12–24 hours. Operations for life- or vision-threatening conditions take priority over laceration repair. Fractures associated with facial lacerations are either repaired at the time of laceration repair or after 3–5 days when the facial swelling resolves. The specific timing for blowout fracture repair will be discussed later. Although facial lacerations rarely become infected, prophylactic broad-spectrum antibiotics, usually a first-generation cephalosporin, are prescribed for 1 week.

In the operating room, the wounds should be injected with local anesthetic containing epinephrine. All foreign bodies should be removed from the wounds. Vigorous cleaning and irrigation should be performed to minimize the chance of infection and tattooing of the skin with foreign materials.

Anterior lamellar repair

Before repair of any laceration, explore the depths of the wound to ensure that deeper injury has not occurred. Any visible orbital fat means that the orbital septum has been violated (Figure 13-5). Make sure that you are not dealing with a potentially more serious injury involving damage to the orbital contents or brain (Figure 13-6). If the laceration occurs perpendicular to the orbicularis fibers and the wound is pulled open, placement of deep absorbable sutures in the muscle will help to approximate the wound edges without tension on the skin closure.

Lacerations parallel to the orbicularis muscle do not require closure of the muscle layer. Placement of interrupted permanent skin sutures that bisect the wound in successive halves prevent the formation of a "dog-ear" (redundant tissue on one side of the wound noted at the completion of closure). A running suture can be used for longer straight lacerations, but this does not permit individual removal of sutures if any infection should occur. Suitable sutures for

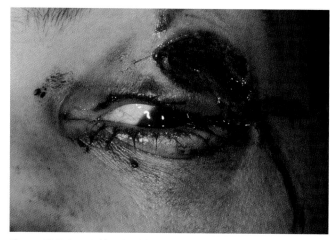

Figure 13-5 Any visible orbital fat means that the septum has been violated. Rule out injury to eye, orbit, or brain and the possibility of the presence of a foreign body.

eyelid skin closure include 6-0 and 7-0 nylon using a reverse cutting needle. Lacerations of the brow in thicker skin can be closed with 4-0 or 5-0 nylon sutures. Blue 5-0 Prolene sutures are especially useful in the brow, where black sutures can easily be confused with eyebrow hairs. A layered closure can be used in the dermis or subcutaneous tissues to remove tension from the skin edges. Do not close the orbital septum. Lagophthalmos may result.

Complex laceration repair

Complex lacerations have many jagged edges and extend into deeper tissue layers. Repair of a complex laceration is like building a jigsaw puzzle. First, you start with pieces of the puzzle that you can identify, the edges and corners, and put them together. Then you fill in the missing areas in the center of the puzzle, looking for less obvious details to guide you.

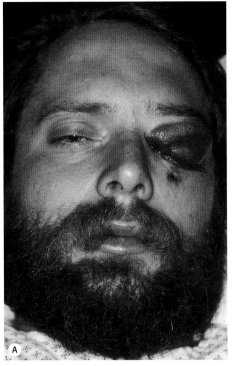

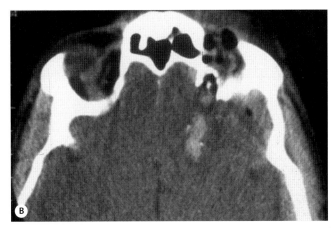

Figure 13-6 Deep orbital penetration through a small skin wound at the inferior orbital rim. (**A**) The patient had a small laceration and ecchymosis after falling on a tree branch. (**B**) Total ophthalmoplegia and no light perception (NLP) vision were noted as a result of penetration of the branch through the orbit and into the brain.

The steps of complex laceration repair are:

1. Clean and inspect the wound (Figure 13-7, A–C)
   A. Rule out deep injury.
   B. Remove any foreign material.
   C. Do not debride any tissue. You will be surprised how well this tissue survives.
2. Repair the deep layer
   A. To begin the laceration repair, identify anatomic landmarks such as the eyebrow, the lid margin, and the canthus (Figure 13-7, D).
   B. Place deep sutures to reposition the anatomic landmarks in proper alignment.
   C. In some cases, temporary "tacking" sutures of large caliber (2-0, 3-0, or 4-0) can be placed full thickness through the skin to help with the orientation of tissues and take tension off the wound while deep layers are being closed. These temporary sutures are removed as the wound comes together.
   D. Start with the deepest layers of closure first, including any posterior lamellar repair of conjunctiva, tarsus, canthal tendons, or levator aponeurosis (Figure 13-7, E).
   E. Close the subcutaneous layer with buried absorbable long-lasting sutures such as 4-0 and 5-0 Vicryl or PDS sutures. In large lacerations extending on the scalp, 3-0 PDS sutures are appropriate. Use a reverse cutting needle for these closures. If you are unhappy with the position of a deep suture, replace it. The final skin closure cannot compensate for poor deep closure alignment.
   F. Complete the deep closure before starting closure of the superficial layer.

3. Close the superficial layer
   A. Approximate the edges of the skin with interrupted sutures (Figure 13-7, F).
   B. Most commonly, 6-0 and 7-0 nylon sutures are used on the eyelids, and 4-0 and 5-0 nylon sutures are used in the thicker periocular skin.
   C. You can use absorbable sutures such as 5-0 or 6-0 fast absorbing gut for the final skin closure (Figure 13-7, G).
   D. Use a topical antibiotic ointment such as erythromycin, placed over the wound.
   E. Dressings are not necessary.

Suture removal should be done between 5 and 10 days after surgery. If you are removing sutures early, you may want to remove every other suture initially and have the patient return a few days later for removal of the remaining sutures. Superficial wound healing occurs within the first week or two. Scar maturation does not occur until 6–12 months after surgery. You need to be supportive during this period. Avoid revisions until all healing is complete and scars are flat and nonerythematous (Box 13-3).

Lid margin repair

You will see lid margin lacerations as isolated minor injuries or in the context of large facial wounds (Figure 13-7, Box 13-4). The technique for repair is the same in either situation. Repair begins with identifying the appropriate anatomic landmarks of the eyelid, especially the landmarks of the lid margin. The strength of the closure is in sutures placed in the tarsal plate. Eyelid margin eversion is necessary to prevent lid notching.

Eyelid margin repair includes:

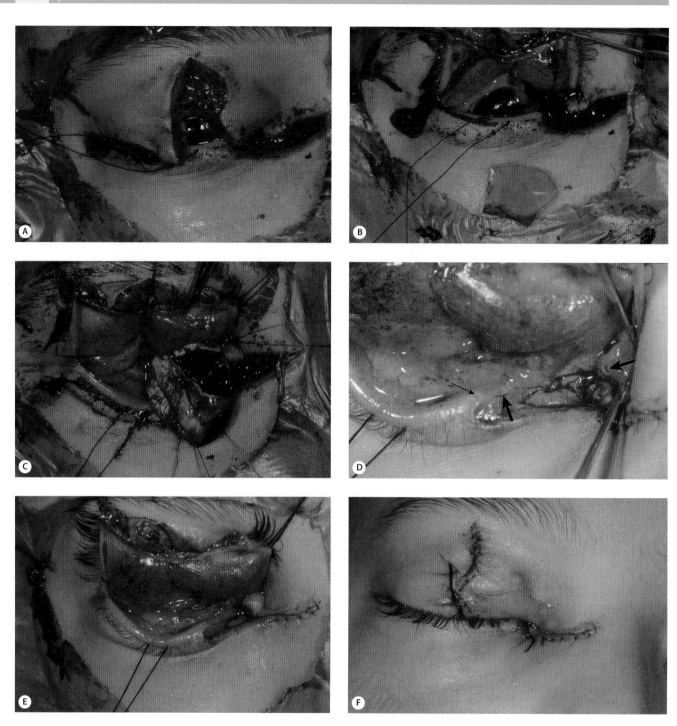

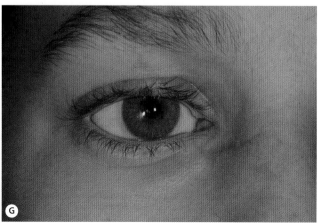

Figure 13-7 Eyelid laceration resulting from an explosion of a bottle containing dry ice. Complex laceration repair series. (**A**) Upper eyelid and medial canthal lacerations. The eye is soft and filled with blood. (**B**) A large piece of glass penetrated the cornea. (**C**) Primary enucleation was performed. (**D**) A canalicular laceration was identified and repaired (small arrow points to punctum; large arrows point to cut ends of canaliculus). (**E**) The posterior lamella and eyelid were repaired. (**F**) The anterior lamella was repaired last. (**G**) Nine months after repair with ocular prosthesis in place.

- Injecting local anesthetic
- Aligning the lid margin
- Suturing the tarsal plate
- Suturing the lid margin
- Closing the skin

The steps of eyelid margin repair are:

1. Inject local anesthetic
   A. Repair can be done with local or general anesthesia.
   B. Instill topical anesthetic drops and inject local anesthetic with epinephrine into the wound.
2. Align the lid margin: Use a 7-0 Vicryl vertical mattress suture passed through meibomian gland orifices to align the lid margin. Keep this suture long for traction (Figure 13-8, A).
3. Suture the tarsal plate: Use two or three interrupted 5-0 Vicryl sutures passed in a lamellar fashion to align the tarsal plate. Traction on the initial lid margin suture will help with the positioning of your tarsal sutures (Figure 13-8, B).
4. Suture the lid margin
   A. Go back to the lid margin and place an additional 7-0 Vicryl vertical mattress suture anterior to the gray line. The vertical mattress sutures should provide eversion of the lid margin wound (Figure 13-8, C).
   B. If you are unhappy with the alignment of the lid margin, replace the sutures.
   C. An additional anterior suture may be used to help the alignment of the eyelashes (Figure 13-8, D).
   D. I prefer to use 7-0 Vicryl sutures for the eyelid margin. Traditional teaching suggests the use of 6-0 or 8-0 silk sutures, which should be left long and require removal later. The 7-0 Vicryl sutures can be cut on the knot and allowed to absorb.
   E. Don't tie the margin sutures very tightly because the tissue may die, resulting in a lid margin notch.
5. Close the skin
   A. The skin can be closed with an interrupted simple or vertical suture using permanent or absorbable sutures (Figure 13-8, D).
   B. If the wound seems to be under tension, you may want to place 5-0 Vicryl sutures through the orbicularis muscle before closing the skin.

Postoperative care is routine. Occasionally, the sutures will rub against the cornea and require removal.

Canalicular reconstruction

Diagnosis of canalicular laceration

Assume that the canaliculus has been cut if there is any injury extending close to the lid margin medial to the puncta of the eyelids (Figure 13-9). If there is any question, confirm the presence of a laceration by passing a probe through the canaliculus. Canalicular lacerations may occur because of a laceration from direct trauma to the canaliculus or, as stated above, as a result of an avulsion from lateral tension on the eyelid. Direct laceration of the canaliculus is easier to fix than an avulsion type injury. Direct lacerations involve the middle portion of the canaliculus, making it easier to find and repair the ends of the lacerated canaliculus. Avulsion type injuries generally tear the canaliculus close to the sac, making visualization of the proximal cut end of the canaliculus difficult. For these injuries, the operating microscope is helpful.

Remember, suspect a canalicular laceration when there is any laceration at or near the medial canthus of the upper or

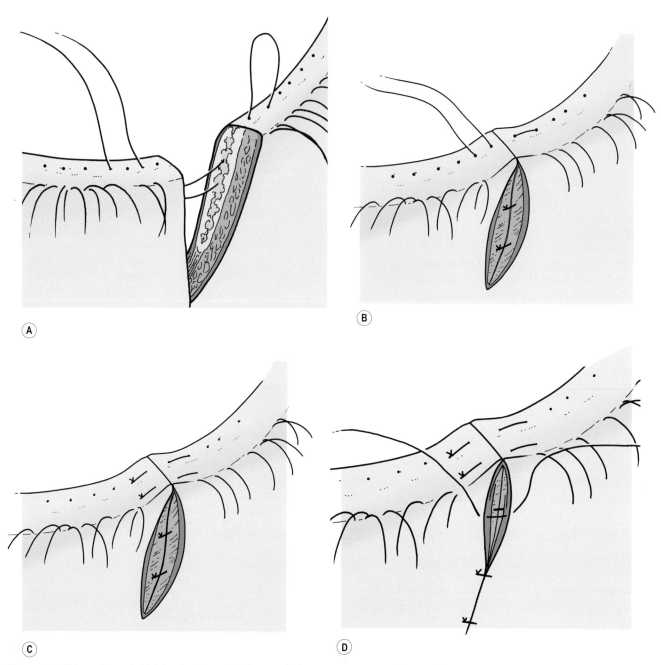

Figure 13-8 Lid margin repair. (**A**) Align the lid margin using a vertical mattress suture passed through the meibomian gland orifices. (**B**) Suture the tarsal plate using two or three interrupted sutures passed in a lamellar fashion. (**C**) Suture the lid margin using an additional vertical mattress suture anterior to the gray line. (**D**) Close the skin.

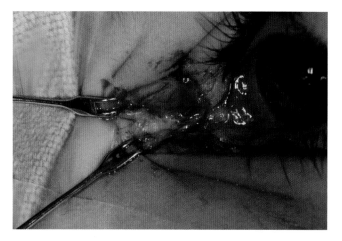

Figure 13-9 Suspect canalicular laceration if there is any trauma medial to the puncta. Note the probe in the torn edge of the canaliculus.

lower lid. Repair of the laceration without special attention to the canaliculus will likely cause occlusion. Approximately 50% of young adult patients will have tearing if one canaliculus is occluded. This percentage is less for older adults. The upper and lower canaliculus contribute nearly equally to the drainage of tears. In most patients, you should attempt to repair the lacerated canaliculus.

Repair of canalicular laceration

> **Box 13-5**
>
> **Canalicular Laceration Repair Using Crawford Stents**
> **Identify cut ends of the canaliculus**
> - A white or pink mucosal ring
> - More difficult to find if lid is avulsed, not cut
> - Operating microscope is helpful
>
> **Pass the stent through the canaliculus**
> - Pass the stent into the punctum and out the distal end of the cut canaliculus
> - Then pass the stent in the cut end of the canaliculus to the sac
>
> **Pass the stent down the nasolacrimal duct**
> - Consider curving the probe in an adult
> - Intubate the opposite canaliculus
> - Retrieve the stent in the nose
>
> **Suture the pericanalicular tissue around the stent**
> - Appose the mucosa with two or three 7-0 Vicryl sutures
> - If the laceration is at the junction of the canaliculus and the sac, it is worth trying to use additional 4-0 Vicryl sutures to reinforce the medial canthal tendon
> - The difficult part of the procedure is over at this point
>
> **Tie the stent in the nose**
>
> **Suture the skin**
>
> **Apply topical antibiotic ointment**

The goal of canalicular laceration repair is to reunite the torn edges of the canalicular mucosa in anatomic alignment. If the wound is deep, the medial canthal tendon will need to be repaired. Use of the operating microscope is helpful for finding the cut ends of the canaliculus and for facilitating repair. The microscope not only provides excellent magnification and illumination, but it also allows both you and your assistant to see the wound without bumping heads in a narrow space. You will pass a silicone stent through the canaliculus as part of the reconstruction to prevent cicatricial changes from closing the canaliculus postoperatively.

Three intubation techniques are used to repair the torn canaliculus:

- Repair using bicanalicular intubation with nasolacrimal duct intubation using Crawford stents
- Repair using bicanalicular intubation with the pigtail probe
- Repair with a monocanalicular stent

The first technique uses standard Crawford stents for intubation of the canaliculi and the nasolacrimal duct (Figure 13-10, A). The second technique requires intubation of only the canalicular system using a pigtail probe (Figure 13-10, B). Several types of monocanalicular stents are available.

Each technique has advantages and disadvantages. You are probably more familiar with intubation of the lacrimal system using Crawford stents. A disadvantage of this technique is that it is difficult to intubate through the duct into the nose using local anesthesia alone. As an alternative to nasolacrimal intubation, you can intubate only the canalicular system using a pigtail probe. The pigtail probe technique has two advantages. First, general anesthesia is not required because no intubation of the nasolacrimal duct is performed. Second, rotation of the pigtail probe through an intact canaliculus will show you the cut proximal end of the canaliculus. The pigtail probe technique has some disadvantages. The probe only works if there is a true common canaliculus. In a small percentage of patients, the upper and lower canaliculi enter the sac independently. In these patients, the pigtail probe cannot be threaded through the system, and Crawford stents are necessary.

You may have been biased by older literature condemning the pigtail probe. Despite its poor reputation, the pigtail probe can be used successfully in all but a small percentage of patients. Intubation of the canaliculi with the pigtail probe is more difficult than using Crawford stents, but no retrieval of the stent in the nose is required. Try to learn both techniques (Box 13-5 and Box 13-6).

Canalicular repair using Crawford stents includes:

- Identifying the cut ends of the canaliculus
- Passing the stent through the torn canaliculus
- Passing the stent into the nasolacrimal duct
- Suturing the pericanalicular tissue
- Passing the other stent through the nose

The steps of canalicular laceration repair using Crawford stents are:

1. Identify the cut ends of the canaliculus
   A. It is easy to identify the cut ends of the canaliculus if the lid margin itself has been directly cut. The mucosa of the canaliculus is visible as a white or pink ring of mucosa (Figure 13-11). It is much more difficult to identify the cut end of the canaliculus if it has been avulsed at the lacrimal sac. A microscope is helpful in all canalicular laceration repairs, but especially for avulsions because the laceration is deep in the medial canthus.
2. Pass the stent through the canaliculus
   A. Thread the stent through the punctum and out the distal end of the lacerated canaliculus (Figure 13-12, A).
   B. Next, thread the stent to the proximal end of the canaliculus.
3. Pass the stent down the nasolacrimal duct (Figure 13-12, B)
   A. This step is similar to all nasolacrimal duct probings. If you are intubating an adult, it is helpful to bend the probe of the stent into a curve to maneuver around a prominent brow. Intubation of adults requires somewhat more manipulation than intubation of children.
   B. Retrieve the stent and pull it out of the nose (use either an Anderson–Hwang grooved director or a Crawford hook; see Chapter 10 for tips on this technique).
   C. Repeat for the opposite canaliculus (see Figure 13-12, B).

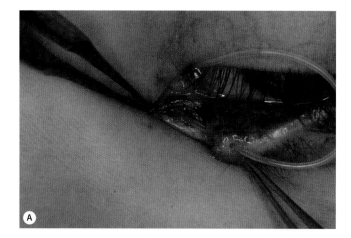

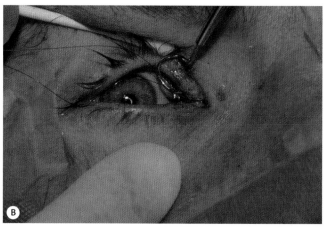

Figure 13-10 Three techniques for canalicular laceration repair. (**A**) Bicanalicular and nasolacrimal duct intubation with Crawford stents. (**B**) The pigtail probe technique for repair of canalicular lacerations, requiring intubation of only the canaliculi. (**C**) Monocanalicular stent being inserted into upper canaliculus.

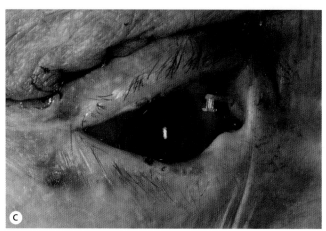

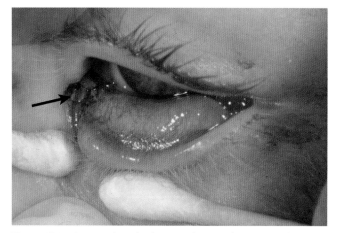

Figure 13-11 Lacerated canaliculus: note the ring of mucosa on the proximal side of the lacerated canaliculus (arrow).

4. Suture the pericanalicular tissue around the stent
   A. If the laceration is at the junction of the canaliculus and the sac, it is worth using additional 4-0 Vicryl sutures (P-2 needle) to reinforce the medial canthal tendon before suturing the pericanalicular tissues (Figure 13-12, C).
   B. Ideally, the mucosal edges of the cut canaliculus should be apposed with suturing. It is not necessary to sew the mucosal edges together, but you should suture the pericanalicular tissue, bringing the mucosal edges together as much as possible. Two or

three 7-0 Vicryl sutures are used for this purpose (Figure 13-12, D). The difficult part of the procedure is over at this point.

5. Tie the stents
   A. Tie the stent in the nose. Be careful not to tie the knot too high so that it retracts into the nasolacrimal duct.
   B. Be careful not to tie the stent too low so that the knot hangs out of the nose.

6. Suture the skin
   A. The skin can be sutured with either an absorbable or a permanent suture, usually 6-0 or 7-0 in size (Figure 13-12, E).

7. Apply topical antibiotic ointment

Canalicular laceration repair using a pigtail probe includes:

- Passing the pigtail probe
- Threading a 6-0 nylon suture through the canalicular system
- Passing the stent through the canalicular system
- Suturing the pericanalicular tissue
- Tying the nylon suture
- Suturing the skin

The pigtail probe technique has been useful for me in many patients. Initially, the technique is somewhat more complex than nasolacrimal duct intubation. Remember that you do not need to use general anesthesia because you do not intubate the nasolacrimal duct.

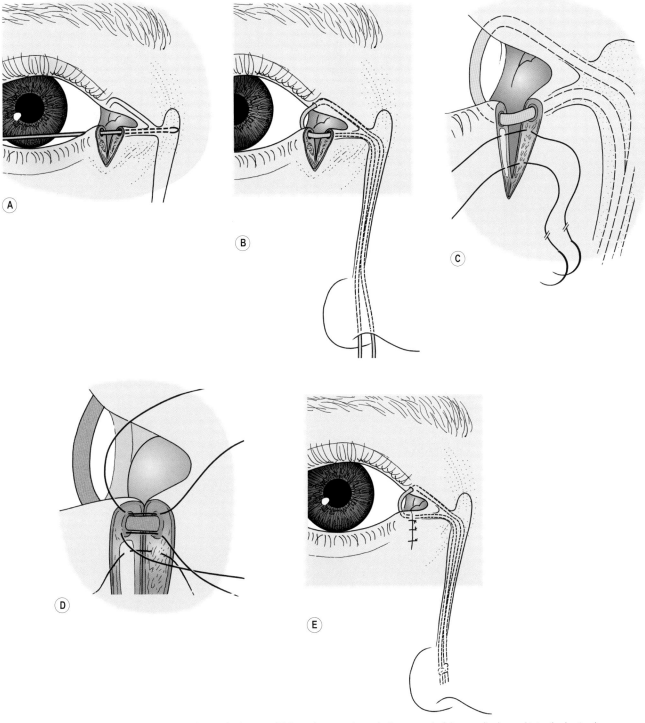

Figure 13-12 Canalicular laceration repair with Crawford stents. (**A**) Pass the stent through the cut end of the canaliculus and into the lacrimal sac. (**B**) Intubate the opposite canaliculus and nasolacrimal duct. (**C**) Reinforce the medial canthal tendon with a 4-0 Vicryl suture. (**D**) Approximate the canalicular mucosa using sutures in the canalicular mucosa or adjacent tissues. (**E**) Use additional sutures in the orbicularis muscle as required to reinforce the wound. Suture the skin. Tie the stents in the nose.

The steps of the canalicular laceration repair using a pigtail probe are:

1. Pass the pigtail probe (Figure 13-13, A)
   A. Use the pigtail probe with a closed needle eye, not an open hook as used several decades ago.

B. Choose the end of the pigtail probe that corresponds to the direction of rotation required. The curves on the ends of the pigtail probe are opposite in direction.

C. Place the tip of the pigtail probe through the intact punctum and rotate it through the normal

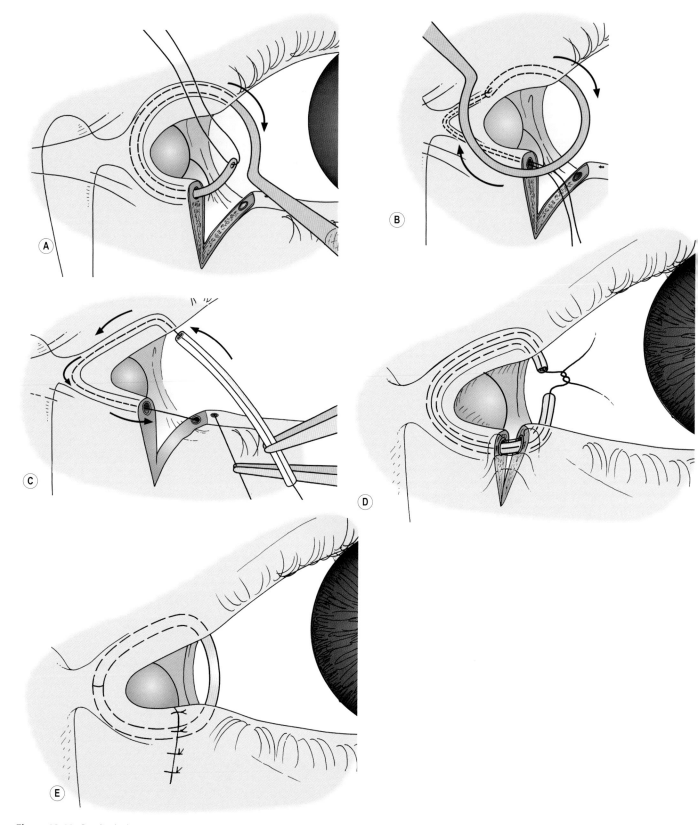

Figure 13-13 Canalicular laceration repair with the pigtail probe. (**A**) Choose the appropriate curve of the probe. Note the closed needle eye. Enter the normal punctum and rotate the probe posterior to the medial canthal tendon. The probe emerges from the cut end of the canaliculus. Thread a 6-0 nylon suture through the eye of the probe. (**B**) Rotate the 6-0 nylon suture through the canaliculus. (**C**) Thread the suture though the remaining canaliculus and punctum. Thread 25 mm of stent material over the suture. Grasp the stent over the suture with a smooth forceps and pull the opposite end of the suture to rotate the stent in place. (**D**) The stent is threaded through the remainder of the cut canaliculus and punctum. Repair the pericanalicular tissues as in **Figure 13-12**. Tie the 6-0 nylon suture with the knot retracting into the stent. (**E**) Rotate the stent "ring," placing the knot in the canaliculus. Close the skin.

canaliculus to the medial canthus. At this point, the handle of the probe should be oriented vertically perpendicular to the coronal plane of the patient.

D. *At the medial canthus, the probe should go posterior to the medial canthal tendon.* You will know that you are in the correct position if you lift the probe toward the ceiling of the operating room and meet resistance at the canthus.

E. Use gentle pressure to guide the pigtail probe through the common canaliculus. The probe should emerge through the cut proximal end of the canaliculus without exerting much pressure.

F. If the probe does not pass easily, try threading the probe through the cut proximal end of the other canaliculus (you lose the advantage of not having to find the canaliculus). If this doesn't work, switch to Crawford stents. You have encountered one of the few patients who does not have a common canaliculus.

2. Thread a suture through the canalicular system (see Figure 13-13, A and B)

A. Thread a 6-0 nylon suture (no needle) through the eye of the probe (see Figure 13-13, A) and rotate the probe out of the intact canaliculus (see Figure 13-13, B).

B. Pass the pigtail probe into the punctum of the torn canaliculus and out the distal end of the cut canaliculus. Thread the suture through the eye of the needle and rotate the probe out the punctum.

C. At this point, the 6-0 nylon suture will be through the upper and lower canaliculus.

3. Pass the stent through the canalicular system (Figure 13-13, C)

A. Cut a piece of silicone tubing 25 mm in length (for kids, slightly shorter).

(1) This tubing can be broken off from a Crawford stent or can be ordered separately (Storz E4251). The silicone stent measures 0.125 mm (inner diameter) by 0.250 mm (outer diameter).

(2) Stent material is also available with a blue Prolene suture prethreaded (FCI Ophthalmics, S1-1900, http://www.FCI-ophthalmics.com).

B. Use your fingers and a smooth forceps to thread the piece of stent over the nylon suture.

C. You will now pull the suture and the stent through the canaliculus. To do so, grasp the silicone stent tightly with a smooth forceps, squeezing the suture within the stent.

D. Pull the opposite end of the 6-0 nylon suture and guide the piece of stent material into the punctum of the intact canaliculus. As you pull, the suture, the stent will travel through the canalicular system and out the cut canaliculus (see Figure 13-13, C).

E. Again, guide the stent through the cut end of the canaliculus and out the punctum. The canaliculi are now intubated.

4. Suture the pericanalicular tissue

A. Use the same technique as that described above for suturing the pericanalicular tissue to appose the mucosa of the cut canaliculus. You may want to place a small hemostat or "bulldog" clamp on the ends of the nylon suture to secure it while you repair the canaliculus.

5. Tie the nylon suture

A. Tie the 6-0 nylon suture with three single throws tight enough to pull the knot into the stent, but not so tight as to kink the circle of stent that you have created. Cut the tails of the knot short so they retract in the tubing (Figure 13-13, D).

B. Rotate the tube moving the knot out of the palpebral fissure into the canaliculus.

6. Suture the skin

A. Use a technique similar to that above to suture the skin (Figures 13-13, E and 13-14).

7. Apply antibiotic ointment

Postoperative care of the repaired canaliculus is routine. Apply topical antibiotic ointment for 1 week. Remove the stent in approximately 6 months. If the stent prolapses after nasolacrimal intubation with Crawford stents, removal of the stent will probably be necessary. A stent placed with a pigtail probe cannot prolapse. To remove a stent placed with a pigtail probe, rotate the knot between the lids and cut the knot. Pull the stent and suture out together.

A third option for repair of a single canalicular laceration is to use a monocanalicular stent. Two styles are available. The Mini Monoko style stent (FCI Ophthalmics, S1-1500u) is a short length of silicone that stents the external two thirds of the canaliculus. It is held in place by a punctal plug type fitting. This is easy to thread as it does not go into the sac or nasolacrimal duct. The Collarette Monoko style stent (FCI Ophthalmics, S1-1710u) has a wire introducer that passes the silicone stent through one canaliculus down the nasolacrimal duct into the nose. It is designed primarily for monocanalicular repair of congenital nasolacrimal duct obstruction, but can be used for a single canalicular laceration repair. Neither of the monocanalicular stents should be used for common canalicular avulsion type injuries.

You will be pleased at how well the tissues heal using any of these techniques. The majority of patients will not have tearing after your repair (Box 13-6).

Useful instruments and supplies for canalicular laceration repair include:

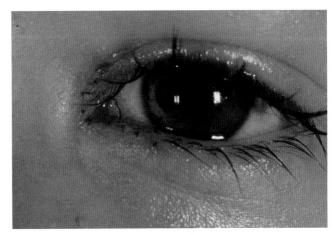

Figure 13-14 Canalicular laceration (see Figure 13-3) after repair with the pigtail probe technique. Note the nylon suture in the stent.

Box 13-6

Canalicular Repair Using the Pigtail Probe

Pass the pigtail probe

- Use the pigtail probe with a closed needle eye not an open hook
- Choose the end of the pigtail probe that corresponds to the direction of rotation required
- Rotate through the intact punctum to the medial canthus
- Go posterior to the medial canthal tendon. Use gentle pressure
- The probe emerges through the cut proximal end of the canaliculus

Thread the suture through the canalicular system

- Thread a 6-0 nylon suture through the eye of the probe and rotate the probe out of the intact canaliculus
- Pass the probe from the punctum of the torn canaliculus out of the end of the cut canaliculus
- Thread the suture through the eye of the needle and rotate the probe and suture out the punctum

Pass the stent through the canalicular system

- Cut a piece of silicone tubing to 25 mm in length
- Thread the piece of stent over the nylon suture
- Squeeze the stent and suture together with a smooth forceps
- Pull the opposite end of the suture, which will guide the stent through the canaliculus

Suture the pericanalicular tissue

- Use two or three 7-0 Vicryl sutures to get the mucosa close together
- Consider suturing the medial canthal tendon

Tie the nylon suture

- Tie the 6-0 nylon suture with three single throws
- Rotate the tube with the knot out of the palpebral fissure

Suture the skin

- Use interrupted 6-0 or 7-0 nylon or 7-0 Vicryl sutures

Apply antibiotic ointment

- Double-end lacrimal dilator, JEDMED Instrument Co. 58-0280, http://www.jedmed.com
- Double-end Bowman probe set, JEDMED Instrument Co. 58-0220, http://www.jedmed.com
- Bicanalicular intubation
  - Crawford intubation set, JEDMED Instrument Co. 28-0185 (without suture), 28-0184 (with suture), http://www.jedmed.com
  - Crawford hook, JEDMED Instrument Co. 28-0186, http://www.jedmed.com
  - Anderson–Hwang grooved director, JEDMED Instrument Co. 28-0189, http://www.jedmed.com
- Pigtail intubation
  - Pigtail probe, Storz instruments E4352 C, http://www.storz.com
  - Silicone stent material, Storz E4251
  - 6-0 nylon suture, Ethicon 1698 P-3 needle
- Monocanalicular intubation
  - Collarette Monoko, FCI Ophthalmics, S1-1710u. This stent has a wire introducer that passes the silicone through the nasolacrimal duct into the nose

  - Mini Monoko, FCI Ophthalmics, S1-1500u. This stent is silicone only and is recommended for repair of a single canaliculus less than two thirds of the distance to the medial canthus

Deep injury

Before we leave this section, I want to re-emphasize that, if you see orbital fat in a wound, you should consider the possibility of deep injury. Make sure that you have adequately evaluated the globe. You may find injury to deeper tissues such as the rectus muscles or the levator muscle. These tissues should be repaired as anatomically as possible. Make sure that you have ruled out the possibility of the presence of a foreign body in the orbit or intracranial penetration. Unless you are absolutely certain that these have not occurred, you should consider obtaining a CT scan.

Canthotomy and cantholysis

If vision is decreased or if there is an afferent pupillary defect in the presence of increased orbital pressure as a result of hemorrhage, consider doing a canthotomy and cantholysis. Check the intraocular pressure and look at the arterial circulation of the optic nerve. Pressure higher than 35–40 mmHg or decreased arterial flow (no flow or pulsing retinal arteries) should make your decision easy.

The canthotomy and cantholysis should be performed as an emergency procedure at the bedside or in the exam chair with local anesthesia.

The steps of the canthotomy and cantholysis are:

1. Inject local anesthetic
   A. Inject a generous amount of local anesthetic with epinephrine under the skin of the lateral canthus and subconjunctivally.
2. Perform a canthotomy
   A. Use Westcott or Stevens scissors to open the lateral canthus for 1 cm. A Colorado microdissection needle works well, but may not be available in an emergency situation.
   B. The canthotomy makes the Y of the lateral canthus into a V (Figure 13-15, A).
   C. The canthotomy *alone* will not decrease the orbital pressure.
3. Perform a cantholysis
   A. Pull the lid under tension toward the ceiling of the room (away from the patient's face). With the scissors turned 90 degrees to the eyelid margin, "strum" the deep tissue to find the crus. Cut this tissue until the lid releases from the rim. You do the same procedure on the lower crus when you do a lateral tarsal strip operation.
   B. The first cantholysis cuts one arm off the V (Figures 13-15, B and 13-16).
   C. You must cut the upper and lower crus of the lateral canthal tendon, cutting both arms off the V.
   D. Hold pressure on the wound. Cauterize as necessary.
4. Recheck the intraocular pressure and retinal blood flow
5. Don't close any wounds (Box 13-7)

- We have covered a large amount of material already. These principles will take care of 99% of soft tissue injuries that you will see.

- The repair of simple lacerations is straightforward. Remember to look for orbital fat and investigate further if you suspect injury to deeper tissues or the presence of a foreign body in the orbit. Check the globe carefully. Order a CT if you think cranio-orbital penetration or a foreign body is a possibility.

- Repair of complex lacerations can be extremely rewarding. Remember to identify landmarks, align the tissues with deep bites, and then close the deep layers and skin. "Tacking" sutures are helpful if you can't figure out how to align the wound. Don't forget to repair any deep injuries, such as the levator aponeurosis.

- Many types of surgeons can repair facial lacerations, but no one can do a better job repairing lid margin and canalicular lacerations than you. Your knowledge of the anatomy and sense of precise alignment of the tissues will give the patient the best result possible.

- Review the anatomy of the lid margin and the placement of the sutures for lid margin repair. Remember to put all the tension on the lamellar tarsal bites and to evert the lid margin with vertical mattress sutures.

- Using the microscope for the repair of canalicular lacerations is not mandatory, but the visualization is great and the repair will be meticulous. Consider using your abilities as a microsurgeon to give the patient the best possible result. Think about the pros and cons of the pigtail probe and the stent techniques. Each is useful.

Examination of the facial skeleton

Signs of facial fracture

The history that you have taken will give you some clues about whether the type and force of injury sustained could cause a facial fracture. You have already asked about diplo-pia and numbness of the infraorbital nerve. Several signs in your examination will point to the possibility of facial fracture. These signs include:

- Limited extraocular motility
- Hypesthesia of the infraorbital nerve
- Enophthalmos
- Epistaxis
- Epiphora
- Subcutaneous emphysema
- Facial deformity
  — Telecanthus
  — Globe ptosis
  — Flattening of the malar eminence
  — Rim discontinuity
- Trismus
- Malocclusion of the teeth

The examination of the patient with facial fractures may be limited if the patient is comatose or uncooperative. Most of the time you will be able to get a reasonable estimate of the degree of injury to the facial skeleton. *Your practical goal is to decide if the patient needs a CT scan.*

Assuming that the patient's condition is medically stable, your first priority is to ensure that the eye has not been damaged. Remember to record the visual acuity. You should be able to explain any asymmetry in acuity from one eye to the other. If the patient is uncooperative, testing for a relative afferent pupillary defect is helpful. Next, check for limitation of ocular motility. Asymmetry of versions suggests either muscle paresis or restriction (caused by tissue swelling or entrapment) and will require further evaluation when the swelling subsides. Epistaxis and subcutaneous emphysema occur when fractures extend into the nose or sinuses. Ask your patient to avoid nose blowing, which can force air into the orbit or other soft tissues (Figure 13-17). The pain of acute injury may predominate over symptoms of infraorbital hypesthesia and tearing, which may cause symptoms later (Box 13-8).

Acute swelling and hemorrhage may prevent you from seeing subtle degrees of facial deformity. Patients with large orbital fractures displacing the floor of the orbit or the body of the zygoma will have enophthalmos or globe displace-

---

Box 13-7

Canthotomy and Cantholysis

Inject local anesthesia

Perform a canthotomy

- Use Westcott or Stevens scissors to open the lateral canthus for 1 cm
- The canthotomy makes the Y of the lateral canthus into a V
- This will not decrease the orbital pressure

Perform a cantholysis

- Pull the lid under tension toward the ceiling (away from the patient's face)
- With the scissors turned 90 degrees to the eyelid margin, "strum" the deep tissue to find the crus and cut
- The first cantholysis cuts one arm off the V
- Repeat for upper and lower eyelids, cutting both arms off the V if necessary
- Don't close any wounds

Box 13-8

Signs of Facial Fracture

- Limited extraocular motility
- Hypesthesia of the infraorbital nerve
- Enophthalmos
- Epiphora
- Epistaxis
- Subcutaneous emphysema
- Facial deformity
  - Telecanthus
  - Globe ptosis
  - Flattening of the malar eminence
  - Rim discontinuity
- Trismus
- Malocclusion of the teeth

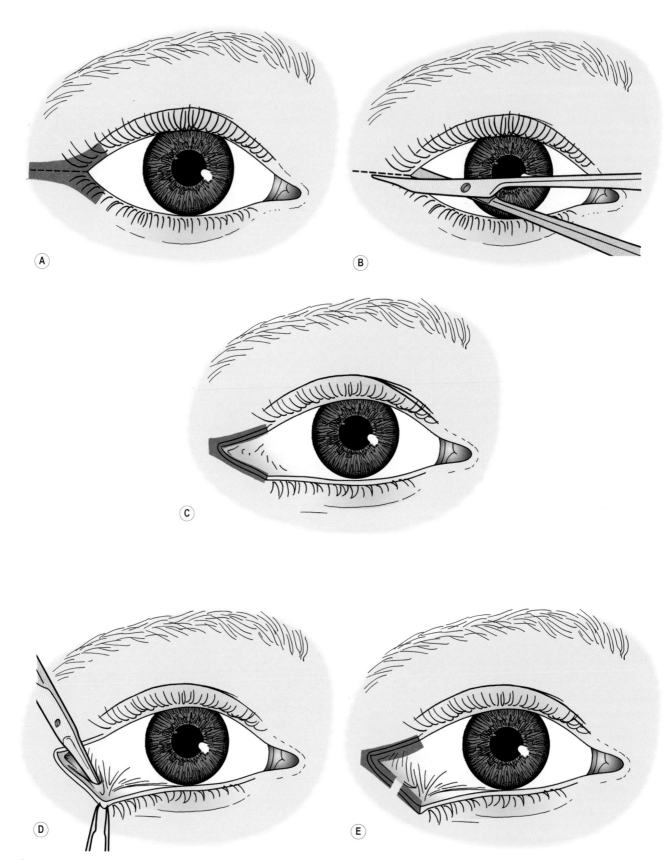

Figure 13-15 Lateral canthotomy and cantholysis. (**A**) The lateral canthal tendon forms a Y. (**B** and **C**) Canthotomy turns the Y into a V. (**D** and **E**) The cantholysis cuts one arm off the V. Pull the eyelid away from the rim and "strain" the tissues. Cut the tight bands, and the eyelid releases from the rim.

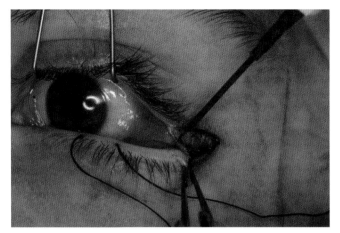

Figure 13-16 Cantholysis of the inferior limb of the lateral canthal tendon releases the lower eyelid from the rim.

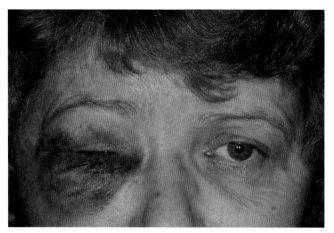

Figure 13-17 Subcutaneous emphysema indicating a fracture into the sinus. Crepitus of the skin is palpable in this patient.

ment. Commonly, enophthalmos may not be visible initially if there is orbital hemorrhage or swelling. Trauma to the bridge of the nose may cause telecanthus (tele-meaning "wide" or "distant") or posterior displacement "telescoping" of the naso-orbital complex. Look at the patient from below to detect the posterior displacement of the zygoma (flattening of the malar eminence) that often accompanies zygomaticomaxillary complex (ZMC) fractures.

Palpate the orbital rims for discontinuity. Specifically, check for a step-off or tenderness at the zygomaticomaxillary and frontozygomatic sutures. Palpate the zygomatic arch for deformity (often "bowing outward") or tenderness. Check for hypesthesia of the infraorbital nerve with a cotton tip applicator. Ask the patient to open the mouth widely. The inability to open the mouth, termed trismus, suggests a depressed zygomatic arch or contusion of the temporalis muscle. Malocclusion of the teeth suggests maxillary or mandibular fractures.

If you have any question about the presence of facial fractures, you should obtain a CT scan.

Fractures of the face

Classification of fractures

For you to get some perspective on orbital fractures, we should talk about fractures occurring anywhere on the head. I like this very simple concept to start with. The bones of the head comprise:

- Cranial bones
- Facial bones
- Jaw bones

Look at the skull (Figure 13-18) in profile. You will notice that the facial bones hang from the cranium. Below the facial bones rests the mandible with the attachment to the skull at the temporomandibular joint. The orbit is made up of bones of both the cranium and the face.

Again in very simple terms, let's discuss this further. Cranial fractures are of interest to the ophthalmologist if they involve the frontal bone. Traumatic optic neuropathy can occur from a blow to the supraorbital rim, with or without fracture. Theoretically, the force of impact is trans-

mitted along the orbital roof to the optic canal. Small vessels where the optic nerve is tethered to the entrance of the optic canal suffer a "shearing injury," resulting in damage to the nerve (see "Traumatic Optic Neuropathy" later in this chapter) (Figure 13-19). Fractures of the superior orbital rim rarely occur, because it is so thick.

Mandibular fractures do not have a direct clinical relationship to the orbit or function of the eyes, so we will not consider them further.

The concept of dividing these fractures into fractures of the cranium, face, and mandible is an important one. With this little bit of new information, you can look at a trauma patient and separate the multiple fractures present into:

- Cranial fractures
- Facial fractures
- Mandibular fractures

You can now start to make some sense of some complicated fractures. You can "ignore" mandibular fractures. You should look for traumatic optic neuropathy when you see cranial fractures involving frontal bone injury. Next we will discuss facial fractures.

Facial fractures

As we said, the orbit is made up of bones from the skull and the face. The orbital roof, apex, and posterior portion of the lateral wall are cranial bones. The rest of the orbit is made up of facial bones. The rest of the orbit is formed by thick, strong bones. Fractures of the orbital rim occur where the thick bones connect, the suture lines, not through the thick orbital bones (usually). You might recall from medical school that the pelvis (the "pelvic ring") always fractures in at least two places. This is true of orbital fractures as well (the orbital rim, also a ring). You will notice this especially in zygomaticomaxillary complex fractures, in which the orbital rims are separated at the frontozygomatic suture and the zygomaticomaxillary suture, allowing the zygoma to separate from the remainder of the face. The zygoma itself (one of those thick orbit bones) can fracture, but that is much less common than a fracture at the suture lines. Understanding where the strong and weak points of the orbit (and the face) are is the key to understanding how fractures occur and how fractures are repaired.

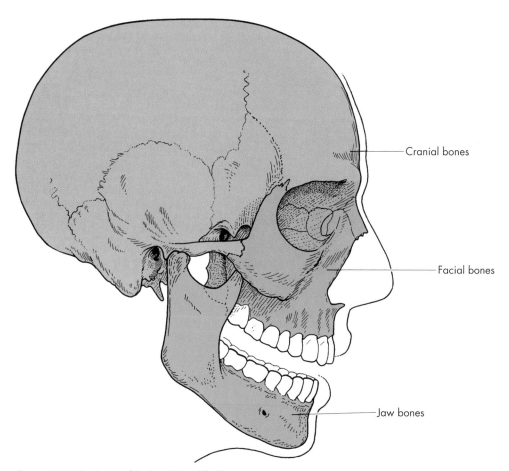

Cranial bones

Facial bones

Jaw bones

Figure 13-18 The bones of the head, "simplified."

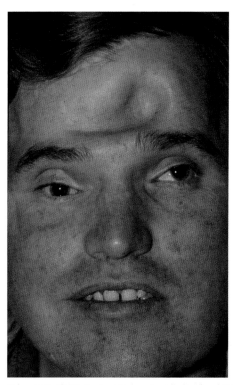

Figure 13-19 Bilateral optic neuropathy after frontal bone fracture in a motorcycle accident. Visual acuity was no light perception OD and count fingers OS.

The strongest rims of the orbit are the superior orbital rim and the lateral orbital rim. Tremendous force is required to fracture these rims other than at the suture lines, in contrast to the medial and inferior orbital rims, which are substantially weaker and commonly sustain comminuted fractures.

The orbital rims are the framework for the orbital skeleton. The medial wall and floor of the orbit span this framework and are less than 1 mm thick. The floor and the medial wall do not contribute to the strength of the facial skeleton. Rather they support the orbital contents. The thin medial wall and floor of the orbit can fracture without disruption of the rims. As these walls blow out, the support of the orbital contents is lost, and tissue is forced into or prolapses into the adjacent sinus. We will discuss the common orbital fractures, including blowout fractures, zygomaticomaxillary complex fractures, and naso-orbital ethmoid fractures, in detail later.

In Chapter 6, we talked about the ideal facial proportions, dividing the face into thirds. The middle third of the facial skeleton, primarily the maxilla, is termed the *midface*. Fractures involving the maxilla and facial portions of the orbit are termed midfacial fractures. *A midfacial fracture that separates the midface from the cranium is termed a Le Fort fracture.* Later in this chapter, we will talk about the classification of these midfacial fractures.

Traumatic optic neuropathy

Traumatic optic neuropathy (TON) is the result of an injury to the optic nerve. The injury can be direct or indirect. A *direct injury* is caused by an object that strikes the optic nerve. The object can be a missile entering the orbit or a fragment of bone. An *indirect injury* is said to occur when concussive forces traumatize the nerve. The most common cause of indirect TON is a blow to the frontal bone (as discussed above). The force of the injury traveling along the orbital roof causes a shearing injury to the nerve. Damage to the microcirculation of the optic nerve results in a loss of vision.

- If the vision is decreased in a trauma patient, rule out injuries to the globe
- If there is no apparent cause for decreased vision and a relative afferent pupillary defect is present, you should diagnose traumatic optic neuropathy

Evaluate the CT scan for a bone fragment that is impinging on the optic nerve, subperiosteal hematoma, or blood within the optic nerve sheath (Figure 13-20). Direct causes of optic neuropathy, such as these, are rare. If present, the fragment should be repositioned or the hematoma drained as soon as possible. In most cases, you will see no fracture or a small nondisplaced fracture of the optic canal. In the absence of any cause of direct optic nerve injury in the presence of a normal eye, you have diagnosed an indirect traumatic optic neuropathy.

The treatment of traumatic optic neuropathy remains controversial. For some 30 years, corticosteroids have been used for head injury patients under the rationale of reducing cerebral inflammation and edema with a presumed protective effect on mortality and other outcomes. This thinking was applied to optic nerve injury in the 1980s and supported by anecdotal reports of improved vision in patients treated with steroids. A treatment scheme with "megadose" steroids (intravenous methylprednisolone (Solu-Medrol) 30 mg/kg followed by a continuous infusion of 5.4 mg/kg) was recommended. Although attempts at proving the success of this treatment have been made, no significant randomized studies have proven the effectiveness of this treatment. In 2004, the results of the CRASH study (Corticosteroid Randomization After Significant Head Injury) showed that head injury patients routinely treated with steroids had a signifi-

cantly increased risk of death compared with the placebo group. Consequently, in the absence of any proven benefit of steroid treatment combined with the results of the CRASH study, we no longer treat traumatic optic neuropathy with high doses of steroids.

The only other suggested treatment for indirect traumatic optic neuropathy has been optic canal decompression. The rationale for this treatment (in some ways similar to the steroids) is that post-traumatic swelling could cause further injury to the nerve. Steroids or surgical decompression could reduce the damage caused by this swelling. Decompression of the optic canal can be approached surgically via craniotomy or through the sphenoid sinus. The sinus route is chosen because of decreased morbidity. You will recall that the lateral wall of the sphenoid sinus is the medial wall of the optic canal. Decompression through the sinus removes the medial wall of the canal. Again, anecdotal reports suggest that improvement may be due to decompression rather than spontaneous recovery but, at this time, there are no controlled studies that confirm the effectiveness of decompression.

In patients with traumatic optic neuropathy, an individualized decision should be made to determine if the benefits of surgical decompression outweigh the risks. A complicating factor is that the patient often has associated injuries that preclude complete examination and informed consent for operation.

New surgical techniques have made optic canal decompression a minimally invasive and relatively safe operation. The advances in the endoscopic surgical technique have allowed better access to the orbital apex for deep tumor biopsy and orbital decompression procedures (see Figure 15-22).

However, due to a lack of evidence that decompression improves the outcome in patients with indirect TON, we do not routinely recommend optic canal decompression. For most patients, the treatment of traumatic optic neuropathy remains supportive care and observation.

You may find yourself in a related trauma situation. You are asked to see a patient with normal vision, who has facial fractures, including nondisplaced apical orbital fractures seen on a CT scan. Your opinion is requested regarding the advisability of fracture repair. The chance of intraoperative optic nerve injury is probably higher than that in a patient who has no apical fractures, but is still low. Cautious repair can be undertaken. The patient should be told about the small risk of blindness associated with surgery, so he or she can give his or her informed consent to the procedure. In the presence of unstable apex fractures involving the canal, manipulation of the orbital fractures should probably not be done.

Blowout fractures

Mechanism

The thin bone of the orbital floor or medial wall is blown out when an impact raises the intraorbital pressure to the point at which the thin bones fracture, pushing the orbital contents into the maxillary sinus or ethmoid sinus. As the intraorbital pressure decreases, the orbital tissues recoil and become "entrapped" in the fracture site, causing a restrictive form of strabismus. The exact mechanism of orbital blowout

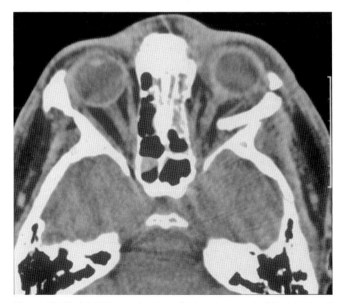

Figure 13-20 Axial CT scan showing a fractured segment of the lateral wall of the orbit impinging on the optic nerve.

fractures has been the subject of debate for many years. Nevertheless, the concept that increased pressure pushes tissue out of the orbit is attractive and seems to explain the clinical signs and symptoms of blowout fractures. The restrictive strabismus after incarceration of orbital tissue is characteristic of small orbital floor fractures. Enophthalmos, resulting from orbital expansion, is the result of larger medial wall and floor fractures. Hypesthesia of the infraorbital nerve occurs because of contusion of the nerve, which is adjacent to, or in, the fracture site.

Diagnosis

The most common complaint of patients who sustain blowout fractures is diplopia. The decreased motility may be in any direction, but is seen most commonly in upgaze (Figure 13-21). The presence of infraorbital nerve hypesthesia accompanying the double vision indicates a floor fracture in almost all patients. Other signs include epistaxis and subcutaneous emphysema. Enophthalmos may be present in patients who have a large floor fracture (Figure 13-22). If you suspect a blowout fracture, you should confirm your impression with a CT scan, including coronal views of the orbital floor.

When you look at a blowout fracture on CT, try to put the fracture in the *large or small* category. Large fractures usually do not entrap tissue, so restrictive strabismus is not likely to be a problem. Large fractures may result in enophthalmos, however. Small fractures are more likely to entrap tissue causing a restrictive strabismus. Smaller fractures tend to occur in younger patients as the bones are more resilient. The classic example is the "white-eyed" blowout fracture occurring in patients usually under 16–18 years of age. We will talk about this type of fracture in more detail later. *This paragraph is important so read it again.* Remember:

- Look for enophthalmos associated with large blowout fractures
- Look for diplopia associated with small fractures

By definition, a blowout fracture implies that the orbital rims are intact. Fractures of the orbital floor often accompany other facial fractures. These fractures are not considered blowout fractures. The floor fracture associated with a ZMC fracture is caused by a different mechanism and presents with different symptoms and signs than a true blowout fracture. We will discuss the ZMC fracture later. Don't describe

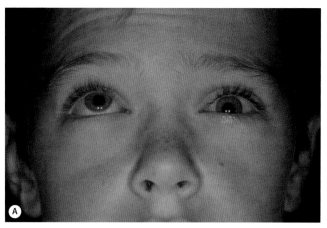
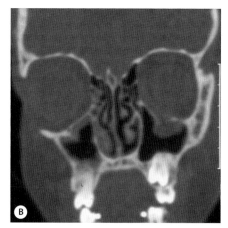

Figure 13-21 "White-eyed" blowout fracture. (**A**) Limited elevation of the eye after a blowout fracture. (**B**) CT scan demonstrating an orbital floor blowout fracture with prolapse of intraorbital contents into the maxillary sinus, resulting in ocular restriction.

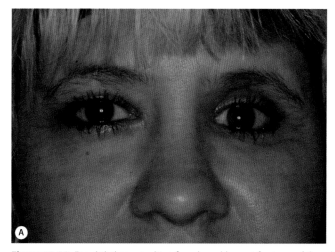
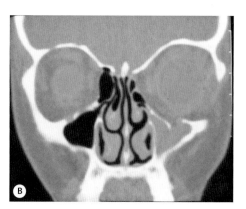

Figure 13-22 Enophthalmos resulting from large blowout fractures of the orbital floor and medial wall. (**A**) Enophthalmos of the left eye after a blowout fracture. (**B**) CT scan showing large blowout fractures of the medial orbital wall and floor with expansion of the orbital volume.

Box 13-9

Signs and Symptoms of a Blowout Fracture
- Diplopia
- Infraorbital nerve hypesthesia
- Epistaxis
- Subcutaneous emphysema
- Enophthalmos
- Intact orbital rim

the floor fracture of your patient with a ZMC fracture as a blowout fracture (Box 13-9).

Indications for repair in adults

The indications for surgical repair of the blowout fracture are:

- Diplopia—restrictive in nature (see Figure 13-21)
- Enophthalmos—greater than 2 mm (see Figure 13-22)

You may have learned that blowout fractures in *adults* should be repaired in 10–14 days. A better way to think of this is that a blowout fracture should be repaired as soon as possible once you know that it needs to be repaired. The presence of a blowout fracture alone is not an indication for surgery, so how do you know which fractures to repair? If you have diagnosed a blowout fracture with diplopia, and no enophthalmos, have your patient return in 5 days to see if the diplopia has resolved. Often as the swelling and hemorrhage within the orbit subside, eye movements will improve and the double vision will resolve. If the diplopia has not resolved, perform forced duction testing (see Figure 13-24, C) to determine if the diplopia is a result of muscle paresis or restriction.

Forced duction testing is performed after instillation of topical anesthetic drops and application of either 4% lidocaine (Xylocaine) or 5% cocaine to the conjunctiva at the inferior rectus insertion and the limbus using a cotton-tipped applicator. Use a small toothed forceps to grasp the conjunctiva at the limbus and manually move the eye in the direction of the deficit (usually upgaze). If you cannot physically move the eye, muscle entrapment or restriction is present. If you can move the eye freely, muscle paresis is present. Compare the left and right eyes for symmetry in forced duction testing if a restriction is suspected, but not obvious.

In the adult patient, if the diplopia is improving and the restriction is minimal, it is reasonable to wait an additional week to see if the diplopia continues to resolve. Surgery may not be required. If the restriction in any patient is pronounced and there has been no subjective improvement as the swelling resolves, the patient should have surgery soon; it is not necessary to wait the 10–14 days in all patients. Surgery is not indicated for muscle paresis.

Diplopia in primary position or in downgaze, shown to be restrictive in nature, is a strong indication for operative intervention. Patients may tolerate diplopia in upgaze or extreme downgaze and may not require surgery.

Rarely, a patient will have enophthalmos on the initial exam. If both the medial wall and the floor have been fractured or if there is a large floor fracture, you can offer surgery to correct the enophthalmos. There is no need to wait longer.

More commonly, enophthalmos will not be present even if a large fracture exists. Swelling and ecchymosis may mask any asymmetry. If the eye movements are full (remember that usually this will be the case), check the patient in 2 or 3 weeks and see if asymmetry in appearance is present. If asymmetry exists and the patient is bothered by it, repair is reasonable. If no asymmetry is present, recheck in a few months. In the past, "delayed" correction of enophthalmos was thought to be dangerous and not likely to succeed. Most orbital surgeons now feel that an adequate repair of enophthalmos is possible even if delayed weeks or months. Furthermore, the clinical observation has been that many patients with large fractures may not develop bothersome enophthalmos.

Infraorbital nerve hypesthesia is not an indication for surgery. Most numbness will resolve over 6–12 months. Infraorbital nerve hypesthesia is usually made worse temporarily after orbital floor repair.

Indications for repair in children: the "white-eyed" blowout

The situation in children and teenagers requires special attention. As we noted above, young patients with blowout fractures often have small fractures that entrap tissue. In fact, in some cases, the fracture can appear to be very small on scan, as the "trapdoor" has slammed almost completely closed. This has been described as the *"white-eyed"* blowout fracture. In the most classic presentation, the child is under 18 years, often receiving a seemingly insignificant trauma, but complains of eye pain or diplopia. The external exam can show little or no apparent trauma (i.e., white-eyed). In some cases, the fracture may have incarcerated tissue so tightly that the patient suffers from vagal symptoms such as nausea or vomiting. Often the patient may be inconsolable, due to discomfort.

You should be suspicious of any child who has an eye movement problem after even a minor trauma. Review the scan yourself. The fracture can be very small and may be overlooked if the radiologist is not well informed and suspicious of a fracture. A small fracture associated with restrictive strabismus should be repaired as soon as possible. The incarceration of the muscle is thought to damage the muscle and lead to fibrosis and permanent restriction. The best chance of a return of full movement is the earlier release of the entrapment—in most cases on the day of diagnosis. The repair technique is similar to adult fractures. The results of urgent surgery in white-eyed blowout cases are greatly improved over the traditional "wait and watch" approach taken prior to understanding the mechanism of restriction in these patients.

The goal of blowout fracture repair is to (Box 13-10):

- Free entrapped orbital tissue
- Return orbital volume to normal

Surgery is performed under general anesthesia. The orbital floor is exposed through either a lower eyelid subciliary or a transconjunctival approach. The most common approach is the "swinging lower eyelid" approach popularized by McCord. This approach combines the transconjunctival inci-

Box 13-10

Indications for Blowout Fracture Repair

Adults

- Diplopia
  - In primary position or downgaze
  - Positive forced duction test results indicating restrictive strabismus
  - Paresis usually improves over 10 days
- Enophthalmos
  - CT shows extensive disruption of orbital floor and/or medial wall
  - Repair if 2 mm or more enophthalmos
    — On initial exam
    — Or developing over time

Children (under 18 years)

- Diplopia
  - CT scan showing small fracture
  - Assume "white-eyed blowout"
  - Urgent repair
- Enophthalmos
  - Rarely occurs

sion with a canthotomy and cantholysis, giving excellent exposure of the orbital floor. This approach was discussed under "Lower Eyelid Blepharoplasty" in Chapter 6 and will be reviewed briefly here.

Orbital floor blowout fracture repair includes:

- Preparation in the operating room
- Dissection in the preseptal plane to the inferior orbital rim
- Elevation of the periosteum at the rim and off the floor
- Freeing the entrapped tissue
- Positioning the implant
- Closing the wound

The steps of orbital floor blowout fracture repair are:

1. Prepare the patient in the operating room
   A. Inject local anesthetic with epinephrine in the conjunctival cul de sac and under the skin adjacent to the inferior orbital rim.
   B. Prepare and drape *both eyes* in the surgical field. You may want to compare forced ductions or orbital volume.
   C. Before making any incision, repeat the forced duction test.
2. Dissect in the preseptal plane to the inferior orbital rim
   A. Place a 4-0 silk traction suture in the lower lid. Use a reverse cutting needle.
   B. Place a 4-0 silk suture through the conjunctiva under the insertion of the inferior rectus. Use a taper needle.
   C. The swinging eyelid approach to the orbital floor begins with a canthotomy and cantholysis (Figure 13-23, A).
   D. Evert the lid margin over a Jaeger lid plate (shoehorn) and make a transconjunctival incision at the inferior margin of the tarsus from the punctum to the lateral canthal incision (Figure 13-23, B).

E. Pull the orbital septum and orbicularis muscle apart with two pairs of Paufique forceps and continue a preseptal dissection to the inferior orbital rim. You will know that you are getting close to the rim when the dissection turns 90 degrees from the plane of the operating table posteriorly toward the orbital rim (Figure 13-23, C).
   F. Palpate the orbital rim and use a Freer elevator to dissect cheek fat away from the periosteum of the rim.
3. Elevate the periosteum off the floor
   A. Place a Jaffe lid speculum in the wound and clamp the attached suture to the drape.
   B. You can use a Desmarres vein retractor for additional retraction.
   C. You will need to wear a headlight for this portion of the operation. Adjust the size of the spot to illuminate only the inside of the wound. Dim the operating room lights to make your headlight illumination more effective.
   D. Cut the periosteum along the inferior orbital rim with a no. 15 blade or the Colorado needle.
   E. Elevate the periosteum off the inferior orbital rim with a Freer elevator in your dominant hand and a Frazier suction tube in your nondominant hand.
   F. Continue the dissection of the periorbita off the orbital floor until you reach the front edge of the fracture (Figures 13-23, D and 13-24, B).
4. Free the entrapped tissue
   A. Most blowout fractures occur medial to the infraorbital canal.
   B. Tease the periorbita off the anterior edge of the fracture. Extend this dissection posteriorly around the perimeter of the fracture site.
   C. You will need to retract the orbital contents with a Sewall or malleable retractor in your nondominant hand. Use a Freer elevator in your dominant hand. If there is bleeding, have your assistant do the retraction and use the suction tube in your nondominant hand.
   D. When the entire perimeter of the fracture has been exposed, try to elevate the entrapped orbital tissue from the broken orbital floor or maxillary sinus mucosa. As this dissection continues, you will be able to gently pry the tissue out of the fracture site.
   E. At this point, the entire perimeter of the fracture should be visible (Figure 13-24, A).
   F. There is no need to elevate the broken bone fragments.
   G. Repeat the forced duction testing at this point. Results should be normal (Figure 13-24, C).
5. Position the implant
   A. There are many materials available to use for implants. I usually use a thin Supramid implant sheet, measuring 0.4 mm in thickness (SupraFOIL® smooth nylon foil, F-SS-04, S. Jackson, Inc., http://www.supramid.com, 0.4 mm sheet). These implants are easy to work with and inexpensive. Thin MEDPOR implants work well also. MEDPOR channel implants are cantilevered implants attached to the anterior orbital rim. This implant provides support for the orbital tissues if there is no posterior

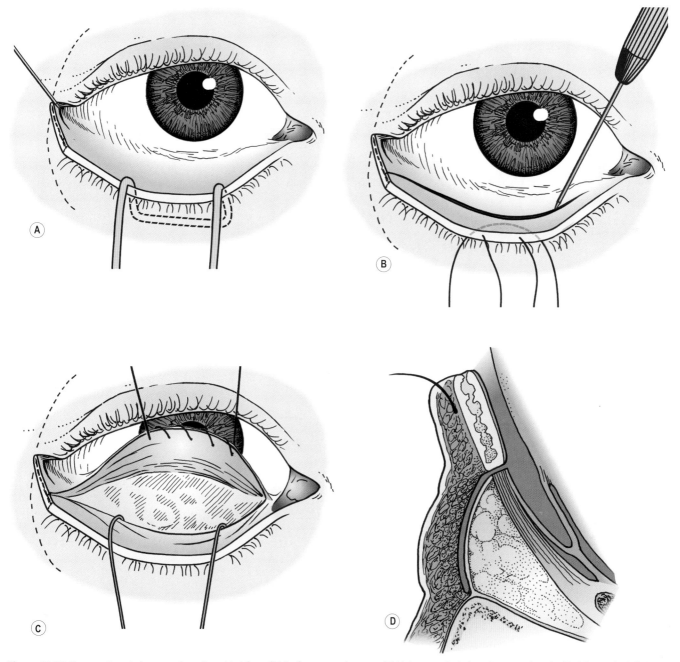

Figure 13-23 Transconjunctival approach to the orbital floor. (**A**) Perform a canthotomy. (**B**) Make a cantholysis and transconjunctival incision at the inferior margin of the tarsus. Place traction sutures in the lid margin and under the inferior rectus insertion. (**C**) Dissect to the inferior orbital rim in the preseptal plane. (**D**) Sagittal view of the dissection plane to the floor fracture. (**E**) Sagittal view of tissue prolapsed into fracture. (**F**) Sagittal view of the implant covering the defect in place. Screws are in place at the rim.

edge of bone to rest a conventional implant on. MEDPOR has recently developed a titanium implant sandwiched between polyethylene (Porex Surgical, http://www.porexsurgical.com). Like the other implants, this comes in a variety of thicknesses. The thin Titan implant holds its shape well and is easy to place. Cut the implant to the size and shape that you feel is necessary. Usually a typical guitar pick shape is used (Figure 13-24, D).

B. Elevate the tissue and place the implant into position with a hemostat. The implant should cover the entire floor defect with the anterior and posterior

edges of the implant resting on solid bone (Figure 13-23, E). Some trimming of the implant may be required to get the perfect fit.

C. If you are having trouble with orbital fat prolapsing around your retractors, cut a second similarly sized piece of Supramid to use as a retractor against the orbital fat. Use your Sewall retractors on the floor side of the retracting implant, and you will have much better exposure to position the floor implant. Remove the retracting implant after you are happy with the shape and position of the floor implant. You might find this little trick very helpful.

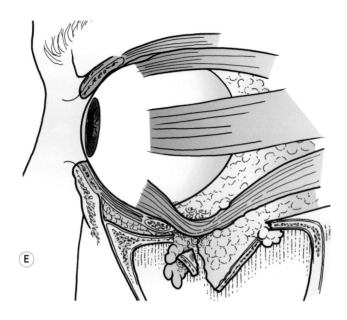

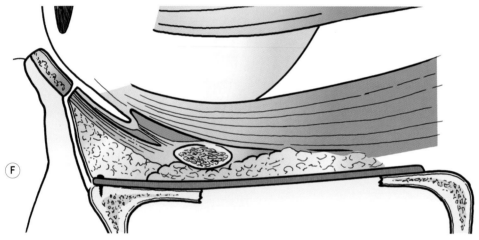

Figure 13-23 Continued.

D. When the floor implant is in good position, elevate the implant with your retractor, and make sure that there is no tissue prolapsing around the implant.

E. Screw the implant into position with two 3 mm microscrews at the inferior orbital rim. Be careful not to screw into the infraorbital nerve (see Figures 13-23, F and 13-24, E).

F. Repeat forced duction tests. If results are positive, the implant may have entrapped tissue and you will need to reposition the implant.

6. Close the wound

A. Close the periosteum with a 4-0 Vicryl suture on a P-2 needle, if possible. Make sure that you do not sew the septum to the periosteum (causes lid retraction).

B. Close the conjunctiva with interrupted 6-0 fast absorbing or 7-0 Vicryl sutures.

C. Reattach the lateral canthal tendon with a 4-0 double-armed Mersilene suture (Figure 13-23, G).

D. Close the canthotomy with the same absorbable suture.

Postoperatively, patients can be hospitalized overnight or observed as an outpatient if a family member or friend can stay with the patient for the first postoperative night. Visual acuity should be checked on a routine basis. Oral steroids can be given to reduce postoperative swelling. Antibiotics should accompany steroid use. The patient should rest with the head of the bed elevated and ice in place. Activity may be resumed over 48 hours. Implant infection or extrusion is rare (Box 13-11).

Useful instruments and supplies for repair of blowout fractures include:

• Implants
  — MEDPOR
• Barrier sheet 1.0 mm (8312), 1.6 mm (9312)
• Barrier channel implant (multiple channels): small size accepts microplate (9532)

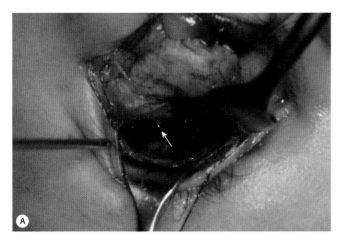

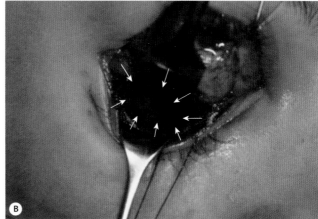

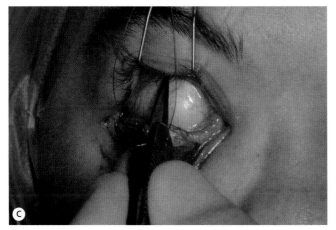

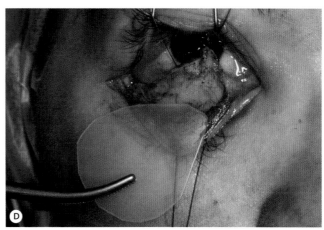

Figure 13-24 Anterior orbitotomy for orbital floor fracture repair. (**A**) Tissue trapped in the fracture site (arrow). (**B**) Tissue freed from the fracture site (arrows point to edge of fracture). (**C**) Free forced duction testing after elevation of prolapsed tissue from the fracture site. (**D**) SupraFOIL implant cut to shape. (**E**) Implant in place, secured to the rim with microscrews.

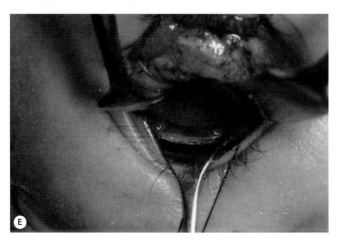

- Titan double BARRIER (BTM™)
- 81024 38 mm × 50 mm × 0.6 mm
- 81026 76 mm × 50 mm × 0.6 mm
  - Supramid implant sheet, measuring 0.4 mm in thickness (SupraFOIL® smooth nylon foil, F-SS-04)

Repair of the medial wall blowout fracture

Medial wall blowout fractures can occur independently or in association with a floor fracture (see Figure 13-22, A and B). The indications and principles of treatment are the same as those for a blowout fracture of the orbital floor. The approach to the medial wall is most commonly done through a con-

junctival incision known as the transcaruncular approach. In this operation, the conjunctiva between the plica and the caruncle is cut with Westcott scissors. Stevens' scissors are used to bluntly dissect through the extraconal fat to the periorbita. The periorbita is elevated off the medial orbital wall until the fracture site is identified. The entrapped tissues are elevated from the fracture and a Supramid implant is placed. The implant is usually screwed in with a single screw or left unsecured. The periosteum is not closed. A simple closure of the conjunctiva is performed. The transcaruncular approach can be combined with a swinging eyelid approach for excellent exposure of the orbital floor and medial orbital wall (Figure 13-25).

Box 13-11

Blowout Fracture Repair

Preparation in the operating room

- General anesthesia
- Local anesthetic injection
- Preparing and draping of both eyes
- Forced duction testing

Preseptal dissection to the infraorbital rim

- Swinging eyelid transconjunctival approach to the floor
- Place a 4-0 silk traction suture in the lower lid margin and under the inferior rectus insertion
- Perform canthotomy and cantholysis
- Make a transconjunctival incision from punctum to lateral canthal incision
- Continue the preseptal dissection to the rim

Elevation of periosteum of floor

- Wear headlight and dim the operating room lights
- Cut periosteum along infraorbital rim
- Elevate periosteum off floor
- Use a Freer elevator in the dominant hand
- Use a Frazier suction tube in the nondominant hand
- Use a Sewall retractor or malleable retractor for exposure

Freeing the entrapped tissue

- Most fractures are medial to the infraorbital nerve
- Elevate the periorbita off the perimeter of the fracture
- Gently pry tissue out of fracture site and repeat forced duction tests

Positioning the implant

- Use Supramid 0.4 mm or MEDPOR (1.0 mm) implant
- Cut to shape
- Position implant over entire perimeter of floor
- Screw implant into place

Closure

- Close the periosteum (4-0 Vicryl sutures)
- Close the conjunctiva (5-0 or 6-0 fast absorbing gut or 7-0 Vicryl sutures)
- Reattach the lateral canthal tendon (4-0 Mersilene)
- Close the canthotomy (5-0 or 6-0 fast absorbing gut sutures)

Postoperative care

- Outpatient or inpatient
- Oral steroids and antibiotics
- Ice and rest

Checkpoint

- What findings on examination suggest a facial fracture?
- Remember that the weak points of the facial skeleton are where fractures occur first:
  — Where are the orbital rims likely to fracture?
  — Where do the orbital walls fracture?
  — Which rim is the strongest?

It takes a tremendous force to fracture the superior orbital rim. Any palpable discontinuity of the rims is diagnostic for an orbital fracture.

- Order a CT scan when you suspect an orbital or facial fracture. You may be surprised that, with a thorough examination and experience, you will be able to predict what the CT scan will look like. After examining a patient with a fracture, try to picture the CT scan in your mind before you look at it.
- Review the general classification of facial fractures. It is so simple that you may be inclined to ignore it, but I guarantee it will help you again and again. You have to understand how the facial bones attach to the cranium.
- You will see many patients with blowout fractures. If you only learn about one type of fracture, learn about blowout fractures. Know the indications for repair:
  — Diplopia, restrictive in nature
  — Enophthalmos
- Know the principles of repair of orbital fractures, taking care to free all restriction possible and restoring orbital volume to normal.
- Compare the blowout fracture management of an adult with diplopia versus a child with diplopia due to a small fracture.

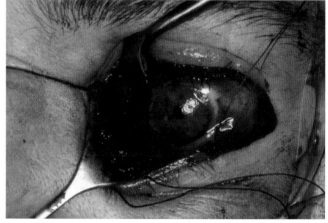

Figure 13-25 Transcaruncular approach to the medial orbital wall (in this case, combined with "swinging eyelid" transconjunctival incision of the lower eyelid).

Zygomaticomaxillary complex fracture—"tripod" fracture

Mechanism

The zygomaticomaxillary complex fracture (ZMC fracture) is usually caused by a blow to the cheekbone, often with a fist. The zygomatic bone is knocked off the rim (Figure 13-26). Fractures occur at:

- The frontozygomatic suture
- The zygomaticomaxillary suture
- The zygomatic arch
- The orbital floor and through the back wall of the maxillary sinus (see Figure 13-26)

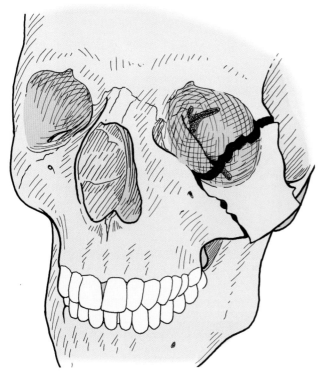

Figure 13-26 Zygomaticomaxillary complex (ZMC) fracture.

The signs and symptoms of a ZMC fracture depend on the amount of displacement of the zygoma. Common findings include:

- Lateral canthal dystopia
- Lid retraction
- Globe ptosis
- Enophthalmos
- Trismus
- Diplopia

Lateral canthal dystopia and globe ptosis occur when the zygoma is displaced inferiorly and posteriorly (Figure 13-27). Because the lateral canthal tendon is attached at Whitnall's tubercle below the frontozygomatic suture, the tendon is pulled inferiorly as the bone is displaced. If the canthus moves more inferiorly than the globe, lid retraction is created. If there is also a large floor fracture, the eye will be displaced inferiorly as well, globe ptosis. If the bone is displaced to a large degree, you may see enophthalmos. Remember that the mechanism of a zygomaticomaxillary complex fracture is different from that of a blowout fracture. There is no increased orbital pressure pushing tissue into the sinus. Diplopia is uncommon. The fracture site on the floor tends to be more lateral than with a blowout fracture.

Trismus occurs because of depression of the zygomatic arch against the temporalis muscle or because of contusion of the muscle itself. Hypesthesia of the fifth nerve may occur, but it is a less obvious finding when compared with the other deformities.

The indications for treatment of zygomaticomaxillary complex fractures include:

- Deformity
  - Globe ptosis
  - Enophthalmos
  - Lid retraction
  - Lateral canthal dystopia
  - Flattening of the malar eminence
- Diplopia
- Trismus

Many patients suffer zygomaticomaxillary complex fractures and seek no treatment with little resulting asymmetry. Minimally displaced ZMC fractures do not require surgery and will cause little or no deformity or functional disability. When bone displacement creates an obvious deformity or the patient has disabling trismus, repair should be undertaken.

The treatment of zygomaticomaxillary complex fractures is open reduction and internal fixation of the displaced zygoma. Periocular incisions (open) are made to gain access to the bone. Soft tissue attachments to the bone are freed, allowing the bone to be moved back into the anatomic position (reduction). Titanium microplates are used to fix the bone in proper position (internal fixation). Typical eyelid incisions include the transconjunctival or subciliary incision to gain access to the inferior orbital rim (Figure 13-28). Oral incisions in the buccal–gingival sulcus allow access to the face of the maxilla. A small incision at the tail of the brow allows access to the frontozygomatic suture. In patients who have minimal displacement of the bone, a small incision at the frontozygomatic suture may be all that is necessary to manipulate the bone into position. In patients with multiple comminuted bone fragments with a large degree of bone displacement, a coronal scalp incision may be required for access to the zygomatic arch.

Naso-orbital ethmoid fracture

Recall that the medial orbital rim is the weakest part of the orbit. Direct trauma to the glabella results in the classic "telescoping" bilateral naso-orbital ethmoid (NOE) fracture (Figures 13-29 and 13-30). The force of impact collapses the bridge of the nose posteriorly, crushing the ethmoid sinus. The nasal bones and frontal processes of the maxilla splay outward, creating telecanthus.

Signs and symptoms typical of naso-orbital ethmoid fractures include:

- Flattening of the nasal bridge (and sometimes the forehead)
- Telecanthus
- Lacrimal injury

Open reduction and internal fixation of the fractures with attention to appropriate reduction of the frontal process of the maxilla soon after injury offers the best chance of successful repair. Later repairs for telecanthus using a transnasal wire are largely unsuccessful.

A unilateral naso-orbital ethmoid fracture occurs when the frontal process of the maxilla and inferior orbital rim on one side are fractured. I think of this as a medial strut, or medial buttress, fracture. Its presentation is less dramatic than that of the more severe bilateral fracture with typical

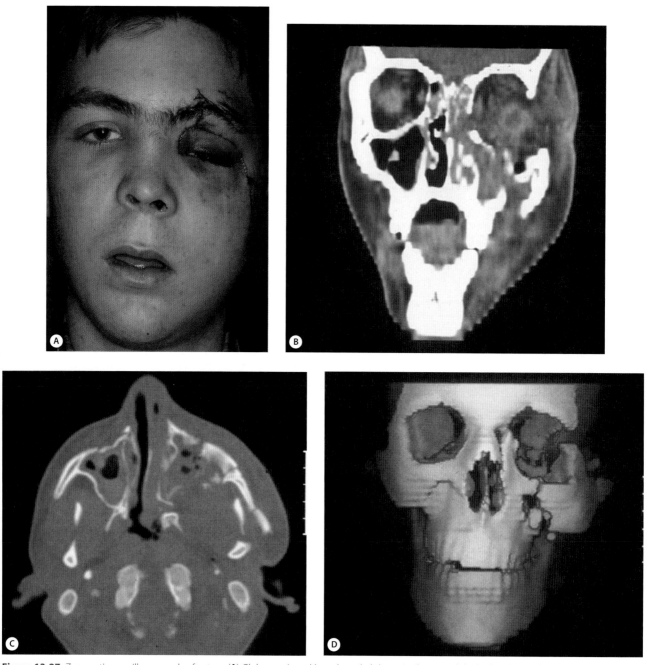

Figure 13-27 Zygomaticomaxillary complex fracture. (**A**) Globe ptosis and lateral canthal dystopia due to widely displaced ZMC fracture. (**B**) Coronal CT scan of a ZMC fracture (soft tissue window). (**C**) Three-dimensional CT scan of a ZMC fracture. (**D**) Axial CT scan of a ZMC fracture (bone window). Note the displaced zygoma and additional fracture of the medial buttress.

telescoping of the nasal bridge. As you might guess, telecanthus and inferior displacement of the medial canthal tendon result (Figure 13-31). Damage to the nasolacrimal duct may result in dacryocystitis or tearing. Treatment of these fractures is similar to that described for zygomaticomaxillary complex fractures in terms of exposure of bone fragments, alignment, and plating.

Le Fort fracture

In 1901, Renee Le Fort used the term pillars of resistance to define the strongest regions of the facial skeleton. Le Fort

noted that facial fractures tended to occur in a characteristic pattern of lines occurring between these pillars (Figure 13-32). These typical patterns of midfacial fracture have been described as Le Fort I, II, and III type fractures (Figure 13-33). In each fracture, the facial skeleton is separated from the cranium by fractures occurring at the pterygoid plates (where the maxillary sinus attaches to the skull). When you evaluate a patient with severe facial fractures, you should look at the axial CT scans to see if the pterygoid plates are fractured (Figure 13-34).

A Le Fort I fracture separates the lower maxilla from the remainder of the midface and the cranium. The main symptom related to Le Fort I fracture is malocclusion. A Le

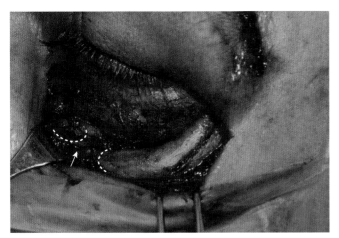

Figure 13-28 Zygomaticomaxillary complex fracture repair through a lower eyelid and a frontozygomatic incision. Note the fracture of the inferior rim at the suture line between the zygoma and maxilla (arrow).

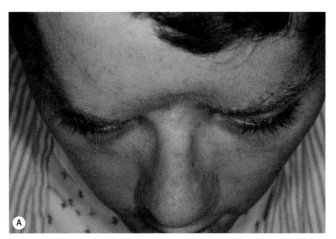

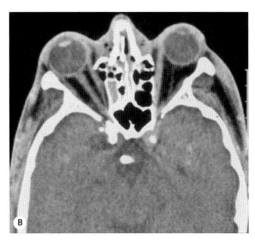

Figure 13-30 Naso-orbital ethmoid fracture. (**A**) Depressed forehead and nasal bridge, viewed from above. (**B**) Axial CT scan showing bilateral naso-orbital ethmoid fractures.

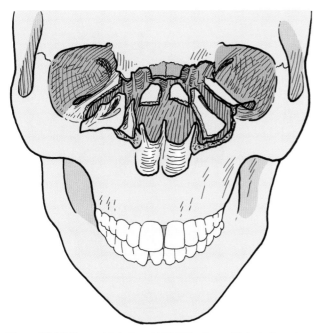

Figure 13-29 Naso-orbital ethmoid (NOE) fracture, with typical nasal flattening and telecanthus.

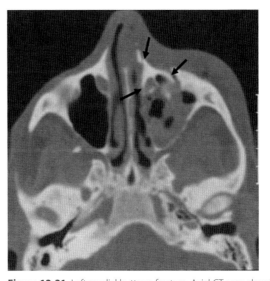

Figure 13-31 Left medial buttress fracture. Axial CT scan showing fracture of the medial buttress (arrows) pushing the nasolacrimal duct posteriorly. Note that the zygoma is intact. The opposite medial buttress is normal.

Fort II fracture involves the anterior orbit and separates the maxilla and medial orbit from the remainder of the midface and cranium (a pyramid-shaped fracture). You can see in Figure 13-33 that the zygoma remains in the normal position. A Le Fort III fracture separates the maxilla and the zygoma from the calvarium.

Le Fort fractures may occur unilaterally or bilaterally. Often there is asymmetry of the fractures. Bilateral Le Fort I and II fractures allow the upper teeth to be moved freely away from the skull. Bilateral Le Fort III fractures separate the entire face from the cranium with fractures extending across the medial canthi through the orbits and frontozygomatic sutures. Like all Le Fort fractures, there is extension posteriorly separating the pterygoid plates from the posterior wall of the maxillary sinus. Bilateral Le Fort III fractures cause a condition known as *craniofacial*

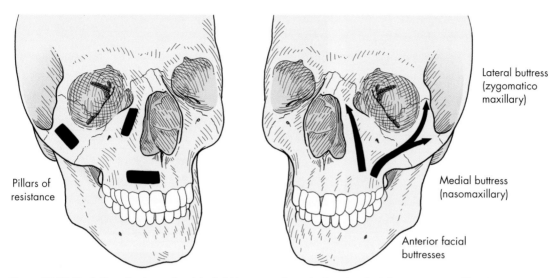

Figure 13-32 The "pillars of resistance" and the facial buttresses. Renee Le Fort described the strong areas of facial bone as pillars of resistance (shown as shaded bars on the left). He noted that facial fractures tended to occur between these pillars. These patterns of fracture have come to be known as Le Fort fractures of the midface. The related facial buttresses (curved arrows) surround and support the structures of the face. Reconstruction of the buttresses is a fundamental concept of facial fracture repair.

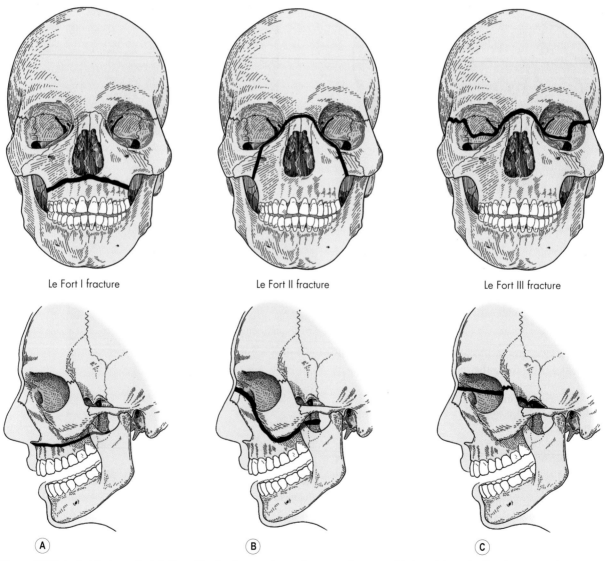

Le Fort I fracture   Le Fort II fracture   Le Fort III fracture

A   B   C

Figure 13-33 Le Fort fractures. By definition, all Le Fort fractures have a fracture at the pterygoid plates (where the "face bones" attach to the "skull bones"). (**A**) Le Fort I fractures separate the maxillary teeth from the upper face (not involving the orbits). (**B**) Le Fort II fractures cross the anterior and inferior orbits, but leave the zygomas intact. (**C**) Le Fort III fractures cross more posteriorly and superiorly into the orbits, separating the zygomas from the skull. If fractures are bilateral, the face bones are separated from the skull bones, a condition known as craniofacial dysjunction.

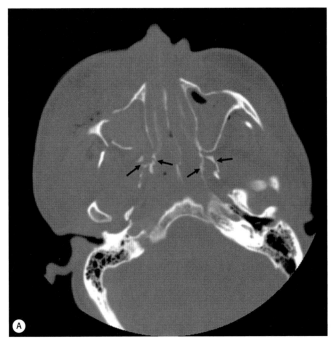

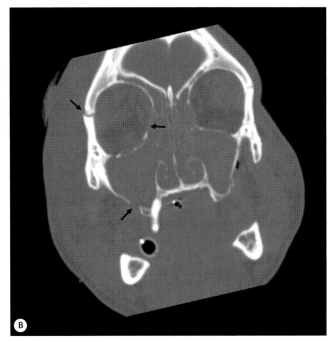

Figure 13-34 Le Fort fractures. (**A**) Axial CT, bone window. Pterygoid plates are fractured from the maxilla (arrows), indicating bilateral Le Fort type fractures. Posterior and anterior walls of the right maxillary sinus are fractured. Anterior wall of the left maxillary sinus is fractured. (**B**) Coronal CT, bone window. Right fractures (arrows) show that the facial bones are fractured off skull (Le Fort III fracture). Left-sided fractures are not all visible, but the frontozygomatic suture is intact. Other views show fractures diagnostic of a Le Fort II fracture

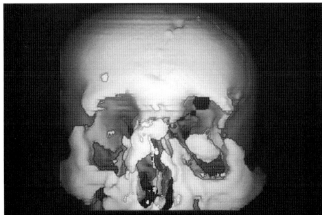

Figure 13-35 Three-dimensional CT scan of a patient with bilateral Le Fort III fractures—craniofacial dysjunction. The facial bones are fractured off the cranium.

Box 13-12

Le Fort Classification of Midfacial Fractures

Le Fort I fracture

- Upper teeth fractured off midface
- Not for ophthalmologists

Le Fort II fracture

- Maxilla separated from the face
- Zygoma intact
- Anterior orbital fractures

Le Fort III fracture

- Maxilla and zygoma are separated from the calvarium; the face is separated from the skull (craniofacial dysjunction)
- Anterior and posterior orbital fractures present

Note that all Le Fort fractures extend posteriorly, breaking the attachment of the face to the skull base at the pterygoid plates

---

dysjunction. An excellent way to understand how the facial bones could be separated from the cranium is by viewing a three-dimensional CT scan of a patient with a Le Fort fracture (Figure 13-35). Reread this section. Understanding these key concepts is the key to understanding midfacial fractures.

The concept of the "pillars of resistance" has been used to describe the bony framework of the face—the anterior and posterior buttresses of the midface (see Figure 13-32). The buttresses are the vertical "columns" that support and surround the structures of the face: the nasal cavity, the orbits, and the sinuses. The anterior facial buttresses include the medial (nasomaxillary) and lateral (zygomaticomaxillary)

buttresses. A posterior buttress is also described that extends vertically along the axis of the pterygoid plates. The concept, not the names, of the facial buttresses is important, because their repair forms the basis of reconstruction of facial features (Box 13-12).

Imaging of facial fractures

When you suspect an orbital or facial fracture, order a CT scan. Plain radiographs are of little use. CT scans should be obtained in both axial and coronal projections. Scans of both soft tissue windows and bone windows should be obtained. Fine cuts measuring 1 mm should be taken through the orbits. New helical CT scanning equipment can obtain axial and coronal views of the orbit in less than 60 seconds of acquisition time. No repositioning of the patient is required.

Three-dimensional CT scans are easy to read, but are expensive and are used only in special cases. You can see from the previous examples that the spatial relationships of the bone fragments are quite dramatically presented and are excellent aids in teaching.

Magnetic resonance imaging is not indicated in the evaluation of facial fractures. Recall that bone is not visualized well with magnetic resonance imaging.

Treatment of facial fractures

Surgical approach

We have covered some of this material already, but I want to review some concepts related to surgical approach, reduction and fixation of bone fragments, and the use of implants. Small periocular incisions can be used to gain access to the bones of the orbit and facial skeleton. Incisions are often combined to gain access to bony fragments from different directions (transoral and transconjunctival). When there are multiple fragments that are widely displaced, access to the entire facial skeleton can be obtained through incisions in the mouth (bilateral buccal–gingival sulcus incisions) in combination with transconjunctival incisions of the lower lid and coronal forehead flaps (facial "degloving"). You can imagine that every bone from the forehead to the upper teeth can be approached through this wide incision.

Reduction and fixation

Reduction starts with reconstruction of the facial buttresses (Figure 13-32). Once the displaced bone is located, soft tissues holding the bone out of position are elevated to allow mobilization of the fragment. After the fragments are mobile,

they can be anatomically aligned using a variety of tools including your fingers, elevators, and various clamps. This is the tough part of fracture repair.

After reduction of the bone fragments, titanium micro- and miniplates are used to secure the bones in anatomic alignment. Fixation starts by plating a fractured bone to a stable (unfractured) bone. The process continues with the adjacent fractured bone being plated to the newly stabilized bone until the anterior facial buttresses are stabilized from above and below. Simultaneously, the horizontal and posterior alignment is set as the plates are positioned. Fixation of smaller fragments follows fixation of larger segments of the buttresses. Multiple plates are often required (Figure 13-36).

Implants and grafts

The facial skeleton is analogous to the wing of an airplane. A strong structural framework provides the support of the wing. Thin sheets of metal span the spaces between the framework. The orbital rims and the buttresses of the face are the framework of the face. The thin bones of the orbital floor, medial wall, and maxillary face span the buttresses. Rebuilding the face starts with anatomic alignment of the orbital rims and buttresses. For patients in whom bone is missing between these structural supports (as in a floor or medial wall fracture), implants can be used to span the gaps.

As we discussed above, several choices for implants of the thin orbital floor are available. One choice is Supramid (SupraFOIL implant). Other alloplastic implants, such as MEDPOR or titanium mesh, are used. Some surgeons prefer the use of autogenous implants such as cartilage or bone grafts. In general, autogenous materials are more difficult to work with and don't significantly improve the final result. Complications with alloplastic implants are minimal, especially when fixed into position with screws. Useful implants and material for repairing facial fractures are listed earlier in this chapter.

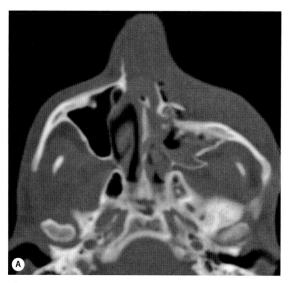
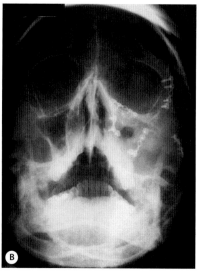

Figure 13-36 Zygomaticomaxillary complex fracture. (**A**) Preoperative CT scan showing a ZMC complex fracture with severe posterior displacement of the zygoma. Note the nasal and medial buttress fractures also. (**B**) Postoperative plain film showing multiple microplates in position.

Checkpoint

- Although you may not be repairing these fractures, learn the concepts in this last section. You should understand and be able to recognize these types of orbital fractures:
  — Blowout fractures
  — Zygomaticomaxillary complex fracture
  — Naso-orbital ethmoid fracture
  — Le Fort fractures
- Recall the difference between the floor fracture occurring in an orbital blowout fracture and a zygomaticomaxillary complex fracture. Recall that diplopia is uncommon in zygomaticomaxillary complex fractures.
- Make sure that you understand the concept of the facial bones being broken "off the cranium" with Le Fort fractures. When you see a severe facial fracture, look at the axial CT scan to see if the pterygoid plates are fractured. If so, the patient has a Le Fort fracture.
- Just as no two eyelid margin lacerations are exactly the same, no two facial fractures are exactly the same.

However, facial fractures do occur in predictable patterns. After you recognize fracture patterns, you will start to understand facial fractures.

- The same is true for the repair of these complex fractures. All fractures are different but all require open reduction and internal fixation. If you decide to treat these fractures, you need to learn:
  — The specific incisions (open)
  — The techniques for alignment (reduction) of the facial buttresses
  — The technique for microplate fixation (internal fixation)
  — Implant or graft placement

There is a huge amount of material in this chapter that is especially demanding from a technical point of view. Learn the concepts. Remember to concentrate on the big picture. The details will fall into place after you learn the concepts. Focus on the details of each particular repair last.

Major points

Look at the organization of this chapter to get an overview:

- General evaluation of the trauma patient
- Examination of the soft tissues
- Repair of the soft tissues
- Examination for fractures
- Classification of fractures
- Principles of fracture repair

When you first see the patient, make sure that his or her medical condition is stable and the eye is not damaged. Take photographs of the facial wounds. Determine how the injuries occurred.

Develop a system for evaluation of the soft tissues

- Evaluate the continuity of the lid margins
  - Rule out a canalicular laceration
- Check the anterior lamella
  - Look for fat in the wound
- Rule out the presence of foreign body or deep injury to the levator, eye, or brain
- Evaluate the surrounding the periocular area, including cranial nerve VII function

Describe the type of injury:

- Contusion
- Abrasion
- Avulsion
- Puncture
- Laceration

Learn the techniques for:

- Simple anterior lamellar repair
- Complex laceration repair
- Lid margin repair
- Canalicular laceration repair

There are three stenting techniques that you can use for canalicular lacerations:

- Bicanalicular intubation
  - Works well for all types of canalicular lacerations
  - Necessary when the upper and lower canaliculi are both lacerated
  - Necessary when the common canaliculus is avulsed
- Pigtail probe intubation
  - Especially helpful when it is difficult to find the cut end
  - Easy to do under local anesthesia
- Monocanalicular intubation
  - Best for a single canalicular laceration within the external two thirds length of the canaliculus

If the patient has an orbital hemorrhage with compromised blood flow to the eye or optic nerve, perform a canthotomy and cantholysis. Remember that a canthotomy alone does not lower the orbital pressure.

Learn the signs of a facial fracture:

- Diplopia and hypesthesia of the infraorbital nerve suggest damage to the orbital floor
- Epistaxis and subcutaneous emphysema suggest a fracture into the nose or sinus
- Look for deformity including:
  - Rim discontinuity or "step-off"
  - Telecanthus
  - Enophthalmos
  - Globe ptosis
  - Flattening of the malar eminence
- Malocclusion of the teeth suggests a mandibular or maxillary fracture
- Trismus suggests a zygomaticomaxillary complex fracture with impingement of the arch on the temporalis muscle and the coronoid process of the mandible

Major points Continued

To understand fractures of the orbit and face you must understand these concepts:

- The head is formed from the bones of the cranium, face, and mandible
- The face "hangs" off the cranium
- The orbit is made of the bones of the cranium and face
- The orbit has a strong framework supporting a thin floor and medial wall
- Fractures of the orbit and face occur in predictable patterns. Orbital fractures most commonly occur:
  - Through thin bones (floor and medial wall)
  - At suture lines

The most common orbital fracture that you will see is a blowout fracture. By definition, the orbital rims are intact. The floor (most commonly), the medial wall, or both are fractured. Signs of a blowout fracture of the floor include:

- Diplopia
- Hypesthesia of infraorbital nerve
- Enophthalmos

Indications for blowout fracture repair are:

- Bothersome diplopia that is proven to be restrictive
- Enophthalmos greater than 2 mm

The goals of fracture repair are to correct the diplopia by freeing the entrapped tissue and to restore the orbital volume by covering the defect in the floor or medial wall with an implant.

Children and young adults with diplopia and small or unrecognized fractures are likely to have a "white-eyed blow out" fracture. Repair should be undertaken urgently.

Two other common orbital fractures occur:

- The zygomaticomaxillary complex (ZMC) fracture
- The naso-orbital ethmoid (NOE) fracture

Entrapment of orbital tissues is uncommon with these fractures. The diagnosis is made by CT scan when typical facial deformity is noted on examination.

- Zygomaticomaxillary complex fractures cause lateral canthal dystopia and flattening of the malar eminence and cause ptosis in severely displaced fractures
- Naso-orbital ethmoid fractures cause telecanthus and flattening of the nasal bridge

Midfacial fractures occur when some or all of the facial bones are separated from the skull base at the pterygoid plates. The Le Fort classification system is used to describe these fractures:

- Le Fort I fracture: Maxillary teeth are off the skull
- Le Fort II fracture: Maxilla is off the cranium; zygoma remains in place
- Le Fort III fracture: Maxilla and zygoma are off the cranium

Evaluation of facial fractures is done with a CT scan. Plain films and magnetic resonance imaging are not used.

Facial fractures are repaired with open reduction and internal fixation (ORIF). Transoral and lower eyelid incisions provide exposure to the facial bones. The bones are put into alignment (reduced) and held in anatomic position using titanium microplates and screws (internal fixation).

Suggested reading

1. Albert DM, Lucarelli MJ: Orbital fractures: diagnosis and management. In *Clinical atlas of procedures in ophthalmic surgery*, pp. 347–359, Chicago: AMA Press, 2004.

2. Alford MA, Nerad JA, Carter KD: Predictive value of the initial quantified relative afferent pupillary defect in 19 consecutive patients with traumatic optic neuropathy. *Ophthal Plast Reconstr Surg* 17:323, 2001.

3. American Academy of Ophthalmology: *Basic and clinical science course: orbit, eyelids and lacrimal system*, sect. 7, pp. 97–108, 184–187, San Francisco: American Academy of Ophthalmology, 2006/2007.

4. Bilyk JR, Shore JW, Ward JB, McKeown CA: Late orbital trauma: diagnosis and treatment. In McCord CD, Tanenbaum M, Nunery WR, eds, *Oculoplastic surgery*, 3rd edn, ch. 18, pp. 553–580, New York: Raven Press, 1995.

5. CRASH trial collaborators: Effect of intravenous corticosteroids on death within 14 days in 10,008 adults with clinically significant head injury (MRC CRASH trial): randomized placebo-controlled trial. *The Lancet* 364:1321–1328, 2004.

6. Gossman MD, Pollock RA: Acute orbital trauma: diagnosis and treatment. In McCord CD, Tanenbaum M, Nunery WR, eds, *Oculoplasty*, 3rd edn, ch. 17, pp. 515–551, New York: Raven Press, 1995.

7. Collin JRO: Eyelid reconstruction and tumour management. In *A manual of systematic eyelid surgery*, 3rd edn, pp. 115–145, Butterworth Heinemann Elsevier, 2006.

8. Green J, Charonis GC, Goldberg RA: Eyelid trauma and reconstruction techniques. In Yanoff M, Duker J, eds, *Ophthalmology*, pp. 720–727, Mosby, 2004.

9. Holck DE, Ng JD: *Evaluation and treatment of orbital fractures*, Saunders, 2005.

10. Nerad J: Eyelid and orbital trauma. In *The requisites—Oculoplastic surgery*, pp. 33–47, St Louis: Mosby, 2001.

11. Nerad JA, Carter KD, Alford MA: Disorders of the eyelid: Eyelid trauma. In *Rapid diagnosis in ophthalmology—oculoplastic and reconstructive surgery*, pp. 62–65, Philadelphia: Mosby Elsevier, 2008.

12. Nerad JA, Carter KD, Alford MA: Disorders of the orbit: Trauma. In *Rapid diagnosis in ophthalmology—oculoplastic and reconstructive surgery*, pp. 242–257, Philadelphia: Mosby Elsevier, 2008.

13. Jordan DR, Nerad JA, Tse DT: The pigtail probe revisited. *Ophthalmology* 97(4):5519, 1990.

14. Jordan DR, St Onge P, Anderson RL, Patrinely JR, Nerad JA: Complications associated with alloplastic implants used in orbital fracture repair. *Ophthalmology* 99(10):1600–1608, 1992.

15. Jordan DR et al: Intervention within days for some orbital floor fractures: the white-eyed blowout. *Ophthal Plast Reconstr Surg* 14(6):379–390, 1998.

16. Bansagi ZC, Meyer DR: Internal orbital fractures in the pediatric age group. *Ophthal Plast Reconstr Surg* 107:829–836, 2000.

17. Linberg JV, Moore CA: Symptoms of canalicular obstruction. *Ophthalmology* 95(8):1077–1079, 1988.

18. Murphy ML, Nerad JA: Complex orbital fractures. *Ophthalmol Clin North Am* 9(4):607–627, 1996.

19. Sauerland S, Maegele M: A CRASH landing in severe head injury. *The Lancet* 364:1291–1292, 2004.

20. Steinsapir KD, Goldberg RA: Traumatic optic neuropathy. *Surv Ophthalmol* 38(6):487–518, 1994.

21. White W, Woog JJ: Disorders of the canaliculus and punctum. In Bosniak S, ed., *Principles and practice of ophthalmic plastic and reconstructive surgery*, vol. 2, pp. 821–833, Philadelphia: WB Saunders, 1996.

CHAPTER 14

The Diagnostic Approach to the Patient with Proptosis

Chapter contents

Introduction

You will see orbital problems in your practice, but most of these problems are rare. My goal for this chapter is to give you a good foundation in approaching the patient with a proptotic eye. You won't be able to diagnose every orbital problem, but you should be able to proceed in a logical fashion and be able to diagnose most causes of proptosis. Orbital disease is the most complex topic in this book. It is easy to get overwhelmed—get an overview initially, and focus on the details during the second or third time through.

Think of all the different tissue types that are found in the orbit—nerves, muscle, veins and arteries, glandular tissue, and connective tissue, to name a few. In addition to these tissues, pigment cells and red and white blood cells are present. A primary orbital neoplasm may arise from any of these tissue types or cells. Now consider the tissues surrounding the orbit—bones of the face and skull, the brain, the sinus and nasal tissues, and the soft tissues of the face. Each of these structures may develop a problem that extends into the orbit as a secondary orbital condition. Given the almost infinite number of processes that can involve the orbit, it is important for you to develop an approach to investigating the patient with a proptotic eye.

Proptosis is the hallmark of orbital disease. When you see a proptotic or displaced eye, you should be able to develop a basic differential diagnosis based on the clues that you find in the history and physical examination. For most patients with proptosis, the diagnostic process will require imaging studies, most commonly a computed tomography (CT) scan. Because of the huge variety of possible problems, a biopsy of the pathologic lesion is often necessary for diagnosis or treatment.

In this chapter, you should:

- Learn to recognize the patient with proptosis
- Learn the approach to taking a basic history and performing a physical examination
- Know when imaging is necessary and what imaging studies are best
- Be able to develop a differential diagnosis based on the history and physical examination and imaging studies

- Become familiar with common orbital problems in adults and children

In all adults with proptosis, you should consider the diagnosis of thyroid orbitopathy first. Thyroid disease is the most common cause of unilateral or bilateral proptosis in adults. Other common causes in adults include lymphoid lesions, idiopathic orbital inflammatory disease, cavernous hemangioma, and metastatic disease. Some orbital neoplasms that are less common, but nevertheless deserve mention, are tumors of the optic nerve and lacrimal gland. You may also see tumors arising outside the orbit that involve the orbit secondarily. Even this small list of orbital problems can be overwhelming. Learn some of the typical features of these processes seen in the history and physical examination and their imaging characteristics. In the beginning, it will be difficult to get the exact diagnosis for each patient. Soon you will be able to develop a sense of the type of problem you are dealing with on a pathogenic basis. Is the problem inflammatory or neoplastic? Is it benign or malignant? Is it congenital or acquired? In a short time, you will be able to recognize the specific diseases that fit.

For the most part, the common causes of proptosis in children are different from those in adults. We will briefly discuss dermoid cyst, capillary hemangioma, orbital cellulitis, rhabdomyosarcoma, lymphangioma, and optic nerve glioma.

The treatment of the proptosis depends on the cause. For some causes of proptosis, such as orbital cellulitis, medical treatment will be initiated without biopsy. For other patients, an incisional biopsy will be required to obtain the diagnosis, for example the biopsy of a suspected lymphoid lesion to determine if the mass is benign or malignant. Often this incisional biopsy will be followed by further medical (chemotherapy or radiation therapy) or surgical (further tumor excision) therapy. In some patients, excisional biopsy or complete removal of the lesion, such as a dermoid cyst, will confirm the diagnosis and complete the treatment at the same time.

Review the basic approach to the patient with proptosis at this point. The presence of proptosis or displacement of the eye suggests an orbital problem. The history and physical examination will give you a differential diagnosis, at least on a pathogenic basis. Imaging studies such as a CT scan are usually required to refine the differential diagnosis. If the diagnosis is not clear at this point, incisional or excisional biopsy will be required to obtain a diagnosis. The plan for treatment is based on the diagnosis.

The normal anatomy and examination of the orbit

Hertel measurements

An exophthalmometer is used to measure the prominence of the eye. The most common exophthalmometer used is the Hertel exophthalmometer (Figure 14-1). The Hertel exophthalmometer measures the anterior projection of the eye, from the lateral orbital rim to the cornea (Table 14-1). When you use the Hertel exophthalmometer, be sure to lightly push the instrument against the lateral orbital rim and make

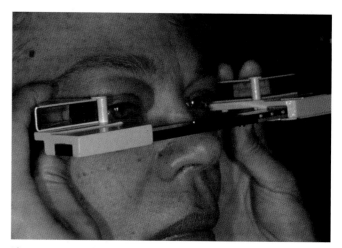

Figure 14-1 Hertel exophthalmometer measures the distance from the lateral canthal angle to the anterior surface of the cornea.

Table 14-1 Average Hertel measurements

Race	Hertel measurement (mm)
Asian	18
White	20
African American	22

the width or base setting of the exophthalmometer as narrow as comfortable for the patient. Try to use the same base setting for an individual patient each time you measure the prominence of the eye. Remember that measurements with the Hertel exophthalmometer are not exact, but you should be able to obtain repeatable measurements within 1–2 mm. When you learn to use the Hertel exophthalmometer, compare your readings with those of a more experienced examiner so that you can make sure you are measuring correctly. As the Hertel exophthalmometer uses the lateral orbital rim at a reference point, any surgery, disease, or trauma that changes the position of the lateral rim will affect the Hertel measurements. In cases where the lateral rim is not in normal position, you can use an exophthalmometer designed by Thomas Naugle. This device uses the forehead and cheek as reference points.

Race and facial bone structure

The normal prominence of the eye in the orbit depends upon the surrounding facial bones. The bony structures vary from individual to individual and among races. The equator of the globe is at the lateral orbital rim in a white patient with average bone structure. You can appreciate the position of the eye relative to the rim during the physical examination by placing your index finger at the lateral orbital rim and pushing against the eye. The average Hertel measurement for a white patient is 20 mm. The Asian face shows less prominent eyes. The average Hertel measurement for an Asian patient is approximately 18 mm. The African American face shows relatively more prominent eyes. The maxilla is shallow compared with white or Asian facial bones. The average Hertel measurement in an African American patient is 22 mm.

Significant measurements: asymmetry and change over time

Because the normal position of the eye in the orbit varies from patient to patient, we are more interested in asymmetry in the prominence of the one eye compared with the other or a change in the globe position on one side that has occurred over time. Proptosis implies an anterior displacement of the globe. An orbital mass not centered within the orbit will displace the eye off axis as well. Globe ptosis is the term used when the eye is pushed down by a mass. As you perform the orbital examination, look for signs of axial and nonaxial globe displacement of the eye that will help you locate the mass that is displacing the globe.

The surgical spaces of the orbit

The orbit is conceptually and anatomically divided into surgical spaces (Box 14-1).

The intraconal space, sometimes called the central surgical space, contains the optic nerve and orbital fat (Figure 14-2). Many tumors arise within the intraconal space or push their way into this space. The most widely discussed tumors of the orbit, optic nerve glioma and optic nerve meningioma, occur in the intraconal space.

The extraconal space, sometimes called the peripheral surgical space, contains the lacrimal gland, the superior oblique muscle and trochlea, and nerves and vessels in the extraconal orbital fat. The lacrimal gland is a common source of orbital pathologic processes. An enlarged lacrimal gland is often palpable in the upper lid and is readily accessible using an anterior orbitotomy through the upper lid skin crease.

A fibrous membrane, the intermuscular septum, extends between the anterior portion of the extraocular muscles, separating the intraconal and extraconal spaces. The muscles can become involved in neoplastic or inflammatory processes. The most common condition is thyroid orbitopathy. Painful inflammation of the muscles, myositis, may also occur. Primary neoplasms of the muscles are very rare, but metastatic lesions occur more commonly.

The subperiosteal space is a potential space between the orbital bones and the periorbita. A hematoma may collect in this space from an adjacent fracture. A collection of pus, a subperiosteal abscess, may collect medially from an adjacent ethmoid sinus infection.

Tenon's space lies between the eye and the fibrous capsule. Tenon's capsule, which surrounds all but the anterior portion of the eye, is the bloodless space in which enucleation and scleral buckle procedures are performed. This space is rarely involved in orbital pathologic processes, the most common lesion being extraocular extension of a choroidal melanoma.

The extraorbital space, or periocular tissue, includes all the structures surrounding the orbit: bone, brain, sinuses, nasal, skin, and conjunctiva. A variety of problems originate

---

Box 14-1

The Surgical Spaces of the Orbit
- The intraconal space
- The extraconal space
- The extraocular muscles
- The subperiosteal space
- Tenon's space
- The extraorbital space

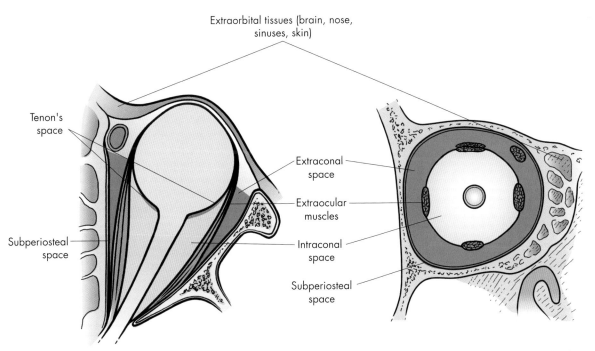

Figure 14-2 The surgical spaces of the orbit: intraconal space (central surgical space); extraocular muscles; extraconal space (peripheral surgical space); subperiosteal space; Tenon's space; the extraorbital space (including periocular tissues, brain, nose, sinuses, bone, and surrounding soft tissues). (**A**) Axial view. (**B**) Coronal view.

Table 14-2 Differential diagnosis based on direction of globe displacement in adults

Displacement	Etiology
(1) Axial displacement	
Enlarged extraocular muscles	Thyroid orbitopathy
Intraconal mass	Cavernous hemangioma
Optic nerve tumor	Optic nerve meningioma
(2) Nonaxial displacement	
(a) Inferior displacement	
(i) Lacrimal gland	Benign mixed or lymphoid tumor
(ii) Frontal sinus	Mucocele
(iii) Orbital roof	Sphenoid wing meningioma
(b) Lateral displacement	
(i) Ethmoid sinus	Abscess or mucocele
(c) Superior displacement	
(i) Maxillary sinus	Carcinoma
(ii) Orbital fat	Lymphoid tumor
(d) Medial (rare)	Benign mixed tumor of lacrimal gland
(3) Enophthalmos	Scirrhous carcinoma of the breast

in these tissues and involve the orbit secondarily. We will talk about some of these conditions at the end of this chapter (Table 14-2).

History

The "P's" of the orbital history and physical examination

Krohel, Stewart, and Chavis described the familiar mnemonic involving the "P's" of the orbital history and physical examination. Although this system is somewhat contrived, it is a useful way to learn the orbital history and conduct the physical examination, providing a checklist of what to consider. The six P's they described are the following:

- Pain
- Progression
- Proptosis
- Palpation
- Pulsation
- Periorbital changes

We will see in a few paragraphs that we should add a seventh P to the list, past medical history.

Pain and progression

Pain and progression are the characteristics of the orbital problems that you will find most helpful in developing the differential diagnosis. Pain is caused by inflammation, infection, acute pressure changes, and bone or nerve involvement. Once you become familiar with the common orbital disorders, you will find that the presence or absence of pain is very helpful in developing a differential diagnosis.

Progression is the other "P" that will refine the differential diagnosis easily for you. As you can imagine, some processes

progress quickly, whereas others take months or years to develop. You can classify progression into:

- Rapid progression, occurring in hours to days
- Intermediate rate of progression, occurring in weeks to months
- Slow progression, occurring in months to years

History as a clue to the pathologic process

It is impossible to diagnose every cause of proptosis based on pain and progression only, but you will be surprised how easy it is to develop a differential diagnosis of a general pathogenesis. Consider the types of pathologic processes that affect the body as a whole. You probably learned these in your medical school pathology course:

- Inflammatory
- Infectious
- Hemorrhagic
- Neoplastic
- Metastatic
- Congenital

Now consider how the symptom of pain fits into the categories. Pain suggests inflammation, infection, hemorrhage, or perhaps a tumor growing into nerves or bone. Neoplasms, in general, do not cause pain until a complication related to the neoplasm arises. You will remember from your general surgery days in medical school that the large bowel tumor sits quietly in the abdomen until there is an obstruction that causes secondary inflammation, infection, or hemorrhage. This is true of orbital tumors as well. The majority of orbital neoplasms do not cause pain until late in their course.

A sudden onset with rapid progression over minutes suggests a hemorrhage (Figure 14-3). Acute processes occurring over hours to days suggest inflammation or infection. Slower processes occurring over weeks to months suggest more chronic types of inflammatory processes such as thyroid disease. Chronic conditions with a vague onset and slow progression over months suggest a benign neoplasm or lymphoma.

Onset and progression of symptoms and signs are related features. Onset identifies a point in time when the problem started and how it manifested itself initially. Progression describes any change in the symptoms (and the rate of change) occurring over the period of time since the onset. For example, an orbital infection may have an onset 3 days after the start of a respiratory infection. The pain and inflammation are minimal initially, but progress rapidly after onset. A contrasting example is the proptosis and globe ptosis resulting from a benign mixed tumor of the lacrimal gland. The progression is so slow, over months or years, that it is difficult for the patient to identify the exact onset of any symptoms. In many chronic conditions, the patient's perception of the onset and the progression of the disorder may not be accurate. In these cases, the patient's perception of onset is often when the proptosis was noted, which may not be when the process actually started. In these cases, the use of the so-called family album tomogram (FAT) scan is useful. The review of these old photos can help to identify the true progression of a disorder.

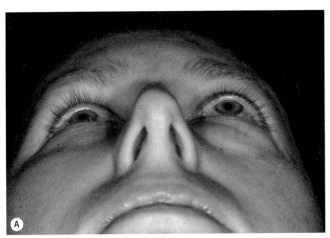
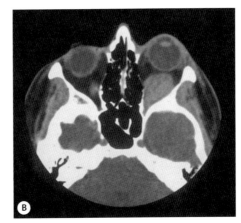

Figure 14-3 Spontaneous orbital hemorrhage. (**A**) Pain and proptosis developed over minutes with no progression after the initial presentation. (**B**) CT scan demonstrates a well-circumscribed mass (based on axial and coronal cuts). Drainage of the hematoma was required because of pain (see **Figure 15-12**). No etiology was determined.

Past medical history

Lastly, we should add past medical history to the list of the original six P's. Any previous diagnosis of neoplasm elsewhere in the body must be noted. Past trauma of the face may have caused some facial asymmetry that may accentuate or diminish the appearance of a proptotic eye. Any history of thyroid disease that has already been diagnosed should be noted. This is perhaps the most important information to solicit. Don't forget to include basic information in the history such as age and sex. You will see that most orbital processes tend to occur at certain ages. The differential diagnoses of childhood and adult orbital disorders don't share many diseases in common. The most common disorder that has a striking sex difference is thyroid disease, which occurs about six times more often in women than in men.

A typical history might be written, "A 65-year-old noted proptosis of the left eye and a mass in the lid 4 months ago. Since that time the proptosis and swelling have progressed slowly. There is no pain. There is no past medical history of trauma or thyroid disease. He was treated for lymphoma in the past. He is currently taking no medications." Are you getting the idea? Already you are thinking about the possibility of orbital lymphoma and will be looking for some fullness of the superior fornix, a little globe ptosis, and a palpably enlarged lacrimal gland during the physical examination.

Physical examination of the orbit

The physical examination "P's"

The "Ps" of the orbital examination are:

- Proptosis
- Palpation
- Pulsation
- Periocular changes

Proptosis

The most important part of the orbital examination is the evaluation of the proptotic eye. An orbital mass or volume-

producing process "pushes" the eye away. The larger the mass is, the more displacement of the globe.

In most cases, when we talk about proptosis, we are really talking about proptosis or an axial displacement of the eye in an anterior direction. When you see axial proptosis, think of thyroid orbitopathy with enlargement of the extraocular muscles. Other intraconal disorders such as optic nerve tumors or a benign cavernous hemangioma may occur within that muscle cone as well and cause axial anterior displacement of the eye. In some conditions, you will see nonaxial displacement of the eye. If you see the eye pushed downward, think of problems arising in the area of the lacrimal gland or, less commonly, defects in the orbital roof due to trauma, encephalocele, or frontal sinus mucocele formation. When you see the eye displaced laterally, there is usually a problem in the ethmoid sinus. The most common situation that displaces the eye laterally is a subperiosteal abscess (an acute process) arising in the ethmoid sinus and extending into the subperiosteal space. Rarely, sinus carcinomas (a slowly progressive process) or mucoceles (a very slowly progressive process) of the ethmoid sinus can cause this type of lateral displacement. You will rarely see the eye being displaced upward. A number of rare conditions can cause this (**Figure 14-4**). Although lymphoid lesions occur most commonly in the superior orbit, lymphoid lesions are so common that they are the most common cause of an inferior orbital mass. Rarely, tumors arising from the maxillary sinus can erode through the orbital floor and push the eye upward. Likewise, it is rare to see the globe pushed medially. If medial globe displacement is present, the eye usually is also being pushed downward by an enlarged lacrimal gland. You can estimate the nonaxial displacement of the eye with a ruler or use an instrument designed for this purpose known as the McCoy Tri-Square (P-3795, Jarit Instruments, http://www.jarit.com) (**Figure 14-5**).

There is an exception to the rule that an orbital mass pushes the eye away from the mass. Scirrhous carcinoma of the breast is an infiltrative sclerosing tumor, which may actually cause an enophthalmos of the eye. You have already asked about past medical history of other carcinomas, so if you heard that the patient has a history of breast carcinoma

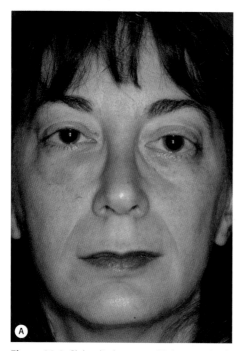
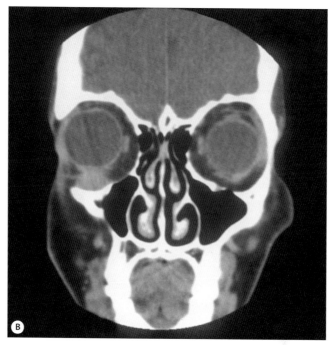

Figure 14-4 Globe displacement. (**A**) Superior displacement of the right eye. (**B**) CT scan shows a well-circumscribed mass, determined to be an unusual mesenchymal tumor after excisional biopsy.

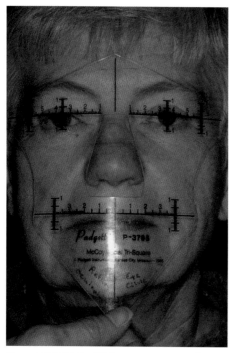

Figure 14-5 McCoy Tri-Square measuring millimeters of globe ptosis.

genital variation may be a cause of the asymmetry. Similarly, a change in the displacement of the eye based on the patient's history or old photographs is an important finding.

Palpation

The next step in the orbital examination is palpation. Start with palpation of the orbital rims and then move toward the eye, palpating the superior and inferior fornix for any anterior masses. If a mass is palpable, you want to note its shape, size, and position. Often, you can tell if the mass has a smooth border separate from adjacent tissues or is infiltrating into adjacent tissues. In some patients, the mass will be fixed to bone or a nearby structure such as an extraocular muscle, suggesting an infiltrative tumor. You should try to determine if there is any tenderness in the area of the lesion as well. Infectious or inflammatory disorders will often cause the skin to be erythematous and warm to touch.

Pulsation

Pulsations of the orbit are rare but, when present, are diagnostic. A classic finding is pulsatile proptosis. This pulsation of the eye suggests either an arterial vascular malformation in the orbit or the absence of orbital bone that allows the normal pulsations of the brain to push on the eye. The most common cause of pulsatile proptosis is the absence of the sphenoid wing seen in neurofibromatosis. If you think you are seeing a case of pulsating exophthalmos, you will find it useful to confirm the globe pulsations using the Hertel exophthalmometer to view the eye from the side. Feel the radial pulse at the same time and you will see that the pulsations are synchronized.

Orbital arterial vascular lesions can pulsate. If the flow is high, you may be able to hear a bruit or feel a thrill. These lesions are rare also. Vascular abnormalities that are prima-

and you note that eye is sunken, think of metastatic breast cancer (Figure 14-6).

We have already talked about the use of the Hertel exophthalmometer to measure the prominence of the eye. Remember that there are normal variations among individuals and races. When you use the Hertel exophthalmometer, asymmetry between the left and right sides is more important than the actual measurement. Any asymmetry measuring more than 2 mm is significant. Don't forget that trauma or con-

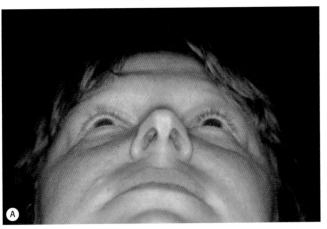
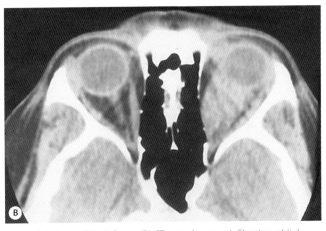

Figure 14-6 Enophthalmos secondary to metastatic breast cancer. (**A**) Note slight enophthalmos of the left eye. (**B**) CT scan shows an infiltrative orbital mass.

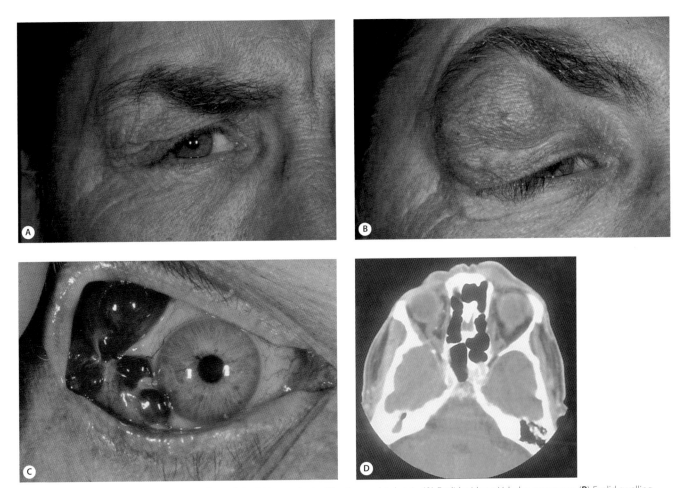

Figure 14-7 Valsalva maneuver causing swelling of the lid in a patient with a large orbital varix. (**A**) Eyelid without Valsalva maneuver. (**B**) Eyelid swelling with Valsalva maneuver. (**C**) Conjunctival varix engorgement with Valsalva maneuver. (**D**) CT scan showing nondiscrete orbital mass. Note phleboliths and enlargement of the superior orbital fissure.

rily venous are more common than arterial lesions. Venous lesions do not pulsate, but they will usually show enlargement with the Valsalva maneuver or with the head in a dependent position (Figure 14-7).

Periocular changes

The last point to note in the orbital examination is periocular changes. These include a variety of abnormalities in the skin, conjunctiva, eye, or surrounding periocular tissues. Some periocular changes that are most useful for diagnosis are the temporal flare of the lateral portion of the upper lid and lid lag seen on downgaze in patients with thyroid orbitopathy (Figure 14-8). Other examples of periocular changes include a conjunctival salmon patch suggesting orbital lymphoma (see Figure 14-18), fullness of the temple suggesting a sphenoid wing meningioma (see Figure 14-22),

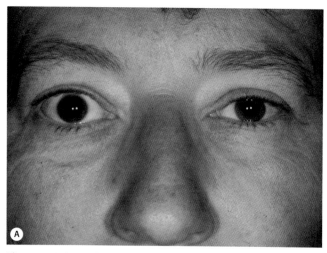
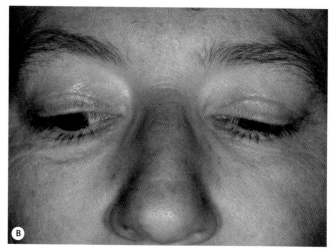

Figure 14-8 Periocular changes associated with thyroid orbitopathy. (**A**) Right upper lid retraction and temporal flare of the lateral upper eyelid, suggesting thyroid orbitopathy. (**B**) Lid lag on downgaze in the same patient.

and periocular skin malignancy suggesting intraorbital spread of cutaneous carcinoma.

At this point, stop and think about the orbital examination and remind yourself of how you will proceed:

- You will start by evaluating the change in the position of the eye in terms of axial and nonaxial displacement, suggesting where a mass might be present and pushing the eye away
- Next you will palpate the orbital rims and soft tissues to see if any abnormality is present
- Then you will check briefly for any pulsations
- Last, you will search for other clues in the periocular area that may give you information to develop a differential diagnosis

Checkpoint

The plan for evaluation of the patient with proptosis is to take the history and perform the physical examination followed by imaging of the orbit. Usually, at this point, you can make a differential diagnosis. You can generally narrow down the choices to one of the general pathologic categories such as neoplasm or infection. Remember thyroid orbitopathy is the most common cause of unilateral, bilateral proptosis. If a mass is diagnosed, incisional or excisional biopsy is usually needed to confirm the diagnosis. Treatment is based upon the pathology results.

Recall the three "Ps" of the history:
- Pain
- Progression
- Past medical history

Recall the four "P's" of the physical examination:
- Proptosis
- Palpation
- Pulsation
- Periocular change

Orbital imaging

Proptosis? Order a CT scan

Almost all patients with proptosis will require orbital imaging. One exception to this may be the patient with findings typical of stable Graves' disease in whom the diagnosis is so apparent that no imaging is needed to confirm your clinical suspicion. CT scanning is used as the primary imaging technique for evaluation of any patient with proptosis. You should order a magnetic resonance imaging (MRI) scan of the orbit in special cases, primarily those situations in which imaging of the orbital apex and chiasm is required.

You are undoubtedly familiar with the CT scan technique. You will recall that CT scanning uses ionizing radiation passed through the tissue to form a computer-generated radiograph. Like other radiographs, excellent views of the bony structure are obtained, making the CT scan the method of choice for viewing bony orbital trauma. Remember that fat is radiolucent (black) on a CT scan. The intraconal fat gives a good natural contrast with adjacent soft tissue structures (shades of gray) without any injection of intravenous contrast agents. For these reasons, the CT scan gives excellent views of the orbital bones and the majority of orbital structures.

CT scan is essential for evaluation of orbital trauma. CT scans are readily available. Helical CT scanners have reduced orbital scanning times to less than a minute per patient. You should order and review axial and coronal projections on all patients. Sagittal views are occasionally helpful. All projections are available without repositioning the patient. You hospital or imaging center should be providing high resolution orbital scans with no more than 1–2 mm cuts. The cavernous sinuses and paranasal sinuses should be included with orbital scans. You will want intravenous contrast agent for evaluation of most tumors. Contrast allergies are not uncommon, so make sure you ask about iodine or fish allergies. CT scanning remains significantly less expensive than MRI.

Magnetic resonance imaging

Generation of images is based on entirely different principles than those used in CT scanning. No ionizing radiation is used. An image is generated based upon the "vibration" of protons in tissue when a patient is placed in the magnetic field and then subjected to a series of radio wave pulses. The radiologist can vary the radio wave pulses so that different tissues generate signals (this is how the standard T1- and T2-weighted scans, and the many other specialized sequences, are generated). Some general imaging characteristics will help you to interpret MRI scans:

- You can recognize a T1-weighted scan because the vitreous is dark
- You can recognize a T2-weighted scan because the vitreous is white ("bright")
- Because the density of the signal depends on the density of protons in the tissue, edema (water, i.e., protons) causes a bright signal on the T2-weighted image
- High vascular flow, such as that in the carotid artery, generates no signal (dark), "a flow void," because the protons are moving too quickly to be imaged
- The protons in bone are too tightly bound to generate a signal, so cortical bone is dark on MRI scans. Marrow spaces will generate a signal

The resolution for MRI is less than for CT. The tissue contrast, however, is better with MRI. As the fat provides a contrast to most other structures, CT can be used as the main screening technique for orbital disease. MRI plays an important role in the evaluation of specific orbital diseases and is sometimes used in addition to CT scan.

The main indication for MRI is to view the orbitocranial junction. If you suspect an optical nerve tumor, you should request an MRI scan. Because bone is not visualized, the bony artifact from the dense bones of the orbital apex seen on CT scans is not present. The soft tissues of the apex are visualized in detail. Some intraorbital organic foreign bodies are seen better with MRI scans than with CT scans. Vascular tumors or other very heterogeneous tumors are often seen more clearly on an MRI scan than on a CT scan, as well. Lastly, any secondary orbital disease originating from the brain or paranasal sinus can often be visualized best by both CT and MRI together. This allows the best view of bone and soft tissue. In the case of sinus neoplasms extending into the orbit, T2-weighted MRI sequences help to distinguish sinus opacity caused mucous retention (bright signal) from that caused by tumor (dark signal).

Most radiology departments have routine imaging sequences that are used under an orbital protocol. In addition, an intravenous contrast material, gadolinium, can be injected to enhance some pathologic processes. An imaging sequence known as fat suppression is used with gadolinium. With this technique, the normally bright orbital fat appears dark. Without fat suppression, you will not see any enhanced orbital structures against the normally bright fat background.

There are many specific sequences that help with imaging certain disease processes; for example, the FLAIR sequence is especially good for identifying optic neuritis due to demyelinating disease. You will want to develop a working relationship with a radiologist interested in orbital disease to help you with these nuances. Similarly, you will find that working with an interventional radiologist can help you understand and deal with vascular flow issues in some of your orbital patients.

In practice, you will be looking at T1 and T2 scans with contrast injection. Use these tips to evaluate an MRI scan:

- Look at the T1-weighted scan for the best anatomic detail
- T2-weighted scans show water as "bright," emphasizing edema or other fluid within a mass
- As you get more familiar with specific disease processes, you can learn the individual characteristics of the T1 and T2 sequences for each process or tumor (don't worry about that now)
- Look at the fat suppression sequence (the fat is dark) on gadolinium-enhanced scans. Enhancement implies a richly vascularized tumor or inflammation (such as sarcoid, often not visible without enhancement)

MRI has several practical disadvantages compared with CT scanning. MRI is still about three times more expensive than CT. Imaging takes significantly longer. Bone is poorly viewed. As we said above, the spatial resolution of MRI is less than that of CT, so detail is not as clear. MRI is not safe for patients who have metallic foreign bodies or aneurysm clips in place. It is difficult, or impossible, to obtain an MRI scan for any patient who requires a ventilator, pacemaker, or cardiac monitor.

Special imaging studies

Special imaging studies are available or can be arranged with consultation with your radiology colleagues.

- CT
  — Three-dimensional (3D) CT
  — Imaging for stereotactic navigation
  — Angiography (CTA)
  — Valsalva
- MR
  — MR angiography (MRA)
- Angiography
- Echography

CT studies for stereotactic navigation are commonly obtained by our ear, nose, and throat (ENT) and neurosurgical colleagues, especially when performing endoscopic operations. You are probably familiar with studies but, if not, you should see the technique in action. By linking the preoperative high resolution images with cameras in the operating room that sense the position of your instruments, you can have real time localization of your position in the patient. This technique is especially useful where the "normal" anatomy is quite variable (paranasal sinuses) and for reoperations where normal landmarks have been altered. It can be helpful for you when you are operating in less familiar areas. For example, I used this when I was less experienced in skull base procedures. CT scanning before and during *Valsalva maneuver* is helpful for detecting the venous flood seen in orbital varies. *3D CT scans* produce amazing pictures (see Figure 14-9). These images are most useful for craniofacial anomalies and extensive facial trauma. 3D scans are valuable

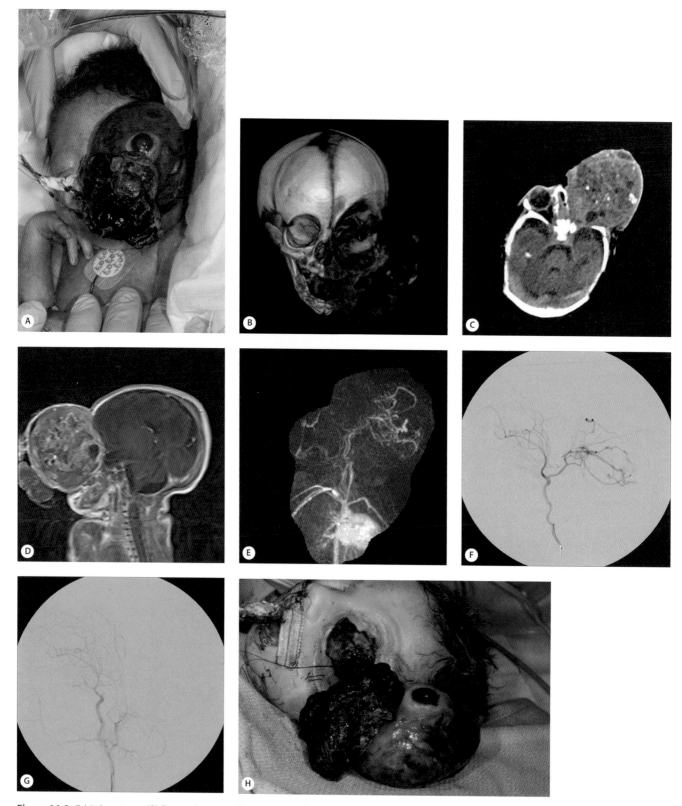

Figure 14-9 Orbital teratoma. (**A**) Extremely rare and large congenital orbital mass in premature infant. (**B**) 3D CT reconstruction demonstrates soft tissue mass and large bony orbit. (**C**) Axial CT scan of head, soft tissue window—shows a large heterogeneous mass in the orbit without extension into the brain. Eye appears to be flattened at the most anterior portion of the mass. (**D**) Sagittal T1 MRI of the head, gadolinium enhanced, shows heterogeneity prompting vascular studies. (**E**) MR angiogram (MRA) demonstrates prominent vascular flow from the internal carotid artery branches. (**F**) Carotid angiography confirmed carotid artery flow. (**G**) Carotid angiography after occlusion of feeding arterial supply. (**H**) Successful tumor excision (orbital exenteration) with minimal blood loss.

for planning a reconstructive operation and are also useful for teaching residents and patients. *CTA and MRA are easy ways to view the blood supply of a tumor.* For a number of reasons, MRA is usually the first choice for our purposes. *Arteriography* remains the gold standard for vascular imaging. At the same time, therapeutic selective occlusion of feeding vessels can cure or decrease vascular flow decreasing or eliminating the problem or, in some cases, making operation safer. Similarly, direct venous puncture and occlusion can be helpful in selected cases of varix or other mixed venous malformations. If your practice includes these patients, you will need a strong working relationship with a neurointerventional radiologist. *Echography* has been used in the imaging of ocular and orbital diseases for many years. In the hands of experienced practitioners, useful information can be obtained. In most centers, CT and MRI have replaced echography in the study of orbital disease.

The information that is available with current imaging techniques and the expertise of our radiology colleagues is incredible. This information can be extremely valuable for diagnosis and surgical planning. A good example is Figure 14-9 which focused our attention on the blood supply of a large congenital mass in a newborn. Vascular studies and embolization made the tumor removal safe for this premature baby weighing only 3 pounds.

Interpretation of orbital imaging

Goals of imaging

As we have already discussed, many patients with proptosis will undergo imaging studies. Orbital imaging serves two purposes:

- Providing diagnostic information (I want to know what the mass is)
- Providing information used to plan orbitotomy (I want to know the best surgical approach to biopsy the mass)

Most times with a quick look at the scan, you will be able to get an idea of what is causing the proptosis. Probably you will see one of two situations:

- An enlarged orbital structure
  — Extraocular muscle(s)
  — Optic nerve
  — Lacrimal gland
  — Eyeball (pseudoproptosis)
- An orbital mass not arising from a specific structure
  — A well-circumscribed mass
  — An infiltrative mass

In a few situations, you may be able to make the diagnosis based upon the scan alone. For example, bilateral enlargement of extraocular muscles indicates thyroid orbitopathy until proven otherwise. More likely, the imaging will give you a few possible diagnoses. For example, an enlarged optic nerve usually indicates meningioma or glioma.

If a mass appears separate from the surrounding structures, the characteristics of the mass may help you put the lesion in a particular pathogenic category, such as neoplasm or inflammation. Based on the location of the mass in the orbit, you can determine the best surgical approach for biopsy.

Remember, the questions we are trying to answer are: "What is it?" and "What is the best surgical approach for biopsy?" Some specific characteristics of an orbital mass will help you with the diagnosis and surgical approach:

- Location
  — What is the tissue of origin?
  — Position of the mass: Which surgical space is involved?
- Imaging clues to the biologic behavior of a mass
  — Relationship to adjacent soft tissues
- A "pusher" (benign)
- An "eater" (malignant)
- Relationship to adjacent bone
  — Fossa formation (benign)
  — Bone erosion (malignant)
- Shape of the mass
- Size of the mass
- Internal characteristics of the mass
  — Homogeneous or heterogeneous
- Contrast enhancement

Location

Tissue of origin

You must be able to describe the location of a lesion. Can you determine the tissue of origin? Does the mass represent an enlargement of a normal orbital structure? The lacrimal gland, the optic nerve, and extraocular muscles can be enlarged, each with a separate differential diagnoses. If the mass represents infiltration of a normal structure, you are likely to be doing an incisional biopsy, rather than removing the structure initially.

Position of the mass: the surgical spaces of the orbit

If you cannot tell whether the mass is derived from a normal structure, you should localize the mass within a specific orbital space and describe its position relative to normal structures within the space. We discussed the surgical spaces of the orbit (see Figure 14-2) earlier in this chapter under "The Normal Anatomy and Examination of the Orbit." The surgical spaces of the orbit are:

- The intraconal space
- The extraocular muscles
- The extraconal space
- The subperiosteal space
- Tenon's space
- The extraorbital space

Knowledge of the surgical space containing the orbital mass is useful for developing a differential diagnosis and choosing the surgical approach for biopsy. The spatial relationship to the optic nerve and the anterior–posterior position within the intraconal space are especially important in choosing the orbitotomy approach. When you operate in the intraconal space, choose a surgical approach so that you do not cross the optic nerve. Approach medial intraconal masses in the anterior portion of the orbit from a medial anterior orbitotomy. Approach lateral intraconal masses in the anterior orbit from a lateral orbitotomy. Masses arising deep in the intraconal space must be approached transcranially. You can see that the location of a mass in the orbit is critical for the diagnosis and biopsy of the mass. We will discuss the surgical approaches to the orbit in the next chapter.

Imaging clues to the biologic behavior of the mass

Relationship to adjacent soft tissue—a pusher or an eater?

This is important. Does the mass push the adjacent structures aside or does it infiltrate the adjacent tissues? Infiltrative lesions are usually malignant. Well-circumscribed lesions with smooth borders are usually benign (Figure 14-10). Think of these lesions as "pushers" or "eaters." Pushers are more likely benign. Eaters are more likely malignant. Is the mass pushing against the optic nerve or growing into the optic nerve (Figure 14-11)? The latter lesion is more likely malignant. The relationship to adjacent structures, or borders, gives you a "snapshot in time" estimate of the biologic behavior of the mass. This concept is simple but extremely important.

Relationship to adjacent bone fossa formation or bone erosion

The relationship of a soft tissue mass to the adjacent bone gives similar information about the biologic behavior of the mass. Slow-growing benign masses "push" the bone or cause fossa formation. Aggressive malignant tumors "eat" the bone or cause bone erosion. When you evaluate a lacrimal gland mass, the presence of fossa formation is typical of a benign slow-growing mixed tumor of the lacrimal gland (Figure 14-12).

You will learn to use the clinical information you obtain during the history and physical examination to complement the imaging studies. A poorly defined mass with indistinct borders presenting without pain is likely to be a malignant neoplasm. A poorly defined mass with indistinct borders presenting with pain is likely to be idiopathic orbital inflammatory disease, rather than any true neoplasm. Hypesthesia of the temple described by the patient with bone erosion adjacent to the lacrimal gland mass (see Figure 14-12) is indicative of the neurotrophic spread typical of the aggressive adenoid cystic carcinoma of the lacrimal gland.

The distinctiveness of the borders helps greatly in determining if the mass can be removed. Infiltrative lesions usually cannot be safely removed (require incisional biopsy). Well-circumscribed masses can often be removed (excisional biopsy).

Shape of the mass

The shape of the lesion is less helpful than the relationship to other tissues in determining its biologic behavior but sometimes suggests the diagnosis. Cavernous hemangiomas are usually "round." Benign mixed tumors of the lacrimal gland are said to be "oval" (see Figure 14-12). Sometimes, a particular feature of the shape will be diagnostic. The "kink" of an enlarged optic nerve (a sharp change in the direction of the nerve) strongly suggests a glioma.

Size of the mass

The size of the lesion doesn't tell us a great deal about the diagnosis. Big is usually worse than small, but a small malignancy is worse than a large benign mass. Combined with clinical information, you may be able to glean something

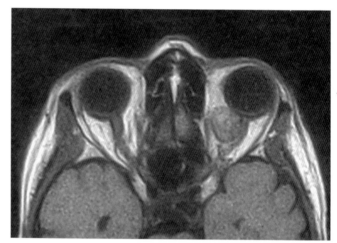

Figure 14-11 MRI scan of intraconal mass, medial to the optic nerve, apparently attached to the nerve. Proven by biopsy to be a metastatic cutaneous melanoma. Smooth shape is not characteristic of most metastatic tumors, which are infiltrative in nature.

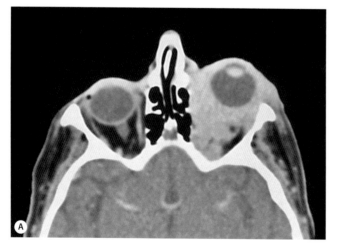

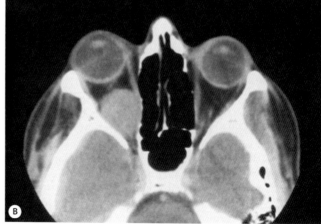

Figure 14-10 Infiltrative mass compared with well-circumscribed mass. (**A**) CT scan of infiltrative lesion shown to be a metastatic breast carcinoma. (**B**) CT scan of a well-circumscribed benign mass, a cavernous hemangioma. Note that the medial orbital wall is bowed outward, but not eroded.

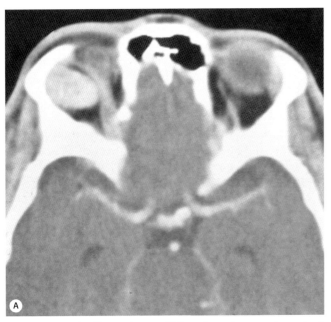

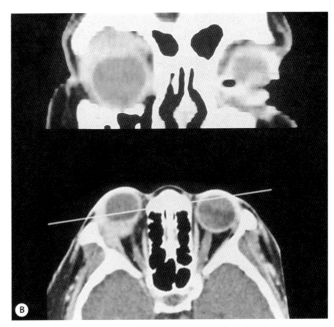

Figure 14-12 Orbital bone changes. (**A**) Fossa formation secondary to benign mixed tumor of the lacrimal gland. Note how the well-outlined mass "pushes" the bone away, creating a smooth fossa. (**B**) Bone erosion secondary to adenoid cystic carcinoma of the lacrimal gland. Note how the infiltrative mass creates an irregular change in the contour of the bone.

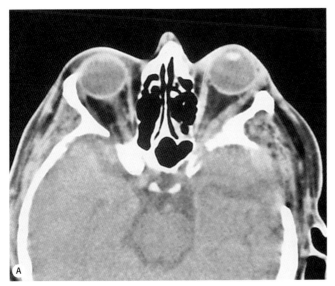

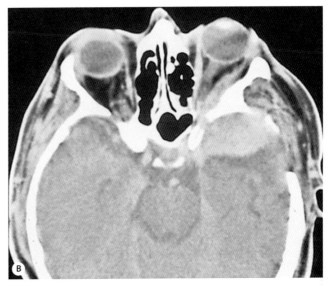

Figure 14-13 Sphenoid wing meningioma. (**A**) CT scan without contrast enhancement. (**B**) CT scan with contrast enhancement.

useful from the size of the mass. A large mass present for a short time (such as a rhabdomyosarcoma) is probably an aggressive tumor. Mass present for many years, large or small (such as a dermoid cyst), is likely to be benign. Make sure you record the size of the mass. Larger orbital masses are easier to find, but more difficult to remove, and you may have to alter your surgical approach if you are planning excisional biopsy.

Internal characteristics of the mass

Homogeneous or heterogeneous

The internal characteristics of a mass can be helpful information. The majority of tumors are homogeneous. Heterogeneous masses may show a diagnostic pattern:

- A combination of solid and cystic components in a child's tumor is typical of lymphangioma
- The layering of fat and keratin debris in a cystic mass is diagnostic for a dermoid cyst
- Small areas of calcification in a soft tissue orbital mass are typical of malignancy
- "Tram tracking" of an optic nerve tumor is diagnostic for an optic nerve meningioma (parallel lines of calcification in the subarachnoid space)
- Hyperostosis of the sphenoid wing is diagnostic for a sphenoid wing meningioma (Figure 14-13)

Contrast enhancement

Intravenous contrast agents are routinely given for CT scan and MRI evaluations of orbital tumors. Although these agents give an estimate of the blood flow to a mass, their main value is for identifying lesions that may not otherwise be seen. Examples are contrast enhancement of meningioma (see Figure 14-13) or rhabdomyosarcoma and inflammatory lesions such as sarcoidosis.

Checkpoint

CT scanning is used as the primary imaging technique for orbital disease.

The main indication for MRI is to view the orbitocranial junction. On an MRI scan, what do the terms bright and dark mean? Is the vitreous on a T2-weighted scan bright or dark? Is cortical bone bright or dark? What is a flow void?

Evaluate the imaging of an orbital mass to answer two questions:

- "What is it?"
- "What is the best surgical approach for biopsy?"
  Consider the following:
- The location of the mass. Can you determine the tissue from which the mass is arising? If not, which surgical space is it in?
- Is the mass a "pusher" or an "eater"? Can you recognize the difference? How does this reflect the biologic behavior? This is one of the most important pieces of information learned from a scan.
- Name three orbital lesions with characteristic imaging features.

Common causes of proptosis in adults

Introduction

There are too many orbital disorders to discuss them all in this text, so I have chosen to describe the most common or most important problems. The "common disorders" are just that, and you will see them most often. Thyroid orbitopathy is an example. As you know, it is the most common cause of unilateral or bilateral proptosis. Thyroid disease is so common that you should consider the possibility of thyroid orbitopathy as a cause of orbital disease in any patient with proptosis. You will be correct in some patients with apparent unilateral proptosis and almost always correct in patients with bilateral proptosis. The "important disorders" are included for a number of reasons. Some are "classic textbook" examples of orbital disease, such as optic nerve tumors. Optic nerve meningioma is an example, a rare problem that you will need to know about, if for no other reason than because it is often a question on board examinations. Other important disorders are included because you should not miss them, usually for a specific reason. Benign mixed tumor of the lacrimal gland is an example. Excisional biopsy should be used for this rare tumor of the lacrimal gland rather than incisional biopsy to prevent a later recurrence, possibly as a malignant tumor. For the more common lymphoid infiltrates of the lacrimal gland, an incisional biopsy of the gland should be performed. Although benign mixed tumors are uncommon, you should at least consider the diagnosis in every patient with lacrimal gland enlarge-

ment before performing an incisional biopsy. Another example is orbital rhabdomyosarcoma in children. In any child with rapidly progressing proptosis, this life-threatening disorder should be ruled out. Early diagnosis results in a cure in greater than 90% of patients with rhabdomyosarcoma of the orbit alone.

Each disorder that we will be discussing is complex in itself. Take the following approach:

- Learn the common presentation—the "P's" of the history and physical examination that will let you make the diagnosis
- Understand what the disease process is
- Recognize the imaging characteristics that help to confirm the diagnosis
- Understand the treatment options

Each topic follows a format that lends itself to learning these points.

Thyroid orbitopathy

Slow progression without pain

The orbitopathy is characterized by an ill-defined onset of progressive orbital inflammation causing lid swelling, proptosis, lid retraction, and strabismus. Unlike other inflammatory conditions, pain is not part of the presentation. Beware of attributing any painful orbitopathy to thyroid disease. Thyroid orbitopathy is the most common cause of unilateral or bilateral proptosis. As we said, at least briefly, consider this diagnosis in all patients with proptosis. Without looking at other signs and symptoms, you will be correct more often with this diagnosis than with any other.

Thyroid orbitopathy affects women five to six times more often than men. The onset is most common in the early 40s and mid-60s. The onset of symptoms is usually gradual, so that patients often cannot recognize when symptoms first appeared. The disease progresses at a highly variable rate with similar variation in severity. In extreme cases, the disease may progress very rapidly. No pain is associated, but discomfort, more like pressure or orbital fullness, is often present. Past medical history often reveals systemic thyroid disease. A family history is common. Smoking is a risk factor.

Bilateral proptosis and associated eyelid findings are diagnostic

The proptosis is usually bilateral, but can be quite asymmetric (sometimes even appearing to be unilateral disease if you don't look carefully for associated lid signs). The proptosis is axial. Hertel measurements vary from normal to off the scale, depending on the severity of the disease. Associated periocular signs are important for making the diagnosis. Look for upper and lower lid retraction, lid lag on downgaze, and "temporal flare" of the eyelid. Temporal flare is the term given to the abnormal contour of the eyelid seen in thyroid disease (see Figures 14-8, A and 14-14). As you recall, the peak of the normal eyelid is just nasal to the pupil. Typically, the lid in a patient with thyroid disease has no obvious peak. The lid just keeps getting higher toward the lateral canthus. If these associated lid signs are present, they will make the diagnosis for you.

Bilateral orbital inflammation with associated thyroid gland abnormalities

Thyroid orbitopathy is an idiopathic inflammatory condition affecting the orbit, primarily the extraocular muscles. The eye is spared from intraocular involvement. Although the exact mechanism is not well known, presumably antibodies attach to tissue in both the thyroid gland and extraocular muscles that are recognized as foreign. The associated immune response stimulates the thyroid gland to produce thyroid hormone. Similarly, the local inflammatory response causes the muscles to enlarge. Most patients will be hyperthyroid at the time of diagnosis of the eye condition. Only a small percentage of patients will remain euthyroid throughout the disease course. Most patients assume that serum normalization of the thyroid levels will help the orbital disease. Reduction in serum thyroid hormone levels is achieved by reducing the output of the thyroid gland by administration of radioactive iodine to destroy the gland, medical treatment to suppress the gland or, rarely, surgical resection of the gland. Few patients will easily understand that treatment of serum thyroid levels has no effect on the orbitopathy. This is something that you will be asked about by many patients.

Imaging may not be necessary

In some patients, the diagnosis is so obvious that no imaging is necessary. If there is any question, order a CT scan with axial and coronal cuts. It is more accurate to judge muscle size on cross-section as seen on a coronal scan than when viewed on an axial scan (Figure 14-15).

Treatment options—active versus chronic stage

If systemic disease has not been diagnosed, order free thyroxine (T4) and thyroid-stimulating hormone (TSH) tests. Probably the T4 level will be high and the TSH level will be low, although in 5–10% of patients, thyroid orbitopathy will be associated with a euthyroid condition. If the patient is not seeing an internist, you should seek consultation.

Treatment depends on the patient's symptoms and stage of the disease. You will learn to quickly sort this out. The severity of the inflammation varies tremendously from patient to patient. Many patients don't know that they are affected and have only a foreign body sensation or mild lid retraction. At the other extreme is rapidly progressive orbital inflammation manifested by lid swelling, lid retraction, proptosis, diplopia and, rarely, compressive optic neuropathy causing vision loss (about 2% of patients) (Figure 14-16, A).

Before initiating any treatment, you must determine where the patient's condition falls in the natural history of the disease. Try to determine if your patient is in the active stage or the chronic stage of the disease. Typically, patients start with an active stage of thyroid orbitopathy, showing signs of progressive acute inflammation (swelling or redness of the orbital, lid, and conjunctival tissues). The eyelids look "wet," as though you could squeeze edema fluid out (see Figure 14-16, A). In patients with less dramatic manifestations, you can recognize active inflammation because eyelid swelling and any diplopia are much worse in the morning. This active inflammatory stage can last a year or more. Once you have determined that the patient has active orbitopathy,

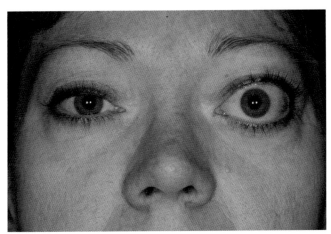

Figure 14-14 Thyroid orbitopathy, in this patient presenting with marked asymmetry. Note the temporal flare in the lesser affected upper eyelid.

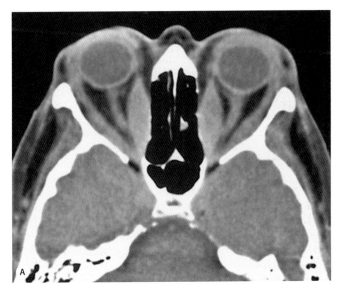

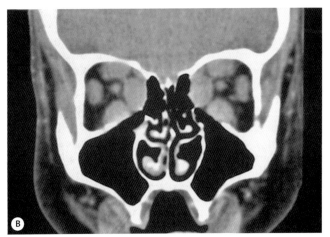

Figure 14-15 CT scan of enlarged extraocular muscles secondary to thyroid orbitopathy. (**A**) Coronal scan. (**B**) Axial scan.

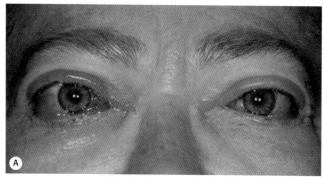
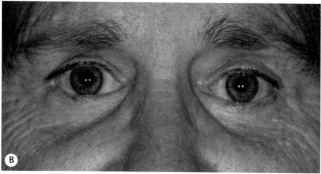

Figure 14-16 Stages of thyroid orbitopathy. (**A**) Active stage with prominent inflammation. Note the swelling and erythema of the lids with associated lid retraction. (**B**) Chronic stage where fibrosis has replaced inflammation. Edema is no longer present. This patient underwent bilateral orbital decompressions for compressive optic neuropathy, and eyelid surgery.

get an idea of how rapidly the inflammation is progressing, or the tempo of the disease. If the symptoms are progressing rapidly, you will need to watch the patient closely. During the active phase, you must monitor the patient's visual function (vision, visual acuity, relative afferent pupillary defect, visual fields, etc.) to make sure there is no sign of optic nerve compression. If the patient's symptoms change drastically, you will need to repeat these tests. It is rare for a patient to develop any optic neuropathy without a striking change in symptoms or signs.

Most patients will require only medical management during the active stage. Follow them for signs of corneal exposure. Treat irritation with lubricating drops and ointment. Elevate the head of the bed using 4 inch blocks to reduce morning swelling or diplopia. Patients will require reassurance during this period. They are uncomfortable and fearful of a loss of vision. You are telling them that their vision is fine and that nothing needs to be done, yet they don't feel that they are making any progress. Perhaps even more significantly, the middle-aged patient (usually a woman) is probably undergoing a change in her facial appearance that may be significant. If the inflammation is progressing rapidly, consider radiation therapy (2000 rads). Optic neuropathy, if severe, is best treated with orbital decompression (enlarging the orbit by removing two or three of the orbital walls). Oral prednisone (80 mg/day) can temporize this situation, but it is not a long-term solution.

The active disease subsides to enter a chronic stage. During this period, there is no progression of symptoms and signs of acute orbital inflammation subside (dry or chronic phase). The morning eyelid swelling and diplopia are gone. Signs of acute inflammation are no longer present. Any remaining proptosis and lid retraction probably will not change.

When you have confirmed that there has been no change over 3–6 months, the patient may want to consider procedures to improve the remaining proptosis, lid retraction, and strabismus. A small percentage of patients (less than 10%) undergoing medial and lateral wall decompression to relieve some of the proptosis will develop strabismus, or the preoperative strabismus pattern will change so decompression should precede any planned strabismus surgery. Similarly, inferior rectus muscle recession may cause or exacerbate lower lid retraction, so strabismus surgery should precede lid surgery. Lower lid retractor extirpation without a spacer elevates the lower lid 1–2 mm. You can use hard palate mucosa to push the lower lid up 3 mm or more. Ear cartilage can be used as a spacer to push the lid margin higher and obtain 3–10 mm of elevation. Upper eyelid recession is the most common procedure performed on patients with thyroid orbitopathy. Lowering the upper lid improves comfort, reduces corneal exposure, and improves the appearance of the retracted lid.

Undoubtedly, you will see many patients with thyroid orbitopathy and will provide them a tremendous service by monitoring for signs of optic neuropathy and managing exposure symptoms. Your reassurance will be especially helpful. Any operation that you perform on a patient with "burned out" or chronic thyroid disease will be technically difficult. Nagging bleeding caused by tissue fibrosis is common. The final result tends to be more unpredictable than similar procedures on patients without thyroid disease. Save these operations until you can perform the easier orbit, lid, and strabismus procedures easily.

Idiopathic orbital inflammatory disease: orbital "pseudotumor" acute onset of pain

When you see a patient with an acute onset of pain, think of idiopathic orbital inflammatory disease. You might consider the presentation of inflammation secondary to pseudotumor to be the opposite of the inflammation seen in thyroid orbitopathy where the onset is gradual and pain is absent. Idiopathic orbital inflammatory disease is just what the name says. For unknown reasons, any of the orbital tissues may become infiltrated with inflammatory cells (dacryoadenitis or myositis). Both young and old people are affected.

The typical presentation is an acute onset of pain with rapid progression occurring over hours to a day or at most two (recall that the inflammation with thyroid orbitopathy has no real pain and has a vague onset with slow progression). Past medical history is only helpful for children in whom a viral syndrome may precede the onset. When you hear a history of upper respiratory infection preceding painful proptosis, you should be thinking inflammation or infection. Patients with bacterial orbital cellulitis may have this severe pain, but the patient is usually sick (febrile, weak, etc.). The onset of orbital cellulitis usually takes place over a few days, and the pain is usually less than with pseudotumor. Another cause of an acute onset of pain is an acute hemorrhage, but the onset is usually more sudden, with

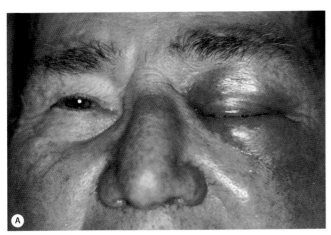
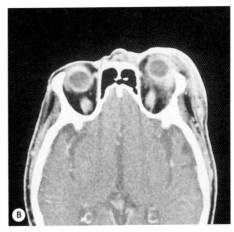

Figure 14-17 Idiopathic orbital inflammatory disease: "pseudotumor." (**A**) Patient with rapid onset of pain resulting from idiopathic orbital inflammatory disease. Note the inflamed periocular tissues (courtesy of the American Academy of Ophthalmology). (**B**) A CT scan shows a diffuse mass in the area of the lacrimal gland. The patient responded to oral prednisone treatment within 24 hours.

progression occurring over a few minutes, rather than hours.

Proptosis is usually present with idiopathic orbital inflammatory disease, but periocular signs of acute inflammation predominate in the physical examination. Lid swelling, chemosis, and limited motility are common. The name pseudotumor comes from the clinical appearance of proptosis without the presence of a true mass. With palpation, you may feel that the tissues are tense and warm, but no distinct mass will be present (Figure 14-17). The inflamed areas are tender to the touch. There are no pulsations.

Clinical diagnosis confirmed with CT scan

The diagnosis can usually be made clinically if the onset and pain are typical. A CT scan should be done. A poorly circumscribed mass may be present in any orbital space. In some patients, a particular tissue will be involved, for example the lacrimal gland (dacryoadenitis) or an extraocular muscle (myositis). Usually the inflammation will spill into adjacent tissues. I prefer to perform a biopsy to confirm the diagnosis, if the involved area is easily accessible, before starting treatment.

Treatment: prednisone

When the inflammation involves the apical orbit or any extraocular muscle, I will institute steroid treatment without a biopsy confirming the clinical diagnosis. A rapid response to oral prednisone (80 mg/day) is characteristic. Treatment should be continued for 6–8 weeks with a tapering schedule. Some surgeons will treat all suspected cases without a biopsy if the clinical picture is typical. I don't recommend not performing a biopsy until you are experienced in making this diagnosis and are familiar with the typical response to treatment. If you are treating without the benefit of a tissue diagnosis, consider biopsy if the response to therapy is not prompt and complete.

Cavernous hemangioma

Painless slow progression of unilateral proptosis

A patient with painless slow progression of unilateral proptosis may have an intraorbital tumor. The most common benign orbital tumor in adults is a cavernous hemangioma. This benign vascular hamartoma is most common around age 40. The cause is unknown. The proptosis is unilateral and axial. Vision is not affected unless the mass pushes directly on the eye causing a hyperopic shift. Rarely, an apical orbital mass can cause optic nerve compression presenting as visual loss, gaze-evoked amaurosis, or disc edema (this is not typical, however). The typical cavernous hemangioma is too far posterior to be palpable. There are no associated periocular signs. Although the lesion is vascular, there is low flow so no pulsations are seen.

CT scan: well-circumscribed intraconal mass

As with most patients with proptosis, you should order a CT scan. A cavernous hemangioma appears as a well-circumscribed oval or round mass, usually in the muscle cone (see Figure 14-10, B). If you are sure that the presentation and imaging are typical of a cavernous hemangioma, observation is an option.

Most of the well-circumscribed masses that I see now are discovered incidentally on an MRI scan of the head as a part of a workup for headache. Although some would say that "observation" is the "conservative" management option, it may be more "risky" to observe a mass than to remove it. You will eventually be wrong by observation. If you choose to observe the lesion, make sure that you have a good orbital CT scan, rather than an MRI scan of the brain using thick cuts. Obtain another scan at 3–4 months or sooner if any visual loss, pain, or change in proptosis occurs. I have personally "observed" an optic nerve meningioma and an orbital metastasis, both well-circumscribed intraconal masses when viewed on an MRI scan of the head, that were thought to be a hemangioma until growth occurred and biopsy proved otherwise.

Removal via orbitotomy is safe

If the diagnosis is uncertain, vision loss is present, or the patient does not want observation, excisional biopsy (removal) is recommended. At orbitotomy, the dissection of the hemangioma away from the surrounding orbital tissues is straightforward, making this tumor a relatively easy deep orbitotomy to do early in your experience.

Lymphoid lesions of the orbit

Painless, slow progression of a unilateral (or bilateral) anterior mass

Lymphoid lesions of the orbit are among the most common orbital tumors that you will see in adults. A gradual onset with slow progression of a painless orbital mass, often anterior and superior, is typical of the orbital lymphoid lesions. About 25% of patients have a previous diagnosis of lymphoma. Lymphoid lesions occur most commonly in elderly patients, but may occur in middle age.

The proptosis can be axial or nonaxial, depending on the position of the mass. In some patients, the disease may present bilaterally (an exception to the rule that orbital tumors are usually unilateral). Most commonly, you will see lymphoid tumors arising in the superior orbital quadrants. The extraconal space, especially with involvement of the lacrimal gland, is a common site. Although the inferior orbit is not the most common site, lymphoid lesions are the most common condition presenting there (not many conditions present inferiorly). You may be able to palpate an orbital mass anteriorly. The lesions are smooth, usually mobile, and firm to the touch. There is no tenderness associated with palpation. The characteristic salmon patch on the conjunctiva is diagnostic for lymphoma (Figure 14-18).

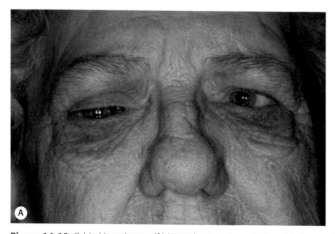

Figure 14-18 The presence of a "salmon patch," the color of salmon flesh, is diagnostic for conjunctival lymphoid tumor.

CT scan: the typical pusher lesion

You can get a good idea that the lesion you see on CT scan is a lymphoid tumor. You will see a smooth mass that is the typical pusher, not eater, of orbital tissues (no infiltration of orbital tissues). The lesion is said to mold to the orbital tissues (Figure 14-19). Bone erosion is rare.

A continuum of malignancy

The goal of classifying lymphoid lesions is to identify characteristics that would predict clinical behavior. Unfortunately, that has not been an easy task. Traditionally, lymphoid lesions were classified histologically as:

- Benign: benign reactive lymphoid hyperplasia
- Malignant: lymphoma
- Indeterminate: atypical lymphoid hyperplasia

We now recognize that classifying lesions as "benign" or "malignant" is not so straightforward. Malignant lymphoid lesions appear to arise from monoclonal populations of abnormal cells. Currently, 70–80% of orbital lymphoid lesions can be classified as malignant based on monoclonal antibody studies. The percentage is as high as 90% based on molecular studies. It turns out that a large percentage of all orbital lymphoid lesions will *eventually* be associated with systemic disease.

You will not be able to predict whether systemic disease is present at the time of diagnosis or will occur based on any clinical or radiological finding. You should have a good idea based upon the imaging that the lesion is lymphoid, however. Remember that lymphoid lesions are the most common, or among the most common, orbital masses seen in adults. Rarely do any other neoplasms present bilaterally. If you suspect a lymphoid lesion, ask specifically about a history of other similar lesions and order a complete blood count (CBC) with a differential count. An incisional biopsy is required to make the final diagnosis. Submit formalin-fixed tissue for hematoxylin & eosin staining and fresh tissue for immunopathologic analysis.

Treatment and survival depend on histological classification

Lymphoid lesions remain poorly understood. Almost all periocular lymphomas are non-Hodgkin type, almost all of

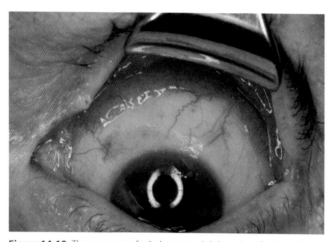

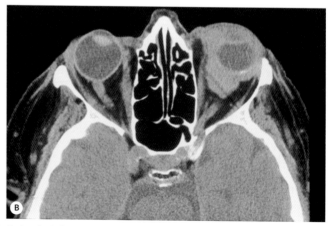

Figure 14-19 Orbital lymphoma. (**A**) Note the superior anterior orbital mass displacing the left eye inferiorly. (**B**) A CT scan shows a typical smooth circumscribed mass that "pushes" orbital tissues away and "molds" its shape around the adjacent orbital structures.

B cell origin. About a quarter of patients will have a history of lymphoma or will have undiagnosed systemic disease at the time of your diagnosis. All patients should undergo an evaluation to rule out systemic involvement. Chest and abdominal CT scans are used to identify abnormal nodes. Bone marrow aspiration is performed to rule out marrow involvement. In the absence of systemic disease, most orbital lesions are treated with radiotherapy at a very high success rate. At least another quarter of patients will develop systemic disease over the next 5 years. Some believe that, given enough time (many years), perhaps all patients would develop systemic disease, but keep in mind that most of these patients are elderly at the time of orbital diagnosis.

The REAL classification system, based on histological characteristics, categorizes lymphoma into one of five categories:

- MALT—mucosal associated lymphoid tumor
- Diffuse lymphoplasmacytic
- Follicle center
- Diffuse large cell
- Rare other lymphomas

The most common periocular lymphoma is the *MALT type* representing over 50% of orbital lesions. The progression of MALT type lymphomas is slow. Rare spontaneous remissions or transformations to a more aggressive type are known to occur.

Systemic lymphoma may or may not be treated initially, depending on the cell type. If the lymphoma is not an aggressive type, the orbital disease will be treated with light to moderate doses of radiation therapy. Local recurrences are rare. Usually, no systemic treatment will be given because these more differentiated tumors are difficult to cure. The course is usually indolent. Recurrent extraorbital disease is treated with further radiation therapy. The patient usually dies of unrelated causes.

Aggressive cell types are usually treated systemically. Chemotherapy can provide a cure for these poorly differentiated types of lymphoma such as large cell and follicular lymphoma. Monoclonal antibody therapy can be used alone and with chemotherapy protocols (commonly CHOP) in some cases. The protein CD-20 is expressed on the surface of all B lymphocytes. *Rituximab* is a monoclonal antibody against CD-20. Rituximab, administered intravenously, binds to the lymphocytes resulting in depletion of both normal and abnormal B cells. New normal B lymphocytes then repopulate the immune system. If the treatment of aggressive lymphoma is unsuccessful, the patient will die of the disease.

One of the more difficult clinical decisions that you will have involves differentiating a lymphoid lesion of the lacrimal gland from a type of lacrimal gland tumor known as a benign mixed tumor. On CT scans, these tumors may look similar. Incisional biopsy is appropriate for a suspected lymphoid lesion. Incisional biopsy of a benign mixed tumor is inappropriate, leaving a curable tumor with a chance of recurrence and malignant degeneration. We will talk more about this later.

Checkpoint

I want you to learn how to differentiate one orbital disease from another. It should be easy to differentiate idiopathic orbital inflammatory disease from a lymphoid lesion. How? Consider the pain and progression. Idiopathic orbital inflammatory disease has an abrupt onset and rapid progression of pain. Lymphoid lesions are slowly progressive and produce no pain. On a CT scan, it would not be difficult to distinguish the poorly defined margins of an inflammatory lesion from the smooth molding shape of a lymphoid lesion. Get the idea?

Now recall the difference between a cavernous hemangioma and a lymphoid lesion. Both have a vague onset, slow progression, and no pain. How can you tell the difference? First, consider the age of the patient. Cavernous hemangiomas occur most commonly in middle-aged patients. Lymphoid lesions occur in the elderly. There could be some overlap on this point because cavernous hemangiomas don't go away as a patient gets older and lymphoid lesions can occur in 40-year-old patients. What about the proptosis? Cavernous hemangiomas are usually intraconal, producing axial proptosis. Lymphoid lesions are usually extraconal and anterior. Any proptosis is often nonaxial. A mass may be palpable anteriorly. Lymphoid lesions may be bilateral, whereas cavernous hemangiomas are almost never bilateral. What about the CT scan? The cavernous hemangioma is usually round or oval and intraconal. The lymphoid lesion is more likely to be lobular or irregular in shape rather than round. Neither of these tumors is infiltrative. If you think the mass is a lymphoid lesion, an incisional biopsy is appropriate. If you think that the mass is a cavernous hemangioma, an excisional biopsy is appropriate.

I hope you are getting the idea. Remember that the presence or absence of pain and the type of onset and rate of progression narrow down the differential diagnosis quickly. Features of the physical examination and imaging studies will help refine the differential diagnosis more. In most patients, you will have made the correct diagnosis before you have done the biopsy.

Metastatic tumors to the orbit

Proptosis with progressive mild pain and inflammation

When a patient is seen with onset of proptosis occurring over a few days to a few weeks, sometimes with mild pain or inflammatory signs, think metastatic tumor and ask about a history of any known malignancy.

Metastatic tumors are relatively uncommon. Lung cancer is the most common metastatic orbital tumor in men. Breast cancer is the most common metastatic orbital tumor in women. The proptosis seen is often nonaxial because the areas infiltrated by tumor are often outside the muscle cone, sometimes eroding the orbital bones. Enophthalmos may actually be seen in patients with metastatic scirrhous breast cancer resulting from fibrosis of the involved orbital tissues. Eyelid swelling and chemosis are often seen with many metastatic tumors. As many as one fourth of metastatic orbital tumors will not have a known primary tumor.

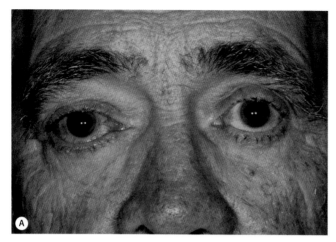
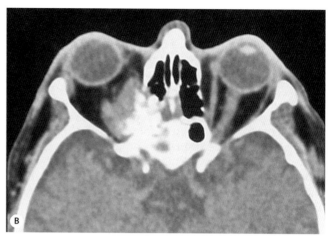

Figure 14-20 Metastatic prostate carcinoma. (**A**) Proptosis of the right eye, fullness of the superior sulcus, and mild globe ptosis in an elderly man with known prostate carcinoma. (**B**) A CT scan shows areas of both osteoclastic and osteoblastic bone involvement. A soft tissue mass is also present in the orbit.

CT scan: infiltrative mass

If you suspect a metastatic tumor, a CT scan should be obtained. An infiltrative mass is usually seen. These tumors are "eaters." Often the tumor extends into more than one of the orbital spaces and infiltrates several orbital structures. Bone erosion is commonly seen with any adenocarcinoma. The diagnosis of metastatic prostate carcinoma can be made on a CT scan alone based on the characteristic combination of both osteoclastic (destroyed bone) and osteoblastic (new bone) changes (Figure 14-20).

Incisional biopsy, systemic workup, and treatment

The definitive diagnosis of a metastatic orbital tumor is made by incisional biopsy. A systemic workup is required to define the extent of disease. If the orbit is the only site of metastasis, radiation therapy may be appropriate. If other areas of metastatic involvement are found, systemic treatment with chemotherapy is usually used. In most patients with systemic disease, the response to chemotherapy is assessed before any radiation therapy is given to the orbit.

Optic nerve tumors

Optic nerve meningioma

Meningioma and glioma are central nervous system (CNS) tumors that can arise primarily from the optic nerve. Optic nerve meningioma is seen most often in middle-aged adults. Patients usually note vision loss. Because the tumor originates in the arachnoid villi of the meningeal sheath of the optic nerve, visual loss caused by compression of the nerve is common before the tumor is large enough to cause much proptosis. The onset of the visual loss is usually not distinct. Progression is very slow over months or years. There is no pain associated.

The proptosis is usually minimal at the time of presentation. If present, the proptosis is axial. No external signs of disease are present. Palpation of the orbit is normal. No abnormal pulsations of the eye are seen. Optic nerve edema may be present. You may see optociliary shunt vessels. (Compression of the central retinal artery can occur so that blood flow is shunted to the retina via the ciliary vessels—the optociliary shunt vessels.)

Most patients with optic nerve tumors will eventually get both CT and MRI scans. A CT scan is usually ordered initially. With meningioma, a CT scan shows enlargement of the optic nerve, which can be fairly subtle. Calcification of the arachnoid is seen in a minority of optic nerve meningiomas (Figure 14-21) but, if it is present on an axial CT scan, you can sometimes see parallel radiodense lines on the sides of the nerve, known as tram tracking. This sign and a radiodense circle on the perimeter of the nerve seen on a coronal projection are diagnostic for optic nerve meningioma. Meningioma involving the orbital apex often shows characteristic hyperostosis of the adjacent bone. When a diagnosis of an optic nerve tumor is made, an MRI scan is usually ordered to see the extent of the tumor into the orbital apex and chiasm. You will be able to see the posterior extent of the tumor without the artifact of the bones in the apex obscuring the soft tissue detail as on a CT scan.

If the diagnosis of optic nerve meningioma cannot be made clinically, an incisional biopsy is performed. Debulking of an optic nerve meningioma cannot be done without damage to the vision, so no attempt to excise is usually done until useful vision is lost or the tumor is extending toward the optic canal as seen on serial MRI examinations. Recall that meningiomas are benign. Damage occurs by adjacent tissue compression, not by distant spread. For excision, you will need a neurosurgical colleague to help you with a transcranial orbitotomy, which gives you good access to the orbital apex. The nerve is usually removed from the chiasm to the posterior surface of the eye. Meningiomas in patients younger than age 35 behave more aggressively, suggesting that earlier excision should be considered.

Sphenoid wing meningioma

Optic nerve meningiomas are rare. More commonly, you will see a meningioma arising from the intracranial side of the sphenoid bone and extending into the orbit secondarily—a sphenoid wing meningioma. Proptosis and downward displacement of the eye precede vision loss, often by years. Hyperostotic bone pushes into the orbit and temporalis fossa. Eventually, bone thickens enough to cause fullness of the temple (Figure 14-22). Advanced meningioma causes disfiguring proptosis and corneal exposure. Vision

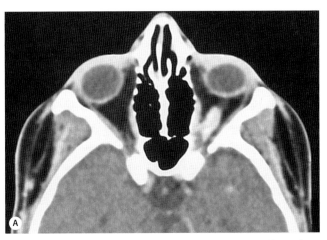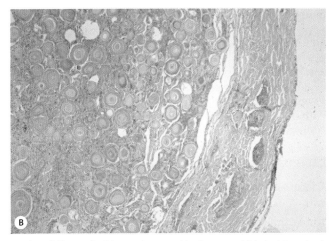

Figure 14-21 Optic nerve meningioma. (**A**) Note calcification of the left optic nerve (parallel lines of calcium or "tram tracking" are not visible in this patient). (**B**) Section of the optic nerve. Note the calcified psammoma bodies in the optic nerve that are responsible for calcification seen on the CT scan.

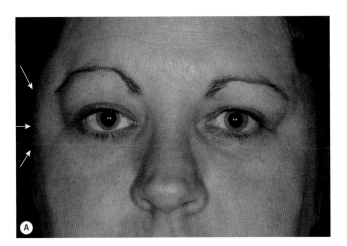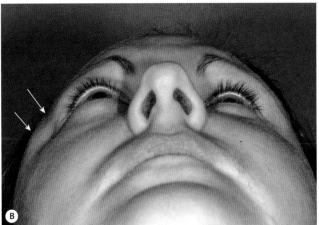

Figure 14-22 Sphenoid wing meningioma. (**A**) and (**B**) Note proptosis of the right eye and fullness of the right temple (*arrows*). (**C**) A CT scan with contrast enhancement shows areas of soft tissue involvement surrounding the hyperostotic sphenoid wing.

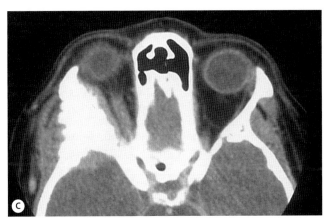

loss develops when optic nerve compression occurs. A CT scan is used to show the areas of hyperostotic bone involvement. A contrast agent is necessary to see the soft tissue portions of the meningioma (see Figure 14-13). An MRI scan is usually performed to view the details of the soft tissues in the orbital apex and around the chiasm. The meningioma can be debulked to relieve compression, but complete removal is never possible. Radiation therapy can be used as adjunctive therapy, although the tumor is not very radiosensitive. Over many years, the meningioma is likely to recur.

Meningioma can occur primarily within the orbital tissues not associated with any normal meningeal structure. This is thought to occur because of a congenital rest of meningeal cells within the orbit. This is extremely rare.

Optic nerve glioma (children)

Optic nerve gliomas occur primarily in children in the first decade of life. In contrast to meningiomas, gliomas originate within the optic nerve tissue itself (recall that glial tissue is the "connective tissue" of the CNS). Consequently, gliomas tend to push the nerve fibers apart rather than compress the nerve. Vision is preserved despite significant proptosis. Progression is extremely slow and painless. Occasionally, rapid progression can occur usually because of mucinous degeneration of the tumor. Most tumors are unilateral. Optic nerve edema may be present. When you see unilateral, slowly progressive, painless axial proptosis in a child, think of a glioma. We will talk about optic nerve glioma later under "Orbital Diseases Occurring in Childhood."

Lacrimal gland tumors

Tumors of glandular tissue or infiltration of the gland with cells?

The lacrimal gland may become enlarged because of one of several disorders, all of which are uncommon. Think of these disorders as one of two processes:

- A neoplasm derived from lacrimal tissue
- An infiltration of abnormal cells into the gland

    Both processes have benign and malignant counterparts:

- Tumors arising from lacrimal tissue
    — Benign mixed tumor (benign)
    — Adenoid cystic carcinoma (malignant)
    — Adenocarcinoma (malignant)
- Infiltration of abnormal cells into the gland
    — Lymphoid tumors
    — Benign reactive lymphoid hyperplasia (benign)
    — Lymphoma (malignant)
    — Atypical lymphoid hyperplasia (indeterminate)
- Sarcoidosis (benign)
- Idiopathic orbital inflammatory disease (benign)

Although most texts devote several pages to the tumors of lacrimal gland origin, these tumors are rare. Infiltration of cells (mainly lymphoid) into the lacrimal gland is the most common cause of lacrimal gland enlargement.

Differential diagnosis based on the findings of the history and physical examination

As we have discussed with the other categories of orbital disease, the "P's" of the orbital history and physical examination are helpful to form the differential diagnosis in the evaluation of lacrimal gland enlargement. True pain is seen only in orbital inflammatory disease. The onset and progression of symptoms become especially important in differentiating adenoid cystic carcinoma from benign mixed tumors (guess which is more slowly progressive). Proptosis occurs relatively late with lacrimal gland masses because the lacrimal gland is anterior to the equator of the eye, tending to cause inferior globe displacement. Proptosis can occur as the tumor enlarges. Fullness or a palpable mass in the superotemporal quadrant is common. If you lift the upper eyelid, you may be able to see an enlarged palpebral lobe of the lacrimal gland.

True neoplasms arising from the lacrimal gland tissue are rare. The most common of these rare problems is the benign mixed tumor of the lacrimal gland. The benign mixed tumor typically occurs in the 40s, but the age of onset is variable. Benign mixed tumors progress very slowly, over a period of years. This slow progression is the key in differentiating this tumor from other causes of lacrimal gland enlargement, so you should pay close attention to this part of the history. The onset is so slow that review of old photos may be the only way to know when the mass started. There is no pain associated. Past medical history is not helpful. As you would expect, initially there is fullness of the sulcus, then globe displacement inferiorly, and finally proptosis (Figure 14-23). You may be able to palpate a smooth firm mass in the lacrimal fossa. There are no pulsations or specific diagnostic periocular signs.

A CT scan shows a round or oval, well-circumscribed mass in the superotemporal quadrant. Often there is adjacent fossa formation in the bone as a result of the long-standing pressure changes. You need to be able to differentiate this bone change suggesting a slowly progressive benign process from an erosive bone change suggesting a more rapidly advancing malignancy. We will talk more about this in the next paragraph. As a benign mixed tumor grows within the lacrimal gland, it compresses adjacent glandular and orbital tissue to form a pseudocapsule ("pseudo" because there is no epithelial lining) separating the tumor from the surrounding tissue. Complete removal of a benign mixed tumor is possible if the pseudocapsule is not broken.

It is important for you to consider the diagnosis of a benign mixed tumor in the evaluation of every lacrimal gland tumor because incisional biopsy of all other lacrimal gland masses is the rule. If you do not consider a benign mixed tumor, you may inappropriately perform an incisional biopsy, increasing the chance of recurrence. Rarely, benign mixed tumors may undergo malignant transformation, appearing as a primary or recurrent malignant mixed cell carcinoma.

The presentation of the most common malignant lacrimal gland tumor, the adenoid cystic carcinoma, is very different from that of the benign mixed tumor. Adenoid cystic carcinoma progresses over a few months; symptoms or signs are almost never present for more than 1 year. There is no pain present, but there is often numbness or paresthesias in the temporal region as a result of typical neurotrophic spread of adenoid cystic carcinoma. Past medical history is not helpful. This tumor also occurs most commonly in the 40s, so age is not diagnostic. The mass effect is similar to that of the benign mixed tumor—fullness, globe displacement, and proptosis—but accelerated in comparison. You may see more motility problems caused by the infiltrative growth pattern. You may be able to demonstrate areas of sensory loss at the lateral orbit, unlike other lacrimal gland masses.

A CT scan will show an infiltrative superotemporal mass extending across the orbital spaces (Figure 14-24). Bone erosion is typical. If you suspect intracranial extension based on the clinical examination or CT scan, order an MRI scan.

The diagnosis of adenoid cystic carcinoma is confirmed by incisional biopsy. Treatment is controversial. Exenteration, including bone removal and craniotomy when necessary, followed by radiation therapy, has been used. Local control can be achieved for many years, but most patients develop late local recurrence. Pulmonary metastases have been reported decades after tumor excision. Many surgeons feel that adenoid cystic tumor is never "cured."

We will discuss the approach to the patient who you suspect has a lacrimal gland mass in more detail later. For now, let's move on to the causes of infiltrative lacrimal gland enlargement. The traditional teaching is that enlargement of

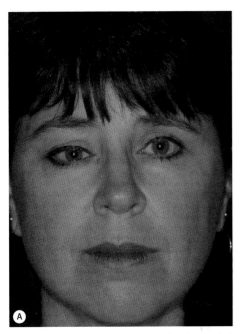

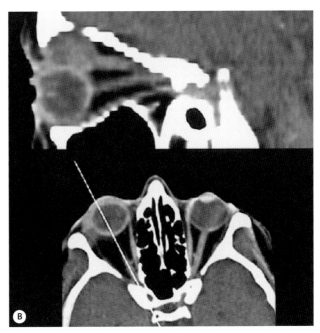

Figure 14-23 Benign mixed tumor of the lacrimal gland. (**A**) Globe ptosis of the right eye present for 2 years in a 42-year-old woman (see **Figure 15-24**). (**B**) CT scan shows an oval mass with bone molding changes. Minimal proptosis is present.

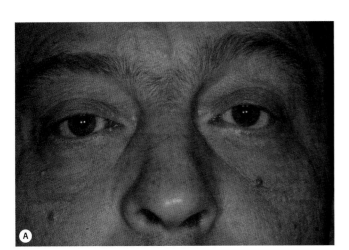

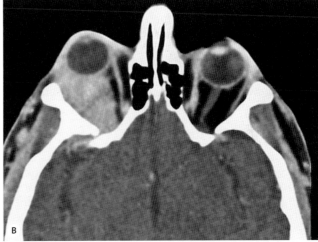

Figure 14-24 Adenoid cystic carcinoma of the lacrimal gland in a 46-year-old man. (**A**) Note proptosis and globe ptosis of the right eye. (**B**) A CT scan shows an infiltrative mass with spread through the superior orbital fissure. Despite radical exenteration with craniotomy and radiotherapy, the patient died of local recurrence in the CNS 8 years after treatment.

the lacrimal gland occurs equally as a result of lacrimal gland neoplasm or infiltrative processes. In my practice, the infiltrative causes are far more common than the primary neoplasms.

You should notice that all the infiltrative disorders involve white blood cells, through either neoplastic or inflammatory processes. Lymphoid tumors fit into the neoplasia category, whereas orbital inflammatory disease and sarcoidosis fall into the inflammatory category. We have talked about lymphoid tumors of the orbit. Many of these will involve the lacrimal gland. Painless, slowly progressive fullness of the superotemporal orbit is the rule. As the mass gets larger and

extends more posteriorly, proptosis and globe displacement inferiorly will occur. An enlarged gland is often palpable.

A CT scan shows well-circumscribed enlargement of the lacrimal gland with the typical molding of the mass to the surrounding tissues (a pusher, not an eater) (Figure 14-25). There are no bone changes. Evaluation of the contralateral gland may show some enlargement. Incisional biopsy is required to obtain a diagnosis, as all of the lymphoid lesions look the same on a CT scan.

Idiopathic orbital inflammatory disease has such a typical onset of acute pain and associated inflammatory signs that the diagnosis is usually obvious. For this reason, many texts

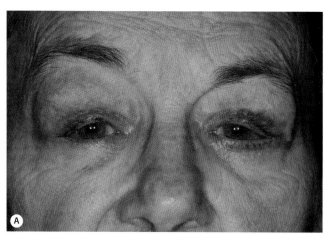
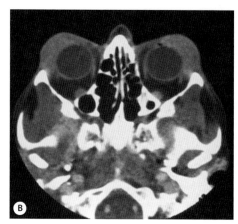

Figure 14-25 Bilateral lymphomas of the lacrimal glands. (**A**) Note fullness of the supratemporal quadrants. (**B**) Axial CT scan shows enlargement of the lacrimal gland with typical "molding" of the tumor around the eye.

do not include idiopathic orbital inflammatory disease in the list of lacrimal gland tumors. At some point, you will see this condition because the lacrimal gland is one of the more common parts of the orbit to be involved with this acute inflammatory process. Diagnosis and treatment are as described earlier.

Sarcoidosis as a cause of lacrimal gland enlargement is rare. There is slowly progressive, painless, periocular swelling and proptosis. Remember that sarcoidosis presents as a chronic low-grade orbital inflammation. No acute inflammatory signs are present. The lacrimal gland is usually palpable. Imaging shows enlargement of the gland with shaggy borders where adjacent tissues are infiltrated. The biopsy shows non-caseating granulomas within the lacrimal tissue. A systemic workup, including pulmonary function tests, serum lysozyme, and angiotensin-converting enzyme measurements, should be done to rule out systemic disease.

Secondary orbital tumors

Secondary orbital tumors include any benign or malignant process arising outside the orbit that grows to invade the orbital tissues. Think about the "surgical space" that we called periocular tissues, and you can name a few of these tumors. We have already talked about sphenoid wing meningioma extending into the orbit from the intracranial space. Other secondary tumors include melanoma growing out of the eye, skin cancers extending through the orbital septum or into orbital bone, and tumors arising from the paranasal sinuses.

Choroidal melanoma

Choroidal melanoma with clinical extrascleral extension is rare, occurring in less than 1% of ocular melanomas. Extension outside the eye is small and usually not seen clinically as proptosis. Echographic examination usually identifies the problem before enucleation. At the time of surgery, Tenon's capsule adjacent to the site of extrascleral extension should be removed. Exenteration is not indicated except in extreme cases. The long-term prognosis is poor.

Skin malignancy

Beware of any patient with previously excised skin cancer who develops proptosis months or years later. Cutaneous

Checkpoint

Let's review for a minute. A patient comes in with globe displacement and proptosis, suggesting a lacrimal gland mass. How do you put all your new information to good use? Probably you will be getting a CT scan and doing a biopsy. So why not just proceed and forget a differential diagnosis? Remember that you should not do an incisional biopsy on a benign mixed tumor. After you clinically diagnose a lacrimal gland mass, the practical task is to make sure you are not missing a benign mixed tumor. Without getting bogged down in every detail below, see if you can answer these questions. From a clinical point of view:

What is the difference in presentation between an adenoid cystic tumor and a benign mixed tumor (Table 14-3)?

It is usually easy to tell these apart clinically. When you determine that the problem has been present more than 1 year and the CT scan shows chronic bone molding, think benign mixed tumor and plan to remove the mass intact.

Distinguishing a benign mixed tumor from a lymphoid lesion is a more common and more difficult question. Consider the clinical points in Table 14-4.

The main characteristic of the benign mixed tumor is its slow progression. This long-standing hard tumor pushes the eye down and molds the bone. It occurs in a younger patient. The lymphoid lesion molds to surrounding structures and has usually been present for a shorter time. You can occasionally be fooled, but this approach works well. If you understand this thinking, it will be easy for you to learn about the other orbital tumors.

malignancy may extend into the orbit under two circumstances. Neglected tumors may extend deeply where appropriate early treatment would have prevented deep extension. This occurs rarely, but is still seen in reclusive patients or those patients in deep denial. The more common situation is an aggressive tumor that recurs deeply after previous excision, most commonly in patients with squamous cell carcinoma or morpheaform basal cell carcinoma (Figure 14-26).

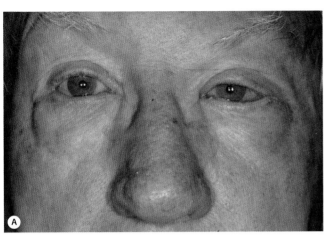
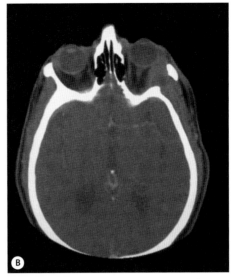

Figure 14-26 Intraorbital extension of squamous cell carcinoma years after excision of the initial tumor from the temple. (**A**) The patient has proptosis, paresthesia, restricted motility, and facial nerve involvement. (**B**) A CT scan. Note bony erosion of the lateral orbital wall and the soft tissue mass extending into the orbit and temporalis fossa.

Table 14-3 Adenoid cystic carcinoma versus benign mixed tumor

Presentation	Adenoid cystic carcinoma	Benign mixed tumor
Progression	Weeks to months	Several months to years
Pain	Vague, numbness	None
Past medical history	Noncontributory	Noncontributory
Age	Middle age	Middle age
Proptosis	Nonaxial initially	Nonaxial initially
Periocular changes	Hypesthesia, some swelling	No hypesthesia or swelling
Palpation	Firm, not smooth	Firm, smooth
Pulsation	None	None
CT scan	Infiltrative bone erosion	Well-circumscribed bony molding, fossa formation

Table 14-4 Lymphoid lesion versus benign mixed

Presentation	Lymphoid lesion	Benign mixed tumor
Progression	Weeks to months	Months to years
Pain	None	None
Past medical history	Possible systemic lymphoma	Noncontributory
Age	Elderly	Middle age
Proptosis	Less likely to cause globe ptosis; palpable anterior mass; can be bilateral	Globe ptosis prominent; usually more posterior; unilateral
Palpation	Soft, more anterior	Firm, larger, more convex, often nonpalpable
Pulsation	None	None
Periocular changes	Lobular enlargement of palpebral and/or orbital lobe; occasional salmon patch	Usually orbital lobe involved; no specific signs
CT scan	Well circumscribed; molds to structures (soft); usually no bone change	Well circumscribed; may indent globe; bony molding, fossa formation

Pain is usually not present. Proptosis and decreased motility may occur. The motility disturbance may be restrictive from the tumor mass or paretic from cranial nerve involvement. A hard, nontender anterior orbital mass is often present. A CT scan shows an infiltrative tumor mass often with bone erosion. Consider an MRI scan if you have any suspicion of neurotrophic spread based on biopsy or the appearance of the superior orbital fissure. If no intracranial extension is found, orbital exenteration is the best chance for cure.

Sinus tumors

Benign or malignant sinus masses can extend into the orbit. A mucocele of the sinus forms when obstruction of the sinus drainage occurs. Painless displacement of the globe occurs over many months or years. The most common site of origin is the frontal sinus. You will see the eye pushed inferiorly and laterally (Figure 14-27; see also Figure 2-49). Usually you can feel a smooth superonasal mass that is nontender. The patient

may or may not have known sinus disease. No pulsations are present. Ethmoid sinus mucocele may cause lateral displacement of the eye, but this is less common than frontal sinus mucocele. A CT scan shows opacification and enlargement of the affected sinus. The chronic benign nature of this process is shown by the loss of any normal sharp contours of the sinus wall with an overall rounding of the sinus. You will see a dome-shaped elevated mass extending into the orbit through

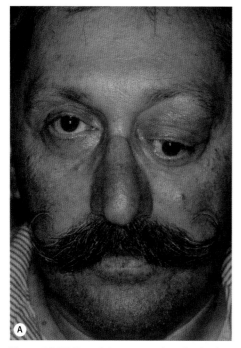
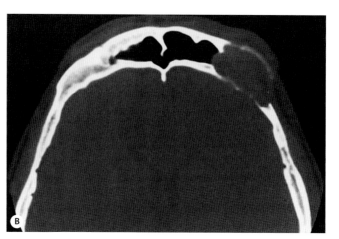

Figure 14-27 Frontal sinus mucocele with orbital extension. (**A**) Note inferior displacement of the globe. (**B**) A CT scan shows opacification and enlargement of the frontal sinus. Coronal scans (not shown) demonstrated a well-outlined soft tissue mass extending into the orbit.

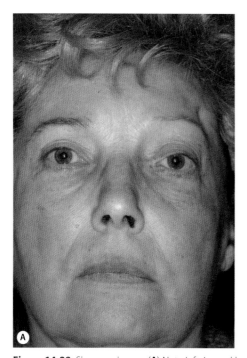
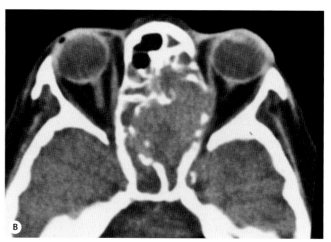

Figure 14-28 Sinus carcinoma. (**A**) Note inferior and lateral displacement of the left eye. (**B**) CT scan shows destruction of the medial orbital wall with a soft tissue mass bulging into the orbit.

a defect in the orbital wall that elevates the periorbita. No orbital soft tissue is infiltrated. Treatment is re-establishment of normal sinus drainage or obliteration of the sinus (removal of the mucosa and packing the sinus with fat or muscle).

Sinus malignancy can extend into the orbit secondarily, as well. The onset of any symptoms is late with sinus carcinoma.

The tumor is usually large before pain or epistaxis appear. No past medical history is significant. Eye findings are variable and reflect the tumor location and extension. Both proptosis and globe displacement laterally, inferiorly, or superiorly can occur (Figure 14-28). Maxillary sinus tumor is one of the rare causes of superior globe displacement (remember lymphoid lesions are the most common cause). A mass is usually not palpable, although tumor in the nose may be visible. Obstruction of the nasolacrimal duct is common. A CT scan shows sinus opacification as in a mucocele, but there is usually bone and soft tissue destruction (see Figure 14-28, B). One or more orbital walls may be eroded but, surprisingly, the periorbita prevents tumor from growing into the orbital soft tissue. An MRI scan is helpful to identify intracranial extension and to distinguish sinus opacification resulting from mucous retention rather than tumor tissue. Treatment varies by cell type, but can include a combination of chemotherapy, radiation therapy, and surgical excision. Despite removal of much of the supporting skeleton for the orbit that occurs with maxillectomy and ethmoidectomy, with appropriate bony reconstructive techniques, the eye and visual function can be preserved in most patients.

Orbital diseases occurring in childhood

Introduction

The common causes of proptosis in childhood overlap little with the common causes in adulthood. Your thought process in developing a differential diagnosis will be similar, however. Pain, progression, and proptosis remain the key features in the history and physical examination. Using these characteristics, as we did with the evaluation of proptosis in adults, you will be able to put the cause of proptosis into a likely pathogenic category (infection, inflammation, tumor, etc.) even before you are familiar with the most common diagnoses. The other "P's" will help you to refine the differential diagnosis further. The common diagnoses, such as dermoid cyst or capillary hemangioma, will not require imaging. If one of these "common diagnoses" appears atypical in any way, you should proceed with a scan, however. If you are not certain of the cause of proptosis, you should order a CT scan. Most patients will require an orbitotomy for the diagnosis or removal of a mass. Patients with infectious disease (orbital cellulitis) may require drainage of an abscess.

As you can see, the process of diagnosis and management of proptosis in children proceeds in the same way as that in adults. Some general differences apply:

- Malignancy is a less common cause of proptosis
- Congenital abnormality, choristoma, and hamartoma are more common causes. (Hamartoma is a congenital abnormality with normal tissue in abnormal quantity, e.g., hemangioma or glioma. Choristoma is a congenital abnormality with normal tissue in an abnormal anatomic location, e.g., dermoid cyst.)
- Thyroid orbitopathy is a rare cause of proptosis in children
- Infection is a common cause of proptosis in children
- Rhabdomyosarcoma must be considered in any child with rapidly progressive proptosis

We will discuss a few of the common causes of proptosis in children: dermoid cyst, capillary hemangioma, and orbital cellulitis. I have included a few of the uncommon, but "have to know about" lesions as well: lymphangioma, rhabdomyosarcoma, and optic nerve glioma.

Dermoid cyst

A choristoma

You will see this lesion in your practice. A dermoid cyst is a choristoma containing skin and skin appendages such as hair and oil glands. In utero, a bit of skin is "pinched" in a suture line where the tissue gradually forms a cyst. The lining of the cyst is normal skin. The contents of the cyst include keratin, oil, and hair. If the cyst wall does not contain skin appendages, it is called an epidermal cyst (although the clinical presentation and management are the same).

Painless mass

The parents notice the cyst in the first few months of life. The cyst can occur at any suture line, but it is seen most commonly at the frontozygomatic suture (frontonasal suture next most common). In most children, the cyst is located on the lateral side of the bone extending into the suture so no proptosis is present. The mass increases in size very slowly. There is no pain associated. On examination, the mass is usually about 1 cm. It is smooth to palpation and can be either freely moveable or attached firmly to the bone (Figure 14-29).

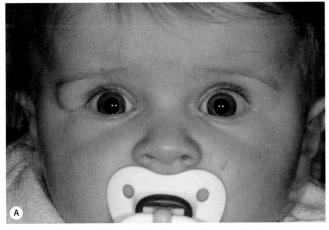
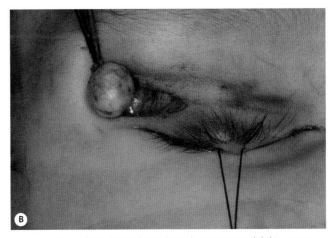

Figure 14-29 Dermoid cyst. (**A**) Typical dermoid cyst at the frontozygomatic suture. (**B**) Excision of the dermoid cyst through an upper eyelid skin crease incision.

Imaging is usually not required

Imaging of the typical frontozygomatic dermoid cyst in an infant is not required if you can feel around the equator of the mass, suggesting that the entire mass is outside the orbital cavity. If the mass is firmly fixed to the bone or you cannot feel around the mass, there may be a component of the cyst extending into the bone or in the orbit itself. Imaging is not absolutely necessary, but it may help you to plan your operation because some bone removal may be required in rare patients. If the mass is nasal, order a scan if you are not absolutely sure that the mass is a dermoid cyst. The differential diagnosis of a mass in this area includes hemangioma and encephalocele, so you should have a low threshold for ordering a scan. A CT scan for a child at this age is easy to do with oral sedation. Probably you will see a well-circumscribed round mass adjacent to the bone. The internal contents of the cyst may have the density of water or oil. Occasionally, you will see an interface between the oil and water layers.

Excisional biopsy

The diagnosis is usually straightforward and excision of the cyst can be performed electively, usually at 1 year of age. If the parents are concerned or you are unsure of the diagnosis, excision can be done at any time. For temporal lesions, the incision can be hidden in the brow or adjacent to the brow. Many temporal lesions can be reached through a skin crease incision (see Figure 14-29, C). This hides the scar nicely, but exposure is more difficult.

Dermoid cyst removal is a great operation to use your best technique of surgical dissection because excision can be easy with proper technique. A good assistant is helpful, as for most orbital operations. You can use a cryoprobe to attach

to the cyst as a "handle." Have your assistant grasp the tissue adjacent to the cyst. Both of you can help to pull the tissues apart. Identify the bands of tissue on stretch and cut them with Westcott scissors. Change positions, working first around the mass superficially and then extending deeper into the wound. Rupture of the cyst may lead to recurrence, so if you are struggling too much, stop, reorganize, perhaps open the wound a little wider, and work again to gently pull the tissues apart to minimize the risk of rupture. Probably you will need to use a Freer elevator to reflect the periosteum off the bone where the cyst is attached. You may see a fossa in the bone that was created by the slow expansion of the dermoid cyst.

Remember that a dermoid cyst can originate at any suture line. Deep orbital dermoid cysts, such as those originating from the sphenozygomatic suture, present later, usually in young adults. Proptosis is the presenting sign for these cysts because the mass is posterior to the eye. Progression is so slow that this congenital lesion takes decades to enlarge to the point that it is noticeable. There is no pain present (in unusual patients, a dermoid cyst may leak spontaneously or after trauma with the presenting sign being inflammation with a little pain). There is no mass palpable. Deep dermoid cysts are usually diagnosed on a CT scan as there are no characteristics in the history or physical examination to make a definitive diagnosis. You will see a large well-circumscribed mass within an area of bone molding to accommodate the slow growth of the cyst (Figure 14-30). Excision of lateral lesions requires a lateral orbitotomy with bone removal.

You recall that *choristomas* are normal tissues in an abnormal place. Dermoid cysts are the most common orbital choristoma. The teratoma (Figure 14-9) is a rare form of

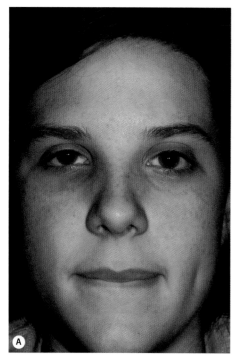
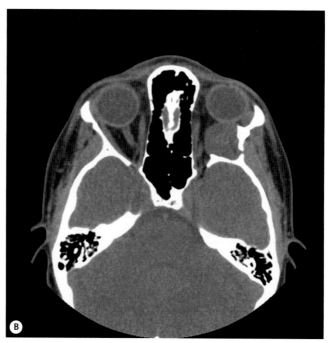

Figure 14-30 Deep dermoid cyst. (**A**) Painless proptosis progressing slowly for many years in teenage girl. (**B**) Axial CT scan—large cystic mass centered at the suture line between the zygoma and sphenoid bones. The typical dermoid cyst presents early in life due to its anterior location. Deeper dermoid cysts present only when large enough to cause proptosis.

choristoma. *Hamartomas* are normal tissues in the normal place, but present in excess amount. Capillary hemangiomas are the most common orbital hamartoma.

Capillary hemangioma

Presentation is diagnostic

The presentation and progression of a capillary hemangioma are so typical that the history is nearly always diagnostic. The usual capillary hemangioma is not present at birth, but appears in the first few months of life. Initially, there is only a blush of red or blue to the skin. Over a few weeks, the vascularization increases to the point where the hemangioma is obvious. The hemangioma may be only cutaneous with little elevation. A subcutaneous hemangioma may develop with no surface vascularization, but a bluish elevation representing deep capillaries. Most capillary hemangiomas have both cutaneous and subcutaneous components. The subcutaneous portion may extend into the orbit causing displacement of the eye or proptosis. Additional lesions may be found anywhere on the body. Most hemangiomas that I see are on the upper lid and forehead. Any large eyelid lesion can cause ptosis or astigmatism so you will need to check for amblyopia and do a cycloplegic refraction. Typically there is no pain present. Pulsations are not present because of the low flow. Slight changes in size occur with crying, probably as a result of vascular engorgement.

Spontaneous involution is the rule

Hemangiomas, if untreated, have three phases:

- Initial growth phase
- Stable phase
- Spontaneous involution phase

During the growth phase, you must follow the patient at appropriate time intervals to observe for any amblyopia. The initial growth phase ends before 6 months of age. There is little change before 1 year when spontaneous involution begins. Involution occurs slowly up until age 8. Initially, the small capillaries close, reducing the red color. Eventually, the majority of the vessels disappear, but often some larger veins will persist. If the lesion is flat, the remaining vessels can be camouflaged with makeup. Cutaneous laser therapy can reduce the remaining vessels significantly. If the hemangioma had significant elevation, a "crepe paper" stretching of the skin may remain. Reconstructive procedures can be used if necessary.

You can imagine the concern most parents will have when an infant rapidly develops the obvious facial "deformity" seen with periocular hemangiomas. Your main job will be to check for amblyopia. The time-consuming part will be educating the parents about the natural history of hemangiomas and reassuring them that involution will occur. It is helpful to have some "before and after" pictures to demonstrate typical resolution (Figure 14-31). Don't put your "best" results in this album, use representative cases. Parents will get many questions from family and friends, all offering friendly advice, so your relationship with the parents is very important. Most patients will not require treatment.

Indications for treatment

Treatment is recommended if amblyopia, astigmatism, or bony orbital asymmetry develops. A superior orbital hemangioma can push the eye inferiorly with long-term globe ptosis as the result. Options for treatment include:

- Intralesional steroid injection
- Oral prednisone
- Surgical excision

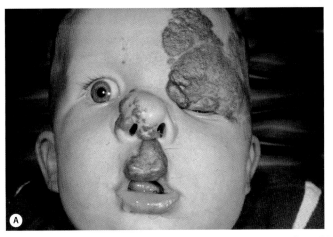
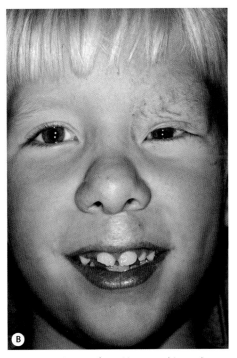

Figure 14-31 Capillary hemangioma. (**A**) Appearance at 4 months of age. (**B**) Appearance at 8 years of age. Note stretching or "crepe paper" skin. This patient was treated with oral prednisone.

You will find that intralesional steroids are very helpful if an upper eyelid mass causes amblyopia. Use a combination of a long-acting steroid (triamcinolone (Kenalog) 40 mg/ml) and short-acting steroid (betamethasone (Celestone) 6 mg/ml) mixed together in a syringe. Inject directly into the lesion with a 23-gauge needle (smaller needles will clog). Make several passes of the needle through the hemangioma as you inject. An alternative is to place the needle in a few single spots, withdraw, and inject. Apply gentle pressure with a gauze sponge to stop any bleeding. There is a minute risk of embolization of the depot material into a vessel, which could cause a central retinal artery occlusion. Regression occurs over a few weeks, sometimes associated with some mild ischemia of the skin (because of the vessels closing). I recheck the patient in 6 weeks. Most hemangiomas will shrink considerably with one injection (Figure 14-32). I will occasionally repeat an injection if the response is not enough.

If a mass is in the orbit causing proptosis or if the hemangioma is very large, it is best to give oral steroids (prednisone 1–2 mg/kg/day). This dose is well tolerated, but it does have the usual steroid side-effects of increased appetite, moodiness, and changes in sleep. Children will be steroid dependent on this dose, so the parents should be counseled about the symptoms of adrenal crisis, such as lethargy or poor feeding. Include the child's pediatrician in this treatment. The full response is usually complete within 6 weeks, and the dose can be tapered. If the child is still in the growth phase, you may see an increase in the size of the mass as the dose is lowered. Recent reports suggest that systemic propanolol can offer significant improvement.

If your medical treatment fails, surgical excision is an option. Large hemangiomas can be safely excised. Although no capsule is present, you can create a fairly bloodless plane of dissection using a Colorado needle. You will have to deal with reconstructing the resultant skin defect. This is advanced surgery.

Orbital cellulitis

Painful, progressive proptosis in a sick child

You are not likely to miss the diagnosis of orbital cellulitis in a child. Infection of the ethmoid sinus spilling into the orbit is the usual cause. The child with orbital cellulitis is seen with proptosis developing over a few days. Pain is present. Recent past medical history usually includes an upper respiratory tract infection, but the symptoms may be mild. Children usually have no history of previous sinus disease like adults with orbital cellulitis. Your physical examination will show mild to advanced signs of orbital inflammation, including proptosis, limited extraocular movements, and chemosis. How does this orbital inflammation look different from the inflammation occurring with idiopathic orbital inflammatory disease? The orbit may look very similar, but the child with orbital cellulitis is "sick"—usually weak, tired, and febrile. At this point, the diagnosis should be clear to you.

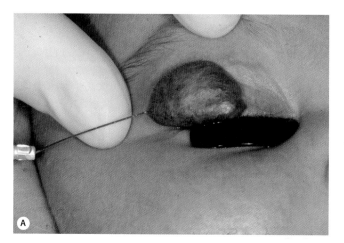

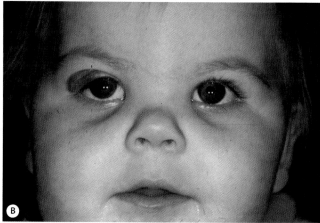

Figure 14-32 Capillary hemangioma. (**A**) Intralesional steroid injection. (**B**) Six weeks after injection. (**C**) Six months after injection.

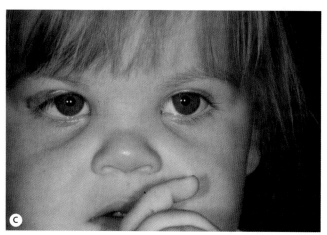

CT scan: orbital inflammation or abscess adjacent to ethmoiditis

Arrange an orbital CT scan. You may want to add views of the sinus, depending on the protocol at your hospital. Take blood cultures and order a complete blood count (which will show an increased white blood cell count with a left shift). When you evaluate the CT scan, you should check to see if there is sinus disease as you suspected. If not, rethink the diagnosis. This will be discussed in more detail below. Most commonly, ethmoid infection will be the cause, spreading into the orbit through the thin lamina papyracea (the "paper plate" of the ethmoid bone). A consultation with an ear, nose, and throat specialist is appropriate. Next, recheck the CT scan to see if there is any abscess forming in the orbit. You will see one of three situations:

- Adjacent inflammation of the orbit and often an enlarged medial rectus muscle
- Subperiosteal abscess
- Intraorbital abscess

Adjacent inflammation of the orbit shows up as a haziness of the medial orbital tissues, sometimes with a thickened medial rectus muscle (Figure 14-33, A). A subperiosteal abscess is present if the periosteum is lifted off the medial orbital wall by pus. The periosteum is tethered at the orbital suture lines so the abscess creates a smooth dome-shaped elevation of periosteum (see Figure 14-33, B and also Figure 2-14). The extraconal fat between the periosteum and the medial rectus muscle retains fat density. An intraconal abscess forms within the orbital fat. On the CT scan, there is opacification of a portion of the orbital fat. Whereas subperiosteal abscess formation is common, the presence of a true intraconal abscess is uncommon.

Treatment

You should start medical treatment immediately. Broad-spectrum intravenous antibiotics and nasal decongestants should be used.

Any intraconal abscess should be drained. In a child younger than 10 years of age, a subperiosteal abscess adjacent to the ethmoid sinus can be treated medically. Improvement should occur within 24–48 hours. If there is uncontrolled pain or any associated vision loss, drainage of the abscess should be performed. If a subperiosteal abscess is present in a child older than 10 years of age or in any adult, drainage should be performed. Any orbital cellulitis arising from the frontal sinus should be drained because of the proximity of the brain and the possibility of meningitis.

Preseptal cellulitis

As you would guess, orbital cellulitis is an infection within the orbit. Preseptal cellulitis is an infection of the eyelids, in the tissue anterior to the orbit. If any "orbital" signs are found (proptosis, decreased motility, or chemosis), the diagnosis of cellulitis is made and a search is done for the cause of the cellulitis. In the absence of orbital signs, you should look for a cause of the preseptal cellulitis. Unless there is an obvious cause for the preseptal cellulitis, such as an insect bite, you should consider the possibility of an ethmoid infection causing the eyelid swelling. In the past, many preseptal infections originated from *Haemophilus influenzae* septicemia resulting from otitis media. Now that the *H. influenzae* vaccine is in widespread use, preseptal inflammation without evidence of a skin wound should be considered sinus in origin until otherwise proven. Order a CT scan to find out.

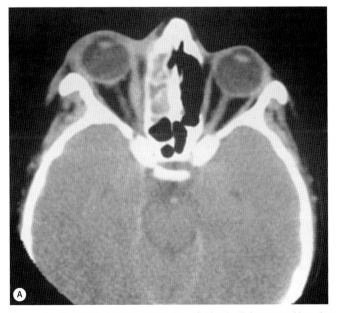
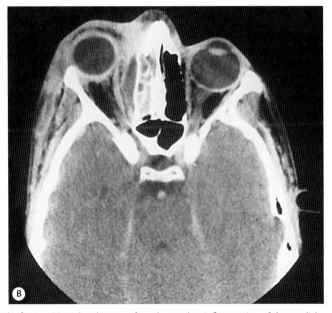

Figure 14-33 Orbital cellulitis. (**A**) CT scan of orbital cellulitis caused by ethmoid infection. Note the absence of an abscess, but inflammation of the medial orbital tissues as demonstrated by enlarged medial rectus muscle. (**B**) A CT scan of orbital cellulitis caused by ethmoid sinus infection. Note the presence of a subperiosteal abscess along the medial orbital wall.

Other causes of orbital cellulitis

What about the opposite situation, in which you have diagnosed an orbital cellulitis, but the scan shows no associated sinus infection? Either your diagnosis of orbital cellulitis is wrong, and the patient has idiopathic orbital inflammatory disease, or there is infection from another source. Consider the other causes of orbital cellulitis:

- Trauma
  - Accidental: rule out foreign body
  - Surgical
- Endogenous
  - From the eye (endophthalmitis)
  - Other adjacent infection (lacrimal sac or dental abscess)
  - Septicemia

Remember that a history of trauma may be forgotten or omitted, especially when dealing with children who don't want to admit some wrongdoing (such as poking a brother's eye with a stick) (Figure 14-34).

Postoperative orbital infections are rare but can occur after an orbitotomy, lid operation, or strabismus procedure. Any infection within the eye or a septicemia can cause an endogenous orbital cellulitis, but this is also rare.

Don't forget that orbital cellulitis can occur in adults. Most adults with bacterial orbital cellulitis have previous sinus disease. Like children, they are also febrile and appear to be ill. On rare occasions, a dental abscess can spread into the orbit, causing orbital cellulitis (Figure 14-35). Remember that the diabetic or immunosuppressed patient (receiving chemotherapy or otherwise immunosuppressed) can develop fungal orbital cellulitis. These patients may have minimal or no signs of inflammation because they do not have a white blood cell response. Similarly, the CT scan will show less opacification (pus) than you would see with bacterial sinusitis.

Optic nerve glioma

Let's look at this tumor type in a real-life clinic situation and see if you are thinking about orbital problems in a systematic fashion. A 10-year-old child is seen with unilateral proptosis. You ask how long the proptosis has been present, and the parents tell you that they just noticed it. You look at old school photos and see that proptosis was present for at least 1 year. You are thinking about the differential diagnosis of slowly progressive painless proptosis in a child. You verify that there is no pain present (not likely or the problem would not have continued unnoticed for 1 year or longer). At this point, based on the slow progression and absence of pain, you have eliminated causes related to infection, inflammation, or a highly malignant neoplasm, leaving you with these possibilities—a slow-growing neoplasm (probably benign), a hamartoma, or a choristoma. You notice that the eye is proptotic without using the Hertel exophthalmometer to measure it, so the proptosis must be at least 2 or 3 mm. The proptosis is axial, suggesting an intraconal mass. It would be too easy if I told you that the vision was down a

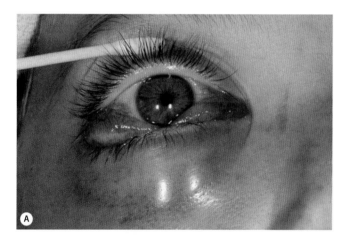

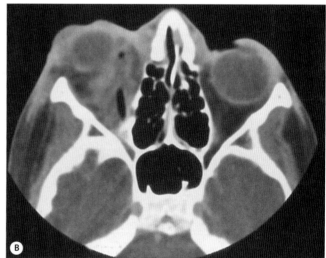

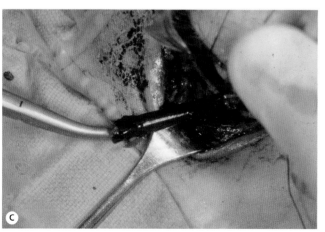

Figure 14-34 Orbital cellulitis caused by a foreign body. (**A**) Orbital inflammation. Note the predominant inferior chemosis. (**B**) A CT scan shows an inferior orbital abscess with "air" in the abscess (actually air in a stick). Note that the sinuses are normal. (**C**) Removal of the intraorbital foreign body (from Reshef D, Ossoinig K, Nerad J: Diagnosis and localization of deep orbital organic foreign bodies, *Orbit* 6(1):3–15, 1987).

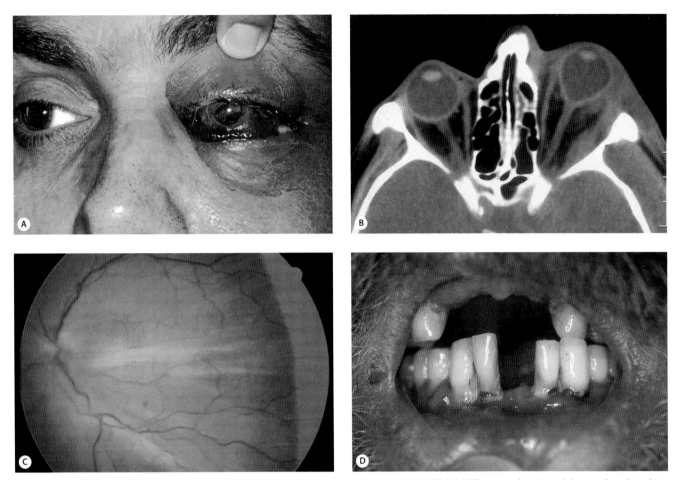

Figure 14-35 Orbital cellulitis of dental origin. (**A**) Proptosis, pain, fever in adult. NLP vision, IOP 55. (**B**) Axial CT scan—subperiosteal abscess along lateral wall. Optic nerve stretched. (**C**) Fundus—CRAO due to high pressure. (**D**) Dental abscess extending into orbit through maxillary sinus, pterygopalatine space, and inferior orbital fissure. Drained, but no return of vision.

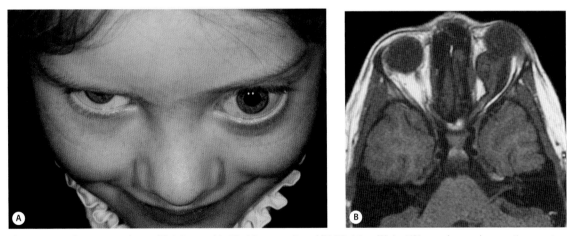

Figure 14-36 Optic nerve glioma. (**A**) A 7-year-old girl with proptosis and 20/20 vision. (**B**) An MRI scan shows a large optic nerve tumor consistent with an optic nerve glioma. A ten year old girl is seen with unilateral proptosis (Figure 14-36, A).

line or two or that the patient has an afferent pupillary defect. You should be thinking glioma. (For extra credit, you look for an associated skin finding.) Imaging is in order. What scan would you order?

Order a CT scan first. You will see an enlarged nerve, often fusiform in shape, usually larger than a meningioma. Sometimes the mass causes eccentric enlargement of the nerve. There is no calcification. As with any optic nerve tumor, you

should order an MRI scan to delineate the posterior extent of the tumor (Figure 14-36, B). The optic nerve tumor is characteristically bright on a T2-weighted scan. Areas of cystic degeneration may be visible (this is likely if there has been a recent progression of proptosis) (Figure 14-36). The chiasm can be involved in up to 50% of cases of optic nerve glioma. There is an association with neurofibromatosis in about 25% of cases (remember the extra credit skin finding you were looking for—café au lait spots). Bilateral optic nerve involvement is diagnostic for neurofibromatosis. Areas of intracranial involvement outside the chiasm can be present and may be lethal, depending on the location.

If the diagnosis is in question, an incisional biopsy can be done. The vast majority of optic nerve gliomas are benign (often considered to be hamartomas), and little or no growth posteriorly along the nerve will be seen over time. You will need only observation for the majority of patients. Serial MRI scans should be performed every 6 months or so. Excision is only recommended for blind eyes with disfiguring proptosis, usually performed through a transcranial orbitotomy, removing the entire nerve. If progression is rapid, rethink the diagnosis—there are malignant forms of "glioma."

Lymphangioma

A rare choristoma

Lymphangioma is a rare choristoma that may not be diagnosed until later in childhood. Lymphatic vessels and collections of lymphoid tissue, not normally present in the orbit, present in one of two ways. Most commonly, a slowly progressive proptosis will be seen. Typically, the proptosis occurs with an upper respiratory tract infection as a result of an increase in the size of the reactive lymphatic tissue (Figure 14-37). There is no pain associated. The second presentation is an acute increase in proptosis associated with pain. This proptosis usually occurs over minutes to a few hours. What are you thinking is likely to be the cause? It is unlikely that an infection or inflammation would progress so quickly. If you are thinking hemorrhage, you are correct. Vessels in the thin wall of lymphatic channels rupture, creating a pocket of blood. Pain results from the rapid distention of the orbital tissues. In some patients, the bleeding occurs chronically over a long period, creating many blood-filled spaces, often visible anteriorly (Figure 14-38).

The physical examination will show proptosis or nonaxial globe ptosis, depending on where the lymphangioma is. There is no mass palpable in most patients. There is no connection with the lymphatic tissue and the blood supply, so there is no pulsation present. Anterior lesions can be seen as cystic dilations within the conjunctiva. You may see associated lymphangiomas on the roof of the mouth (Figure 14-39).

CT scan: heterogeneous infiltrative mass

When you look at the CT scan of a lymphangioma, you will see an infiltrative mass that can extend across the orbital spaces into many tissues (Figure 14-40). The tumor may have some associated heterogeneity with alternating areas of lymphatic cysts, hemorrhage, and lymphatic tissues. If hemorrhage has occurred, you may be able to see a cystic space. An MRI scan is useful to show the heterogeneity if the diagnosis is in question.

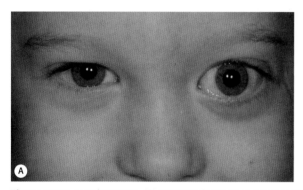
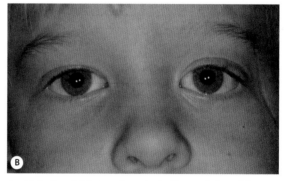

Figure 14-37 Lymphangioma. (**A**) Proptosis during an upper respiratory tract infection. (**A**) Reduced proptosis after resolution of the upper respiratory tract infection.

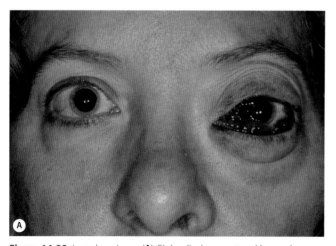
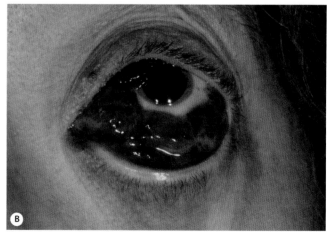

Figure 14-38 Lymphangioma. (**A**) Globe displacement and hemorrhage caused by lymphangioma. (**B**) Chronic bleeding into the potential lymphatic spaces, creating a "bloody" appearing chemosis.

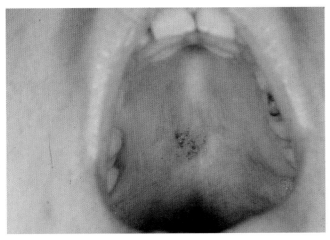

Figure 14-39 Lymphangioma on the roof of the mouth associated with an orbital lymphangioma.

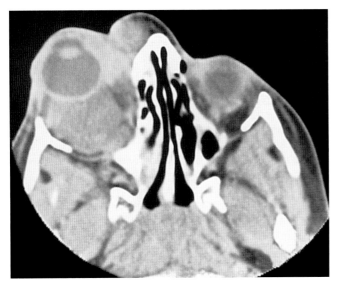

Figure 14-40 A CT scan of a lymphangioma. Note the infiltrative pattern with the orbital mass involving all the orbital spaces. Expansion of the orbit is a typical finding with a childhood orbital mass.

Treatment

There is no medical treatment for lymphangioma. Complete excision of a lymphangioma is not possible because of its infiltrative pattern of growth. After hemorrhage, drainage of "blood cysts" is possible if pain is uncontrolled or if there is vision loss. Fortunately, the growth of most lymphangiomas is self-limited. As you might imagine, because there is no medical or surgical treatment, the few tumors that continue to grow can get unsightly.

Rhabdomyosarcoma

Progressive proptosis in a child

The child with an onset of painless proptosis over a period of several days to a few weeks is considered to have rhabdomyosarcoma until proven otherwise. You will see few instances of this, but its recognition is important. Without treatment, rhabdomyosarcoma is lethal. Seventy percent of these tumors occur in the first decade of life, but a wide range in age may be seen (birth to seventh decade). Often there is a vague history of trauma that may delay bringing the child in for evaluation. Typically, the proptosis is relatively advanced, somewhat out of scale to the short duration of symptoms. The proptosis is often nonaxial, with the superonasal quadrant being involved most commonly (Figure 14-41). Often you will be able to palpate a smooth mass in the anterior orbit, sometimes fixed to bone. There are no abnormal pulsations. The tumor may involve facial structures outside the orbit so look for masses elsewhere, including in the nose. You may find enlarged preauricular or cervical lymph nodes.

CT scan: mass with bone destruction

Obtain a CT scan. Often the orbital mass is well circumscribed, but with associated bone destruction. If the mass extends outside of the orbit, you will see extensive soft tissue involvement and bone destruction. If any of the cranial bones are involved, an MRI scan will be necessary to determine the extent of intracranial involvement. The imaging studies will help you determine the appropriate surgical approach for biopsy.

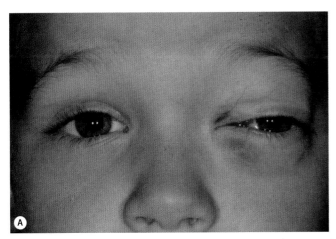
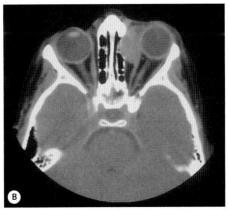

Figure 14-41 Rhabdomyosarcoma. (**A**) Rapidly progressive, painless proptosis in a 5-year-old boy. Notice the nonaxial proptosis with the globe being pushed laterally. The left eye cannot adduct well. (**B**) A CT scan shows a superonasal orbital mass displacing the globe laterally. Note erosion of the medial orbital wall. Because the mass is firm, it may distort the shape of the eye.

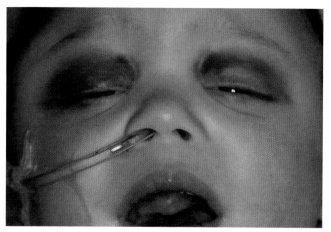

Figure 14-42 Neuroblastoma, metastatic to orbit. Bilateral periocular ecchymoses are typical. Note mass extending from right orbit into temple.

Hematology oncology consultation

Obtain an early oncology consultation. After biopsy, these colleagues will manage the patient. They may want to do a bone marrow biopsy at the time of your orbitotomy. After completion of the systemic workup, a combination of chemotherapy and radiation therapy will be used to control the disease. This tumor treatment is an example of the advances made in the treatment of pediatric cancers. Thirty years ago, rhabdomyosarcoma metastatic to the orbit was treated with exenteration. Now, if the tumor is isolated to the orbit, the cure rate is greater than 90% without any disfiguring surgery.

Fortunately, metastatic disease to the orbit in children is uncommon. Although you may never see a metastatic neuroblastoma, the presentation of bilateral periocular ecchymosis is so typical I have included an example (Figure 14-42).

Checkpoint

Remember the general differences in the causes of proptosis in children compared with those in adults:
- Malignancy is a less common cause of proptosis
- Congenital abnormality, choristoma, and hamartoma are more common causes
- Thyroid orbitopathy is a rare cause of proptosis in children
- Infection is a common cause of proptosis in children
- Rhabdomyosarcoma must be considered in any child with rapidly progressive proptosis

A small cystic mass above the lateral canthus in a child is almost always a dermoid cyst. Remove this on an elective basis.

Remember the natural progression of the capillary hemangioma. If amblyopia, astigmatism, or facial deformity occurs, consider treatment. Recall the options for treatment.

Make sure you know the signs of orbital cellulitis. Image and treat urgently. Be reluctant to diagnose preseptal orbital cellulitis in a child without an obvious cause (why?).

Compare the clinical and imaging characteristics of optic nerve glioma with those of optic nerve meningioma.

Progression of proptosis in a child over days to weeks suggests a diagnosis of rhabdomyosarcoma. How would this presentation differ from the presentation of orbital cellulitis?

Go through the "P's" of the history and physical examination.

What are the clues to the pathogenic categories of neoplasm versus infection or inflammation?

Don't forget about the usefulness of pain as a symptom.

Major points

Proptosis is the hallmark of orbital disease.

Thyroid disease is the most common cause of unilateral or bilateral proptosis. The diagnosis can usually be made by clinical examination.

The approach to the proptotic patient with a suspected orbital mass can be summarized as:

- An orbital mass displaces the eye away from the mass
- Almost any tissue type can form an orbital tumor
- History and physical examination are used to:
  - Place the disease process into a pathogenic category
  - Develop a differential diagnosis
- Imaging is required in most cases to:
  - Refine the differential diagnosis
  - Plan incisional or excisional biopsy
- Biopsy of an orbital mass is often required to establish or confirm a diagnosis

The Hertel exophthalmometer is used to measure proptosis of the globe:

- The equator of the globe is at the lateral orbital rim in a white patient with average facial bone structure
  - The average Hertel measurement for a white patient is 20 mm
  - The average Hertel measurement for an Asian patient is 18 mm
  - The average Hertel measurement for an African American patient is 22 mm
- Asymmetry (2 mm or more) or a change in a Hertel measurement is more significant than the absolute measurement
- Remember to use the same base measurement each time on an individual patient

Proptosis means anterior displacement of the eye. Globe ptosis is the term used when the eye is pushed down by a mass.

The orbit is conceptually and anatomically divided into surgical spaces:

Major points Continued

- The intraconal space
- The extraocular muscles
- The extraconal space
- The subperiosteal space
- Tenon's space
- The extraorbital space

The "P's" of the history are:

- Progression
- Pain
- Past medical history

Pain and progression are characteristics of the orbital problem that you will find most helpful to develop the differential diagnosis.

- Ask about the presence or absence of pain as one of the first questions in the history
  - Pain implies infection or inflammation
  - Neoplasms usually don't cause pain
- The progression will give an idea of how quickly the disease is progressing, the tempo. Record both the onset of the symptoms as well as the pace of the progression

Using pain and progression, you should be able to develop a differential diagnosis for the proptosis based on the pathogenic process involved:

- Inflammatory
- Neoplastic
- Metastatic
- Congenital (malformation, hamartoma, and choristoma)
- Infectious
- Vascular (hemorrhagic)

This seems basic, but you will find this very helpful, especially when you are learning.

Add past medical history to the list of "P's" from the history. Include:

- Trauma
- Thyroid disease
- Neoplasm

The "P's" of the physical examination are:

- Proptosis
- Palpation
- Pulsation
- Periocular changes

The direction of the proptosis is the most important of the physical findings. Is the proptosis axial? Is the globe displaced up, down, or to the side? Tumors push the eye away. You should be able to develop a basic differential diagnosis based on the direction of globe displacement.

Common causes of proptosis in adults include:

- Thyroid orbitopathy
- Lymphoma
- Cavernous hemangioma
- Pseudotumor (idiopathic orbital inflammatory disease)
- Metastatic tumor

Common orbital diseases in children include:

- Dermoid cyst
- Capillary hemangioma
- Orbital cellulitis

Unless there is an obvious cause for the "preseptal" cellulitis, such as an insect bite, you should consider the possibility of an ethmoid infection causing the eyelid swelling (actually a subclinical orbital cellulitis).

Rhabdomyosarcoma should be considered in any child with proptosis progressing over days or weeks.

Suggested reading

1. American Academy of Ophthalmology: *Basic and clinical science course: orbit, eyelids, and lacrimal system*, sect. 7, pp. 63–96, San Francisco: The American Academy of Ophthalmology, 2006/2007.

2. Augsburger et al: Metastatic cancer to the eye. In Yanoff and Duker, eds, *Ophthalmology*, Philadelphia: Mosby, 2004.

3. Dortzbach RK, Kronish JW, Gentry LR: Magnetic resonance imaging of the orbit, Part I. Physical principles, *Ophthalmic Plast Reconstr Surg* 5(3):151–159, 1989.

4. Dortzbach RK, Kronish JW, Gentry LR: Magnetic resonance imaging of the orbit, Part II. Clinical applications, *Ophthalmic Plast Reconstr Surg* 5(3):160–170, 1989.

5. Freedman MI, Folk JC: Metastatic tumors to the eye and orbit: patient survival on clinical characteristics, *Arch Ophthal* 105:1215–1219, 1987.

6. Dutton JJ, Orbital imaging techniques. In Yanoff and Duker, eds, *Ophthalmology*, pp. 649–654, London: Mosby, 2004.

7. Dutton JJ: *Atlas of clinical and surgical orbital anatomy*, Philadelphia: WB Saunders, 1994.

8. Dutton JJ: Gliomas of the anterior visual pathway, *Surv Ophthalmol* 38(5), 1994.

9. Dutton JJ: Optic nerve sheath meningiomas. *Surv Ophthalmol* 37(3), 1992.

10. Dutton JJ: Clinical anatomy of the orbit. In Yanoff and Duker, eds, *Ophthalmology*, pp. 641–648, London: Mosby, 2004.

11. Dutton JJ, Haik BG, eds: *Thyroid eye disease*, New York: Marcel Dekker, 2002.

12. Garrity JA, Henderson JW, Cameron, JD: *Henderson's orbital tumors*, 4th edn, Philadelphia: Lippincott Williams and Wilkins, 2007.

13. Gorman CA, Garrity JA, Fatourechi V et al: A prospective, randomized, double blind, placebo-controlled study of orbital radiotherapy for Graves' ophthalmopathy, *Ophthalmology* 108:1523–1534, 2001.

14. Harris GJ: Subperiosteal inflammation of the orbit: a bacteriological analysis of 17 cases, *Arch Ophthal* 106:947–952, 1988.

15. Harris GJ: Subperiosteal abscess of the orbit. Age as a factor in the bacteriology and response to treatment, *Ophthalmology* 101(3):585–595, 1994.

16. Harris GJ, Sakol PJ, Bonavolonta G, DeConcilis C: An analysis of thirty cases of orbital lymphangioma: pathophysiologic considerations and management recommendations, *Ophthalmology* 97(12):1583–1592, 1990.

17. Krohel G, Steward W, Chavis R: *Orbital disease, a practical approach*, New York: Grune & Stratton, 1981.

18. Nerad J: The diagnostic approach to the patient with proptosis. In *The requisites—Oculoplastic surgery*, pp. 348–386, St Louis: Mosby, 2001.

19. Nerad JA, Carter KD, Alford MA: Disorders of the orbit: orbital imaging. In *Rapid diagnosis in ophthalmology—oculoplastic and reconstructive surgery*, pp. 154–157, Philadelphia: Mosby Elsevier, 2008.

20. Nerad JA, Carter KD, Alford MA: Disorders of the orbit: infections, inflammations, neoplasms, vascular abnormalities. In *Rapid diagnosis in ophthalmology—oculoplastic and reconstructive surgery*, pp. 160–239, Philadelphia: Mosby Elsevier, 2008.

21. Rootman J: *Diseases of the orbit*, Philadelphia: JB Lippincott, 1988.

22. Rootman J, Stewart B, Goldberg RA, eds: Orbital anatomy. In *Orbital surgery, a conceptual approach*, ch. 7, pp. 79–146, Philadelphia: Lippincott-Raven, 1995.

23. Rootman J: *Orbital disease—present status and future challenges*. Boca Raton: Taylor and Francis, 2005.

24. Vaphiades MS, Horton JA: MRA or CTA, that's the question, *Surv Ophthalmol* 50:406–410, 2005.

25. Weiss RA: Orbital disease. In McCord CD, Tanenbaum M, Nunery WR, eds, *Oculoplastic surgery*, 3rd edn, ch. 15, pp. 417–476, New York: Raven Press, 1995.

26. Wobig JL, Dailey RA, eds: *Oculofacial plastic surgery: face, lacrimal system, and orbit*, pp. 192–254, New York: Thieme, 2004.

Surgical Approaches to the Orbit*

Introduction

Orbital tumors are rare. Biopsy for removal or diagnosis is often necessary. From our discussion in the last chapter, you have a good idea about which tumors should be removed (excisional biopsy) and which tumors should be sampled (incisional biopsy). In this chapter, you will learn the logic in choosing the most appropriate surgical approach for anterior and deep orbital masses. Understanding the surgical spaces of the orbit will help you with an anatomic approach that will guide your choice of procedure as well as help you navigate in the orbit itself. Many tumors can be approached from the front of the orbit through an anterior orbitotomy. Tumors deeper in the orbit require more advanced procedures.

Before orbitotomy, you must prepare the patient, the operating team, and the operating room. A preoperative

medical workup and review of medications, especially those with anticoagulation effects, are necessary. The surgical plan should be coordinated with any additional surgical teams and the pathologist. Once in the operating room, the procedure should be reviewed with the scrub team, and the equipment and instruments need to be organized. We will review some of the specialized equipment, instruments, and surgical techniques used in orbital surgery. Proper illumination, magnification, exposure, orbital dissection, and hemostasis are necessary for a successful outcome to the orbitotomy.

Because many of the orbital processes that you will see occur in the anterior orbit, you should be most familiar with the anterior orbitotomy approaches. You should learn to do the following three anterior orbitotomy approaches:

- The upper lid skin crease approach
- The lower lid transcutaneous approach
- The lower lid transconjunctival approach

Because you are likely to be doing these procedures, I will describe them in detail.

Deep tumors in the orbit are more difficult to expose. Deeper tumors in the medial aspect of the orbit are espe-

*Many of the line drawings in this chapter are based on Kersten RC, Nerad JA: Orbital surgery. In Tasman W, Jaeger EA, eds, *Duane's clinical ophthalmology*, rev. edn, vol. 5, ch. 86, pp. 1–36, Philadelphia: Lippincott Williams & Wilkins, 1998.

cially difficult to reach. Specialized anterior orbitotomy techniques can be used to approach deeper tumors; however, you may not want to perform them until you master the more basic procedures. Because these procedures are used less often, I have included less detail for you. Nevertheless, you should know that they exist.

Deep lateral and apical orbital tumors may require removal of one or more walls of the orbit. These procedures include:

- The lateral orbitotomy
- The transcranial orbitotomy

Deep tumors lateral to the optic nerve are usually approached using the lateral orbitotomy with bone removal. This is the classic orbitotomy, the "work horse" for deeper orbital tumors, so I will describe this technique in detail, as well.

Tumors in the orbital apex must be approached using the transcranial orbitotomy. This approach requires elevation of the brain and removal of the orbital roof. The transcranial orbitotomy can be combined with other intracranial approaches to the optic canal, the chiasm, and the sphenoid wing. The procedure requires coordination between the ophthalmology and neurosurgery teams. You should understand the indications for this procedure. If you have the opportunity to assist with a transcranial orbitotomy, you will see some incredible orbital anatomy.

Approach to the patient with proptosis

In the last chapter, we discussed the evaluation of the patient with proptosis. As you recall, the diagnosis begins with a history and physical examination utilizing the "P's" of the orbital examination. Most patients with proptosis will undergo a computed tomography (CT) scan as the primary diagnostic imaging test. A magnetic resonance imaging (MRI) scan is used as a secondary test and is especially useful for evaluating the orbitocranial junction. Some cases will require both CT and MRI. Using the information obtained from the history and physical examination and imaging tests, you will arrive at a differential diagnosis. In a few patients, you will know the exact cause of the proptosis is (e.g., thyroid orbitopathy). In other patients, you will base a differential diagnosis on the tissue involved (e.g., optic nerve tumor). In the remaining patients, you will only be able to arrive at a pathogenic diagnosis (e.g., inflammation or neoplasm). In a small number of patients, you will be able to initiate medical treatment without further testing (e.g., antibiotic treatment for orbital cellulitis). Most patients will require a biopsy.

The orbital biopsy will be either incisional or excisional. As a general rule, infiltrative processes suggest malignancy and will require an incisional biopsy. The exact nature of a malignancy or benign infiltrative disorder will be identified based on the incisional biopsy. Usually, additional medical or surgical therapy is required. Well-circumscribed or cystic masses tend to be benign and amenable to complete removal or excisional biopsy. The ovoid mass of a benign mixed tumor of the lacrimal gland is an example of a well-circumscribed benign tumor for which an excisional biopsy is indicated (a tumor rarely seen clinically, but commonly seen in questions on board examinations). Incomplete removal may allow eventual recurrence of a malignant form of lacrimal tumor. There are exceptions to these rules, the most common being the well-circumscribed mass that is diagnosed histopathologically as a malignant lymphoid process. Incisional rather than excisional biopsy should be used for lymphoid tumors, even though they are well circumscribed. The malignant and benign forms of lymphoid infiltrate cannot be distinguished clinically. Neither form is treated with excision; both are treated with either radiation therapy or medication.

Choosing the surgical approach

There are several factors to consider in choosing the surgical approach:

- Anterior or deep location
- Position relative to the optic nerve
- The surgical space occupied
- The goal of biopsy
  - Incisional
  - Excision

Based on these factors, the safest and most practical approach to reaching the orbital tumor is chosen. In most patients, the skin incision will be chosen to provide optimal scar camouflage by placing it in a skin crease, hiding it on a posterior surface of the eyelid, or placing it adjacent to prominent anatomic landmarks such as the eyebrow or eyelashes (Figure 15-1).

Anterior versus deep tumors

The anterior–posterior position of an orbital mass within the orbit is the most important factor to consider in choosing a surgical approach. Tumors anterior to the equator of the eye are most commonly approached from the front of the orbit using a type of anterior orbitotomy. Tumors posterior to the equator of the eye require more advanced deep surgical approaches. The choice of orbitotomy for deep tumors is related to the relationship of the tumor to the optic nerve.

Relationship to the optic nerve

A fundamental principle of orbital surgery is:

- Choose an orbitotomy approach that avoids crossing the optic nerve

Following this guideline, deep orbital tumors lateral to the optic nerve are approached with a lateral orbitotomy approach. Removal of the lateral orbital wall provides excellent access to these tumors.

Deep tumors medial to the optic nerve are more difficult to reach because there is no bone that can be easily removed to provide good exposure and access. The surgical spaces of the medial orbit can be reached through deep medial orbitotomy approaches, through either the eyelid or the conjunctiva. Access to the apical medial orbit from these anterior orbitotomy approaches is limited. In unusual situations, the medial orbital wall may be removed and limited access to the deep medial orbit can be obtained (Figure 15-2).

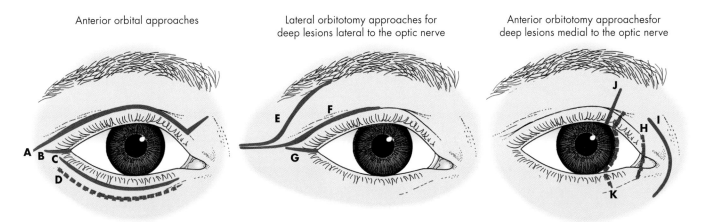

Anterior orbital approaches

Lateral orbitotomy approaches for deep lesions lateral to the optic nerve

Anterior orbitotomy approachesfor deep lesions medial to the optic nerve

Figure 15-1 Surgical incisions for orbitotomy. *Anterior orbital approaches:* (**A**) Upper lid skin crease incision. (**B**) Lateral canthotomy incision. (**C**) Lower lid transcutaneous incision. (**D**) Lower lid transconjunctival incision. *Lateral orbitotomy approaches for deep lesions lateral to the optic nerve:* (**E**) Stallard–Wright lateral orbitotomy incisions. (**F**) Upper lid skin crease incision with lateral canthal extension. (**G**) Modified lateral canthotomy incision. *Anterior orbitotomy approaches for deep lesions medial to the optic nerve:* (**H**) Transcaruncular incision. (**I**) Frontoethmoidal Lynch incision. (**J**) Vertical lid split incision. (**K**) Transconjunctival medial orbitotomy incision.

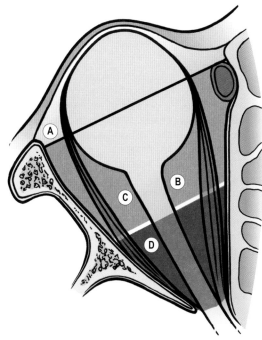

Figure 15-2 The choice of orbitotomy approach is based on the position of the mass. (**A**) Anterior to the equator of the eye: anterior orbitotomy. (**B**) Posterior to the globe and medial to the nerve: deep medial anterior orbitotomy. (**C**) Posterior to the globe and lateral to the nerve: lateral orbitotomy. (**D**) Involving the posterior one third of the orbit: transcranial orbitotomy.

Box 15-1	
Surgical Approaches to the Orbit	
Anterior to the equator of the eye	Anterior orbitotomy
Posterior to the globe and lateral to the nerve	Lateral orbitotomy
Posterior to the globe and medial to the nerve	Deep medial anterior orbitotomy
Posterior one third of orbit, optic canal, chiasm	Transcranial orbitotomy

otomy or a lateral orbitotomy approach. Excision of the entire optic nerve, however, requires a much wider area of exposure, usually provided only by a transcranial orbitotomy approach. You can see that the intent of the operation is a factor in your choice of orbitotomy approach (Box 15-1).

The surgical spaces of the orbit

You will recall that the surgical spaces already discussed in Chapters 2 and 13 are (Figure 15-3):

- The intraconal space
- The extraocular muscles
- The extraconal space
- The subperiosteal space
- Tenon's space
- The extraorbital space

You should already know these spaces. This section is intended as an illustration of how you will begin to think of the spaces of the orbit and their relationship to the orbitotomy approach. Don't memorize the specific pathologic processes and approaches mentioned here. We will talk about them again later in this chapter. Just start to get an idea of how you are going to choose the orbitotomy

Type of biopsy

The surgical approach may be influenced by the goal of the operation. It is easier to perform an incisional biopsy through a small incision than it is to perform an excisional biopsy. For example, an incisional biopsy of the optic nerve can be performed through either a transconjunctival anterior orbit-

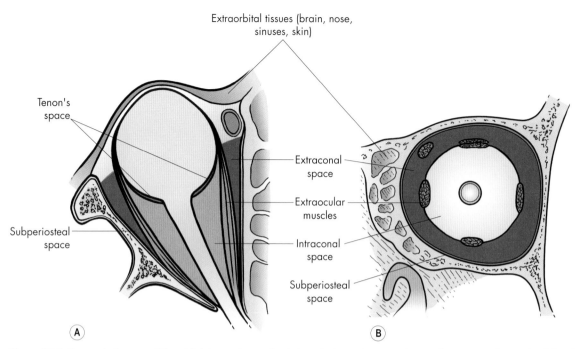

Extraorbital tissues (brain, nose, sinuses, skin)

Tenon's space

Subperiosteal space

Extraconal space

Extraocular muscles

Intraconal space

Subperiosteal space

(A)

(B)

Figure 15-3 The surgical spaces of the orbit: intraconal space (central surgical space); extraocular muscles; extraconal space (peripheral surgical space); subperiosteal space; Tenon's space; the extraorbital space (including periocular tissues, brain, nose, sinuses, bone, and surrounding soft tissues). (**A**) Axial view. (**B**) Coronal view.

approach, based on the position of the pathologic process and what you have already learned in this chapter.

The extraconal space contains the lacrimal gland, the superior oblique muscle and trochlea, and nerves and vessels in the extraconal orbital fat. An enlarged lacrimal gland is often palpable in the upper lid and then is readily accessible through an anterior orbitotomy using the upper lid skin crease approach. Lymphoid tumors are among the most common orbital masses. Because lymphomas tend to occur in the lacrimal gland or elsewhere anteriorly in the extraconal fat, anterior orbitotomy approaches to the extraconal space are commonly used. When a lacrimal gland mass is not palpable (mostly posterior to the globe), a lateral orbitotomy, usually with bone removal, is required. The superior oblique muscle and trochlea are in the medial portion of the extraconal space, but rarely require biopsy. Schwannoma of the frontal nerve may be seen in the superonasal quadrant and can be approached anteriorly, but if the mass extends into the apex, a transcranial approach may be necessary for removal. The anterior portion of the superior ophthalmic vein lies in the extraconal space, but it almost never requires surgical intervention.

The intermuscular septum lies between the anterior portion of the extraocular muscles, separating the intraconal and extraconal spaces. The muscles may become involved in neoplastic or inflammatory processes. The most common condition is thyroid orbitopathy. Painful inflammation of the muscles, myositis, may also occur. Primary neoplasms of the muscles are very rare, but metastatic lesions do occur. Although biopsies are not often performed on the extraocular muscles, the muscles can be approached surgically through anterior orbitotomy incisions if the pathologic lesion is anterior. If the enlargement of the muscle is posterior, you can decide on the best approach for incisional biopsy following the principles described in the previous section. The extraoc-

ular muscles are important surgical landmarks to guide your surgical dissection. During lateral orbitotomy approaches, the intraconal space is usually entered between the lacrimal gland and the lateral rectus muscle. We will discuss this dissection technique further in the section "Approach to Deep Lateral Lesions: The Lateral Orbitotomy."

The subperiosteal space is the potential space between the orbital bones and the periorbita. A hematoma may collect in this space from an adjacent fracture. A collection of pus, a subperiosteal abscess, may collect medially from an adjacent ethmoid sinus infection. For drainage of a subperiosteal abscess, you will usually approach the medial subperiosteal space anteriorly through the skin and conjunctiva with elevation of the periorbita from the orbital rim and dissection posteriorly along the medial orbital wall (frontoethmoidal and transcaruncular anterior orbitotomy). Repair of orbital floor fractures begins with surgical approaches to the subperiosteal space using transconjunctival or transcutaneous lower eyelid anterior orbitotomy techniques. Similarly, you can approach medial wall fractures using the transcaruncular anterior orbitotomy technique.

Tenon's space lies between the eye and the fibrous capsule, Tenon's capsule, which surrounds all but the anterior portion of the eye. Probably you have already operated in this space when performing an enucleation or scleral buckle procedure. Although we usually don't think of it, these operations start with a transconjunctival anterior orbitotomy. Tenon's space is rarely involved in pathologic processes; one example is the extraocular extension of a choroidal melanoma.

The extraorbital space includes all the tissues surrounding the orbit: bone, brain, sinus, nasal, skin, and conjunctiva. You are already familiar with some of the many problems that originate in these tissues and involve the orbit secondarily. The surgical approach to many of these tissues is obvious, whereas others involve areas of overlap with other surgical specialties for which interdisciplinary cooperation is essential to the success of the operation.

We will talk about the orbital spaces in the context of the orbitotomy procedures again and again throughout this chapter, so start thinking of these spaces in the context of orbitotomy approaches.

Names of orbitotomy approaches

There is no consistent nomenclature or classification of orbitotomy approaches. Most of the names used in this text and by other surgeons are descriptive. You shouldn't memorize these terms because they can mean different things to different people. Some commonly used descriptive terms and my interpretation of them are:

- *Anterior orbitotomy* means that the approach is from the front of the orbit, usually through the eyelid or conjunctiva. In general, an anterior orbitotomy approach does not involve bone resection.
- *Lateral orbitotomy* means that the approach is from the lateral side of the orbit. In general, the term lateral orbitotomy implies that the lateral rim will be removed. We will see later that a lateral orbitotomy can be performed through a small skin incision at the lateral canthus without any bone removal.
- The terms *anterior* and *deep* are opposite. The term superficial orbital tumor is not used. Anterior tumors are palpable and accessible by the "anterior" approaches. Deep is usually used to describe posterior tumors in the orbit.
- Anatomy accessible only via *transcranial orbitotomy* includes the posterior one third of the orbit, superior orbital fissure, sphenoid wing, and chiasm.
- *Deep tumors* are posterior to the globe. I use the term deep medial anterior orbitotomy for approaches to intraconal tumors medial to the nerve. As we discussed above, the lateral orbitotomy is used for approaches to deep tumors lateral to the nerve.
- *Apical* implies the posterior one third of the orbit. I use the term orbitocranial to describe tumors involving the orbital apex and optic canal, chiasm, superior orbital fissure, or other intracranial structures. The transcranial orbitotomy is used to approach apical or orbitocranial tumors. The terms superotemporal orbitotomy and panoramic orbitotomy are sometimes used interchangeably with the term transcranial orbitotomy.

Checkpoint

Review the "P's" of the orbital examination and the approach to the patient with proptosis. You should know the "P's" by memory. You should also understand the flow from history and physical examination to imaging to differential diagnosis and, finally, to biopsy or treatment.

State in your own words how each of these factors influences the choice of orbitotomy:

- Anterior or deep location
- Position relative to the optic nerve
- The surgical space occupied
- Goal of biopsy, incisional or excisional

Preoperative considerations

Before orbitotomy, the patient should have a general medical examination with an emphasis on the cardiopulmonary system to receive clearance for surgery. Blood pressure should be optimally controlled before orbitotomy. All anticoagulants including warfarin (Coumadin), aspirin products, and nonsteroidal anti-inflammatory agents should be discontinued before surgery, if possible.

Preoperative informed consent should be obtained. Damage to important neurovascular structures is possible, but rarely occurs. Postoperative swelling, diplopia, and upper eyelid ptosis are common, but usually resolve. In rare patients, blindness may occur because of intraoperative injuries to the optic nerve or postoperative hemorrhage. Patients undergoing deep orbitotomy procedures are usually hospitalized overnight. The visual acuity is checked every 2 hours for the first 12–24 postoperative hours. Death is an extremely unlikely occurrence during an orbitotomy procedure.

If the orbitotomy is part of a multidisciplinary procedure, the division of responsibilities among the various surgical subspecialists should be clearly outlined. If you anticipate an unusual diagnosis, preoperative discussion with the pathology team is appropriate.

Intraoperative considerations

Room setup

You should have a plan for the setup of the room and any specialized equipment that will be required. If you anticipate using an operating microscope, it should be positioned and adjusted while the patient is being prepared. Any pathology requisitions should be filled out before you start the surgery. You should discuss the plan for operation with the nursing staff before beginning the procedure.

Orbital instruments

Specialized orbital instruments are used (Box 15-2). Retraction of skin is necessary, using small (Storz double-fixation forceps) or large (Joseph) skin hooks and suture retractors (4-0 silk). Retraction of the orbital fat is facilitated with Sewall and malleable ribbon retractors of various lengths. Neurosurgical cottonoids placed under the retractors prevent fat prolapse into the surgical wound. A variety of periosteal elevators should be available, including Freer, Joseph, and Dean elevators. Bone removal equipment including a power saw, drill, and bone rongeurs are necessary if deep orbitotomy procedures with bone removal are anticipated. A microplating system is useful to repair complex orbital bone cuts. A Freer elevator or a long cotton-tipped applicator is a useful orbital dissection tool. Small neurosurgical dissectors can be helpful.

As we discussed in Chapter 1, scissors and forceps for deeper orbital procedures are usually longer than eye instruments for routine procedures. Bayonet-type handles allow comfortable hand position without blocking visualization in deep surgical wounds, especially when an operating microscope is used. Yasargil neurosurgical scissors (which look like long-handled Westcott scissors) with curved or

---

Box 15-2

Instruments of Special Interest for Orbital Surgery

Retractors

- Skin
  - 4-0 silk traction suture, reverse cutting (Ethicon 783G G-3 single-armed cutting needle)
  - 4-0 silk, taper needle for bridle sutures under extraocular muscles (Ethicon K-871 RB-1 needle)
  - Joseph skin hooks: large double-pronged skin hooks (Storz N4730)
  - Storz double-fixation hooks: small double-pronged skin hooks (Storz E0533)
- Orbital
  - Sewall retractors
    - — 52 mm blade (Storz N3321)
    - — 51 mm blade (Storz N3322)
    - — 50 mm blade (Storz N3323)
    - — 67 mm blade (Storz N3324)
  - Malleable ribbon retractors (brain spatula)
    - — Codman Ribbon retractor
      - —— 5/8 × 8 in (Codman 50-5638)
      - —— 3/4 × 8 in (Codman 50-5639)
      - —— 1/4 in special order
- Neurosurgical cottonoids

Periosteal elevators

- Freer septal elevator: light elevator (Storz N2348)
- Joseph periosteal elevator: heavy, but narrow elevator (Storz N4610)
- Dean periosteotome: heavy elevator (Jarit *JSO2848)

Bone instruments

- Kerrison rongeur (upbiting)
  - Extra small (Storz N1950)
  - Small (Storz N1951)
  - Medium (Storz N1952)
- Leksell laminectomy rongeur (large bone rongeur)
  - Regular curve (Storz NLS 3268 TIN)
  - Full curve (Storz NLS 3270 TIN)
- Spurling Kerrison rongeur (similar to Hardy sella punch: smaller bone rongeur)
  - Angled, 3 mm bite (Storz NLS3299 3 TIN)
  - 90 degree, 3 mm bite (Storz NLS3301 3 TIN)
- Hall microsagittal saw
- Hall Surgairtome (air drill)
- Bien drill (electric drill)

Dissectors

- Freer elevator (Storz N2348)
- Cotton-tipped applicator, 6 inch
- Neurosurgical dissectors (Rhoton)

Scissors

- Westcott tenotomy scissors, curved right, blunt tips (Storz E3320 R)
- Titanium bayonet scissors, curved, fine tip (Yasargil type) (Storz NLS4050)

Forceps

- Gruenwald nasal dressing forceps, delicate bayonet (Storz N2862)
- Storz ear forceps (alligator type) (Storz X0240)
- Storz sinus cup forceps: small cup biopsy forceps, useful for biopsies and retraction of friable tumor tissue (Storz N2898)
- Takahashi nasal forceps: ethmoidectomy forceps (Storz N2997)
- Hartman–Herzfeld 3 mm cup forceps: small upbiting angled forceps (Storz N0965)
- Wilde nasal forceps for ethmoidectomy procedures
  - Straight (Storz N2980)
  - Upturned (Storz N2982)
  - Blakesly nasal forceps: smaller forceps for ethmoidectomy procedures (Storz N2990)

Cautery

- "Colorado" microdissector needle
- Bipolar cautery (jeweler tips for anterior dissection)
- Bipolar cautery (long bayonet tips for deep dissection)
- Microbipolar cautery, long bayonet tips (Yasargil) (Storz S2050 38D)

Hemostatic agents

- Bone wax
- For improving platelet aggregation
  - Gelfoam (absorbable gelatin sponge)
  - Surgicel (oxidized regenerated cellulose)
  - Avitene (microfibrillar collagen)
- For improving clotting
  - Thrombogen (thrombin)
  - Thrombin and Gelfoam
  - FloSeal
  - Tisseal (fibrin "glue")

Suction

- Baron suction tube, 5 French (Storz N0610)
- Frazier suction tube, 9 French (Storz N2421)
- Yankauer tonsil suction tube (Storz N7550)

---

straight blades are good for deep dissections. Westcott scissors are used in anterior orbitotomy procedures. Most eyelid forceps (Paufique forceps) work well for anterior orbital approaches. Myringotomy forceps or any of a variety of small cup biopsy forceps are useful for grasping tissue in deep or tight spaces. The cup forceps or a small "nasal bead" forceps (Hartman–Herzfeld 3 mm cup forceps) is useful for small biopsies of friable tumor tissue. A variety of cautery forceps are helpful, especially microbayonet bipolar forceps (Fischer or Yasargil bipolar forceps) for deep procedures.

Illumination and magnification

You will need excellent illumination to visualize the orbital structures. You can perform anterior orbitotomy procedures with standard operating room lights. You'll find a fiberoptic headlight helpful for any deeper orbitotomy procedures. The coaxial lighting and view provided by the operating microscope is the only way that both the surgeon and the assistant can see deeper orbital structures at the same time.

Magnification using surgical loupes is standard for anterior orbitotomy procedures. Loupes (2.5 power) from Designs for Vision (Ronkonkoma, NY) are expensive, but great. For deep orbitotomy procedures, you should use the operating microscope for magnification and illumination. The optimal microscope for orbital surgery is mounted on a counter-weighted stand that allows the microscope to be positioned in any direction in three-dimensional space. These stands are commonly used by your neurosurgical colleagues. The gold standard is operating microscopes made by Zeiss. A variety of configurations are available, but opposing microscope heads are ideal for lateral orbitotomy procedures. A 300 mm objective lens provides an adequate distance between the patient and the microscope to move the longer orbital instruments in and out of the operating field without hitting the microscope. An attached video camera and monitor are important for keeping the operating room staff involved.

Body mechanics and posture

This is a good place to remind you to pay attention to your posture and body mechanics as a surgeon. If you are lucky, you will spend many hours a week for many years in the operating room (so far for me, over 20,000 hours!). In your early years as a surgeon, it is easy to abuse your body, often operating in awkward positions, craning your neck to see the field or pass a suture. Over time, operating with the microscope presents its own set of problems, especially for your neck. Combined with your many hours of study, you will find that, if you are not careful, your posture will slump and your neck will start to grow from your chest, not on your shoulders. It is easy to ignore this in your early career, but all you have to do is look at the posture of your senior staff to recognize that the "hanging head" position is an occupational risk. Long cases will start to take a toll on your aging body. So make it a habit to adjust the table and seat height for each case. Set the microscope to be comfortable with your arms and head in a natural position. I recently found I could order a slight tilt (the "dental angle") on my loupes that prevents me from having to hang my head down all day while operating. Consider stretching breaks during the day. Try to keep fit. It will pay off over time.

Exposure and intraorbital dissection

Adequate surgical exposure begins with well-chosen surgical incisions. You should choose a hidden, or camouflaged, incision as close to the orbital mass as possible. If you choose an incision that will produce a minimal scar, your resistance to making an incision that is long enough to give adequate exposure will be decreased. When the skin and muscle layers of a transcutaneous approach are opened, use 4-0 silk suture retractors to hold the wound edges apart.

Remember that, as you dissect deeper into the orbit, you should make the deep portions of the surgical wound at least as wide, or wider, than the initial skin incision (make the wound A shaped rather than V shaped). Use a hand-over-hand dissection technique with the orbital retractors to move into deeper orbital tissues (Figure 15-4). As with dissections elsewhere, the key to an effective dissection is to gently spread or pull the involved tissues apart. When you get to a point where you cannot pull the layers apart with the Sewall or malleable retractors, ask your assistant to hold

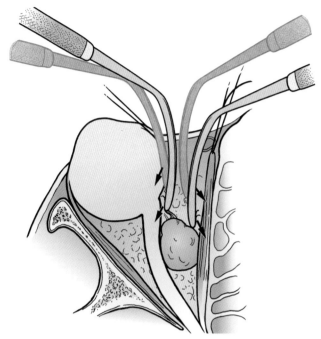

Figure 15-4 Hand-over-hand dissection technique to visualize deeper orbital tissues.

the retractors, keeping the tissue on stretch. You can then use additional blunt dissection with the Freer elevator or cotton-tipped applicator. You can use cautious sharp dissection with a Westcott or Yasargil scissors to open the connective tissue planes of the orbit if blunt dissection through a plane of tissue is too difficult. When the plane is open, use the hand-over-hand technique with the retractors until you reach the structure you are looking for. If you get lost, put your finger in the wound and reorient yourself. It is easy to pass by a smaller lesion.

No doubt there will be times when you are very close, but you cannot see what you are looking for. Palpation can be very helpful for showing you where you are in relation to where you want to be. Once you have identified the mass, gently place dampened neurosurgical cottonoids (1 inch by 3 inches) into the wound using a bayonet forceps. Reposition the retractor over the cottonoid to push the fat behind the retractor and to prevent the orbital fat from prolapsing around the retractor. You may remember the analogous general surgical technique of packing the bowel off with a lap sponge to allow exposure of the abdominal surgical wound. Repeat this using three or four cottonoids to expose the wound (Figure 15-5). With the cottonoids in place, you can remove or reposition the retractors without the surgical wound collapsing on itself.

You will need to follow surgical landmarks to find the area of the orbit that you are interested in. For example, to find the optic nerve during an intraconal dissection:

- Use your finger to palpate the optic nerve and the back of the eye. Note the orientation of your finger
- Strum the optic nerve with the Sewall retractors
- Keep the retractors against the back of the eye as you dissect into the orbit toward the optic nerve

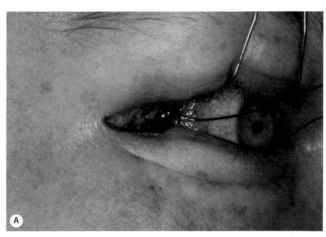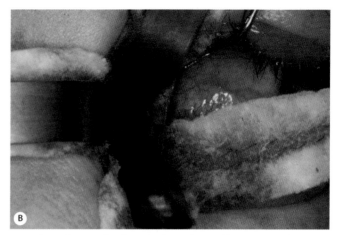

Figure 15-5 Neurosurgical cottonoids. (**A**) Lateral canthotomy approach to fenestrate the optic nerve. Small canthotomy incision. (**B**) Neurosurgical cottonoids under malleable and Sewall retractors are essential to prevent the orbital fat from prolapsing around the retractors. Note that the optic nerve is faintly visible in the depth of wound.

- When you are close to the nerve, you will see the color of the posterior ciliary vessels through the connective tissue
- If you become lost, palpate the orbit again and start over. Remind yourself not to dissect past the nerve. There will be times when you unknowingly go past the nerve and see the medial rectus. Palpation will help you avoid this

You will learn to use the visible or palpable landmarks to navigate through the orbital tissues.

If you find that exposure is poor, inspect the wound. There may be a band of periorbita or other tough tissue resisting your retraction. Don't be afraid to lengthen your incision if visualization is poor or you are struggling with lack of room. Consider an alternative or additional orbitotomy approach if you cannot safely obtain the goal of the orbitotomy with the original plan (see "Combined Orbitotomies" below).

Learn to use orbital retractors safely. Remember to have your assistant release the pressure on orbital tissues intermittently to maintain blood flow to the orbital tissues. With cottonoids in the wound, you can relax the retractors without "losing your place." Avoid toeing in on the orbital retractors to prevent damage to the orbital tissues. Suture retractors or self-retaining retractors, such as the Jaffe lid speculum, are safe for retraction of the skin and muscle, but self-retaining retractors should not be used deep in the orbit.

As we discussed in Chapter 1, you cannot underestimate the help that an experienced assistant can give you, especially in a deep orbitotomy. The anticipation and facilitation of the assistant provide you with a third and fourth hand. This is necessary because it is not possible for the surgeon alone to retract the deep wound open and perform a dissection or biopsy. If you are dissecting out an orbital mass:

- The assistant should use a retractor to pull the fat away from the mass as you pull the mass away from the fat with your nondominant hand. You can use a forceps, a cotton-tipped applicator, a suction tube, or a retractor

- You can then use your dominant hand to bluntly or sharply separate any bands of tissue on stretch between the fat and the tumor. You can use a pair of scissors or a Freer elevator

This is a basic and important technique for you to know and use for all surgical dissections. If you don't understand this, ask an experienced surgical colleague to explain it to you. You must understand this technique to function effectively as a surgeon (Figure 15-6). When I am having trouble with an orbital dissection, I remind myself of this basic concept. Probably the tissues are not being pulled apart by either me or my assistant.

Hemostasis

Intraoperative hemostasis begins with preoperative preparation. Have the patient discontinue any medications with an anticoagulant effect. Aspirin and other platelet-inhibiting medications are very common and should be stopped prior to most orbital cases, if possible. Some herbal remedies have an anticoagulant effect (the 3 G's—garlic, ginkgo and ginseng—and high doses of vitamin E). Make sure that blood pressure is controlled. Intraoperatively, place the patient in the reverse Trendelenburg position. Inject local anesthetic containing epinephrine into the location of the proposed skin incision before prepping and draping the patient. Intraoperatively, control of the blood pressure is important.

You must learn how to cauterize tissues if you are planning to do any orbital surgery. Short and long nonstick bipolar cautery works well in the orbit (Stryker bipolar silver guide). Long microbipolar forceps with fine tips are best. Turn the power down on the cautery control unit when cauterizing in the orbit. Minimize the amount of cautery that you use. In the past, surgeons were taught not to use monopolar cautery in the orbit. I, and many other surgeons, have used the microdissection needle without any problems, especially for excision of fat during orbital decompression. I am not aware of any study that testifies to its danger or safety, however.

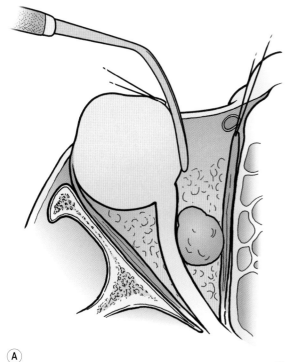

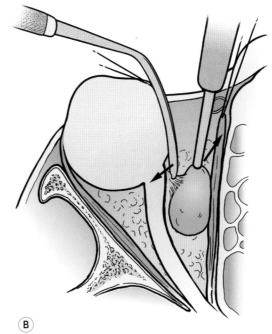

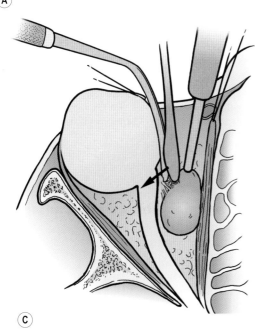

Figure 15-6 Orbital dissection technique. (**A**) Globe and medial rectus are removed. (**B**) As the assistant "pulls the orbital fat away from the mass" with an orbital retractor, the surgeon "pulls the mass away from the fat" with the nondominant hand. (**C**) The surgeon then frees any tissue on stretch between the mass and the fat with the dominant hand using a dissecting tool such as a Freer elevator.

Small amounts of blood in the surgical wound can be evacuated with cotton-tipped applicators. Larger amounts of blood require the use of a small suction tube such as a Baron suction tube. Hold the suction in your nondominant hand. Avoid closing the hole in the suction tube near your finger to prevent orbital fat from being sucked into the tubing. Suctioning over a neurosurgical cottonoid will also prevent fat from being sucked into the tubing.

Bleeding from bone or diffuse orbital oozing is not easily treated with bipolar cautery. Bone wax should be used to stop bleeding from the orbital bones. Several materials are

available to promote coagulation when oozing occurs in orbital tissues. Products that promote platelet aggregation include Gelfoam (absorbable gelatin sponge), Surgicel (oxidized regenerated cellulose), and Avitene (microfibrillar collagen). The coagulation effect occurs early in the clotting cascade so the latter parts of the cascade must be functional. Topical thrombogen (thrombin) works a step later in the cascade stimulating the conversion of fibrinogen to fibrin. A favorite technique of mine is to use pieces of Gelfoam soaked with thrombin. This combination stimulates two parts of the clotting sequence. These products are useful to stop lesser degrees of bleeding in the orbit when no point source responsible for the bleeding can be identified. All are absorbable over days and weeks. All swell so should be used with caution in the orbital apex. For troublesome bleeding, especially around the dura, FloSeal and Tisseal are especially helpful. FloSeal contains bovine thrombin suspended in gelatin granules so the mechanism is similar to the Gelfoam/thrombin combination. The mix sticks to wet tissue and does not swell to the degree that Gelfoam does. Tisseal (a "fibrin glue") contains human fibrinogen, bovine thrombin, and an antifibrinolytic agent (to stabilize the clot). FloSeal tends to be more useful for cranio-orbital applications, but you should know about both. Your neurosurgical and ENT colleagues can give you tips on how to use these materials.

Intraoperative flexibility

The ability to modify your surgical plan intraoperatively is a sign of an experienced and mature surgeon. You may determine that the lesion is not what you expected it to be. You may need to change the goal of the operation from an excisional to an incisional biopsy or vice versa. You may need to increase the surgical exposure by lengthening the initial incision. You may choose an additional or alternative surgical approach if necessary. You must learn to think on your feet while operating.

Handling biopsy specimens

The goal of many orbitotomies is incisional biopsy of an unknown orbital mass. To obtain an accurate diagnosis, you must learn how to provide the best tissue sample possible. Choose a biopsy site that appears to be representative of the entire tumor. If the tumor varies in appearance, consider more than one biopsy site. Avoid damaging the specimen with forceps or cautery.

Provide as large a tissue sample as practical. If you are unsure whether the sample is representative of tumor or large enough for analysis, you may want to send a portion of the sample for frozen section analysis. It is not reasonable to expect the pathologist to give you the final diagnosis based on a frozen section, but the pathologist can assure you that the tissue is adequate in size and quality. You may want to leave the operating room and look at the frozen section with the pathologist.

Prevent desiccation of the specimen by placing the tissue in the proper fixative as soon as possible. For routine permanent tissue analysis, place the tissue in formalin. If you suspect a lymphoid tumor or an unusual diagnosis, you should submit fresh tissue in dampened gauze to be frozen for later immunopathologic examination. In all but the most rare of situations, immunopathologic examination has replaced electron microscopic examination. Genetic testing can be done on some primitive tumors, such as rhabdomyosarcoma. If you think you are dealing with an unusual tumor, it is worthwhile to let your pathologist know ahead of time, to make sure that no additional testing or unusual handling of the specimen might be helpful.

Checkpoint

Think about how you can give a preoperative patient adequate information about a procedure that you will be doing so he or she can give informed consent. The goal is to let the patient know all the possible side-effects and complications without scaring him or her away from surgery. Put the risks into the appropriate perspective ("it is possible to die or go blind from any operation around the eye, but that is very unlikely with your type of operation," etc.). Think of the consent as a part of the patient's education about the medical problem. The patient will appreciate the fact that you have his or her best interest in mind.

When you are learning a new operation, make a checklist of things to do when you get to the operating room. Write down the instruments and sutures that you plan to use. You may even want to give this list to the staff. The operating room staff will appreciate your planning and thoroughness. Your operating room time will be used much more efficiently.

Look through the instrument trays for your procedures. Ask about the names and uses for the instruments that you are unfamiliar with. The operating room nurses may know how other surgeons use instruments with which you may be unfamiliar.

Invest in a good pair of surgical loupes.

Be an interested surgical assistant. Anticipate and facilitate. Ask how you could do a better job if you are unsure what is needed.

As the surgeon, learn how to dissect the tissues, pulling the layers apart with your nondominant hand and cutting with your dominant hand. Aim to gain accuracy and speed with the cautery tips.

Approach to anterior orbital lesions: anterior orbitotomy techniques

As I stated earlier, I use the term anterior orbitotomy to mean a surgical approach to the orbit from the front or anterior surface of the orbit. The majority of anterior orbitotomy techniques are used for the biopsy of palpable masses that are in the extraconal space of the orbit anteriorly. We will talk about the special anterior orbitotomy techniques that are used to approach deeper orbital tumors occurring medial to the optic nerve in the next section.

Many anterior orbitotomy procedures can be done under local anesthesia. The patient usually does not require inpatient hospitalization after surgery.

Upper eyelid skin crease approach

The upper eyelid skin crease approach for anterior orbitotomy gives excellent access to palpable orbital masses in the superior extraconal space of the orbit (Figure 15-7). The majority of these lesions involve the lacrimal gland (Figure 15-8). You should already be familiar with this technique because it uses the same incision and approach as upper eyelid ptosis surgery.

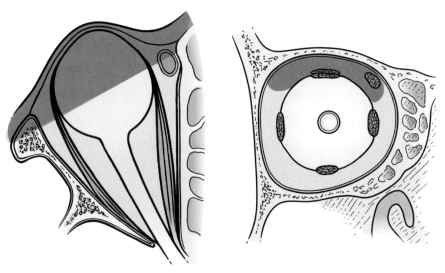

Figure 15-7 Orbital spaces accessible through an upper eyelid skin crease anterior orbitotomy approach.

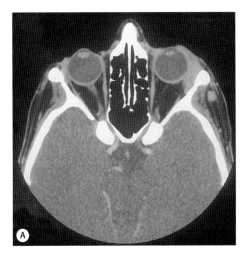

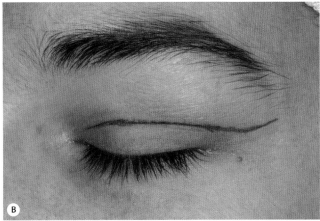

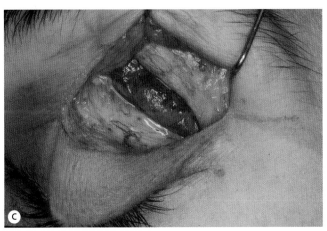

Figure 15-8 Anterior orbitotomy: upper lid crease approach. (**A**) A CT scan showing a lacrimal gland mass. (**B**) Mark the skin crease incision. (**C**) Repeat the steps of an anterior approach ptosis repair: skin crease incision, open the orbicularis muscle to the septum, dissect superiorly anterior to the septum until you find orbital fat, and then open the septum. If the mass is not visible, let palpation guide the dissection. After exposure, perform a biopsy and close in a single running layer. In this case, the mass was a lymphoid lesion.

The upper eyelid skin crease approach to anterior orbitotomy includes:

- Marking the skin
- Injecting local anesthetic
- Making the skin incision
- Performing the orbital dissection
- Obtaining the biopsy specimen
- Closing the skin

The steps of the upper eyelid skin crease approach to anterior orbitotomy are:

1. Mark the skin
   A. Mark an upper eyelid skin crease incision from the punctum to the lateral canthus.
   B. Extend the mark laterally in a "laugh line" (Figure 15-8, B).
2. Inject local anesthetic
   A. Inject a local anesthetic mixture of 2% lidocaine (Xylocaine) with 1:100,000 epinephrine in combination with 0.5% bupivacaine (Marcaine) directly under the skin.
3. Make the skin incision
   A. Prepare and drape the patient.
   B. Place a 4-0 silk suture through the upper lid margin for traction.
   C. Use a no. 15 blade or Colorado microdissection needle to make a skin incision.
   D. Continue the incision through the orbicularis muscle using Westcott scissors or the Colorado needle.
4. Perform the orbital dissection
   A. Identify the orbital septum and open it using Westcott scissors.
   B. If the mass is not visible, palpate the wound to locate the mass.
   C. Separate the orbital fat from the mass with blunt dissection, pulling the tissues apart (Figure 15-8, C).
5. Obtain the biopsy specimen
   A. Obtain either an incisional or excisional biopsy specimen using the principles outlined earlier under "Handling Biopsy Specimens."
   B. Obtain hemostasis with bipolar cautery before closing.
6. Close the skin
   A. Do not close the orbital septum.
   B. Close the skin with a running 5-0 fast absorbing gut or 7-0 nylon suture.
   C. Apply topical antibiotic ointment to the wound.

Routine postoperative care is required. Use topical antibiotic ointment three or four times a day for 1 week. Use ice packs for 24–48 hours. No oral antibiotics are necessary. Restrict activity in the first 24 hours.

Lower eyelid transcutaneous approach

Palpable masses in the inferior extraconal space of the orbit can be approached through the lower eyelid using either a transcutaneous or a transconjunctival approach. The choice of incision is largely up to the surgeon (Figure 15-9).

The inferior anterior orbitotomy (Figure 15-10) using the lower eyelid transcutaneous approach includes:

- Marking the skin
- Injecting local anesthetic
- Making the skin incision
- Performing the orbital dissection
- Obtaining the biopsy specimen
- Closing the skin

The steps of the inferior anterior orbitotomy using the lower eyelid transcutaneous approach are:

1. Mark the skin
   A. Mark a subciliary incision 2 mm below the lash line from the punctum to the lateral canthus.
   B. Extend the mark superiorly in a laugh line.
2. Inject local anesthetic
   A. Inject a local anesthetic mixture of 2% lidocaine with 1:100,000 epinephrine in combination with 0.5% bupivacaine directly under the skin.
3. Make the skin incision
   A. Place a 4-0 silk suture through the lid margin for superior traction on the lower eyelid.
   B. Use a Colorado needle or no. 15 blade to incise the skin.
   C. Use a Westcott scissors to cut the orbicularis muscle.
   D. Cauterize as needed.
   E. Form a skin muscle flap inferiorly to the orbital rim, attempting to keep the orbital septum intact.
   F. If the mass is not visible, palpate the orbit to locate the mass.

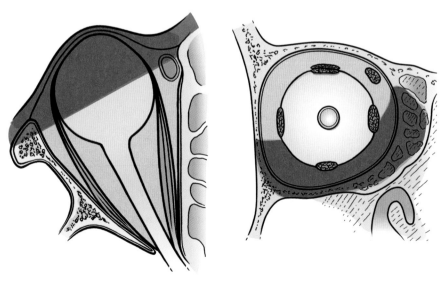

Figure 15-9 Orbital spaces accessible through a lower anterior orbitotomy.

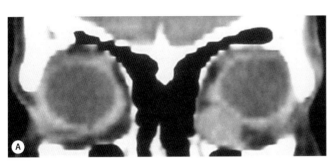
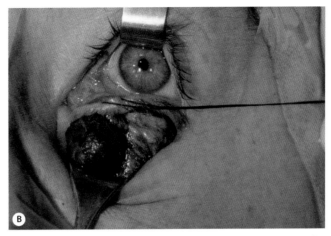

Figure 15-10 Transcutaneous inferior anterior orbitotomy. (**A**) Well-outlined inferior anterior orbital mass. (**B**) Exposure of the mass for excisional biopsy of a blood-filled cyst.

4. Perform the orbital dissection
   A. Open the orbital septum.
   B. Dissect the mass free from surrounding orbital tissues (Figure 15-10).
5. Obtain the biopsy specimen
   A. Obtain either an incisional or an excisional biopsy specimen using the principles outlined earlier under "Handling Biopsy Specimens."
   B. Obtain hemostasis with bipolar cautery in the orbit.
6. Close the skin
   A. Do not close the orbital septum.
   B. Close the skin with a running 5-0 fast absorbing gut or 7-0 nylon suture.
   C. Apply topical antibiotic ointment.

Routine postoperative care is required. Use topical antibiotic ointment three or four times a day. No oral antibiotics are necessary.

Lower eyelid transconjunctival approach

The lower eyelid transconjunctival approach will place you in the same position as the transcutaneous approach (Figures 15-11 and 15-12, A).

The transconjunctival incision can be combined with a lateral canthotomy and cantholysis to provide excellent exposure to the inferior and lateral orbit. There is no visible skin incision. Lower lid retraction is less likely. The lower lid can be tightened horizontally upon closure.

You can extend the transconjunctival incision into a transcaruncular incision. The inferior oblique muscle can be elevated from its attachment at the inferior orbital rim to provide excellent access to the inferior and medial subperiosteal spaces, orbital floor, and medial wall.

The lower eyelid transconjunctival approach to inferior orbitotomy includes:

- Injecting local anesthetic
- Performing a canthotomy and lower cantholysis
- Making a transconjunctival incision
- Performing the orbital dissection and obtaining the biopsy specimen
- Closing the wounds

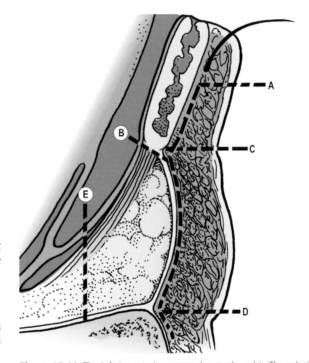

Figure 15-11 The inferior anterior approaches to the orbit. The subciliary incision (**A**) and the subtarsal transconjunctival incision (**B**) end up at the same point and preserve the orbital septum. The skin crease incision (**C**) and rim incision (**D**) are not recommended because they tend to leave a visible scar. The fornix approach (**E**) gives quick access to the orbital fat, but it can be difficult to control exposure because of fat prolapsing around retractors.

The steps of the lower eyelid transconjunctival approach to inferior anterior orbitotomy are:

1. Inject local anesthetic
   A. Inject lidocaine and epinephrine into the inferior and lateral conjunctival cul de sacs.
   B. Inject additional local anesthetic under the skin inferior to the lashes and at the lateral canthus.

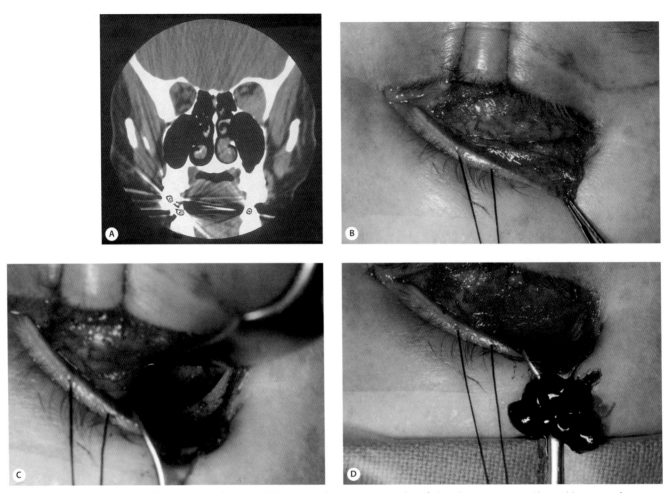

Figure 15-12 Transconjunctival inferior anterior orbitotomy. (**A**) A CT scan showing a mass in the inferior orbit in a woman with a sudden onset of proptosis. (**B**) Perform a canthotomy and cantholysis with a Westcott scissors or a Colorado needle. Dissect a myocutaneous flap to the inferior rim. (**C**) Enter the orbit (in this case, the extraconal space). (**D**) A hematoma was drained from the extraconal space and inferior rectus muscle (spontaneous orbital hemorrhage, cause never identified) (see also **Figure 14-3**).

2. Perform a canthotomy and lower cantholysis
   A. Place a 4-0 silk suture through the lower lid margin.
   B. Perform a canthotomy using Westcott scissors, a no. 15 blade, or a Colorado needle.
   C. Perform a lower cantholysis, detaching the lateral portion of the lower lid from the orbital rim (**Figure 15-12, B**).
3. Make a transconjunctival incision
   A. Evert the eyelid over a Jaeger lid plate ("shoehorn").
   B. Make a transconjunctival incision with a no. 15 blade. Be extremely careful if you use a Colorado needle, because the eye is not protected well. Consider using a corneal shield.
   C. Dissect a plane between the orbicularis muscle and the orbital septum to the inferior orbital rim.
   D. You can facilitate this by placing a suture through the lower lid retractors to lift the conjunctiva, the retractors, and the septum superiorly and away from the orbicularis muscle.
   E. A Desmarres retractor or Jaffe eyelid speculum can be used for retraction of the lid margin and anterior lamella.

4. Perform the orbital dissection and obtain the biopsy specimen
   A. Open the orbital septum or periorbita (**Figure 15-12, C**).
   B. If the mass is not visible, palpate the orbital tissues to locate the mass.
   C. Dissect the mass away from the normal surrounding tissue (**Figure 15-12, D**).
   D. Obtain the biopsy specimen using the principles outlined earlier under "Handling Biopsy Specimens."
   E. Cauterize as needed.
5. Close the wounds
   A. Close the conjunctival wound with either interrupted or running absorbable sutures of 5-0 fast absorbing gut or 6-0 chromic.
   B. Reattach the lateral edge of the eyelid to the periosteum on the inner aspect of the lateral orbital rim using 4-0 Mersilene on a P-2 needle.
   C. Close the canthotomy with two interrupted absorbable sutures.
   D. Place topical antibiotic in the conjunctival cul de sac and on the lateral canthal wound.

E. Postoperative care is routine. Apply a topical antibiotic three times daily. No oral antibiotics are necessary.

Approach to deep medial lesions

Before computed tomography (CT) and scanning magnetic resonance imaging (MRI), the patient with proptosis was evaluated by clinical examination and plain x-ray films. Most orbital tumors were approached through a generous lateral orbitotomy with bone removal in hopes of finding the tumor. With the currently available sophisticated imaging techniques, the exact size and location of an orbital mass can be determined preoperatively. Refinements in orbital surgical techniques and the use of the operating microscope have made it practical to approach many deeper tumors through the anterior approach without bone removal. The spaces medial to the optic nerve are particularly well suited for these techniques because there is no easy access from the medial side of the orbit. We will discuss these techniques briefly. As you gain more experience in the simpler anterior orbitotomies, you can start to use these techniques for approaching the deeper medial spaces of the orbit.

Transconjunctival medial anterior orbitotomy

The transconjunctival medial anterior orbitotomy is used for access to Tenon's capsule, the medial intraconal space, and the anterior one third of the optic nerve on the medial side (Figure 15-13). The main uses of this procedure are:

- Optic nerve sheath fenestration (decompression of the subarachnoid space of the optic nerve in patients with idiopathic intracranial hypertension)
- Optic nerve incisional biopsy for glioma or meningioma
- Medial rectus muscle biopsy
- Medial intraconal mass biopsy

The orbitotomy is performed under general anesthesia. A 180 degree conjunctival peritomy is performed at the medial limbus. Radial relaxing incisions of the bulbar conjunctiva can be made to improve exposure. Tenon's capsule is bluntly separated from the sclera with Stevens scissors. Sewall and 1/4 inch malleable retractors are used to spread through Tenon's capsule to enter the intraconal space. In a young patient, careful sharp dissection through Tenon's capsule can

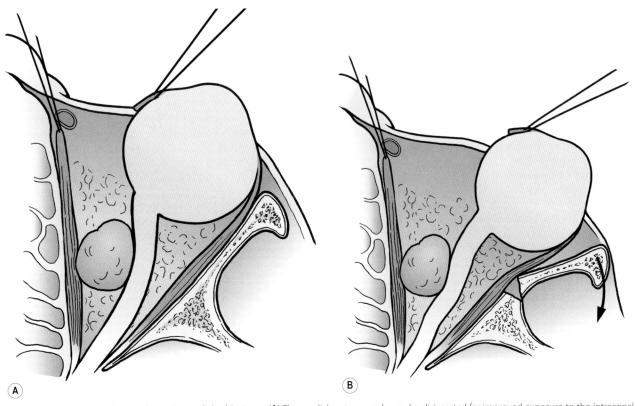

(A)

(B)

Figure 15-13 The transconjunctival anterior medial orbitotomy. (**A**) The medial rectus muscle can be disinserted for improved exposure to the intraconal space. (**B**) Exposure to the mesial intraconal space can be improved without fracture of the lateral wall.

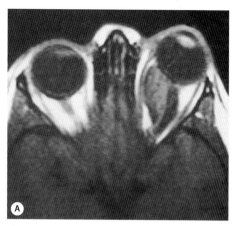
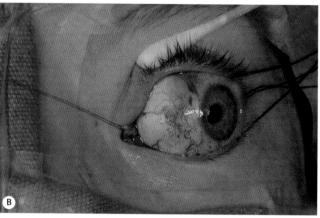

Figure 15-14 Transconjunctival medial orbitotomy for biopsy of presumed optic nerve glioma. (**A**) An MRI scan showing enlargement of the optic nerve. Note that the prechiasamal intracranial optic nerve appears normal. (**B**) Intraoperative view of the orbitotomy. Note that the medial rectus is detached from the eye.

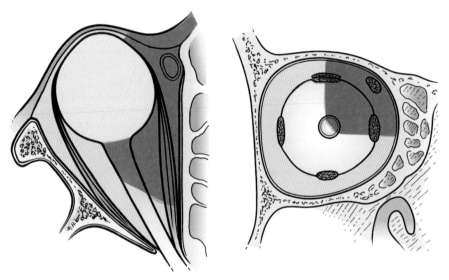

Figure 15-15 The areas of the orbit that can be approached using the vertical upper lid split approach to anterior orbitotomy.

speed up the dissection. Palpation of the base of the wound is not possible. If a deep intraconal dissection is anticipated, the medial rectus should be disinserted from the eye to improve exposure (Figure 15-14).

The operating microscope is used for magnification and illumination. After the abnormal anatomy is found, neurosurgical cottonoids are used to pack the wound open. If exposure is limited, a lateral orbitotomy can be combined to provide more room medially (see below). Once the biopsy is complete, the medial rectus is sewn back on the globe and the conjunctiva is closed with absorbable sutures. This approach provides good exposure of medial orbital tumors in the anterior half of the intraconal space. Apical medial intraconal tumors are usually better approached using a transcranial orbitotomy.

Vertical upper lid split anterior orbitotomy

It is difficult or impossible to reach beyond the equator of the eye using the standard upper lid crease anterior orbitotomy approach. The vertical lid split approach allows you to reach the deeper areas of the extraconal and intraconal spaces of the medial orbit (Figure 15-15). A vertical incision line is marked on the upper eyelid at the junction of the medial one third and the lateral two thirds of the lid. A scalpel blade is used to incise the margin, and a Stevens scissors is used to extend the wound full thickness through the eyelid. The cut extends above the tarsus, dividing the levator aponeurosis, Müller's muscle, and the conjunctiva. The upper portion of the sclera is usually visible. Dissection into the intraconal space is possible using standard dissection techniques. This technique is particularly well suited for removal of intraconal cavernous hemangiomas (Figure 15-16). The posterior one third of the medial intraconal space cannot be reached easily using this technique.

Upper eyelid skin crease medial anterior orbitotomy

An incision in the medial half of the upper eyelid skin crease can be used to gain access to the medial side of the optic nerve, most commonly for optic nerve sheath fenestration. The skin and muscle incision is followed by a superior preseptal dissection similar to a ptosis surgery. You will then

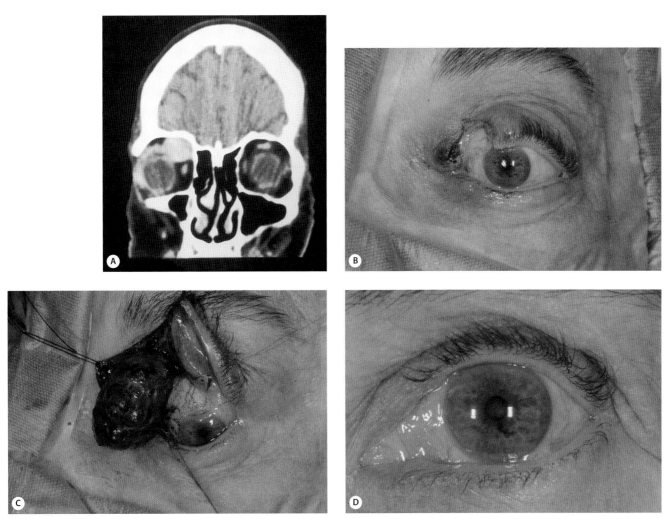

Figure 15-16 Vertical upper lid split approach for anterior orbitotomy. (**A**) A CT scan showing a superior nasal orbital mass. (**B**) Vertical upper lid incision extending into the conjunctival fornix. (**C**) Excisional biopsy of cavernous hemangioma. (**D**) Patient 6 weeks after the operation.

open the septum, dissect superior to Whitnall's ligament, and enter Tenon's capsule between the medial edge of the levator muscle and the medial edge of the superior muscle (you are posterior to the superior oblique tendon). Stay close to the sclera and dissect over the eye toward the optic nerve. When you see the color of the posterior ciliary vessels, you know you are near the optic nerve.

The exposure for fenestration of the nerve is good from this approach. Opening the sheath on the medial side has some potential advantages over a lateral fenestration. The ciliary ganglion and the papillomacular bundle of the optic nerve are both on the lateral side of the nerve. Allegedly, pupil and accommodation problems are less frequent. The vast majority of fenestrations that I have performed are from the lateral side, so I cannot comment from personal experience. Both routes have limited exposure and require a microscope for illumination and magnification. You will want to master some simpler orbitotomies before taking either of these procedures on.

Transcaruncular anterior orbitotomy

The transcaruncular anterior orbitotomy provides access to the extraconal and subperiosteal space of the medial orbit

(Figure 15-17). The main uses of this orbitotomy approach are:

- Repair a medial wall fracture
- Perform an ethmoidectomy as a part of orbital decompression

The orbitotomy is performed under general anesthesia. An injection of local anesthetic with epinephrine is given in the medial bulbar conjunctiva and plica. A Westcott scissors is used to cut between the plica and the caruncle. Stevens scissors are used to bluntly dissect a plane to the medial orbital wall, and 4-0 silk retractor sutures can be used on each side of the wound. Additional retraction is required with a Desmarres vein retractor and a narrow Sewall retractor. In most patients, the goal of the orbitotomy is to gain access to the bony medial wall, so the periorbita is cut and elevated with a Freer elevator. While the assistant holds the retractors, the surgeon uses a suction tube in the nondominant hand and a Freer elevator in the dominant hand to expose the bone.

A fracture may be repaired, an ethmoidectomy performed, or a hematoma drained (Figure 15-18). The closure does not require periorbital sutures. Only one or two absorbable conjunctival sutures are required. Drainage of medial subperiosteal abscesses secondary to ethmoid infections is usually performed by a transcutaneous frontoethmoidal anterior orbitotomy approach to leave a drain in position.

Transcutaneous frontoethmoidal anterior orbitotomy

The transcutaneous frontoethmoidal anterior orbitotomy or Lynch incision is used for access to the medial extraconal and subperiosteal spaces when the transcaruncular approach does not provide adequate exposure or a drain to the skin is required (Figure 15-19).

The orbitotomy is performed under general anesthesia. An arched incision is placed midway from the medial canthal angle to the bridge of the nose, extending from the inferior to the superior orbital rim in the concavity of the medial canthus (Figure 15-20). Local anesthetic with epinephrine is injected. A skin incision is made. The subcutaneous tissues are incised with a Colorado needle or other cutting cautery tool.

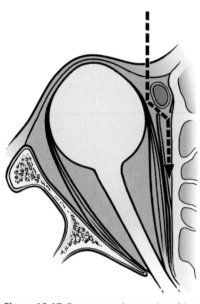

Figure 15-17 Transcaruncular anterior orbitotomy. Path of dissection starting between the plica and the caruncle, extending medial to the medial rectus muscle. Most often the dissection is carried to the medial wall in the subperiosteal space where a fracture repair or decompression is performed.

The periosteum of the inferior and medial orbit is reflected. With this reflection, the lacrimal sac is elevated. Suture retractors in the subcutaneous tissues and Sewall retractors in the orbit allow a clear view of the medial orbital wall. The anterior and posterior ethmoidal vessels can be cauterized or clipped and cut, if necessary, to provide additional exposure of the subperiosteal and extraconal spaces of the orbital roof.

Drainage of the subperiosteal space for abscess or hematoma can be performed through this skin incision. A Penrose or a "rubber band" drain is placed to allow postoperative drainage of blood or pus. Intranasal endoscopic ethmoidectomy and the transcaruncular approach to the medial wall have largely replaced this approach for drainage of medial subperiosteal abscesses. Extensive fractures of the medial orbital wall or frontal process of the maxilla (as in naso-orbital ethmoid fractures) can be repaired with this orbitotomy approach. Lower lid incisions combined with a bicoronal forehead incision allow somewhat less visualization of fractures in the medial canthus but do not cause significant postoperative scarring.

For the most part, this approach is used only when other routes do not give adequate exposure. Although this approach provides excellent exposure, the postoperative scar is visible and prone to webbing across the medial canthus. The frontoethmoidal anterior orbitotomy is still used for resection of large ethmoid and frontal sinus carcinomas that extend toward the orbit (see Chapter 16). Lacrimal sac tumors can be removed with this approach in combination with an incision along the side of the nose to remove the bony nasolacrimal duct (medial maxillectomy).

Transnasal endoscopic access to the apex

Endoscopic surgical techniques have advanced tremendously over the past few years. Functional endoscopic sinus surgery (FESS), once a complicated and risky operation, is now routine. New instrumentation, image-guided intraoperative navigation, and experience have opened a whole new area of "maximally invasive" endoscopic surgery. Using these techniques, the skull base can be approached from a number of different directions with some incredible visualization. If you have not seen examples of these procedures, such as endoscopic clivus resection, you should check it out. These

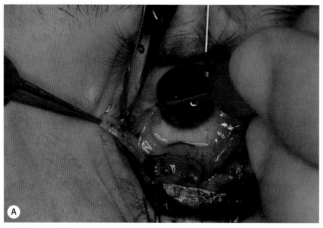

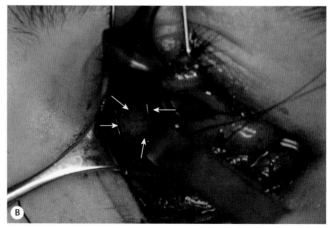

Figure 15-18 Transcaruncular approach to the medial orbital wall. (**A**) A conjunctival incision between the plica and caruncle (in this case, combined with transconjunctival inferior anterior orbitotomy incision). (**B**) Spreading through the extraconal fat to the medial wall using Stevens scissors. Use Sewall or malleable retractors to retract the orbital fat. The periorbita is elevated with a Freer periosteal elevator. Note the fat herniating into the ethmoid sinus in this medial wall and floor blowout fracture (arrows).

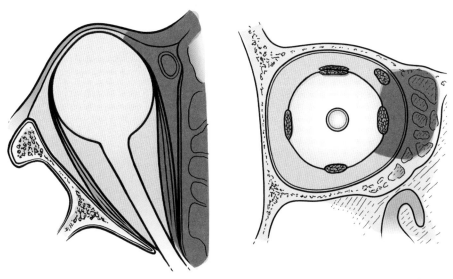

Figure 15-19 The areas of the orbit that can be approached by the transcutaneous frontoethmoidal anterior orbitotomy.

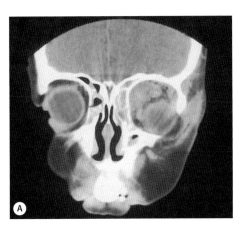
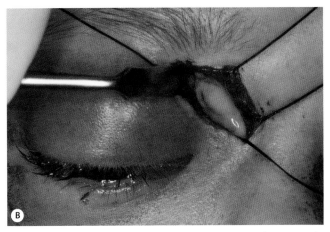

Figure 15-20 Orbital cellulitis: the transcutaneous frontoethmoidal anterior orbitotomy (Lynch incision). (**A**) A CT scan showing a subperiosteal abscess secondary to ethmoid and frontal sinus infection. (**B**) Intraoperative view showing drainage of a subperiosteal abscess.

refined endoscopic skills have given us new opportunities to approach the medial orbit and optic canal.

For several years, optic canal decompressions have been performed through endoscopic ethmoidectomy and sphenoidectomy approaches (remember that the lateral wall of the sphenoid sinus is the medial wall of the optic canal; Figure 15-21). New drills make this a safer and faster operation. The Stryker Saber drill, with its long thin guide, is a great help for this approach. You will find it useful for your endoscopic dacryocystorhinostomy (DCR) procedures also. You have probably heard of transnasal endoscopic orbital decompression where the lamina papyracea is removed endoscopically. This technique is very atraumatic.

Endoscopic techniques have improved to the point that apical orbital lesions can be approached safely. The need for these approaches is not frequent. It is unlikely that you would do these surgeries without the help of an experienced endoscopic surgeon, but you should be aware of this rapidly changing technology. Figure 15-22 shows an optic canal tumor that was endoscopically excised in a young woman with severe vision loss. No doubt more and more sophisticated orbital surgeries will be performed with the aid of the endoscope.

Approach to deep lateral lesions: the lateral orbitotomy

Lateral orbitotomy with removal of the lateral orbital wall

Lateral orbitotomy with removal of the lateral wall of the orbit provides excellent access to the extraconal and intraconal spaces of the orbit lateral to the optic nerve (Figure 15-23). This approach is commonly used for removal of intraconal tumors and incisional biopsy of the optic nerve. Lacrimal gland masses requiring incisional biopsy that cannot be palpated anteriorly are biopsied through this approach. Lacrimal gland masses requiring excisional biopsy are always approached through the lateral orbitotomy with bone removal (Figure 15-24). Access to the orbital apex is limited using the lateral orbitotomy. Tumors in the orbital apex should be approached through a transcranial orbitotomy.

The lateral orbitotomy with bone removal includes:

- Anesthesia and room preparation
- Exposing the lateral orbital rim
- Making the bone cuts

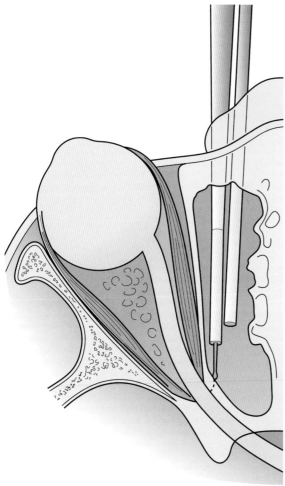

Figure 15-21 Frontoethmoidal transcutaneous anterior orbitotomy, ethmoidectomy, and sphenoidectomy for optic canal decompression.

- Drilling holes to reposition the bone
- Out-fracture and removal of bone
- Performing the intraorbital dissection
- Replacing the lateral orbital wall
- Closing the soft tissues in layers

The steps of the lateral orbitotomy with bone removal are:

1. Administer anesthesia and prepare the operating room
   A. Lateral orbitotomy is performed with general anesthesia. Place the patient in 10 degrees of a reverse Trendelenburg position. Turn the head slightly to the side with the lateral orbit facing toward the ceiling.
   B. While the patient is being prepared for general anesthesia, you should ready the room and balance the operating microscope.
   C. After the patient is asleep, mark an upper lid skin crease incision with an extension laterally into a lateral canthal skin crease (Figure 15-24, B).
   D. Inject local anesthetic with epinephrine into the wound. Inject additional local anesthetic into the lateral conjunctival cul de sac to the periosteum. Inject an additional 2 ml of local anesthetic into the temporalis muscle posterior to the lateral orbital rim.

2. Expose the lateral orbital rim
   A. Wear a headlight and surgical loupes for this portion of the procedure.
   B. Place a 4-0 silk suture through the lateral rectus muscle for traction.
   C. Make a skin incision with a no. 15 scalpel blade or Colorado needle. Cut through the orbicularis muscle down to the orbital septum in the lid. At the lateral canthus, incise the soft tissues overlying the lateral rim.
   D. Expose the periosteum of the lateral orbital rim with blunt dissection using a Dean periosteal elevator. Place 4-0 silk traction sutures in the subcutaneous layer to provide exposure to the lateral orbital rim.
   E. To elevate the periosteum off the external side of the lateral orbital rim, incise the periosteum 2 mm posterior to the lateral orbital rim and dissect it off the rim posteriorly toward the temporalis fascia. Open the temporalis fascia posteriorly for 1 or 2 cm to allow access to the temporalis fossa. Now elevate the temporalis muscle out of the temporalis fossa with a Dean periosteal elevator. Stay close to the bone as you direct the elevator around the posterior edge of the lateral rim to get between the temporalis muscle and the bone. This elevation requires some effort. As you elevate the muscle, pack two 2 inch gauze sponges between the temporalis muscle and the bone of the temporalis fossa to help with hemostasis and prevent injury to the muscle when you perform the bone cuts. The external aspect of the lateral orbital wall is now exposed (Figure 15-24, C).
   F. To elevate the periorbita on the inner aspect of the orbit, turn the head slightly toward you to see along the lateral wall. Elevate the periorbita using a Freer elevator in your dominant hand and a Sewall retractor or suction in your nondominant hand. You may need bipolar cautery and bone wax at the sites of bleeding corresponding to the zygomaticotemporal and zygomaticofacial vessels.

3. Make the bone cuts
   A. Next choose sites for your bone cuts. Plan on removing a 3–4 cm piece of bone. The exact position of the bone cuts depends on the goal of the procedure. Generally, the superior bone cut is at or above the frontozygomatic suture and the inferior bone cut is at the junction of the zygomatic arch to the lateral orbital rim. You will need to use a power saw such as a Hall microsagittal saw.
   B. To make sure that you don't enter the anterior cranial vault during the superior bone cut, look on both the inside and the outside of the lateral orbital wall to judge the thickness of the bone you are about to cut. You will be able to tell where the bone expands superiorly to become the floor of the anterior cranial fossa. While your assistant protects the periorbita with a Sewall or malleable retractor, make the superior bone cut using the power saw. Stop when the saw blade reaches the thicker sphenoid bone posteriorly.
   C. Make the inferior cut at the junction of the lateral orbital rim and the zygomatic arch. You may need

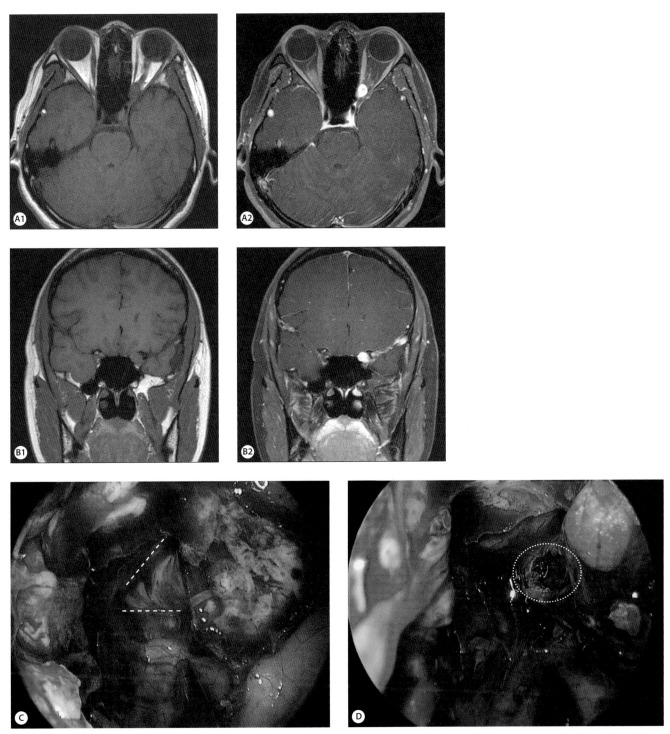

Figure 15-22 A 28-year-old woman with painless sudden loss of vision in the left eye several months previously. Optic nerve was pale. (**A1** and **A2**) Axial MRI without and with gadolinium showing apical orbital mass extending into the optic canal. (**B1** and **B2**) Coronal MRI without and with gadolinium showing easy access through sphenoid sinus. (**C**) Trans-sphenoidal view of optic canal (dotted lines) and carotid artery (at suction tip). (**D**) Intracanalicular biopsy of mass showing schwannoma (see circle).

to work quickly because you are likely to see some bleeding during the bone cuts that is difficult to control until the bone is out.

4. Drill holes to reposition the bone

   A. Use a Bien drill or Hall Surgairtome to drill 1 mm holes through the rim on both sides of your bone incisions. You will use these holes to pass sutures to secure the bone back into position. Alternatively, if you are planning to reposition the rim with a microplate, you can use the plate to predrill the screw holes at this time. My preference has been to use sutures to secure the bone because they are much less expensive than the microplates. The microplates are more secure, however.

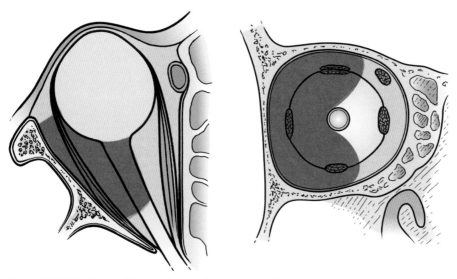

Figure 15-23 The lateral orbitotomy. Spaces of the orbit accessible with the lateral orbitotomy.

5. Out-fracture and remove the bone
    A. Out-fracture the bone with a Leksell angled laminectomy rongeur. The bone will break free, and you can then remove it and place it in a saline-soaked gauze pad (Figure 15-24, D).
    B. Remove the remaining posterior portion of the lateral orbital wall with a Leksell laminectomy rongeur. Stop removing the bone when you reach bleeding points in the cancellous bone of the sphenoid wing. Pack small pieces of bone wax to stop the bleeding at the rongeur and bone saw sites.
6. Perform the intraorbital dissection
    A. Next, open the periorbita in a T-shaped incision with the leg of the T parallel to the lateral rectus muscle. You will see the lacrimal gland and the extraconal fat.
    B. If you are planning an optic nerve biopsy or superior intraconal space operation, enter the intraconal space between the lacrimal gland and lateral rectus. If you are planning a dissection of a more inferior mass, enter between the lateral and inferior rectus muscles.
    C. Use blunt dissection with Sewall retractors or a Freer elevator to spread or pull the tissues apart.
    D. Before proceeding more deeply, palpate the orbit using your finger to identify the orbital mass, optic nerve, or other landmarks to get your positioning.
    E. Move the operating microscope in for the necessary illumination and magnification of the deep dissection. The coaxial view provided by the microscope will be necessary to allow you and your surgeon to see simultaneously in the operating site.
    F. You will need to follow surgical landmarks to navigate within the orbit (review the section above, "Exposure and Intraorbital Dissection"), for example to find the optic nerve.
    G. In older patients, you will be able to move through the orbit using blunt dissection only. In a younger patient, occasional sharp dissection through a tissue plane will be necessary.
    H. Gently spread or pull the layers apart using the retractors. After the orbital mass is identified, use

neurosurgical cottonoids to prevent the orbital fat from slipping around the retractors. When removing an orbital mass, a cryoprobe can be attached to the mass for traction.
    I. Once the mass is removed, be sure to obtain adequate hemostasis before closing (Figure 15-24, E).
7. Replace the lateral orbital wall
    A. You do not need to close the periorbita.
    B. Place the bone into position. Use two pieces of 3-0 Prolene suture without a needle to secure the bone into position. Alternatively, you can use microplates as described above (Figure 15-24, F).
8. Close the soft tissues in layers
    A. Close the periosteum over the bone using 4-0 Vicryl sutures.
    B. Close the subcutaneous tissues with 5-0 Vicryl sutures.
    C. Close the skin using a running 6-0 nylon suture (Figure 15-24, G).
    D. Apply topical antibiotic ointment in the eye and on the suture line.

In selected patients, the lateral orbitotomy can be performed without removal of the lateral orbital rim. This approach provides more limited exposure of the orbit. The anterior portion of the lacrimal gland can be visualized reasonably well, especially if the patient has prominent eyes. The intraconal space can be entered and the anterior portion of the optic nerve exposed. This is the approach that I favor for optic nerve sheath fenestration. Although this approach is simpler in that the bone is not removed, the orbital dissection is more difficult because there is less exposure and little room to manipulate the instruments. If you try this approach and need more exposure, you can always change plans and remove the bone.

Give patients undergoing lateral orbitotomy 60 mg of prednisone 1 day before the operation. Use an intraoperative intravenous dose of 10 mg of dexamethasone (Decadron) and 1 g of cephalexin (Keflex). Patients are hospitalized on the first postoperative night with frequent vision checks. Prescribe 5 days of 60 mg of prednisone and 7 days of cephalexin postoperatively.

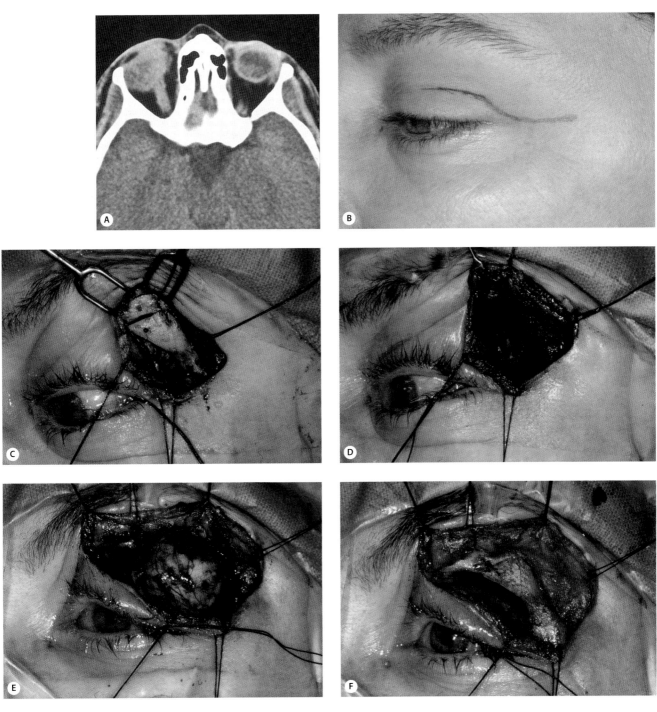

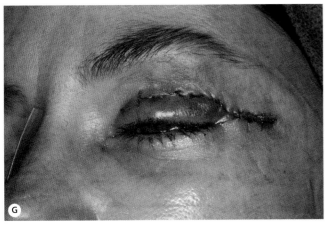

Figure 15-24 The lateral orbitotomy. (**A**) A CT scan showing a lacrimal gland mass thought to be a benign mixed tumor. (**B**) Mark an upper lid skin crease incision extending beyond the lateral canthus. (**C**) Dissect to the periosteum and place suture retractors in the wound. Elevate the periosteum and periorbita off the lateral wall and dissect the temporalis muscle out of its fossa. In this patient, the superior bone cut is made superior to the frontozygomatic suture to gain access to the lacrimal gland fossa. The inferior bone cut is at the floor. Be sure to make the drill holes before removing the bone. (**D**) Using a Leksell laminectomy rongeur, rotate the bone outward to fracture the lateral wall and remove the bone. You can see that the periorbita is intact. Palpate the lacrimal gland. (**E**) Dissect the mass away from normal tissue, usually removing a cuff of normal lacrimal gland and periorbita attached to the mass. (**F**) Suture or plate the bone back into position. Close the periosteum and temporalis fascia over the bone. (**G**) Close the orbicularis muscle with interrupted sutures. Close the skin with a running 6-0 nylon suture.

Complications are rare. Discomfort with chewing is common postoperatively due to contusion of the lateral rectus muscle. Lateral rectus palsy is not uncommon initially. Skin sutures are removed 1 week postoperatively (Box 15-3).

Approach to the orbital apex: transcranial orbitotomy

Transcranial orbitotomy

Anterior and lateral orbital approaches can provide a limited view of the apex, which can be useful for specific intents. A transcutaneous anterior orbitotomy provides exposure to the anterior half of the superior orbit only. The vertical lid split allows access to the intraconal space and will permit excision of a large hemangioma extending into the apex. The lateral orbitotomy provides exposure to the anterior two thirds of the lateral orbit, but the superior orbital fissure prevents access to the apex. The transcaruncular and frontoethmoidal approaches provide a limited view of the orbital apex even with removal of the ethmoid bone and air cells. The transethmoid endoscopic approach is useful to provide access to the medial portion of the apex, usually for incisional biopsy or decompression, as described earlier.

The transcranial orbitotomy provides the greatest access to the orbital apex. Three transcranial approaches are used to approach the orbit.

- Frontal transcranial orbitotomy
- Pterional craniotomy
- "Eyebrow" craniotomy

During the *frontal transcranial orbitotomy* (termed the *panoramic orbitotomy* by Rootman), a frontal bone flap, created by a neurosurgeon, is removed. The superior orbital rim and the anterior portion of the orbital roof are broken free with the flap exposing the periorbita of the superior orbit (Figures 15-25 to 15-27). The frontal lobe of the brain is elevated, and the posterior portion of the orbital roof is removed to the optic canal with a rongeur. This approach can be used for:

- Deep orbital tumors, especially those medial to the optic nerve
- Removal of the optic nerve in conjunction with optic canal unroofing and exploration of the chiasm for meningioma and glioma
- Debulking of an extensive sphenoid wing meningioma
- Extensive orbitocranial extension of any tumor, especially involving the orbital roof

The orbital portion of a tumor can be removed by opening the thin periorbita without opening the dura (an extradural approach). Any orbital bone involvement can be excised without opening the dura as well. Any remaining cranial portion of an orbitocranial neoplasm (most commonly optic nerve meningioma and glioma) is explored by opening the periorbita and the dura (intradural approach) (Figure 15-27).

Box 15-3

The Lateral Orbitotomy with Bone Removal

Anesthesia and room preparation

- Use general anesthesia
- Place the patient in 10 degrees of the reverse Trendelenburg position
- Mark an upper lid skin crease incision with an extension laterally into a lateral canthal skin crease. Inject local anesthetic with epinephrine

Exposure of the lateral orbital rim

- Wear a headlight and surgical loupes
- Use 4-0 silk suture through the lateral rectus muscle for traction
- Make a skin incision and dissect to septum and orbital rim
- Expose the periosteum of the lateral orbital rim
- Pass 4-0 silk sutures to retract the edges of the wound
- Elevate the periosteum and muscle out of the temporalis fossa
- Elevate the periorbita on the inner aspect of the bone

Bone cuts

- Plan on removing a 3–4 cm piece of bone
- The superior bone cut is above the frontozygomatic suture
- Don't enter the anterior cranial vault
- The inferior bone cut is at the junction of the zygomatic arch to the lateral orbital rim

Drill holes to reposition the bone

Out-fracture and remove the bone

- Use a Leksell laminectomy rongeur to fracture the rim outward
- Remove the bone
- Remove the remaining posterior portion of the lateral orbital wall with a Leksell laminectomy rongeur

Intraorbital dissection

- Open the periorbita in a T-shaped incision to expose the lacrimal gland and the extraconal fat
- Enter the intraconal fat above or below the lateral rectus muscle
- Use blunt dissection to "pull" the tissues apart
- Palpate the orbit using your finger
- Use the operating microscope for the necessary illumination and magnification
- Follow surgical landmarks to navigate within the orbit
- Obtain adequate hemostasis before closing

Lateral orbital wall replacement

- You do not need to close the periorbita
- Secure the bone into position using two pieces of 3-0 Prolene suture

Layered closure of the soft tissues

- Close the periosteum over the bone using 4-0 PDS sutures
- Close the subcutaneous tissues with 5-0 Vicryl
- Close the skin using a running 6-0 nylon suture
- Apply topical antibiotic ointment in the eye and on the suture line

An important anatomic consideration in deep orbital dissections is the position of the superior orbital fissure. Because the cranial nerves enter the orbit lateral to the optic nerve, it is safest to enter the orbital apex medial to the optic nerve (Figure 15-28). When the optic nerve is being removed, any damage to the trochlear nerve (along the medial orbital roof) resulting in torsional movement deficit will be relatively inapparent. You can see that excellent exposure of the superior, lateral, and medial apex is obtained with the transcranial orbitotomy. Rare tumors of the inferior portion of the orbital apex must be approached from a temporal craniotomy approach, often combined with a lateral orbitotomy.

After the surgery, the bone flap is returned to its natural position, repairing the orbital roof. Early postoperative ptosis and extraocular muscle paresis are usually seen, but they generally resolve. Enophthalmos, globe ptosis, pulsations of the globe, and temporalis wasting can be permanent.

The *"eyebrow" craniotomy* is a mini frontal craniotomy that gives access to the anterior orbital roof and soft tissues. It has limited application, but can be useful in selected cases (Figure 15-25 and 15-29). A 3–4 cm incision is made above the eyebrow hairs, the frontal bone is exposed, and a small window of bone is removed to gain access to the frontal lobe and anterior orbit. The procedure is relatively fast and recovery is rapid.

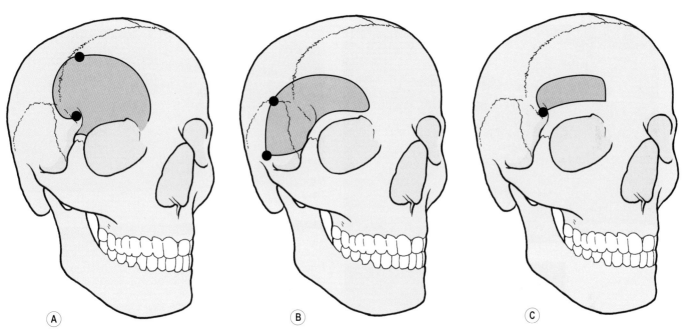

(A) (B) (C)

Figure 15-25 Transcranial approaches to the orbit. (**A**) Bone flap for "panoramic" transcranial orbitotomy, used most commonly to remove optic nerve tumors or other large intraconal tumors, especially apical and superior. (**B**) Pterional craniotomy—lateral approach to sphenoid wing and optic canal. (**C**) "Eyebrow" craniotomy—approach for anterior and superior orbital roof masses.

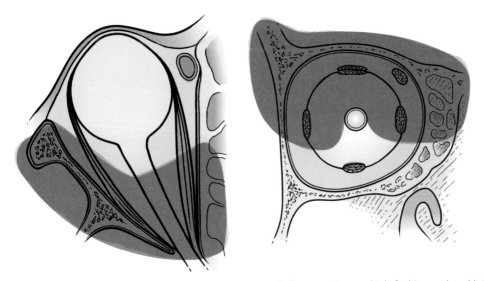

Figure 15-26 Spaces accessible via transcranial orbitotomy including posterior one third of orbit, superior orbital fissure, sphenoid wing, and chiasm.

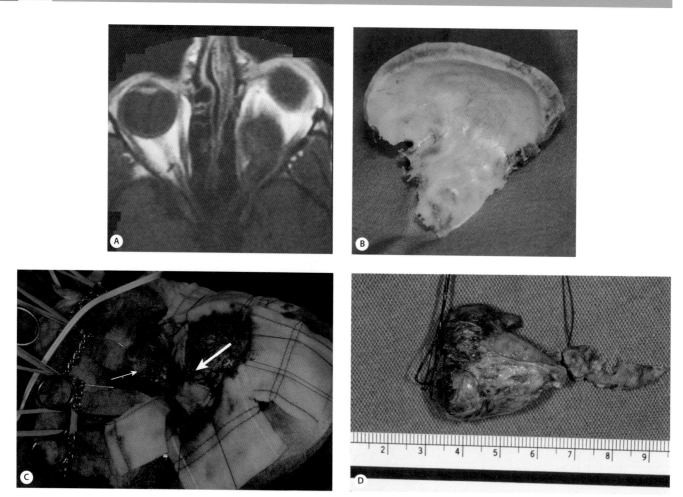

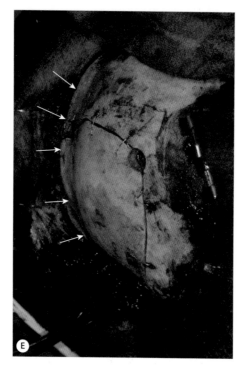

Figure 15-27 Transcranial orbitotomy. (**A**) An MRI scan showing a large optic nerve tumor. The tumor extends into the optic canal. The eye was blind. (**B**) Frontal bone flap removed to gain access to superior orbit. Note that the thin triangular portion of the bone is the orbital roof. The thicker bone anteriorly (top of photo) is the frontal bone superior to the superior orbital rim. (**C**) Exposure of the superior orbit and dura. A coronal scalp flap has been raised and is shown retracted to left of photo. Bone flap has been removed. Note that cottonoids have been placed between the dura (large arrow) and the periorbita (small arrow). Remaining frontal bone is covered with large cottonoids on right-hand side of photo. (**D**) Optic nerve glioma removed from the globe to the chiasm (proximal end of nerve is on right-hand side of photo). (**E**) Frontal bone flap sutured back into position. Note normal curve of superior orbital rim has been restored (arrows). Clips are seen on edge of scalp incision on right-hand side of photo.

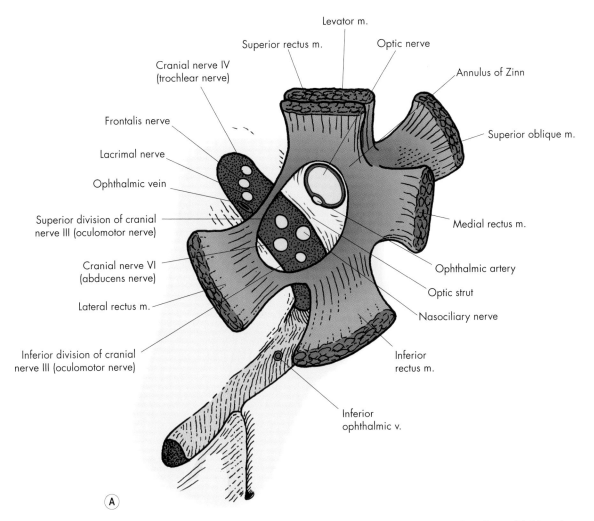

Levator m.

Superior rectus m.

Optic nerve

Cranial nerve IV
(trochlear nerve)

Annulus of Zinn

Frontalis nerve

Superior oblique m.

Lacrimal nerve

Ophthalmic vein

Superior division of cranial
nerve III (oculomotor nerve)

Medial rectus m.

Cranial nerve VI
(abducens nerve)

Ophthalmic artery

Lateral rectus m.

Optic strut

Nasociliary nerve

Inferior division of cranial
nerve III (oculomotor nerve)

Inferior
rectus m.

Inferior
ophthalmic v.

(A)

Figure 15-28 Orbital apex. (**A**) Anterior view of right orbit. Note that it is safest to approach the optic nerve from the medial side as the superior orbital fissure is lateral (after Housepian). (**B**) Superior view of right orbit. Note that the ophthalmic division of trigeminal nerve V1 is the most obvious nerve when viewed from above (terminating anteriorly as the frontal nerve). The trochlear nerve is medial to the optic nerve and difficult to avoid when dissecting medially.

The *pterional craniotomy* is a neurosurgical approach that your neurosurgical colleagues are very familiar with. From our point of view, this approach gives excellent exposure of the lateral and apical portions of the orbit. It is used most commonly for removal of sphenoid wing meningiomas. The bone around the superior orbital fissure can be removed. During this "skeletonization" of the fissure, you will remove the optic strut and the anterior clinoid process, both part of an optic canal decompression. The roof and lateral wall of the optic canal can be removed to complete the decompression.

Obviously, these are advanced surgeries. As you gain experience, adding these and other skull base procedures to your practice epitomizes the team approach that you can be a part of with your other surgical colleagues. The anatomy is fascinating and the results can be very gratifying.

Combined orbitotomies

Lateral and medial orbitotomies

As we saw earlier with lid reconstruction procedures, as your familiarity with individual orbital approaches grows, you will learn to combine procedures for additional or safer exposure to involved areas of the orbit. An example of a combination of orbitotomies is the addition of a modified lateral orbitotomy to the transconjunctival medial orbitotomy procedure. The lateral wall is exposed in the usual manner, and the lateral wall is cut and out-fractured but not removed. This provides space for the orbital contents to shift laterally, making exposure in the medial orbit much better.

Orbital decompression for thyroid eye disease

A combined lateral and medial orbitotomy is used as the technique of choice for orbital decompression to relieve optic neuropathy or decrease proptosis resulting from thyroid eye disease. The orbital volume is expanded by:

- A transcaruncular medial orbitotomy for ethmoidectomy
- A lateral orbitotomy with out-fracture of the lateral orbital wall
- Burring away of the body of the sphenoid wing

The lateral wall is held in an "out-fractured" position using microscrews to prevent the bone from rotating back

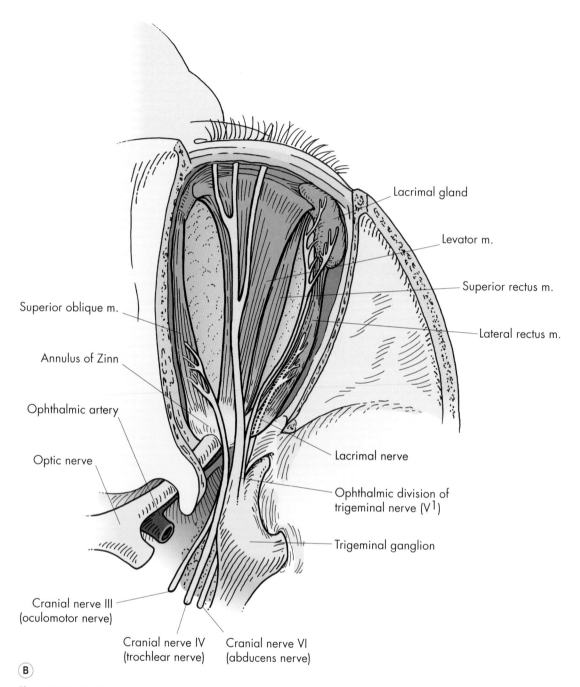

Lacrimal gland

Levator m.

Superior rectus m.

Lateral rectus m.

Superior oblique m.

Annulus of Zinn

Ophthalmic artery

Optic nerve

Lacrimal nerve

Ophthalmic division of trigeminal nerve (V^1)

Trigeminal ganglion

Cranial nerve III (oculomotor nerve)

Cranial nerve IV (trochlear nerve)

Cranial nerve VI (abducens nerve)

(B)

Figure 15-28 Continued.

into normal position (Figure 15-30). Some surgeons leave the lateral rim and remove the thin bone posterior to the rim. The outer cortex and cancellous bone of the sphenoid wing are burred away through the lateral orbitotomy incision. This approach reduces proptosis by 2–4 mm. This so-called "balanced" two-wall decompression is not associated with the high rates of postoperative diplopia that often resulted after decompression by removal of the orbital floor and medial wall. Globe ptosis and infraorbital nerve hypesthesia are eliminated with this operation. If additional reduction of proptosis is desired, the orbital floor can be removed at a later operation, creating a three-wall decompression.

Removal of orbital fat for orbital decompression was first proposed by Olivari several years ago. Many surgeons have enthusiastically embraced this technique alone or in addition to expanding the orbital bony volume. Intraconal fat can be safely excised from the inferotemporal quadrant. In some cases, fat will also be excised from the infero- and superonasal quadrants as well (Figure 15-31). The strongest indication for a large amount of fat removal is in the uncommon patient who has significant proptosis, often with the optic nerve on stretch, but has only thin muscles. For the majority of decompression cases, I still consider bony decompression as the first choice, but may resect a conservative amount of fat for a supplemental effect.

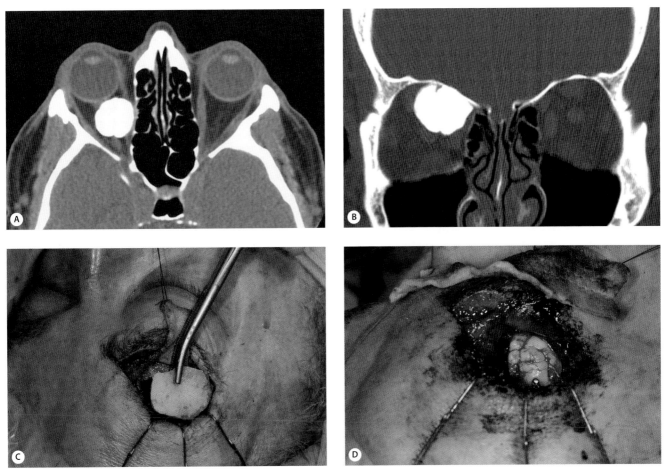

Figure 15-29 Eyebrow craniotomy. (**A**) and (**B**) Axial and coronal CT scans showing large bony mass attached to orbital roof. (**C**) Small bone flap removed through eyebrow incision. (**D**) Osteoma removed with the aid of a screw placed in the bony lesion. Patient was discharged on postoperative day 1.

Eyelid surgery for thyroid eye disease

In the last chapter, we talked about the approach to treatment of the patient with thyroid orbitopathy. We discussed the important distinction between active and chronic disease and the goals of preservation of vision, comfort, and appearance. Medical treatment consists mainly of lubricants. If surgery is necessary, decompression precedes eyelid surgery and eyelid surgery precedes any strabismus surgery.

Although this chapter is about orbital surgery, I thought that I might fill in a few gaps in the book regarding eyelid surgery for thyroid eye disease. We discussed *recession of the lower eyelid* and spacer grafts used to raise the eyelid for exposure related to poor closure in the chapters discussing ptosis, facial nerve palsy, and lower lid retraction after blepharoplasty. The technique and indications for exposure related to lower eyelid retraction are the same. Recession of the retractors will raise the eyelid 1–2 mm. Recession and a spacer will raise the lower eyelid more (even more than 5 mm using ear cartilage).

Upper eyelid recession is similar to a reverse ptosis repair procedure. The anatomy is the same, but the technique is much more difficult due to more bleeding and a higher degree of unpredictability in the final result. The results of recession in a patient with proptosis are much better when the proptosis is reduced with decompression. The high skin crease and "duck bill" appearance of a recessed eyelid over a proptotic eye is not a natural look. Upper eyelid recession should be done under local anesthesia. Start with marking a crease incision at the top of the tarsus, and then use the usual local anesthesia injection. Prep and drape.

The Colorado microdissection needle works well to decrease the bleeding. Often the preaponeurotic fat will be difficult to find if the eye is proptotic, so take some extra care to avoid damage to the aponeurosis. Depending on the amount of retraction, the progression of the next steps is:

- Recess the levator aponeurosis
- Cut the lateral horn
- Excise Müller's muscle
- Possibly release conjunctiva
- Reattach the aponeurosis at the eyelid peak, if necessary

If the retraction is minimal, proceed slowly with the aponeurotic recession. That may be all you need. If the height is good medially, but flared temporally, *cut the lateral horn*, by sliding Westcott scissors around the horn and cut it until the aponeurosis is free from the rim. If the general height is still too high, excise Müller's muscle, by sharply dissecting it free from the underlying conjunctiva. Again

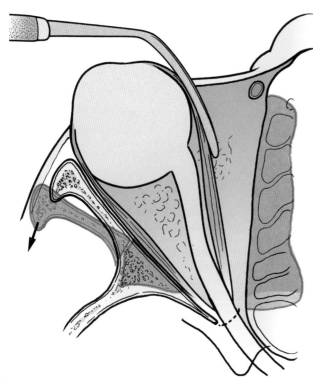

Figure 15-30 Combined orbitotomy procedures: the "balanced" orbital decompression for thyroid orbitopathy. Transcaruncular anterior orbitotomy for ethmoidectomy combined with lateral orbitotomy for rotation of the lateral wall and excavation of the sphenoid wing.

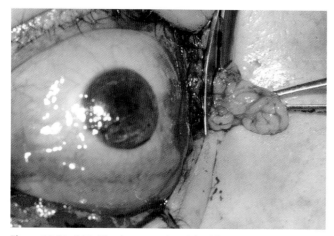

Figure 15-31 Orbital fat decompression. Orbital fat can be removed to augment the effect of bony orbital decompression. The most common quadrant to remove the fat is the inferotemporal quadrant. Fat can also be removed from the inferonasal or superonasal quadrant (as shown here). In cases where the muscles are thin, fat decompression may be the only treatment required.

check the height. If the eyelid is still too high, you may need to cut through the conjunctiva (you will be seeing eyeball) (Figure 15-32). If the retraction was severe, you may be leaving only a narrow bridge of conjunctiva intact at the peak. Eventually, the eyelid height will be about where you want it. If the height is okay, but the contour flat, reattach a bit more conjunctiva or advance the aponeurosis toward the

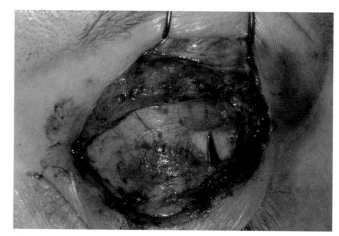

Figure 15-32 Upper eyelid recession. Graded recession of levator aponeurosis, lateral horn release, excision of Müller's muscle, and conjunctival incision. Note tip of Westcott scissors visible through full-thickness eyelid incision.

tarsus with a "hang back" suture. Eventually, you will get a reasonable contour with the final leaving the lid about 1 mm low. You can see, this can be a bit complicated.

A simpler approach has been recommend recently. After a crease incision, a full-thickness blepharotomy is performed across the eyelid where needed to get the height and contour correct. This is essentially what I described above, but not proceeding in a layer-by-layer approach. In some cases, this can be simple and very effective. The main contribution of this newer technique is the recognition that conjunctival recession may be required and that it is well tolerated.

A blepharoplasty can be done at the same time, but be *very conservative* (Figure 15-33). Eyelid surgery on these patients is difficult and unpredictable even for experienced surgeons. The reoperation rate is high, around 25%, so save these cases until you are ready for the challenge.

Medial and inferior orbitotomies for fracture repair

Fractures involving both the medial orbital wall and the orbital floor can be approached with combined anterior orbitotomies using transcaruncular and inferior trans-conjunctival incisions. Imagine each approach individually with the subperiosteal space of the floor exposed through the lower eyelid and the subperiosteal space of the medial wall exposed through the transcaruncular incision. With these combined incisions, it is possible to slide a large MEDPOR or SupraFOIL implant into position, covering the floor and extending up on the medial orbital wall (see Figures 15-17 and 15-18). Even better exposure is obtained if you connect the conjunctival incisions and elevate the inferior oblique muscle with the periosteum of the rim and periorbita of the floor. This gives the same orbital wall exposure as the frontoethmoid anterior orbitotomy, but without a visible scar.

As you can imagine from our discussions in this chapter, the combinations of orbitotomies that you can use are limited only by sound surgical technique and your creativity.

Checkpoint

The deep and combined orbitotomies are more difficult than the anterior procedures. There is less space to work in and exposure is more difficult. In most cases, you will need a microscope.

Rather than focus on the steps of these orbitotomies, emphasize the choice of orbitotomy based on the surgical space involved and goal of the operation.

Review the orbital apex anatomy after you have read about the transcranial orbitotomy.

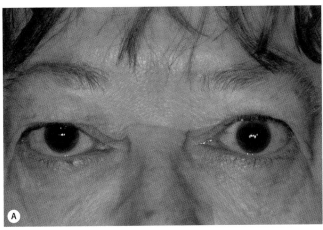
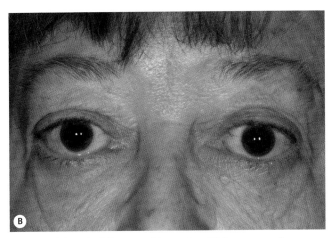

Figure 15-33 Thyroid eyelid retraction. (**A**) Left upper eyelid retraction and mild proptosis. Bilateral mild lower eyelid retraction. (**B**) Appearance after bilateral upper eyelid blepharoplasty and recession of left upper eyelid. Note that the upper eyelid height and contour are symmetric, but the left skin crease is high from the recession.

Major points

Remember the approach to the proptotic patient:

- History and physical examination
- Differential diagnosis
- Imaging, usually a CT scan, to refine the differential diagnosis
- Most patients will require orbitotomy, for biopsy, either incisional or excisional

Your choice of orbitotomy is based on:
Anterior or deep location

- The position relative to the optic nerve (medial or lateral)
- The surgical space occupied
- The goal of biopsy
  - Incisional
  - Excisional

The anterior–posterior position of an orbital mass within the orbit is the most important factor to consider in choosing a surgical approach. Biopsy specimens for palpable anterior lesions are obtained by an anterior orbitotomy approach.

For deep orbital tumors, you should choose an orbitotomy approach that avoids crossing the optic nerve.

Following this guideline, deep orbital tumors lateral to the optic nerve are approached with a lateral orbitotomy approach, usually with removal of the lateral wall.

Deep orbital tumors medial to the optic nerve are approached via specialized anterior orbitotomy procedures through the eyelid or conjunctiva:

- Transconjunctival medial anterior orbitotomy
- Vertical upper lid split anterior orbitotomy
- Transcaruncular anterior orbitotomy
- Transcutaneous frontoethmoidal anterior orbitotomy

Apical orbital lesions are usually approached through a transcranial orbitotomy. The surgical spaces of the orbit are:

- The intraconal space
- The extraocular muscles
- The extraconal space
- The subperiosteal space
- Tenon's space
- The extraorbital space

Learn to describe a mass on a CT scan with regard to the surgical space involved.

Intraoperatively, learn to navigate through these spaces to reach the area of interest.

Once you have made the decision to operate, you will need to do some preoperative planning:

- Arrange a general medical examination
- Have the patient stop all medications with anticoagulant effects

Major points Continued

- Obtain preoperative consent with the goals and risks of the procedure clearly outlined
- Coordinate the surgical plan with any other subspecialists involved. For unusual cases, consult with your pathologist preoperatively

Organize the operating room setup while the patient is being anesthetized.

Learn the specialized orbital instruments well:

- Retractors
  - Tyrell and Joseph skin hooks
  - Suture retractors
  - Sewall and malleable orbital retractors
  - Neurosurgical cottonoids
- Periosteal elevators
  - Freer
  - Joseph
  - Dean
- Power saws and drills
- Bone rongeurs
  - Leksell laminectomy and Kerrison
  - Microplating systems
- Forceps
  - Bayonet
  - Myringotomy
  - Small cup biopsy forceps
- Scissors
  - Yasargil
  - Westcott
- Dissectors
  - Cotton-tipped applicators
  - Freer elevators
  - Neurosurgical dissectors (Rhoton)

You will need excellent illumination and magnification to visualize the orbital structures. Consider using:

- Fiberoptic headlight
- Surgical loupes
- Operating microscope

Exposure and dissection of the orbital tissues requires:

- Well-chosen surgical incisions
- 4-0 silk suture retractors for the skin and muscle layers
- Hand-over-hand dissection to pull the tissues apart
- Gentle retraction with Sewall or malleable retractors; avoid prolonged retraction or toeing in with the retractors
- Palpation to get oriented
- Neurosurgical cottonoids placed to keep the fat out of the wound

You must understand the basic, but extremely important, concept of pulling the tissues apart with retractors using your assistant and your nondominant hand to "put the tissues on stretch." Use your dominant hand to separate the tissues off the tumor.

Developing your skills to obtain hemostasis is essential for orbital surgery.

- Use low suction against a cottonoid to evacuate moderate amounts of blood. Use cotton-tipped applicators for small amounts of blood. Learn to use these cautery tools:
  - Colorado needle (for outside the orbit)
  - Bipolar cautery (jeweler tips for anterior dissection)
  - Bipolar cautery (long bayonet tips for deep dissection)
  - Microbipolar cautery (Fisher long bayonet tips)
- Use bone wax for bleeding from the bony foramina or for areas of cortical bleeding
- Consider additional hemostatic agents when no point source for the oozing can be identified:
  - Gelfoam (absorbable gelatin sponge)
  - Surgicel (oxidized regenerated cellulose)
  - Avitene (microfibrillar collagen)
  - Thrombogen (thrombin)

Maintain intraoperative flexibility. Don't be afraid to change your plan intraoperatively, if necessary. Your ability to think "on your feet" will make you a better surgeon.

Prepare intraoperative specimens carefully. The goal of many orbitotomies is incisional biopsy. Your surgical expertise is only as good as the specimen is.

Although personal goals vary, I would suggest:

- Emphasize learning the reasons for choosing a particular orbitotomy approach
- You should be able to perform most anterior orbitotomy approaches. The steps are described in detail for you to learn. Start with these approaches before tackling others
- The lateral orbitotomy with bone removal is the next operation to learn. If you know anterior and lateral approaches, you can take care of most orbital problems. The steps of the lateral orbitotomy are presented in detail for you
- When you are an expert in exposure, hemostasis, and biopsy techniques, you can work on the deep medial approaches. I have provided a general description of how to do these procedures
- As your orbital practice and skills increase, develop a relationship with a neurosurgeon and a head and neck surgeon whom you can work with and learn to do transcranial orbitotomies and other combined facial approaches together

Suggested reading

1. American Academy of Ophthalmology: *Basic and clinical science course: orbit, eyelids, and lacrimal system*, sect. 7, pp. 63–96, San Francisco: The American Academy of Ophthalmology, 2006/2007.

2. Bonavolonta G: Anterior, medial, lateral and combined surgical approaches to orbital tumor resection. In Bosniak S, ed., *Principles and practice of ophthalmic plastic and reconstructive surgery*, vol. II, ch. 102, pp. 1060–1069, Philadelphia: WB Saunders, 1996.

3. Bonavolonta G: Surgical approaches to the orbit. In Bosniak S, ed., *Principles and practice of ophthalmic plastic and reconstructive surgery*, vol. II, ch. 100, pp. 1050–1055, Philadelphia: WB Saunders, 1996.

4. Dutton J: *Atlas of ophthalmic surgery. Volume II: oculoplastic, lacrimal, and orbital surgery*, St Louis: Mosby, 1992.

5. Dutton J: *Atlas of clinical and surgical orbital anatomy*, Philadelphia, WB Saunders, 1994.

6. Dutton J: Clinical anatomy of the orbit. In Yanoff M, Duker J, eds, *Ophthalmology*, pp. 744–751, London: Mosby, 2004.

7. Dutton JJ, Haik BG, eds: *Thyroid eye disease*, New York: Marcel Dekker, 2002.

8. Elner V, Hassan A, Frueh B: Graded full-thickness anterior blepharotomy for upper eyelid retraction, *Trans Am Ophthalmol Soc* 101:67–75, 2003.

9. Elner V, Hassan A, Frueh B: Graded full-thickness anterior blepharotomy for upper eyelid retraction, *Trans Am Ophthalmol Soc* 101:67–75, 2003.

10. Garrity JA, Henderson JW, Cameron, JD: Henderson's orbital tumors, 4th edn, Philadelphia: Lippincott Williams and Wilkins, 2007.

11. Housepian EM: Microsurgical anatomy of the orbital apex and principles of transcranial orbital exploration, *Clin Neurosurg* 25:556, 1978.

12. Jane JA, Park TS, Pobereskin LH, Winn HR, Butler AB: The supraorbital approach: technical note, *Neurosurgery* 11:537, 1982.

13. Kazim M, Trokel SL, Acaroglu G, Elliott A: Reversal of dysthyroid optic neuropathy following orbital fat decompression, *Br J Ophthalmol* 84(6):600–605, 2000.

14. Kersten RC: The eyelid crease approach to superficial lateral dermoid cysts, *J Pediatr Ophthalmol Strabismus* 25:48–51, 1988.

15. Kersten RC, Kulwin DR: Optic nerve sheath fenestration through a lateral canthotomy incision, *Arch Ophthalmol* 111:870, 1993.

16. Kersten RC, Nerad JA: Orbital surgery. In Tasman W, Jaeger EA, eds, *Duane's clinical ophthalmology*, rev. edn, vol. 5, ch. 86, pp. 1–36, Baltimore: Lippincott Williams & Wilkins, 1998.

17. Krohel GB, Stewart WB, Chavis RM, eds: *Orbital disease, a practical approach*, ch. 9, pp. 95–116, New York: Grune & Stratton, 1981.

18. McCord CD, Cole HP: Surgical approaches to the orbit. In McCord CD, Tanenbaum M, Nunery WR, eds, *Oculoplastic surgery*, 3rd edn, ch. 16, pp. 477–514, New York: Raven Press, 1995.

19. McNab AA: *Manual of orbital and lacrimal surgery*, 2nd edn, Oxford, England: Butterworth and Heinemann, 1998.

20. Nerad J: The diagnostic approach to the patient with proptosis. In *The requisites—Oculoplastic surgery*, pp. 348–386, St Louis: Mosby, 2001.

21. Olivari N: Transpalpebral decompression of endocrine ophthalmopathy (Graves' disease) by removal of intraorbital fat: experience with 147 operations over 5 years, *Plast Reconstr Surg* 87:627, 1991.

22. Rootman J, Stewart B, Goldberg RA: *Orbital surgery, a conceptual approach*, Philadelphia: Lippincott-Raven, 1995.

23. Rootman, J: Orbital surgery. In Rootman J, ed., *Diseases of the orbit*, ch. 16, pp. 579–612, Philadelphia: JB Lippincott, 1988.

24. Shorr N, Baylis H: Transcaruncular–transconjunctival approach to the medial orbit and orbital apex. Oral presentation at the American Society of Ophthalmic Plastic and Reconstructive Surgeons, 24th Annual Scientific Symposium, Chicago, November 13, 1993.

25. Wobig JL, Dailey RA, eds: *Oculofacial plastic surgery: face, lacrimal system, and orbit*, pp. 192–254, New York: Thieme, 2004.

26. Wojno TH: Indications for orbital surgery. In Bosniak S, ed., *Principles and practice of ophthalmic plastic and reconstructive surgery*, vol. II, ch. 98, pp. 1046–1047, Philadelphia: WB Saunders, 1996.

27. Wojno TH: Operative principles and instrumentation. In Bosniak S, ed., *Principles and practice of ophthalmic plastic and reconstructive surgery*, vol. II, ch. 99, pp. 1048–1049, Philadelphia: WB Saunders, 1996.

28. Zide BM, Jelks GW: *Surgical anatomy of the orbit*, New York: Raven Press, 1985.

29. Zide BM, Jelks: *Surgical anatomy around the orbit: the system of zones*, Philadelphia: Williams & Wilkins, 2006.

CHAPTER 16

Enucleation, Evisceration, and Exenteration
The Care of the Eye Socket

Chapter contents

Introduction

For many ophthalmologists, the enucleation of an eye is the end of a series of medical or surgical failures resulting in the loss of the eye. The procedure may bring an end to a long relationship between the ophthalmologist and the patient because there is "nothing else that can be done." This is far from the truth. The removal of the eye starts a lifelong relationship between the ophthalmologist and the patient centered on maintaining a healthy socket for the patient. The good news is that most patients undergoing enucleation today can expect to wear an ocular prosthesis that will be comfortable and not apparent to the public at large. The purpose of this chapter is to give you the tools to prepare for that relationship. Remember: if you don't know how to take care of the socket, who will?

We will start this chapter with the indications for removing an eye. The option of a *scleral shell* is often overlooked for blind and disfigured eyes in patients without pain. If pain cannot be controlled medically, enucleation or evisceration is an option. We will talk about the indications and steps for each procedure in detail.

We will review the normal examination of the socket. Many residents don't get training in how to deal with common socket problems. We will cover the *discharging socket, implant exposure, extrusion and migration, the superior sulcus syndrome*, and *the stock eye syndrome*. If you don't already have a working relationship with a well-trained ocularist, consider a visit to the ocularist's laboratory. You will find the ocularist's experience and insight into the anophthalmic patient's problem extremely valuable. The better you know each other, the better off your patient will be.

Unfortunately, some patients have tumors extending into the orbit secondarily, which require removal of the entire socket and sometimes the surrounding tissues. The most common causes are tumors extending into the orbit from the sinuses or eyelids. We will discuss the technique of orbital exenteration in general terms. We will touch on some orbital prostheses and some advanced socket procedures that can prevent loss of the eye.

I hope you will put this information to good use. Don't be the ophthalmologist who doesn't remove the prosthesis to look at the socket. Learn about the normal socket and the common problems that can occur. Your expertise as the surgeon removing an eye and as the physician providing the long-term care of the socket will be greatly appreciated by your patient.

When to remove the eye

The scleral shell

When a patient comes to you with a blind eye requesting removal of the eye, the first question to ask is, "Does the eye cause you pain?" If the answer is no, consider a scleral shell. A scleral shell is a thin ocular prosthesis that fits over the blind eye (Figure 16-1). The shell provides a natural appearance and is comfortable for most patients. No surgery is

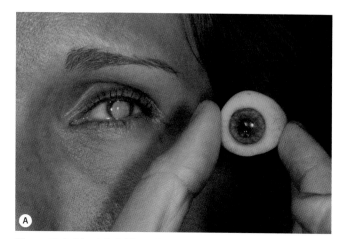

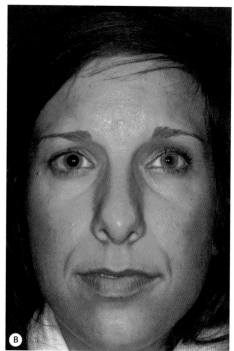

Figure 16-1 Scleral shell. (**A**) Painless small eye is a good choice for a scleral shell. (**B**) Comfortable scleral shell in place with natural appearance and reasonable symmetry.

required to treat the patient. Patients who are ideal candidates for wearing a scleral shell are those with:

- No pain
- Decreased corneal sensation
- Slight enophthalmos or phthisis
- No intraocular tumor
- Blind eye

Patients with severe pain probably will require enucleation or evisceration. You can sometimes treat patients for the mild aching pain that may accompany phthisis with prednisone ophthalmic (Pred Forte 1%) and atropine drops to control any intraocular inflammation. Undoubtedly, your enthusiasm for a scleral shell decreases as the complexity of any treatment to minimize pain increases. For many patients, removal of the eye is better than long-term treatment with drops and a shell, but at least consider the option of controlling mild pain medically. Most patients can tolerate the fit of a shell even with normal corneal sensation. Although the scleral shell sits over the eye, the posterior face of the shell is vaulted to sit off the cornea. If there is any question about pain, consider a trial period with a custom conformer. This prosthesis is custom-made to fit the shape of the socket, but does not have any color applied. The cost of the custom conformer is only 10–20% that of a completed prosthesis, so a trial is worth the cost if doubt exists that the shell will be tolerated. Although the scleral shell can be thin, an element of enophthalmos or phthisis makes it easier to get symmetry (Figure 16-1). Don't recommend fitting a scleral shell if you think that the eye is continuing to shrink. In a few months, the shell will not fit and time and money will have been wasted. Obviously, enucleation should be considered for an eye with an intraocular tumor. Most patients wearing a scleral shell are

blind in the eye that is covered. A patient with normal vision cannot see through the shell. For any patient with a disfigured iris who has good vision, a cosmetic contact lens (a special contact lens painted with matching iris details) should be considered.

Enucleation or evisceration?

Once the decision has been made to remove the eye, there are two options:

- Enucleation
- Evisceration

The enucleation operation removes the eyeball in its entirety. The extraocular muscles are cut off the eye, and the optic nerve is severed. The orbital contents are otherwise undisturbed. The evisceration procedure "eviscerates" or removes the contents of the eye. The sclera is opened, and the intraocular contents are scooped out. The extraocular muscles and optic nerve are left attached to the sclera.

The *indications for enucleation* are:

- Blind, painful eye
- Intraocular tumor

Most of the eyes that you are likely to remove will have been damaged by *trauma*. Occasionally, eyes may have been blinded by *infection* (endophthalmitis or corneal ulcer) or glaucoma. *Choroidal melanoma* is the most common intraocular tumor in adults requiring enucleation. *Retinoblastoma* is the most common intraocular tumor in children requiring enucleation.

Blind, painful eyes may be considered for evisceration instead of enucleation. Contraindications for evisceration are:

- Intraocular tumor
- Phthisis

Evisceration does not permit a complete, controlled removal of an intraocular tumor. Surgical margins are impossible to evaluate. Eyes that are shrunken as a result of phthisis should not undergo evisceration because the sclera cannot hold an adequate-sized implant.

In the absence of tumor or phthisis, either enucleation or evisceration can be performed. So how do you choose? More and more, it has become the surgeon's choice. It used to be said that the incidence of sympathetic ophthalmia was much higher with evisceration than with enucleation. This swayed the decision in favor of enucleation for eyes blinded by trauma or those having exposure to the S antigen through surgery or perforating corneal ulcer in an attempt to prevent sympathetic ophthalmia. Since that time, it has become increasingly apparent that the incidence of sympathetic ophthalmia is exceedingly low after evisceration.

Factors favoring evisceration over enucleation are theoretically better eye movements and less chance of postoperative enophthalmos, both owing to less disruption of the orbital tissues. Evisceration requires less operating time as well. For these reasons, many surgeons now perform evisceration in all patients without intraocular tumor or phthisis. It is said that evisceration does not eliminate pain in all patients because the posterior ciliary nerves are not cut. I don't know if this is true. In my practice, a large percentage of the eyes that are removed are for choroidal melanoma, so we perform many more enucleations than eviscerations. The majority of eyes that meet the indications for evisceration are enucleated as well, mainly because of habit.

An important use for evisceration is for the blind, painful eye with severe conjunctival scarring, as in an alkali burn. Evisceration requires less conjunctival dissection than enucleation. This allows a more normal-sized prosthesis to be fit because the fornices are not shortened by tearing the conjunctiva when you try to free it from the eye.

You should know that many of my trusted colleagues have switched to evisceration whenever possible.

The enucleation operation

Preoperative considerations

Goals

The goals of the enucleation operation are:

- Remove the eye
- Restore the orbital volume
- Provide movement to the ocular prosthesis

Removal of the eye is carried out in a routine fashion by severing the attachments of the extraocular muscles and optic nerve from the eye. The technique for controlled enucleation with minimal bleeding is described below. You must be careful when removing an eye with an intraocular tumor not to penetrate the eye with any needle. The goal of restoring orbital volume is usually met by placing an orbital implant. The majority of implants placed today fit within Tenon's space in the same position as the eye. No doubt, many times the implant will be pushed posteriorly into the intraconal space as it is placed. You should minimize the manipulation of the orbital fat to avoid postoperative fat atrophy. The movement of the implant and the conjunctival

fornices pushes the prosthesis to provide natural eye movements within the "conversational range" (10–15 degrees).

The volume of the orbit is approximately 30 ml. The volume of the eye is 7.5 ml. The volume of the eye must be replaced with volume provided by the combination of the implant and the prosthesis. A 16 mm sphere replaces 2 ml of volume. A 20 mm sphere replaces 4–5 ml of volume. An average-sized prosthesis can make up for the additional 2.5 ml of volume lost during enucleation. In general, patients receive implants that are 20 mm in diameter. Occasionally, a 22 mm implant can be placed without undue tension on the closure.

Remember that any surgical trauma, such as retraction and cautery, can cause additional loss of orbital volume (the fat atrophy we mentioned above). Any loss of orbital volume occurring due to enucleation that is not replaced creates an enophthalmic appearance to the prosthesis, usually apparent as a hollowing of the superior sulcus. A larger than average prosthesis provides only a temporary solution because the lower eyelid cannot support the additional weight of the prosthesis and eventually sags. We will discuss this problem later under "Superior Sulcus Syndrome."

Timing of the operation

When enucleation is planned for removal of an intraocular tumor, the procedure should be carried out as soon as possible after a systemic workup to rule out metastatic disease. When enucleation is planned after trauma to the eye, surgery should be carried out within 10 days. The risk of sympathetic ophthalmia following enucleation is close to zero if enucleation is carried out within 10 days.

Choice of implant

With the introduction of the hydroxyapatite implant in 1985, a resurgence of interest in orbital implant design has occurred. Implants can be classified as:

- Buried or exposed
- Muscles attached or unattached
- Integrated or nonintegrated
- Porous or solid

A *buried implant* implies that the entire implant is covered with a closure of conjunctiva. *Exposed implants* were used primarily in the 1940s when a portion of the implant was allowed to project through an opening in the conjunctiva. This exposed portion of the implant was physically linked or "integrated" to the prosthesis. These implants failed because of chronic infection and eventual extrusion. Almost all implants in use today are covered with conjunctiva or buried.

To provide the maximum motility of the ocular prosthesis, *the extraocular muscles should be attached to the implant at the time of enucleation.* The point of attachment may be directly to the implant or indirectly by suturing the muscles to a covering over the implant such as human sclera or fascia, or Vicryl mesh. Some surgeons feel that a significant amount of movement of the ocular prosthesis is provided by movement of the conjunctival fornices. These surgeons often attach the extraocular muscles directly to the fornix rather than to the implant.

The term *integrated implant* was originally used to describe the attachment of a prosthesis to the implant. As was stated earlier, exposed implants were integrated directly to the prosthesis through an opening in the conjunctiva. This integration provided excellent motility of the ocular prosthesis. Experimentation with different shaped implants led to the development of the quasi-integrated implant (the Iowa and the universal implants). These buried implants had an irregular anterior surface, projecting mounds on the surface of the conjunctiva. An ocular prosthesis was fit with impressions on its posterior surface to "mesh" or "quasi-integrate" with the prosthesis. These implants provide good motility, but they require more time to place and are sometimes associated with migration or rotation of the implant.

Materials used in implant construction can be either *porous* or *solid*. Porous materials include hydroxyapatite (HA) and MEDPOR (a high-density polyethylene material). The most common solid material for implant design is polymethylmethacrylate (PMMA). Porous implants have gained favor in recent years.

The idea of a porous implant that would allow vascular ingrowth and support "integration" of the prosthesis and implant brought a renewed interest in the anophthalmic socket in the late 1980s. During this same decade, oculoplastic surgery, as a specialty, flourished. Both these factors have benefited patients wearing prosthetic eyes, who had, more or less, been ignored by all but a few surgeons.

The idea of an "integrated" implant was borrowed from the earlier exposed integrated implants of the 1940s and 1950s that we have just talked about. The vascular ingrowth has mistakenly been called "orbital integration" by the makers of hydroxyapatite implants. This term should not be used because it creates confusion with the descriptive term "integration" with regard to the attachment of the ocular prosthesis to the implant. With a porous implant, an integration of the implant with the prosthesis could be accomplished while at the same time having a buried implant not predisposed to infection.

As you probably know, after satisfactory vascular ingrowth into hydroxyapatite implants (usually after 6 months), a hole can be drilled into the implant. Conjunctiva will migrate into the hole and the vascular ingrowth will support a conjunctival epithelium, which lines the drill hole. A peg can be attached to the ocular prosthesis, which then fits into the hole in the implant. This "lock and key" fit provides a firm attachment between the prosthesis and the implant that provides great movement. Because this implant is covered with conjunctiva, it is truly a buried implant. In theory, the best of all worlds is achieved—a truly integrated implant and prosthesis providing great movement with a covered implant not likely to get infected.

Unfortunately, for many patients, the epithelium over the peg site is not able to withstand the pressures of the peg against the implant created by the eye movements. Not infrequently, exposure and problems with granulation tissue occur at the junction. Several revisions of the integration have not solved these problems. Consequently, most surgeons have abandoned any attempts at pegging or "integrating" an HA implant with the prosthesis.

Porous polyethylene spheres (MEDPOR) were introduced as an alternative to hydroxyapatite. Tissue ingrowth prevents implant migration, as with other porous implants. MEDPOR implants appear to have a lower exposure rate than HA, perhaps due to a smoother anterior surface. A titanium screw integration system was introduced, but did not gain wide

acceptance. A new magnetic coupling device has been introduced more recently.

Synthetic hydroxyapatite and other ceramic materials continue to be tested as implant materials. A few surgeons still peg these implants with reasonable success due to diligent attempts at revisions as needed.

There is no perfect anophthalmic socket implant. Everyone agrees that the implant should restore adequate orbital volume requiring at least a 20 mm sphere. Most surgeons would agree that the extraocular muscles should be reattached to the implant. There are differing opinions regarding whether porous or solid implants are best. My current personal choice for an ocular implant is a 20 mm MEDPOR SST sphere. This implant has predrilled holes that allow easy attachment of the muscles, and the anterior surface of the implant is smooth, so that exposure is an infrequent problem (MEDPOR PLUS SST porous polyethylene spheres: 16 mm #80046, 18 mm #80048, 20 mm #80050, 22 mm #80052, http://www.porexsurgical.com). We use no integration of the implant and the prosthesis. Movement is good in the conversational range (within 10–15 degrees of primary position).

We can all look forward to new implant designs in the future as this area of surgery continues to evolve. For the most part, the problem of migration, sometimes seen with nonporous implants, is solved. Replacing the orbital volume is reasonable with current implants. If a deficit remains, additional orbital volume can be added later. There remain issues with an exposure rate that should be reduced. Likely, a better tolerated integration system will be devised that will give even better movement of the prosthesis.

Enucleation operation

Anatomy

The eye sits within Tenon's space. This fibrous capsule covers the anterior and posterior surfaces of the eye. As the rectus muscles extend anteriorly from the orbit, they penetrate Tenon's capsule to attach to the eye. This point of penetration is the arbitrary division of the anterior and posterior Tenon's capsule. The optic nerve enters the eye through the posterior Tenon's capsule. The enucleation operation is performed within the relatively bloodless space of Tenon's capsule. The rectus muscles are detached from the eye without disruption of the attachments of the muscle to Tenon's capsule. The optic nerve is severed posterior to the globe, sometimes leaving a hole in the posterior Tenon's capsule. The majority of ocular implants are placed within Tenon's capsule in the normal anatomic position of the eye. The eye muscles are attached in a near anatomic position to the surface of the implant or a covering over the implant. A layered closure of anterior Tenon's capsule and conjunctiva "buries" the implant.

Enucleation procedure

Enucleation of the eye is most commonly performed under general anesthesia. In selected patients, the procedure can be performed using local anesthetic and sedation.

The enucleation procedure using a MEDPOR SST spherical implant includes:

- Patient preparation
- Detaching the extraocular muscles
- Severing of the optic nerve

- Inserting the implant
- Attaching the muscles to the implant
- Closing in layers

The steps of the enucleation operation with placement of a MEDPOR PLUS SST spherical implant are:

1. Prepare the patient
   A. Develop a preoperative routine ensuring that you will remove the correct eye.
      (1) Unless the eye is obviously abnormal, leave preoperative instructions to dilate the eye to be removed.
      (2) Before surgery, visit the patient to make sure you know which eye will be operated on. Place a mark on the patient's forehead on the side that will be operated on. Tell the patient why you are placing the mark.
      (3) In the operating room, confirm which eye will be operated on (a "time-out").
      (4) And lastly, look into the dilated eye to ensure that there is a pathologic process present (Figure 16-2, A).
      (5) This may seem like a lot of trouble, but you must be sure in every case. Figure out the system that will work for you.
   B. Administer anesthesia
      (1) The majority of patients will be under general anesthesia.
      (2) Inject local anesthetic with epinephrine under the conjunctiva for hemostasis before you scrub (Figure 16-2, B).
2. Detach the extraocular muscles
   A. Begin the procedure with a 360 degree peritomy using Westcott scissors (Figure 16-2, C).
   B. Dissect Tenon's capsule away from the eye using curved Stevens scissors, spreading in each quadrant between the rectus muscles (Figure 16-2, D).
   C. Hook the extraocular muscles using a smooth von Graefe muscle hook followed by a Green muscle hook from the opposite direction to make sure that you have hooked the entire muscle.
   D. Pass the typical von Pirquet suture through the muscle insertion. I use 5-0 Vicryl on a spatula needle (Ethicon J571, S-14 needle) (Figure 16-2, E). I find the traditional strabismus technique in which the surgeon holds the muscle hook in one hand and the needle holder in the other hand to be cumbersome. This technique may be important for a strabismus surgeon where the muscle is sutured and cut in a precise position, but is not important for enucleation surgery. I would suggest you try one of two options. Either (1) hold the muscle hook yourself and have your assistant load the second arm of the needle back-handed for you on an additional needle holder; or (2) have your assistant hold the muscle hook, leaving you two free hands to load the needle and manipulate the tissues.
   E. Now cut the muscle off the eye, leaving a bit of muscle tendon on the eye, especially at the horizontal rectus muscle insertions, so you can place traction sutures at the horizontal muscle insertions later (Figure 16-2, F).
      (1) Detach all four rectus muscles in the same way.
      (2) Tape the sutures to the drape as you proceed.
   F. Hook the oblique muscles and cut them from the eye (near Tenon's capsule, not at the eye) (Figure 16-2, G). Hook the inferior oblique muscle in the inferior and temporal quadrants with the tip of the muscle sweeping from posterior to anterior toward the muscle as it leaves the lower lid retractors heading for the eye. Cauterize the inferior oblique muscle before cutting it.
   G. Place 4-0 silk traction sutures at the muscle insertions of the medial and lateral rectus muscles. If you have left some muscle at the insertion, this is quite easy. By all means, do not penetrate the eye with a needle if you are removing a choroidal melanoma.
3. Sever the optic nerve
   A. Give traction on the globe, prolapsing it out of the conjunctiva.
   B. Use Sewall retractors to retract the posterior Tenon's capsule away from the globe, exposing the optic nerve. Wearing a headlight is essential for this portion of the procedure.
   C. Use a long hemostat to clamp the optic nerve approximately 1 cm posterior to the eye.
      (1) To apply the clamp, insert the hemostat with the blades closed. Tap the optic nerve from the inferior side. Next, tap the optic nerve from the superior side. Open the blades to surround the nerve and tap each side of the nerve with the open blade. Once you are sure that you are around the nerve, close the hemostat (Figure 16-2, H).
   D. Cutting the optic nerve can be done in the same way.
      (1) Tap the nerve from below and above. Open the blades and tap the nerve from above and below again.
      (2) As you apply upward traction on the eye, push the scissors posteriorly and cut the nerve (Figure 16-2, I).
      (3) If the clamp is in the proper position, there will be no bleeding.
      (4) Any soft tissues clinging to the back of the eye can be cut with the enucleation scissors.
   E. Before releasing the clamp, retract the tissues around the optic nerve with the Sewall retractors and visualize the cut end of the optic nerve in the clamp.
   F. Use a Bayonet bipolar cautery to cauterize the optic nerve.
   G. Slowly release the clamp. In most patients, there will be no bleeding.
   H. Put a damp gauze pad into the wound.
4. Insert the implant
   A. Most patients will require a 20 mm spherical MEDPOR implant. Open the sterile wrap and color the side of the smooth side of the sphere with a marker. Put the implant in sterile saline.
   B. It is important to fill the implant with saline. Take the end off a 35 cc syringe and drop it into the barrel of the needle as a spacer. Then place the implant in the

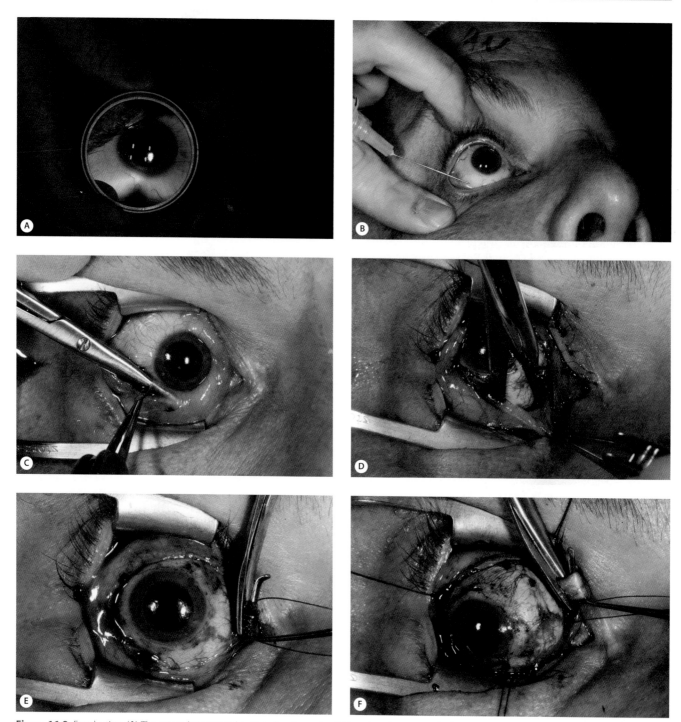

Figure 16-2 Enucleation. (**A**) The eye to be removed is dilated and examined. Note that the operated side is marked with the surgeon's initials. (**B**) Local anesthesia with epinephrine is injected under the conjunctiva. (**C**) 360 degree peritomy. (**D**) Stevens scissors spreading in each quadrant. (**E**) Von Pirquet sutures are passed through the rectus muscle insertions and the muscles are removed from the eye. (**F**) The superior oblique tendon is cut from the eye. (**G**) The inferior oblique muscle is cut from the eye. (**H**) The optic nerve is clamped. (**I**) The optic nerve is severed and the eye is removed. (**J**) Tenon's space exposed. (**K**) The MEDPOR PLUS SST implant is placed in the introducer. (**L**) The introducer is pushed into the socket. (**M**) The introducer is removed with the implant in Tenon's space. (**N**) The rectus muscles are sewn onto the implant. (**O**) Tenon's capsule and the conjunctiva are sewn closed. (**P**) Antibiotic ointment and a conformer are placed in the socket.

syringe and aspirate saline. Expel any air from the implant with repeated "washes" of the implant.

C. Place the implant "colored side up" in the introducer (Figure 16-2, K). With upward traction on the rectus muscle sutures, push the introducer deep into Tenon's space (Figure 16-2, L).

D. After placing your index finger on the implant, slowly withdraw the introducer (Figure 16-2, M). Inspect the position of the implant. Using a "hand-over-hand" technique with Paufique forceps, pull Tenon's capsule anteriorly over the sides of the implant to insure that the implant is deeply placed.

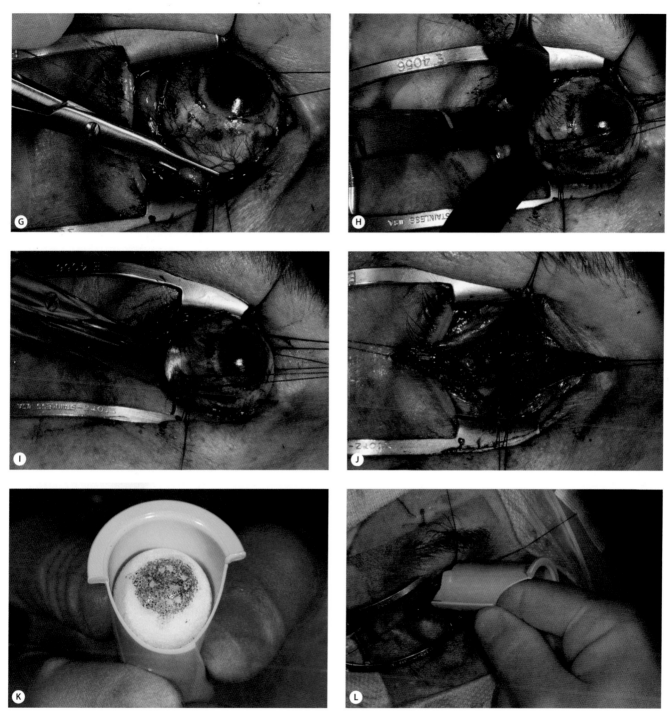

Figure 16-2 Continued.

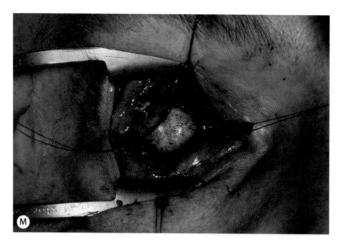

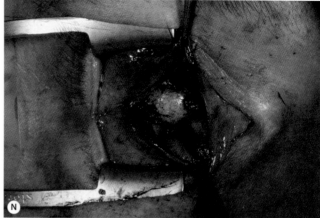

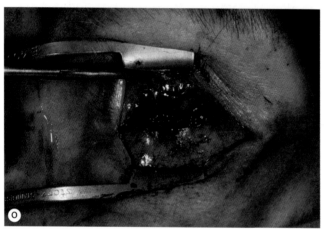

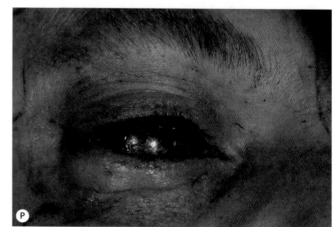

Figure 16-2 Continued.

The edges of Tenon's capsule should meet over the implant with little tension.

E. If there appears to be tension on the closure, remove the implant and try again. If tension remains, you will need a smaller implant.

5. Attach the muscles to the implant

A. Suture each of the rectus muscles to the implant by passing the needle backwards through the implant (Figure 16-2, N). The coloring on the face of the implant should help you see the holes.

6. Close Tenon's capsule and the conjunctiva

A. Close the anterior Tenon's capsule using the same 5-0 Vicryl suture from the muscle sutures. Use interrupted sutures.

B. Close the conjunctiva using a running locking 7-0 Vicryl suture (Ethicon TG140-8) (Figure 16-2, O).

C. Inject local anesthetic with bupivacaine (Marcaine) into the retrobulbar space for postoperative pain relief.

7. Provide postoperative care

A. Place topical ointment and a conformer in the conjunctival fornix (Figure 16-2, P).

B. Tape a pressure patch over the eye. Leave the patch on for 24–48 hours.

C. In the recovery area, explain that a conformer is in place and that it may rarely come out. Offer to "fog" the patient's lens with 2 inch translucent tape to cover the socket without drawing the attention of a pirate patch.

D. Inpatient or outpatient care is appropriate. Narcotic pain medications are appropriate for 24–48 hours. After removing the patch, the patient should use topical antibiotic ointment tid.

The patient should return in 1 week for inspection of the socket. A custom-fit prosthesis should be made when the swelling has totally subsided, usually 6 weeks after surgery. Sometimes it is helpful to have the patient and family visit the prosthetic lab at this time, so they know what to expect (Box 16-1).

Secondary implant

In the United States and most developed countries, an implant is placed into the socket after enucleation for almost every patient. In rare patients with severe endophthalmitis or hemorrhage, an implant cannot physically be placed into the socket because of swelling. In a small percentage of patients, the implant will extrude after surgery. In these unusual instances, an implant can be inserted in a separate operation. The term *secondary implant* is used when an implant is placed into the socket during an operation other than the initial enucleation procedure.

During a secondary implant procedure, the extraocular muscles can be found and attached to the implant, especially if the procedure is done with local anesthetic administered

Enucleation

Patient preparation
- General anesthesia
- Create a routine to ensure operating on the correct eye

Detaching the extraocular muscles
- Use a 360 degree perimetry
- Dissect Tenon's capsule away from the eye
- Hook the rectus muscles
- Place von Pirquet sutures
- Detach the rectus muscles from the eye
- Hook the oblique muscles and cut free
- Use traction sutures at the horizontal rectus insertions

Severing the optic nerve
- Place traction on the globe prolapsing it forward
- Use Sewall retractors to retract Tenon's capsule from the globe laterally
- Identify the nerve
- Clamp the nerve
- Cut the nerve
- Remove the eye
- Cauterize the stump
- Remove the clamp

Preparing the implant
- Use a 20 mm MEDPOR PLUS SST implant no. 80050
- Hydrate the implant
- Use the introducer to place the implant

Attaching the muscles to the wrapped implant
- Suture each of the rectus muscles to the wrap

Closing Tenon's capsule and the conjunctiva
- 5-0 Vicryl closure of Tenon's capsule
- 7-0 Vicryl closure of conjunctiva

Postoperative care
- Place a conformer
- Place a patch

in small amounts. If the patient is cooperative, voluntary movements of the eye with sight will help you to locate the muscles in the enucleated socket. When you have found the muscles, open Tenon's capsule to provide a space for the implant. You may need to use blunt dissection through the posterior Tenon's capsule into the retrobulbar space to make adequate room for the implant. After the implant is in place, you can reattach the muscles to the implant using von Pirquet sutures, as in a primary enucleation. Closure is routine.

Implant exchange

Occasionally, an older implant will be exchanged for a new implant. Four situations exist in which an implant exchange should be considered:

- To improve motility
- To increase orbital volume
- To reposition a migrated implant
- To replace an exposed implant for a smaller or new type of implant

In many patients, before 1990, implants were placed into the socket without any extraocular muscle attachment. If the eye movement is unsatisfactory to the patient, some improvement is possible by placing a new implant and attaching the muscles to the implant. The technique requires dissection of the original implant and identification of the muscles as described above. In some patients, a large implant can replace a smaller implant. In most patients, the placement of a subperiosteal implant on the orbital floor is preferred, if an orbital volume increase is the main goal. If an implant migrates or rotates into a position that does not allow a well-fitting prosthesis to be made, the original implant can be removed and a new implant placed. This procedure is easiest if the muscles were attached to the original implant. Lastly, if an implant becomes exposed and cannot be repaired surgically, the old implant can be removed and a new implant repositioned. These procedures can be tedious, requiring a lengthy dissection to identify the muscles and free the implant.

The evisceration operation

Options for evisceration

The evisceration operation has gained popularity in recent years. Two standard types of evisceration are performed:

- Evisceration with the cornea left in place
- Evisceration with keratectomy

If the cornea is healthy, it may be preserved. In these patients, the superior rectus is cut off the eye and an incision through the sclera is made posterior to the superior rectus insertion. After the intraocular contents are removed, an implant is placed into the eye and the scleral wound is closed. The superior rectus is reattached.

The more common type of evisceration operation begins with a complete keratectomy for access to the intraocular contents. This procedure is described below.

The evisceration operation

The evisceration with keratectomy includes:

- Patient preparation
- Conjunctival peritomy
- Keratectomy
- Removal of the intraocular contents
- Placement of an implant
- Closure in layers

The steps of evisceration with keratectomy are:

1. Prepare the patient
   A. Most procedures are performed under general anesthesia. Evisceration can be performed with retrobulbar anesthesia alone, if necessary (Figure 16-3, A).
   B. Take the same precautions mentioned earlier to correctly identify the eye to be removed.
2. Perform conjunctival peritomy
   A. Do a conjunctival peritomy using Westcott scissors. You should dissect only a few millimeters posterior to the limbus (Figure 16-3, B).

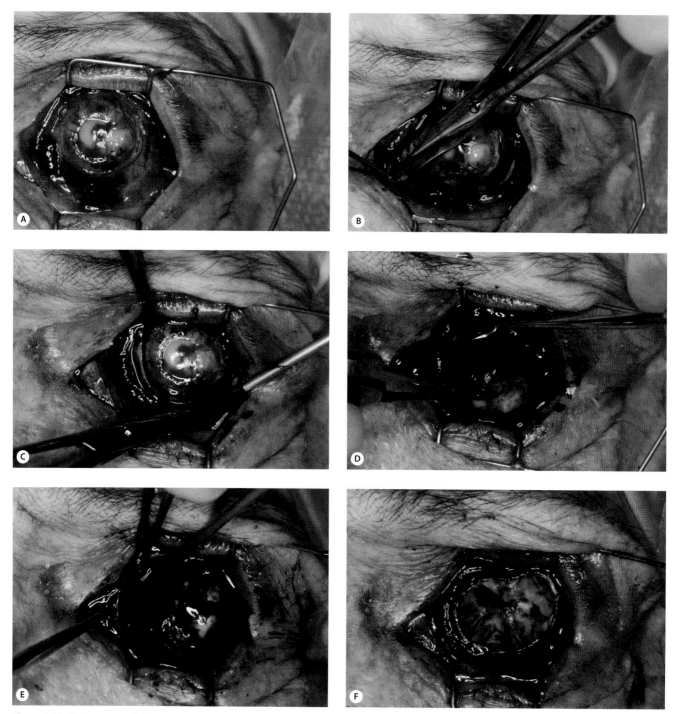

Figure 16-3 Evisceration with keratectomy. (**A**) Endophthalmitis secondary to ruptured fungal corneal ulcer after penetrating keratoplasty. Inject local anesthetic with epinephrine under the conjunctiva before you scrub. (**B**) Perform a peritomy and 5 mm dissection away from the limbus. (**C**) Use a no. 15 blade to enter the eye at the limbus. Complete the keratectomy with a Westcott scissors. (**D**) Place the evisceration spoon between the uvea and the sclera. (**E**) Sweep the spoon along the sclera and remove the intraocular contents. (**F**) View of the eviscerated sclera. (**G**) Make four radial incisions through the posterior scleral wall. (**H**) Cut relaxing incisions in the limbal wound at 3 and 9 o'clock. Push an 18 mm PMMA ball into the sclera, extending into the intraconal space (can use a MEDPOR implant alternatively). (**I**) Overlap and close the sclera with interrupted 5-0 polyester sutures. (**J**) Close the conjunctiva with a running locking 7-0 Vicryl suture. Inject retrobulbar bupivacaine (Marcaine).

3. Complete a keratectomy
   A. Make a stab wound through the cornea at the limbus.
   B. Use the Westcott scissors to make a full-thickness cut through the cornea for 360 degrees (Figure 16-3, C).
   C. Remove the cornea with a toothed forceps.

4. Remove the intraocular contents
   A. Use an evisceration spoon to remove the internal contents of the eye (Figure 16-3, D).
   B. Place the spoon between the choroid and the sclera and deliver the contents of the eye (Figure 16-3, E and F).

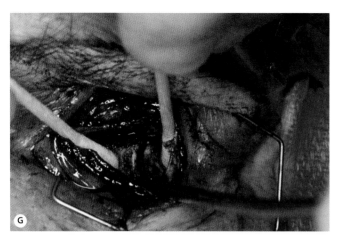

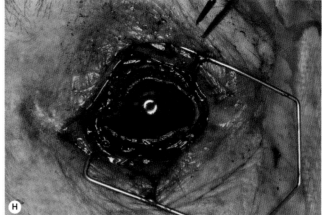

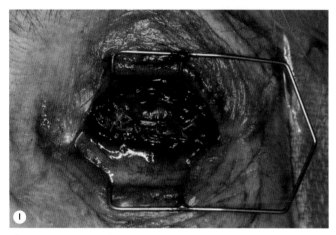

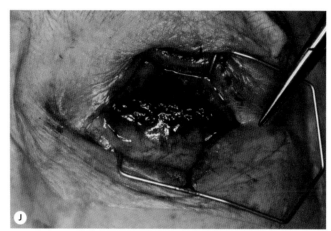

Figure 16-3 Continued.

5. Place an implant
   A. Your implant of choice can be placed. PMMA, MEDPOR, or hydroxyapatite implants can be used.
   B. An 18 mm or 20 mm spherical implant can be placed if you open the sclera posteriorly using four radial incisions that allow the implant to move into the retrobulbar space (Figure 16-3, G).
   C. To put the implant in the eye, you will need to make anterior radial relaxing incisions from the limbus posteriorly.
   D. Push the implant into the sclera (Figure 16-3, H).
6. Close in three layers
   A. Overlap the edges of the sclera and close with permanent sutures such as 5-0 Dacron or polyester (5-0 polyester, Davis and Geck 2828-23 D-1 spatula needle) (Figure 16-3, I).
   B. Pull the edges of Tenon's capsule together and close with interrupted 5-0 Vicryl sutures.
   C. Close the conjunctiva with running locking 7-0 Vicryl sutures (Figure 16-3, J).
   D. Inject local anesthetic with bupivacaine into the retrobulbar space for postoperative pain relief.
7. Provide postoperative care
   A. Place topical ointment and a conformer in the conjunctival fornix.
   B. Tape a pressure patch over the eye as with enucleation.
   C. Inpatient or outpatient care is appropriate. Use narcotic pain medications for 24–48 hours.

The patient should return in 1 week for inspection of the socket. Remember to discuss the role of the conformer and offer to "fog" the lens. Fit for a prosthesis in 6–8 weeks (Box 16-2).

Checkpoint

At this point in the chapter, you should understand the indications for enucleation and evisceration.

Don't forget to consider a scleral shell in a patient with a disfigured, blind, but not painful eye. Remind yourself of the characteristics of the ideal patient for a scleral shell.

What are the contraindications for evisceration?

What are the advantages of evisceration? Remember that scarred conjunctiva is a well-accepted indication for evisceration.

The purpose of an orbital implant after enucleation or evisceration is to restore the orbital volume and provide movement to the prosthesis. Usually porous implants are used. Implants are rarely integrated or "pegged." Do you recall why?

You should be able to remember the steps of both evisceration and enucleation procedures (Box 16-3).

Box 16-2

Instruments of Special Interest for Enucleation, Evisceration, and Exenteration

Exposure

- Eye speculum
  - Barraquer eye speculum, adult, wire (Storz E4106 H)
  - Barraquer eye speculum, pediatric, wire (Storz E4107)
  - Lancaster eye speculum, solid blades (Storz E4056)

Isolating the muscles

- Westcott tenotomy scissors, curved right, blunt tips, used for the conjunctival peritomy and disinsertion of the muscles (Storz E3320 R)
- Stevens tenotomy scissors, curved to dissect in Tenon's capsule (Storz E3562)
- Von Graefe strabismus hook to isolate the extraocular muscles (Storz EO592)
- Green strabismus hook to isolate the extraocular muscles (Storz EO588)
- Sterile tape or Steri-Strips to tape the von Pirquet sutures to the drapes

Removing the eye

- Sewall retractors
  - 7 × 52 mm blade (Storz N3321)
  - 9 × 51 mm blade (Storz N3322)
  - 11 × 50 mm blade (Storz N3323)
  - 13 × 67 mm blade (Storz N3324)
- Malleable ribbon retractors 1/4 inch
- Fiberoptic headlight
- Kelly hemostatic forceps, longer than "mosquito" forceps used to clamp optic nerve (Storz N5511)
- Bipolar cautery with bayonet forceps
- Storz curved enucleation scissors (Storz E3650)

Implant placement

- 20 mm MEDPOR PLUS SST implant no. 80050 (enucleation)
- 16–18 mm MEDPOR PLUS SST implant (16 mm no. 80046, 18 mm no. 80048) or PMMA sphere implant (evisceration)
- Bunge evisceration spoon (Storz E3740)

Closure

- Sutures for enucleation and evisceration
  - 5-0 Vicryl suture for von Pirquet sutures on muscles (Ethicon J571 S-14 needle)
  - 4-0 silk reverse cutting needle (Ethicon 783 P-3 needle) or 5-0 Vicryl with spatula needle (Ethicon J571 S-14 needle) for traction on globe
  - 5-0 polyester suture to suture wrap around the implant (Davis–Geck 2820-23 D-1 needle)
  - 7-0 Vicryl suture for conjunctival closure (Ethicon TG140-8)
- Conformer
- Patch tape

Box 16-3

Evisceration

Patient preparation

- General anesthesia

Conjunctival peritomy

Keratectomy

- Stab wound at limbus
- 360 degree full-thickness cut through limbus
- Remove the cornea

Remove the intraocular contents

- Place the evisceration spoon between the choroid and the sclera
- Deliver the contents of the eye

Place an implant

- Four posterior radial relaxing incisions
- Two anterior relaxing incisions
- 16 mm MEDPOR PLUS SST (no. 80046) or PMMA sphere implant in sclera
- 18 mm MEDPOR PLUS SST (18 mm no. 80048) or PMMA sphere implant into sclera and retrobulbar space (through posterior relaxing incisions)

Closure

- Overlap the edges of the sclera and close
- Close Tenon's capsule and the conjunctiva

Postoperative care

- Place a conformer
- Patch

Care of the socket

Normal wear and care

After the removal of the eye, most patients will wear a prosthesis that looks normal in the primary position and moves naturally in conversation. No prosthesis moves in synchrony with the natural eye at extreme gaze positions. Most of your patients will require minimal or no daily care of the prosthesis. You should encourage your patients to minimize handling of the prosthesis. Advise against daily removal of the prosthetic eye or cleaning. Your patients should sleep with the prosthesis in place.

Your patient may find that the eye will be somewhat more comfortable with lubrication. Several options are available. Artificial tears or contact lens rewetting solution will be helpful for many patients. Your patients may find vitamin E oil a longer lasting alternative for lubrication.

Annual eye examination

As part of your patient's annual eye examination, you should examine the artificial eye. Remember: don't be the ophthalmologist who totally ignores the patient's prosthetic eye and socket. Ask your patient about the daily comfort and appearance of the eye. Inquire about the presence of any discharge.

Start your physical examination of the prosthetic eye with the general external appearance. The prosthetic eye should be well centered within the socket and at the same horizon-

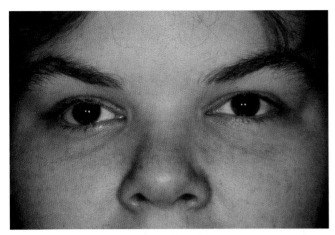

Figure 16-4 A natural appearing prosthesis following enucleation of the left eye. Note the edge of the prosthesis adjacent to the plica.

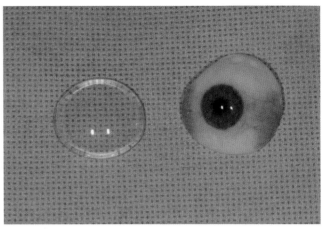

Figure 16-5 Normal prosthesis and postoperative conformer. Note that the superior portion of the prosthesis is not colored, the medial portion of the prosthesis is pink to simulate the plica, and superonasally there is a notch to provide for the superior oblique muscles.

tal level as the natural eye. The prominence of the prosthetic eye should match the natural eye. A small amount of superior sulcus deepening is common, as a reflection of slightly decreased orbital volume (Figure 16-4). Evaluate the patient's lower lid. Commonly, the lower lid will sag with time. A lower lid horizontal tightening may improve the fit and comfort of the eye.

The prosthesis should have a high gloss, wet shine. The eyelid should blink naturally. The eye should close without lagophthalmos. Evaluate the ocular movements within the conversational range of 10–15 degrees. The well-fitting prosthesis should make quick darting movements in synchrony with the natural eye. Don't expect that your patient will have comitant eye movements at the extreme gazes.

Next, do a slit lamp examination of the prosthesis and socket. The surface of the prosthesis should have a minimal number of scratches and be free from any debris on the eye. The tears should coat the prosthesis evenly. If any surface problem on the prosthesis exists, the patient should be referred to an ocularist for polishing of the eye.

Remove the prosthesis. Pull the lower lid down and the inferior edge of the prosthesis will tip forward and the prosthesis will come out. Examine the conjunctival mucosa. The mucosa should be healthy without any erythema or signs of giant papillary conjunctivitis. The implant should be well centered and the conjunctival fornices should be deep. Compare the back of the prosthesis to the front of the socket. They should appear to fit together. Just as elsewhere, the shape of the socket will change over time.

Reposition the prosthesis. You will be able to orient the prosthesis easily if you look at a few details (Figure 16-5):

- The superior nasal edge of the prosthesis is usually cut out to accommodate the trochlea
- The medial edge of the prosthesis is usually "pinker" than elsewhere to simulate the plica and caruncle
- The superior one third of the prosthesis is usually not painted because it will be hidden under the upper eyelid (Box 16-4)

Box 16-4

Examination of the Discharging Socket

Evaluate the fit of the prosthesis

Palpate the lacrimal sac

At the slit lamp:

- Evaluate the anterior surface of the prosthesis
- Remove the prosthesis and evaluate the conjunctiva of the socket
- Evert the upper lid, looking for giant papillary conjunctivitis (GPC)
- Compare the shape of the prosthesis with the shape of the socket

---

Examine the normal eye

Safety glasses: polycarbonate lenses

Of course, you should do a complete examination of the normal eye. Remind your patients that they should be wearing their polycarbonate lenses at all times through the day.

The role of the ocularist

Encourage your patients to see the ocularist annually. The ocularist will polish the eye and make minor adjustments in the fit of the eye. The average ocular prosthesis lasts 7–8 years before replacement is necessary. If you haven't developed a professional relationship with a good ocularist, consider doing so. You will find the technical and artistic expertise of the ocularist to be impressive. Their experience and insights into problems related to comfort and fit of the eye will be invaluable to both you and your patients.

Common problems

Discharge

A discharging socket is the most common complaint among prosthetic eye wearers. In most patients, you will not find anything during the examination, and the problem will be

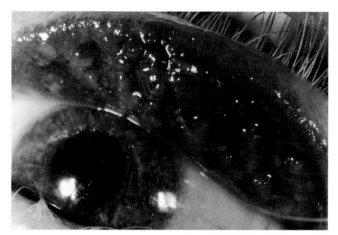

Figure 16-6 Giant papillary conjunctivitis. Note the "cobblestone" appearance of the conjunctiva on the superior tarsal plate and the lifelike appearance of the iris.

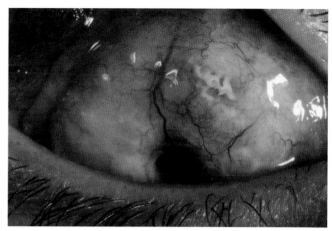

Figure 16-7 Exposure of a hydroxyapatite implant.

related to a lack of lubrication. Before you recommend a lubricant, consider some other less likely possibilities.

The eyelid, conjunctiva, and lacrimal system of the anophthalmic socket is susceptible to the same causes of inflammation as the natural eye. Bacterial or viral conjunctivitis may be present with the typical discharge. Dacryocystitis may occur as a result of nasolacrimal duct obstruction.

The other causes of a discharging socket are specific to the anophthalmic socket. If the discharge is white and ropy, look for giant papillary conjunctivitis (GPC). Typically, large papillae (greater than 1 mm) are present on the conjunctiva of the superior tarsal plate (Figure 16-6). The cause is unknown, but it is thought to be an immunologic reaction to the plastic of the prosthesis. If the prosthesis is scratched or has debris adhering to it, polishing may help relieve the symptoms, because there may be a mechanical component to the conjunctivitis. If the prosthesis is more than 7–8 years old, it should be replaced. The condition will improve in most patients with a tapering schedule of prednisone ophthalmic drops or nonsteroidal anti-inflammatory drugs. Cromolyn sodium drops can be used alternatively or in combination with the steroid drops if the problem is persistent.

Other causes of discharge include exposure of the implant or tumor recurrence, so be sure to remove the prosthesis to examine the socket. Accumulation of mucus in a dead space behind a poorly fitting prosthesis can cause a collection of mucus to move from behind the eye with eye movements. Compare the shape of the prosthesis with the shape of the socket. If the shapes don't match, the implant may have moved or rotated. Ask the ocularist to check the fit of the prosthesis.

If you cannot identify a cause for the discharge, ask the patient to use repeated doses of an ocular lubricant. Artificial tears or contact lens rewetting solution can be used for mild discharge. Vitamin E oil with aloe vera is often helpful if the teardrops are not enough. Patients with extremely dry sockets, producing almost no tears, can use a silicone-based oil (Sil-Ophtho). This drop is not immiscible with water, so it is not a good general lubricant. You should be able to keep your patient comfortable with minimal discharge by following these guidelines (Box 16-5).

Box 16-5

Causes of the Discharging Socket

General problems
- Bacterial or viral or viral conjunctivitis
- Dacryocystitis

Socket problems
- Lack of lubrication (most common)
- Giant papillary conjunctivitis
- Poorly fitting eye: dead space
- Extrusion, exposure
- Tumor recurrence

Exposure and extrusion

If the conjunctiva and Tenon's capsule break down over an implant, exposure is said to occur (Figure 16-7). If the implant falls out, extrusion is said to occur. Both events should be rare in your practice, occurring at a rate of less than 5%. Exposure or extrusion of an implant can occur early or late in the postoperative course. Early exposure or extrusion suggests inadequate surgical technique or infection. Exposure or extrusion can occur many years after the initial enucleation, usually for unknown reasons. A poorly fitting prosthesis can sometimes be implicated as the cause.

If you see an exposure in the first week or two postoperatively, you may be able to close the wound. You can try to patch a small exposure of a nonporous implant (around 5 mm) by placing a piece of sclera under the edges of Tenon's capsule. The conjunctiva may grow across the scleral "scaffold." If this fails, you will need to exchange the implant. Exposure of a nonporous implant will eventually lead to extrusion if not repaired.

Exposure of hydroxyapatite implants is more common than exposure of PMMA implants (as high as 10% in my cases). Exposure of MEDPOR implants occurs less often. In either case, exposures don't usually lead to extrusion because the fibrous ingrowth holds the implant in place. Very small exposures can heal spontaneously, but areas larger than 2–3 mm rarely close spontaneously. It is almost impossible to mobilize the conjunctiva and Tenon's capsule over a porous implant without creating a larger defect. For this reason, I

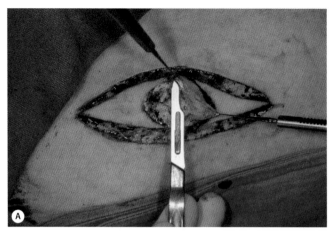
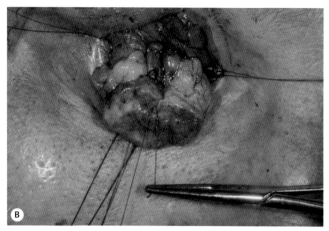

Figure 16-8 Dermis fat graft. (**A**) Harvest a fat graft from the buttocks. Remove the epidermis and a split layer of dermis from the central plug of tissue. Excise redundant skin for closure. (**B**) Suture the dermis fat graft to the edges of the conjunctiva.

usually burr away the face of an exposed porous implant until the overlying tissues can be closed primarily. This decreases the size of the implant by 30–50%. If large areas of conjunctiva are lost as a result of exposure or extrusion, a dermis fat graft can be used to replace the volume of the prosthesis and to add tissue to cover the face of the socket.

A *dermis fat graft* is harvested from the buttocks. The epidermis is removed from the surface of a 20 mm circle of skin leaving bare dermis. A plug of dermis with underlying subcutaneous fat is removed and transferred to the bed in the anophthalmic socket. The eye muscles and edges of the conjunctiva are sewn to the perimeter of the graft (Figure 16-8). Over several weeks, the conjunctiva will migrate over the face of the graft. Shrinkage of the fat occurs in every patient over the following months, so you should try to overcorrect the volume. Dermis fat grafts are seldom required, but they provide a useful solution to a tough problem.

Migration

Migration of anophthalmic implants occurs less commonly with porous spherical implants than with PMMA implants. If the implant is off center in the socket, the shape of the prosthesis can be modified. If movement is compromised or a satisfactory fit cannot be obtained, an implant exchange is indicated.

Superior sulcus syndrome

Volume deficits in the orbit show up first in the superior sulcus. Some deepening of the sulcus is commonly seen in patients after enucleation. If your patient develops a deep superior sulcus after wearing a prosthetic eye for some period of time, consider the diagnosis of the superior sulcus syndrome (Figure 16-9). This syndrome consists of:

- Deep superior sulcus
- Globe ptosis
- Lax lower eyelid

The weight of an ocular prosthesis is supported by the lower eyelid. If there were no lower eyelid, the prosthesis would fall out. With time, the weight of the prosthesis and the blinking of the eye cause the lower eyelid to sag, which manifests itself as globe ptosis and a deep superior sulcus.

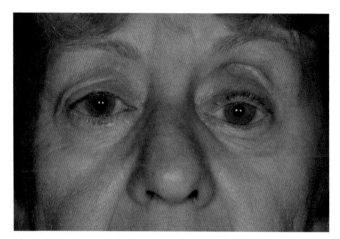

Figure 16-9 Superior sulcus syndrome. Note the deep superior sulcus, globe ptosis, and the lax lower eyelid.

Rather than increasing the size of the prosthesis to fill the sulcus, it is better to tighten the lower eyelid. This will lift the prosthesis into a normal position, filling the sulcus and correcting the globe ptosis. Before the recognition of this syndrome, many patients received a larger prosthesis. The larger prosthesis temporarily fixed the sulcus problem, but added more weight on the lower lid, eventually making the problem worse.

If your patient has a deep sulcus, but does not have a lax lower eyelid, the orbital volume is inadequate and one of two causes is present. If the eye was lost as a result of trauma, there may be an *unrecognized orbital fracture* present or ongoing orbital fat atrophy. Alternatively, *an adequate orbital implant may not have been placed at the time of enucleation or may have extruded.* If you think a fracture is possible, order a computed tomography (CT) scan to evaluate the orbital rims and floor. Repair of the fracture will improve the volume problem. In some patients, additional orbital volume, as described later, will be required for complete filling of the superior sulcus. If no anophthalmic implant is present in the socket, you should place a secondary implant as described earlier. If an implant is in place, any orbital fracture has been fixed, and the sulcus is still hollow, consider a subperiosteal floor implant to add orbital volume.

A variety of subperiosteal implant materials can be used. My two current choices are the preformed MEDPOR implants (enophthalmos shapes, http://www.porexsurgical.com) or cadaver costal cartilage. The MEDPOR implant comes in a large and regular size for each of the right and left sides. The costal cartilage, available from the local tissue bank, can be shaped to fit.

The floor is approached through the standard transcutaneous anterior approach (subciliary incision). A myocutaneous flap is formed down to the inferior orbital rim. The periosteum along the rim is sharply incised and the periorbita is elevated to create a subperiosteal pocket. The implant is sized to provide a slight overcorrection and placed into the pocket (usually a regular sized MEDPOR enophthalmos shape is used) (Figure 16-10). In some patients, you will need to excise some tissue from the inferior orbital fissure to slide the implant into position. The greatest volume of the implant should be placed posterior to the equator of the implant to push the eye anteriorly rather than superiorly. Push the implant deep in the orbit so that you do not inadvertently fill the inferior fornix making a fit difficult. Check to make sure that you have not pushed the spherical implant too high against the orbital roof. The enophthalmos shapes should be anchored to the inferior rim using microscrews. The periosteum does not require suturing. The skin is closed with a continuous running suture.

The procedure is the similar for costal cartilage. You can customize the shape and size. When larger amounts of volume are required, additional cartilage can be placed in a subperiosteal pocket along the medial orbital wall. It is difficult to anchor with screws, so you should try to close the periosteum to prevent anterior migration.

"Stock eye syndrome"

I use the term stock eye syndrome to describe the characteristic cicatricial changes that occur when a patient has worn a poorly fitting eye for many years. This situation used to occur more commonly when patients wore prosthetic eyes that were chosen "off the rack" rather than custom fit using the current impression-fitting techniques. These eyes induced a gradual inflammatory process that led to posterior lamellar shortening with the eyelashes pulled inward or against the prosthesis (Figure 16-11). Lid reconstruction using posterior lamellar mucous membrane grafts is required to lengthen the posterior lamellae and reorient the eyelashes. A new prosthesis is then custom made for the patient.

Lesser degrees of cicatricial entropion may be encountered. In these patients, modification of the prosthesis or marginal rotation procedures (tarsal fracture or terminal tarsal rotation, see Chapter 5) can be used to correct the eyelash malposition. If you encounter a patient with cicatricial entropion related to the fit of the prosthesis, consult with your ocularist to plan correction.

Contracted socket

A severe cicatricial process, known as socket contraction, may occur spontaneously (Figure 16-12). The resultant scarring can obliterate the conjunctival fornices entirely. The cause is unknown. The popular belief is that, if the patient goes without the prosthesis for a night or several days, the process can begin. This seems unlikely to me, but my colleagues tell me they have seen it happen.

Once under way, there is no treatment to halt the progressive scarring that occurs with socket contraction. Once the

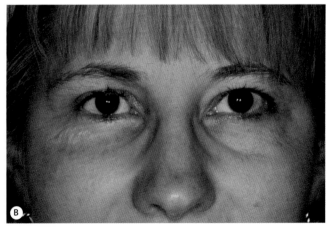

Figure 16-11 "Stock eye syndrome." Note the characteristic cicatricial entropion with the eyelashes against the prosthesis.

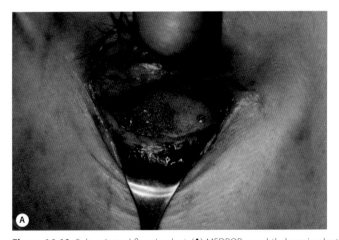
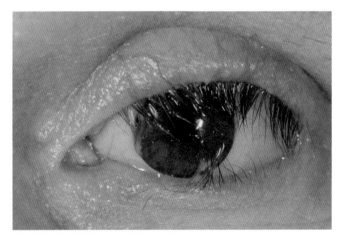

Figure 16-10 Subperiosteal floor implant. (**A**) MEDPOR enophthalmos implant in the subperiosteal space. (**B**) Postoperative appearance with no superior sulcus defect.

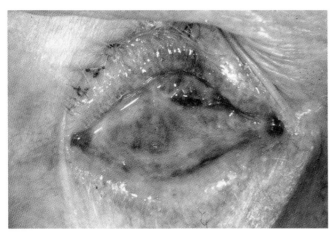

Figure 16-12 Socket contraction. Note that there are no fornices to retain the prosthesis.

scarring has halted, the socket can be relined with mucous membrane grafts. Large amounts of buccal mucous membrane may be required, and often the results are not optimal. Contracted sockets resulting from radiation treatment of retinoblastoma are particularly difficult to repair. Some success can be obtained using temporoparietal or free tissue flaps to provide a healthy nonirradiated bed for the mucous membrane grafts.

Ptosis of the upper eyelid

Ptosis of the upper eyelid of the anophthalmic patient can be caused by a loss of the support of the levator muscle complex. Your ocularist may be able to supply this support by modifying the curve of the prosthesis. In some patients, the lift will not be complete or may cause lagophthalmos and drying of secretions on the prosthesis. If this is the case, you can correct the ptosis surgically (Figure 16-13). If a new prosthesis is required, the ocularist can provide you with a wax model of the proposed prosthesis with a properly positioned iris to help you adjust the eyelid height and contour. Don't forget that the ptosis may occur for any of the same reasons as ptosis occurring in a seeing eye, as well.

Orbital exenteration

Indications

Exenteration of the orbital contents is indicated when a malignant tumor grows into the fat or other orbital tissues. In these patients, complete excision of the tumor with tumor-free surgical margins cannot be guaranteed because of the formless nature of the orbital fat. Exenteration is considered the only alternative to preserve the patient's life. In most cases in which exenteration is performed, any smaller excision of the tumor and orbital tissue would make the eye nonfunctional regardless, usually because of a loss of motility secondary to restriction or direct damage to one or more extraocular muscles.

Two situations where exenteration should be considered are:

- A primary orbital malignancy is diagnosed
- A periocular malignancy extends into the orbit secondarily, most commonly
  — A cutaneous malignancy
  — A sinus malignancy

Orbital malignancies requiring exenteration are rare. Probably the most common type is the adenoid cystic carcinoma of the lacrimal gland. Although a controversial treatment, exenteration is often used to remove this deadly tumor. More commonly, malignant tumors originating from the sinus or skin invade the orbit (Figure 16-14). Squamous cell carcinomas of the sinus or skin are the most common types of secondary orbital tumors requiring orbital exenteration.

Rarely, choroidal melanoma will extend outside the eye. Usually, this extrascleral extension is microscopic or extends minimally beyond the sclera without gross involvement of the Tenon's capsule or orbital fat. In these cases, Tenon's capsule overlying the tumor is excised. Orbital exenteration has not been shown to improve survival. When there is obvious extension into the orbital fat, exenteration is performed only if no other form of palliation can be used.

Exenteration may be required when a fungal infection extends from the sinus into the orbit. Infections caused by fungi such as mucormycosis or, less commonly, aspergillosis cause thrombosis of the vessels perfusing the infected tissues. Intravenous antifungal medications cannot penetrate the orbital tissues. Extensive debridement of the tissues, sometimes including orbital exenteration, may be required as a life-saving step to control the spread of infection.

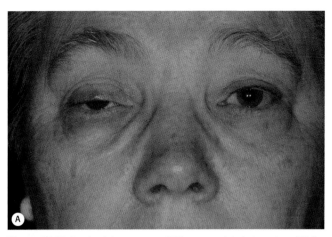

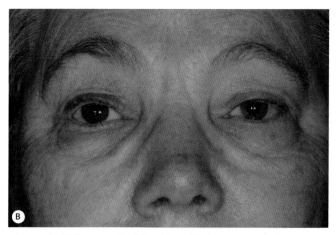

Figure 16-13 Ptosis of the upper eyelid in an anophthalmic patient. (**A**) Preoperative ptosis. (**B**) Postoperative lid position with the new prosthesis.

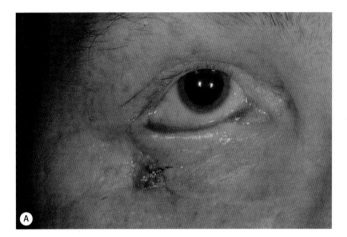

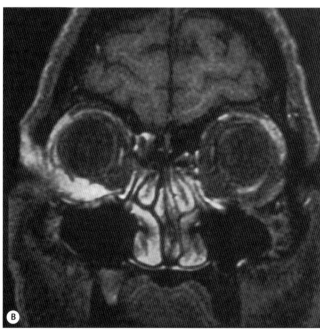

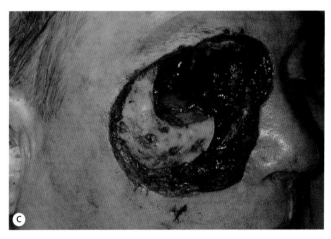

Figure 16-14 Recurrent cutaneous squamous cell carcinoma extending into the orbit. (**A**) Preoperative clinical photo. (**B**) Preoperative MRI scan showing the mass extending into the orbit attached to the orbital floor. (**C**) Exenterated socket with inferior rim osteotomies.

The exenteration operation

Orbital exenteration is performed under general anesthesia. An incision line is drawn around the orbit on the orbital rim (Figure 16-15, A), and 4-0 silk traction sutures are placed through the lid margins. The skin and orbicularis muscle are incised to the periosteum (Figure 16-15, B). The periorbita is incised and elevated off the orbital walls (Figure 16-15, C). The tissues in the inferior and superior orbital fissures are cauterized and cut. A right-angled clamp is placed across the apex tissue. A curved enucleation scissors is used to cut across the orbital tissues (Figure 16-15, D). The eye and the orbital tissues are delivered out of the socket (Figure 16-15, E). A bayonet bipolar cautery forceps is used to apply cautery to the bleeders in the orbital apex. A split-thickness skin graft is harvested from the thigh,

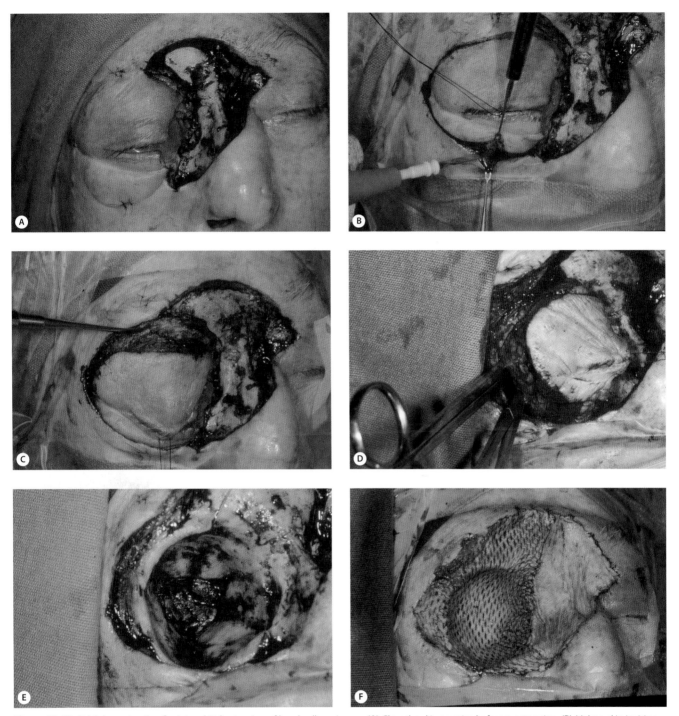

Figure 16-15 Orbital exenteration for intraorbital extension of basal cell carcinoma. (**A**) Clear the skin margins before exenteration. (**B**) Make a skin incision with the cutting cautery tool. (**C**) Elevate the periorbita off the orbital walls with a Freer periosteal elevator. (**D**) Cut the tissue out of the inferior and superior orbital fissures, and then cut the orbital apex and deliver the contents of the orbit. (**E**) View of the socket. (**F**) Apply a split-thickness meshed skin graft in the socket. In this patient, a split-thickness unmeshed graft was laid over the bare bone in the medial canthus.

meshed (1:2), and placed into the socket (Figure 16-15, F). The meshing allows the graft to contour to the orbit without overlapping. The orbit is packed with a sponge wrapped in Telfa. The packing is removed after 1 week. The socket heals over 4–6 weeks. The socket can be allowed to granulate; however, healing time is delayed.

Oculofacial prosthetics

Orbital exenteration is a disfiguring operation. A difficult psychological adjustment must take place over time. Most patients keep the wound covered with a gauze bandage during the healing phase. A pirate patch, Opticlude adhesive patch, or a "fogged" eyeglass lens can be used to cover the

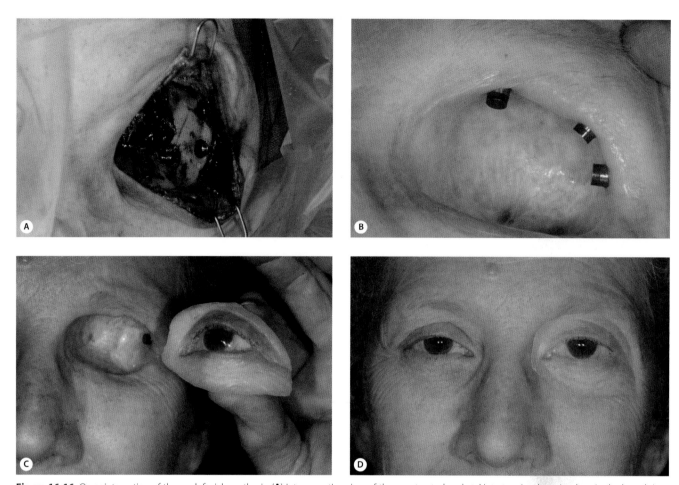

Figure 16-16 Osseointegration of the oculofacial prosthesis. (**A**) Intraoperative view of the exenterated socket. Note two implants in place in the lateral rim. (**B**) Rare earth magnets attached to abutments screwed into the osseointegrated implants are used to retain the prosthesis. (**C**) The prosthesis easily inserts into the socket in perfect alignment without retention problems commonly encountered with tape or glue fixation. (**D**) The prosthesis in place.

socket for an indefinite time. Some patients prefer to wear an oculofacial prosthesis to cover the socket. Although the prosthetic eye does not move and the eyelids do not blink, the prosthesis allows most patients to move relatively unnoticed in public.

A frustration for many patients with oculofacial prostheses is difficulty with alignment and retention. These prostheses are usually held in place with adhesives or double-sided tape, which can provide unreliable fixation. Exact alignment is often difficult for elderly patients to achieve. Unfortunately, many patients abandon the use of the prosthesis.

The osseointegration technique can be used to retain the oculofacial prosthesis (Figure 16-16, A). You may know patients who have teeth held in place with this technique. Titanium implants "bond" with bone or osseointegrate. A titanium abutment, attached to the bone implant, protrudes through the skin. This abutment will provide the point of attachment for the prosthesis (Figure 16-16, B). A biologic barrier to infection between the skin and titanium forms, preventing infection or extrusion of the titanium. Rare earth magnets are attached to the abutments and the posterior surface of the prosthesis. The prosthesis is "pulled" into perfect position and retained securely by the magnetic forces (Figure 16-16, C and D). The osseointegration technique is a big confidence booster for the patient after exenteration. The patient no longer has to worry about the alignment and

retention of the prosthesis. Patients rarely abandon the use of an oculofacial prosthesis retained by the osseointegration technique.

Craniofacial excision

Large tumors arising from the sinuses or the skull base can infiltrate the bones of the orbit. If the periorbita is not violated, the orbital contents may be preserved. With contemporary reconstructive procedures, normal function can be retained even if one or more orbital walls are removed (Figure 16-17, A and B). Excised portions of the orbital rims can be reconstructed using bone grafts. The orbital walls can be reconstructed with titanium mesh or other implant materials. The medial and lateral canthal tendons can be reattached in the anatomic position to the orbital rims using titanium microplates and screws. The lacrimal drainage system can be maintained using silicone stents (Figure 16-17, C).

In patients whose periorbita is invaded and orbital tissues are infiltrated, exenteration is required. Free tissue transfer grafts (latissimus dorsi, rectus abdominus, or other muscle flaps) can be used to fill in large areas of tissue loss including the orbit. In some patients, the eyelids and conjunctival cul de sacs can be preserved over a free flap, filling the socket (Figure 16-18).

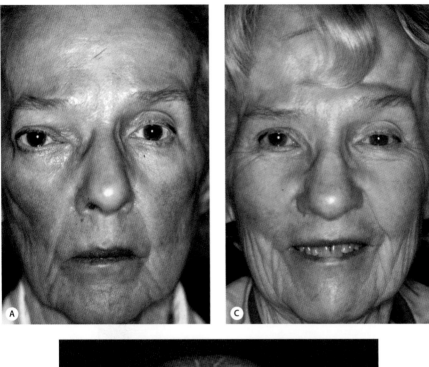

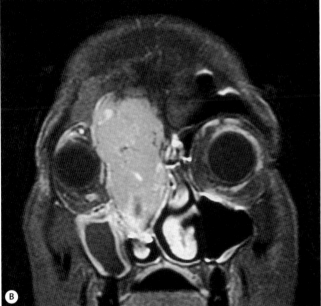

Figure 16-17 Craniofacial excision adenocarcinoma of sinus. (**A**) Sinus carcinoma extending into the orbit. Note that the right eye is displaced inferiorly and laterally away from the tumor. (**B**) A magnetic resonance imaging scan showing a large tumor requiring removal of the orbital floor, medial wall, and roof via orbitotomy and craniotomy. (**C**) Postoperative appearance. Preservation of the eye using reconstruction of the orbital skeleton with bone grafts for the orbital rim and a titanium mesh sheet implant for the orbital walls.

Checkpoint

Orbital exenteration is indicated when removal of the contents of the orbit is necessary to save the patient's life. Primary orbital malignancies (adenoid cystic carcinoma of the lacrimal gland) or secondary orbital malignancies arising from the skin or sinuses are the usual indications for orbital exenteration.

Oculofacial prosthetic devices can be anchored to the orbital rims using osseointegrated implants. The prosthesis is easily positioned and alignment is automatic. Retention is perfect.

Advanced reconstructive procedures can maintain the position of the globe even after significant removal of the facial skeleton.

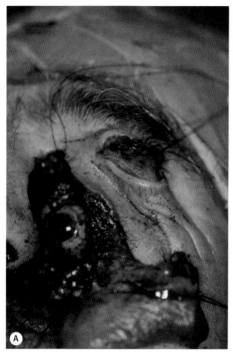

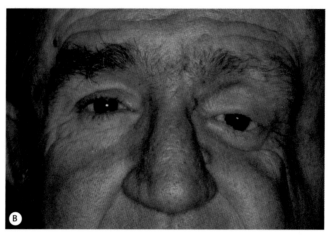

Figure 16-18 Apical orbital extension of squamous cell carcinoma of the sinus. (**A**) Intraoperative view of orbital exenteration with preservation of eyelids and conjunctiva later used for reconstruction of the socket. (**B**) Patient after reconstruction. The orbit has been reconstructed over a myocutaneous free flap with mucous membrane grafts and preserved conjunctiva and eyelids, allowing the patient to wear an ocular prosthesis.

Major points

Don't be the ophthalmologist who doesn't remove a prosthesis to look at the socket.

If you don't already have a working relationship with a well-trained ocularist, consider a visit to the ocularist's laboratory.

When a patient comes to you with a blind eye requesting removal of the eye, the first question to ask is, "Does the eye cause you pain?" If the answer is no, consider a scleral shell.

Characteristics of the ideal patient for wearing a scleral shell are:

- No eye pain
- Decreased corneal sensation
- Slight enophthalmos or phthisis
- No intraocular tumor
- A blind eye

When the decision has been made to remove the eye, there are two options:

- Enucleation: removal of the entire eyeball
- Evisceration: removal of the contents of the eye

The indications for enucleation are:

- Blind, painful eye
- Intraocular tumor

Contraindications for evisceration are:

- Intraocular tumor
- Phthisis

In theory, factors favoring evisceration over enucleation are:

- Better eye movements
- Less chance of postoperative enophthalmos
- Less operating time

The main indication for evisceration, as far as I am concerned, is for the eye with severe conjunctival scarring, where enucleation without destroying a large amount of conjunctiva is difficult.

The goals of the enucleation operation are:

- Remove the eye, obtain a specimen
- Restore the orbital volume
- Provide movement to the ocular prosthesis

The average orbital implant used today is a 20 mm sphere providing 5 ml of volume (the eye contains about 7.5 ml of volume). The prosthesis must restore the remaining volume to prevent enophthalmos.

The risk of sympathetic ophthalmia after enucleation is close to zero if enucleation is carried out within 10 days after trauma.

There are many implant designs and materials available.

- All surgeons agree that an implant should be placed at the time the eye is removed
- Most, if not all, believe that the muscles should be attached to the implant
- The type and size of implant used vary among surgeons

Major points Continued

An implant may be placed after the initial enucleation. This is known as a secondary implant. With some experience, you can find and attach the extraocular muscles. In rare patients, an implant may be removed and a new one placed. This is known as an implant exchange.

Two standard types of evisceration are performed:

- Evisceration with the cornea left in place
- Evisceration with keratectomy (most commonly performed)

Wait 6–8 weeks after enucleation or evisceration to fit a prosthesis.

Discourage handling of the prosthesis. Encourage lubrication for any signs of irritation.

Examination of the prosthesis and socket includes:

- General external appearance
  - Superior sulcus depth
  - Lower lid position and tension
  - Evaluation of conversational eye movements

- Slit lamp examination
  - Surface shine of the prosthesis
  - Health of the conjunctiva

Socket problems include:

- Discharge (caused by lack of lubrication, bacterial conjunctivitis, GPC, dacryocystitis, poorly fitting prosthesis, implant exposure, or tumor recurrence)
- Exposure and extrusion of the implant
- Migration of the implant
- Superior sulcus syndrome
- "Stock eye syndrome"
- Contracted socket
- Ptosis of the upper eyelid

Suggested reading

1. Albert DM, Lucarelli MJ: Aesthetic and functional surgery of the eyebrow and forehead ptosis. In *Clinical atlas of procedures in ophthalmic surgery*, pp. 378–395, Chicago: AMA Press, 2004.

2. American Academy of Ophthalmology: *Basic and clinical science course: orbit, eyelids, and lacrimal system*, sect. 7, pp. 119–129, San Francisco, The American Academy of Ophthalmology, 2006/2007.

3. Anderson RL, Gordy DD: The tarsal strip procedure, *Arch Ophthalmol* 97(11):2192–2196, 1979.

4. Chen WP-D: Enucleation, evisceration and exenteration. In McCord CD, Tanenbaum M, Nunery WR, eds, *Oculoplastic surgery*, 3rd edn, ch. 19, pp. 581–608. New York: Raven Press, 1995.

5. Collin JRO: Enucleation, evisceration and socket surgery. In *A Manual of systematic eyelid surgery*, 3rd edn, pp. 203–228, Butterworth Heinemann Elsevier, 2006.

6. Dortzbach RK, Woog JJ: Choice of procedure: enucleation, evisceration, or prosthetic fitting over globes, *Ophthalmology* 92:1249, 1985.

7. Dutton JJ, ed.: *Atlas of ophthalmic surgery*, vol. II, pp. 306-325, St Louis: Mosby, 1992.

8. Ferrone PJ, Dutton JJ: Rate of vascularization of coralline hydroxyapatite ocular implants, *Ophthalmology* 99:376, 1992.

9. Gion GG: Orbital prostheses. In Bosniak S, ed., *Principles and practice of ophthalmic plastic and reconstructive surgery*, ch. 108, pp. 1134–1149, Philadelphia: WB Saunders, 1996.

10. Green WR, Maumenee AE, Sanders TE, Smith ME: Sympathetic uveitis following evisceration, *Trans Am Acad Ophthalmol Otolaryngol* 76:625, 1972.

11. Heinz GW, Nunery WR: Anophthalmic socket: evaluation and management. In McCord CD, Tanenbaum M, Nunery WR, eds, *Oculoplastic surgery*, 3rd edn, ch. 20, pp. 609–637, New York: Raven Press, 1995.

12. Jordan DR, Anderson RL: The lateral tarsal strip revisited: the enhanced tarsal strip, *Arch Ophthalmol* 107:604–606, 1989.

13. Karesh JW, Dresner SC: High-density porous polyethylene (MEDPOR) as a successful anophthalmic socket implant, *Ophthalmology* 101:1689, 1994.

14. Kostick DA, Linberg JV: Evisceration with hydroxyapatite implant: surgical technique and review of 31 case reports, *Ophthalmology* 102(10):1542–1548, 1995.

15. Linberg JV, Tillman WT, Allara RD: Recovery after loss of an eye, *Ophthal Plast Reconstr Surg* 4(3):135–138, 1988.

16. Migliori ME: Evaluation and management of the anophthalmic socket. In Bosniak S, ed., *Principles and practice of ophthalmic plastic and reconstructive surgery*, ch. 106, pp. 1105–1126, Philadelphia: WB Saunders, 1996.

17. Nerad JA, Carter KD, Alford MA: Disorders of the orbit: Anophthalmic socket. In *Rapid diagnosis in ophthalmology—oculoplastic and reconstructive surgery*, pp. 260–267, Philadelphia: Mosby Elsevier, 2008.

18. Nerad J: Enucleation, evisceration, and exenteration: the care of the eye socket. In *The requisites—Oculoplastic surgery*, pp. 419–443, St Louis: Mosby, 2001.

19. Nerad JA: Osseointegration for the exenterated orbit. In Bosniak S, ed., *Principles and practice of ophthalmic plastic and reconstructive surgery*, ch. 109, pp. 1150–1160, Philadelphia: WB Saunders, 1996.

20. Nerad JA, Carter KD, LaVelle WE, Fyler A, Branemark PI: The osseointegration technique for the rehabilitation of the exenterated orbit, *Arch Ophthalmol* 109:1032, 1991.

21. Nerad JA, Hurtig RR, Carter KD, Bulgarelli D, Yeager DC: A system for measurement of prosthetic eye movements using a magnetic search coil technique, *Ophthal Plast Reconstr Surg* 7:31, 1991.

22. Nunery WR, Hetzler KJ: Dermal-fat graft as a primary enucleation technique, *Ophthalmology* 92:1256, 1985.

23. Tanenbaum M: Enucleation, evisceration and exenteration. In Yanoff M, Duker J, eds, *Ophthalmology*, pp. 752–760, Mosby, 2004.

24. Wobig JL, Dailey RA: Enucleation and exenteration. In Wobig JL, Dailey RA, eds, *Oculofacial plastic surgery: face, lacrimal system, and orbit*, pp. 255–266, New York: Thieme, 2004.

Index

Notes: Pages numbers suffixed by 'f' indicate figures: page numbers suffixed by 't' indicate tables: page numbers suffixed by 'b' indicate boxed material.

Z